RADIOLOGY OF THE SMALL BOWEL

SERIES IN RADIOLOGY 2

Other volumes in this series:

Series ISBN: 90-247-2427-9

RADIOLOGY OF THE SMALL BOWEL

Modern Enteroclysis Technique and Atlas

JOHAN L. SELLINK, M.D.

X-Ray Department, Westeinde Hospital, The Hague, The Netherlands
(Visiting Professor at Indiana University School of Medicine, Indianapolis, Indiana, U.S.A., 1977)

and

ROSCOE E. MILLER, M.D.

Distinguished Professor and Chief of Gastrointestinal Radiology
Indiana University School of Medicine, Indianapolis, Indiana, U.S.A.

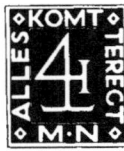

1982

MARTINUS NIJHOFF PUBLISHERS

THE HAGUE / BOSTON / LONDON

Distributors:

for the United States and Canada

Kluwer Boston, Inc.
190 Old Derby Street
Hingham, MA 02043
USA

for all other countries

Kluwer Academic Publishers Group
Distribution Center
P.O. Box 322
3300 AH Dordrecht
The Netherlands

Library of Congress Cataloging in Publication Data

Sellink, J. L.
    Radiology of the small bowel.

    (Series in radiology ; 2)
    Includes bibliographies and index.
    1. Intestine, Small--Radiography--Atlases.
2. Contrast media. I. Miller, Roscoe E. II. Series.
RC804.R6S45   616.3'407572   81-9531
                                   AACR2

ISBN-13: 978-94-009-7432-6   e-ISBN-13: 978-94-009-7430-2
DOI: 10.1007/978-94-009-7430-2

Photography: C.T. Ruygrok and M. Popkes, Leiden.
Translation: G.P. Bieger-Smith, Wassenaar.

Softcover reprint of the hardcover 1st edition 1982

CONTENTS

PREFACE

This atlas is a selection of roentgenograms of patients who visited the radiology departments at the University Hospital in Leiden between 1970 and 1978, the Free University Hospital in Amsterdam in 1979, and the radiology department at the Indiana University Medical School in Indianapolis in 1977. The most common radiological abnormalities of the small intestine are illustrated clearly, unhindered by flocculation or segmentation of the contrast fluid. The authors believe this book is a definite contribution to the goal of precise early small bowel diagnosis. However, the key to good diagnosis is not only a superb examination technique, but also the knowledge, the character, and the personal perfectionism of the physician. If these factors are optimal, then the best possible roentgenographic series will be obtained – at least as far as the technique is concerned. All patients illustrated here were examined by using the enteroclysis technique. With this method of small bowel examination, the contrast fluid is administered via an infusion directly into the duodenum instead of orally. The infusion method has added a new dimension to the usual radiological examination of the small intestine. This method is also especially suited for the comparative evaluation of motility, and the study of disturbed motility. Throughout the course of the examination, the technique can be adapted to special situations at any given moment and can be modified to produce precise diagnostic roentgenograms and diagnosis. Each new enteroclysis examination can be a source of considerable satisfaction to the physician, since it – more than any other gastrointestinal examination – demands his constant attention and all of his skills, all in a relatively short period of time. The publication of the first atlas in 1976 resulted in a meeting between the two authors in Leiden in 1976. This was followed by a longer association in Indianapolis in 1977. In the first instance, the bond between the two authors became particularly strong because of their profound interest in the common problems surrounding this most important tool for diagnosis of the small bowel. One of their problems was the barium suspension – which as yet has still not been completely solved to our satisfaction. It soon became apparent that the goal of both of us, each a teacher of digestive tract diagnosis, was above all to obtain results that are optimum, including routine examination. It subsequently became evident, partly through character and partly due to a deep appreciation of each other's work, that each was able to accept the frequent and relentless criticism of the other without rancor and to profit from it. As a result, the foundation was laid for fruitful collaboration and thus for this second edition. The changes in this book with respect to the first atlas can be grouped into four categories:

1) Adaptation to terminology commonly used in the USA to indicate the concentration of the barium suspension, as well as how to dilute the barium suspension to obtain the desired specific gravity; finding an infusion system made up only of parts readily available in the USA; determining the various heights of the contrast fluid with respect to the top of the examination table so as to obtain the desired rate of flow.

2) Numerous visits to other clinics and confrontation with the problems and results of others have proven that it is certainly possible to achieve little or nothing with a poor enteroclysis examination. These bad results are due without fail to superficial reading of the text, and failure to adhere to the procedures described in this book. Furthermore, some examiners tried to introduce variations immediately although they lacked experience and understanding, and thus they obtained poor results. In a separate chapter (chapter 16), a number of the most common errors and their solutions are described.

3) For many radiologists, the enteroclysis examination of infants appears to cause considerable difficulty. The approach is slightly different from that used for adults and was not included in the first edition. The procedure for infants is described in a separate chapter (chapter 15) in this edition.

4) The chapters in which the pathology of the small intestine is described and illustrated (chapters 9–14) have been expanded to include a number of interesting cases as well as cases that increase the total range of possibilities.

Numerous colleagues who studied in the Department of Radiology at Leiden mastered the enteroclysis technique in the past seven years and, as a result of their great enthusiasm, many became interested in a particular aspect of small intestine pathology. The authors of this atlas were able to benefit from their experience and have been given permission to use their data that generally have been published elsewhere.

We wish to thank the following for their cooperation: J.R. Achterberg – drug-induced atony; C.A. van Hees – Meckel's diverticulum; W.F. Muller – celiac disease (awarded the Boris Rajewski Medal at the AER Congress in Edinburgh in June 1975, and thesis in 1978); J.Th. Schlangen – radiation enteritis; W.H.B. Tuynman – melanoma metastases; P.J. van Wiechen – *Yersinia enterocolitica* infections; and C.J.L.R. Vellenga – aspecific ulcerations.

In addition to the members of the photography section of the Department of Radiology at the Leiden University Hospital, who handled an enormous amount of work, we wish to thank Prof. Dr. J.R. von Ronnen and Prof. A.J.Ch. Haex for their highly stimulating influence and encouragement during the first 'years of life' of the enteroclysis technique, and Mrs. S.M.L. Sellink-Cowan, who did the typing for both editions of this atlas.

JOHAN L. SELLINK, M.D.   ROSCOE E. MILLER, M.D.

1. INTRODUCTION

Although there has been some improvement over the past few years, the radiological examination of the small intestine must still be regarded as a stepchild of radiology and even of the examination of the digestive tract. The net gain of a transit examination of the small intestine has been disappointing for so many years that the negative attitude on the part of many radiodiagnosticians is certainly understandable. Gradually, however, steady improvement has changed this somber situation and presently an adequately performed roentgenological examination of the small intestine is definitely worthwhile. Its contribution to diagnosis is considerable.

Early in the fifties, Golden showed that even if the examination techniques are not at an optimum and the contrast fluids are not the best, good results can be achieved if the radiologist himself at least approaches the examination enthusiastically.

Somewhat later in the same decade, Marshak pointed out that better results are obtained if larger amounts of contrast fluid are used. Then not only is there better filling of the intestinal loops so that abnormalities are not as easily overlooked, but in addition an examination carried out in this manner is more efficient since more inestinal loops are visualized per exposure. Furthermore, the examination as a whole is shorter. An even shorter examination as well as an improvement in the mucosal patterns are achieved by using drugs to accelerate passage.

Bodart, in the past ten years, has demonstrated effectively that smaller abnormalities of the mucosa need not escape the attention of the physician, if he studies the intestinal loops carefully by using fluoroscopy and the compression technique in combination with detail spot films.

More recently as a result of the introduction of the enteroclysis technique, the many meters of small intestine have become much more accessible for radiodiagnosis. With this method, optimum filling of the intestinal loops is obtained and the fear of malabsorption, a misdiagnosis in the conventional transit examination, has disappeared.

To a certain extent the enteroclysis technique demands more of the radiologist since this examination must be executed properly in every respect. Neglecting one or more of the various factors, which will be discussed in detail, leads without fail to disappointment and often to a return to less adequate procedures. Because of the rather high degree of filling achieved with enteroclysis, careful compression of the superimposed intestinal loops has become essential. Otherwise, as before, numerous abnormalities will be overlooked.

Unfortunately it has also become clear that the diagnostic output of the radiological examination of the small intestine, even more than that of other examinations, can vary greatly, depending upon the technique used and the care and skill with which the examination is carried out.

Although the radiological examination of the small intestine has always been referred to the general radiologist – and this will continue to be true because of the high frequency of abdominal complaints – it may be to the advantage of many patients if the examination is carried out by a gastrointestinal radiologist especially interested or specialized in this aspect of radiodiagnosis.

The scala of radiologically demonstrable abnormalities has by now become quite extensive; furthermore, diseases of the small intestine appear to occur much more frequently than previously assumed.

In addition to complaints such as abdominal pain, unexplained high fever, blood loss in the digestive tract, diarrhea, and diseases accompanied by malabsorption, all of which clearly require radiological evaluation of the small intestine, this type of examination must also be carried out in the event of unexplained hypoalbuminemia, whether accompanied by edema in the lower extremities or not. Since a well-executed enteroclysis examination is the best possible method of examination, every conceivable aspect and pitfall of this procedure have received special attention in this atlas.

2. ANATOMY

1. Normal mucosa in the small intestine

For correct interpretation of the roentgenogram, it is more important to have a thorough knowledge of the anatomical structure of the wall of the small intestine than for the technical execution of the examination. However, it is difficult to differentiate between a precise examination and interpretation because the radiologist is actively involved in both phases as is also the case for gastric and colon examinations.

The wall of the small intestine, shown schematically in fig. 2.1, consists of the following layers, starting from the outside:

1) The serosa.
2) The tunica muscularis, which consists of an outer longitudinal layer and an inner circular layer.
3) The submucosa, which contains many blood and lymphatic vessels in a loose connective tissue so that the tunica muscularis can move freely with respect to:
4) The mucosa; this layer is made up of three parts:
   a) The muscularis mucosae which, like the tunica muscularis, consists of an outer longitudinal layer and an inner circular layer. The muscular strands of this inner circular layer extend into the folds of Kerkring and some even extend through the tunica propria into the villi that cover the surface of the mucosa. The villi vary in number from 10 to 40/mm^2; they are 0.2–1.0 mm high and contain a centrally located, blind-ended lymphatic vessel. Between the villi are the crypts of Lieberkühn.
   b) The tunica propria, like the submucosa, consists of a loose connective tissue containing blood and lymphatic vessels as well as nerve fibers. Occasionally conglomerates of lymphocytes are found in this layer.

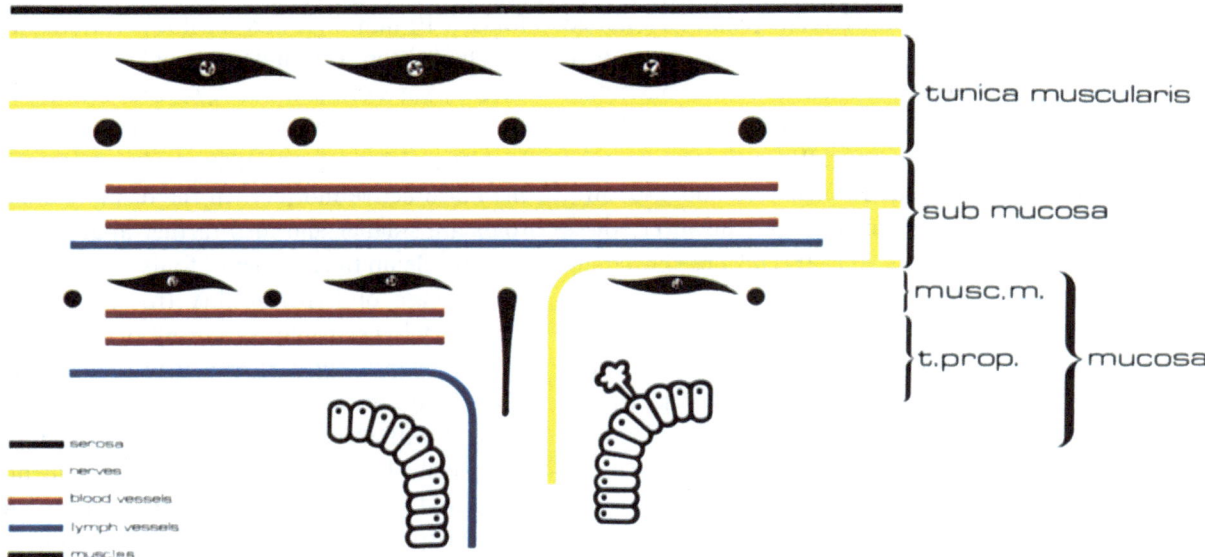

serosa
nerves
blood vessels
lymph vessels
muscles

tunica muscularis
sub mucosa
musc.m.
t.prop.
mucosa

Fig. 2.1. Schematic drawing of a cross section of the intestinal wall.

4

c) A layer of simple columnar epithelial cells which can move freely with respect to the tunica propria. The surface of each epithelial cell is covered with hundreds of microvilli, which are 0.2–1.0 mm high and together form the so-called 'brush border'.

Although several studies have been published concerning the length of the small intestine, the definitive answer has yet to be found. Most handbooks list values varying between 5 and 7 m and the small intestine is assumed to be $\frac{3}{5}$ of the total length of the digestive tract. The distance from nose or mouth to the duodenojejunal flexure varies only slightly; a length of 90 cm is assumed here. It is known that the length as well as the diameter of the small intestine is highly dependent upon its tone, so that the results of measurements taken postmortem or under anesthesia are too high. A length of 12 m is not unusual for American Negroes and natives of India. X-ray films of the small intestine occasionally show that individual variations can be enormous. However, when several measurements are taken of the same patient, the results appear to differ at the most by only 10% [90]. Underhill [235] obtained postmortem values of 4.7–9.7 m with an average length of 6.9 m. Unfortunately she took some measurements several hours after death and others after the body had been stored for several days.

Hirsch et al. [93] report that, shortly after death, contraction of the smooth musculature causes the intestine to shorten; autolysis later causes a renewed increase in length. They took measurements in vivo by having patients swallow a rubber tube 3.5 mm in diameter; their values then varied between 220 and 270 cm from mouth to anus. When they used a tube 2 mm in diameter, the results were 400–540 cm – considerably longer. Postmortem, however, these values turned out to be 800–900 cm! The shortening of the intestine around an ingested tube is called the 'telescope effect'.

Some authors state that an asthenic will have a slightly longer small intestine than a pyknic. In fact we have almost never encountered problems of superposition of convoluted ileal loops in the small pelvis in our pyknic patients.

For the jejunum, the diameter is normally assumed to be 2.5–3.0 cm and for the ileum 2.0–2.5 cm. Values have also been reported of 1.0 and 0.5

inch, respectively, which are probably a closer approximation of the diameter in vivo and during a conventional transit examination. During an enteroclysis examination, as a result of the more active peristalsis, the diameter of the loops of the small intestine is generally greater and more variable than during a conventional examination. With infusion of 600–900 ml and a flow rate of 75 ml per minute, as used in our departments, the maximum diameter of the proximal jejunal loops will be 4 cm in normal cases. Generally the diameter of the distal ileal loops depends to a large extent on the counter-pressure caused by a fecal-filled cecum. A diameter of 3 cm for those segments that are in a resting phase is normal in this region. During a conventional transit examination, the diameter of the contrast column in the distal ileum depends partly on the degree of increased viscosity of the contrast fluid, which in turn is determined by the length of the examination. At the transition between the jejunum and the ileum, the diameter of the intestinal lumen differs only slightly from the standard values for a conventional transit examination. Of course with a greater flow rate, an increased amount of contrast medium, or other transit-retarding factors, the diameter of the intestinal lumen will increase.

The folds of Kerkring begin 3–5 cm beyond the pylorus; in the proximal part of the jejunum, they are 3–6 mm high and 1–6 mm apart. Occasionally folds 7–10 mm high and local separations of 7–12 mm have been seen under normal conditions in an enteroclysis examination. A separation of 1 mm is encountered only when the tone of the intestine is high (fig. 2.2AB) or in children (fig. 2.2C); there is then also active motility. In the distal jejunum the folds are smaller and also farther apart.

In the ileum the number of folds can vary greatly. In the case of hypermotility (fig. 2.2B) or compensatory hypertrophy as a result of atrophy of the jejunal mucosa (fig. 2.3), there can be as many folds as there are in the jejunum. On the other hand, in patients with atony of the bowel, fold relief may be completely lacking in the ileum. Even in normal cases fold relief can be barely visible (fig. 2.4). In comparison with a conventional examination of the small intestine, the height of a fold may therefore be somewhat less on an enteroclysis film; but the

5

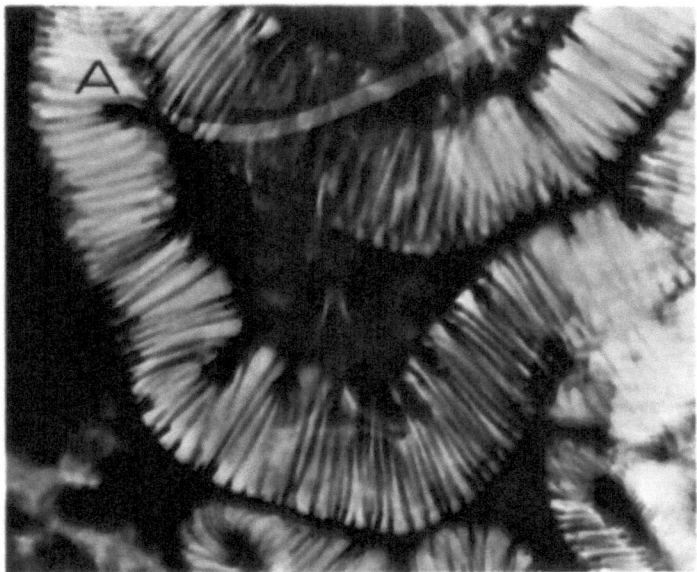

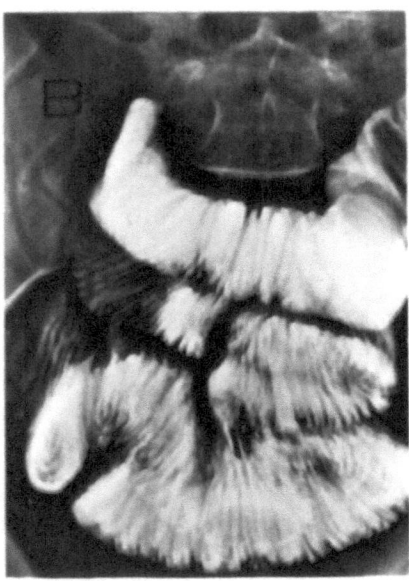

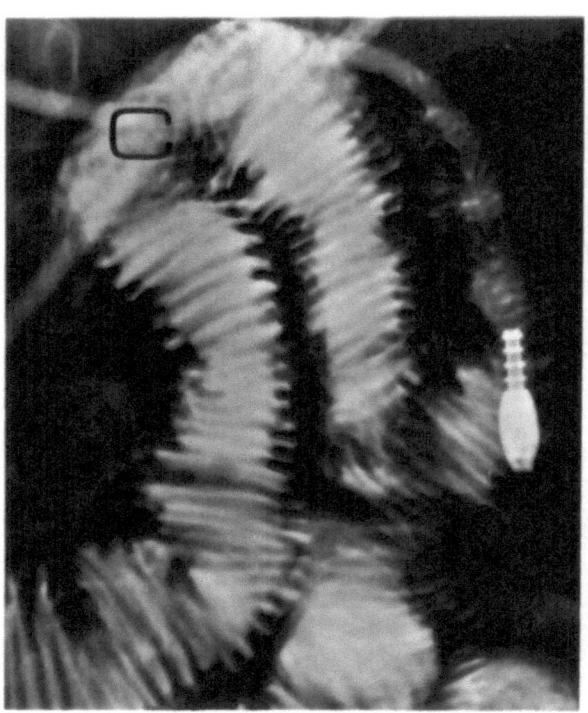

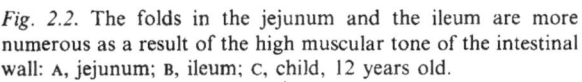

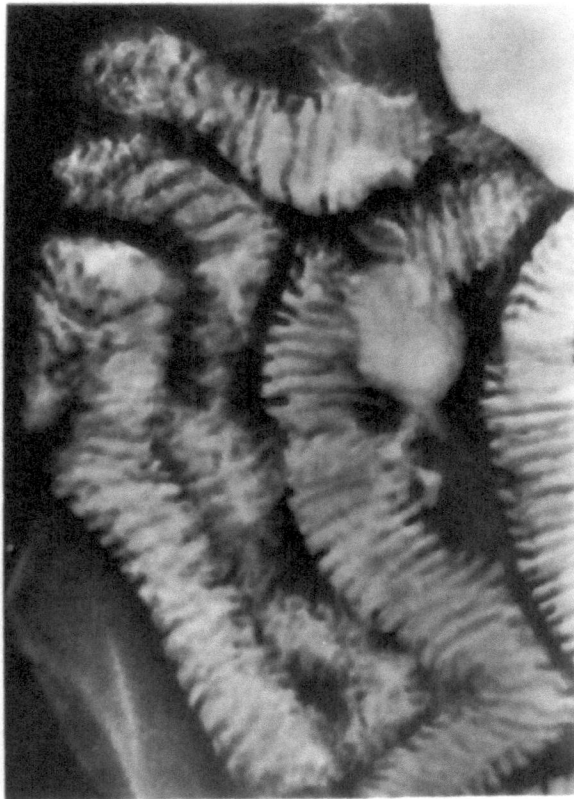

Fig. 2.2. The folds in the jejunum and the ileum are more numerous as a result of the high muscular tone of the intestinal wall: A, jejunum; B, ileum; C, child, 12 years old.

Fig. 2.3. Increased number of folds in the ileum ('jejunization') in a patient with atrophy of the jejunal mucosa as a result of celiac disease.

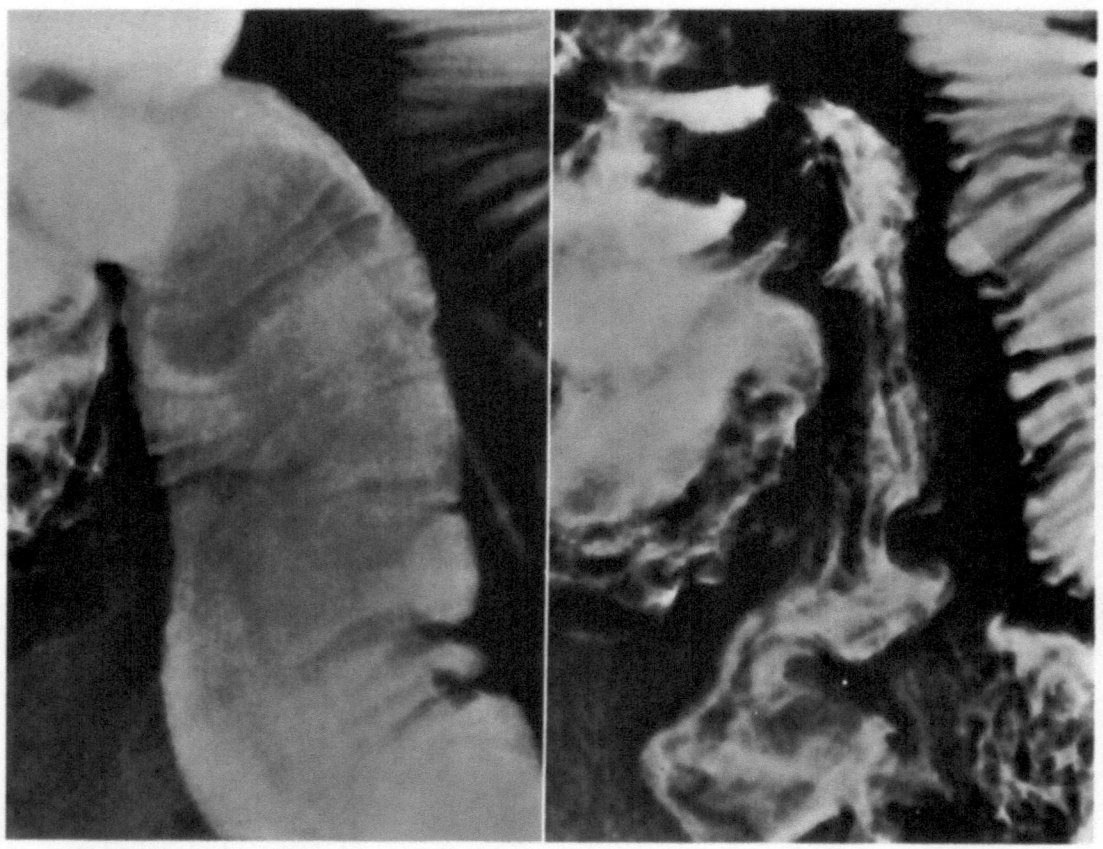

Fig. 2.4. When the ileum is stretched, the fold relief is barely visible.

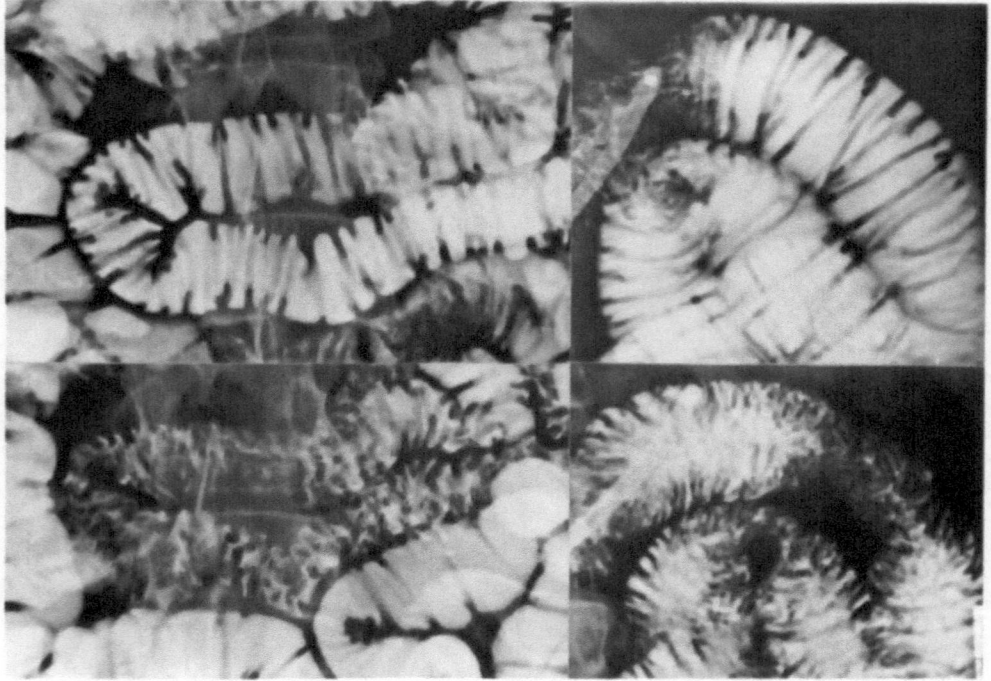

Fig. 2.5. Circular course of the mucosal folds in the proximal part of the jejunum. Evaluation is much easier when the intestine is stretched than during the rest phase (bottom).

thickness will barely change. Evaluation of the height of a fold is much easier with enteroclysis because the more active peristalsis induces stronger contractions as well as more pronounced dilatations during the rest phases (fig. 2.5). When the intestine is in a state of dilatation, the folds are stretched and quite orderly with respect to one another so that they are easy to measure. In addition, minor anatomical abnormalities are less likely to be overlooked (fig. 2.6).

The margins of a normal fold of Kerkring extend in parallel into the intestinal lumen; the transition from fold to intestinal wall can best be described as a rounded corner (fig. 2.7). On the roentgenogram, the space between two intestinal loops is 2–3 mm, depending upon the phase of contraction; the thickness of the intestinal wall is therefore only $1-1\frac{1}{4}$ mm.

In the proximal half of the jejunum, the folds lie in a more or less circular configuration (fig. 2.8), but in the distal half of the jejunum and the proximal half of the ileum, the course becomes

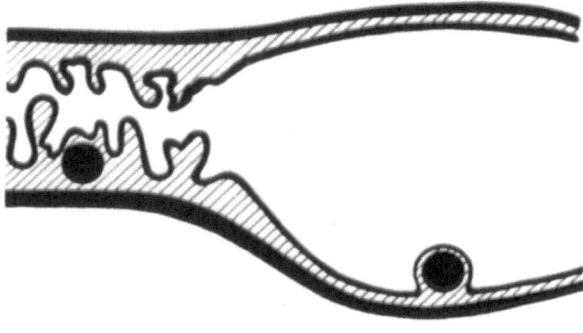

*Fig. 2.6*A. An abnormality of the mucosa is more clearly visible when the intestine is in a state of dilatation than in a state of contraction.

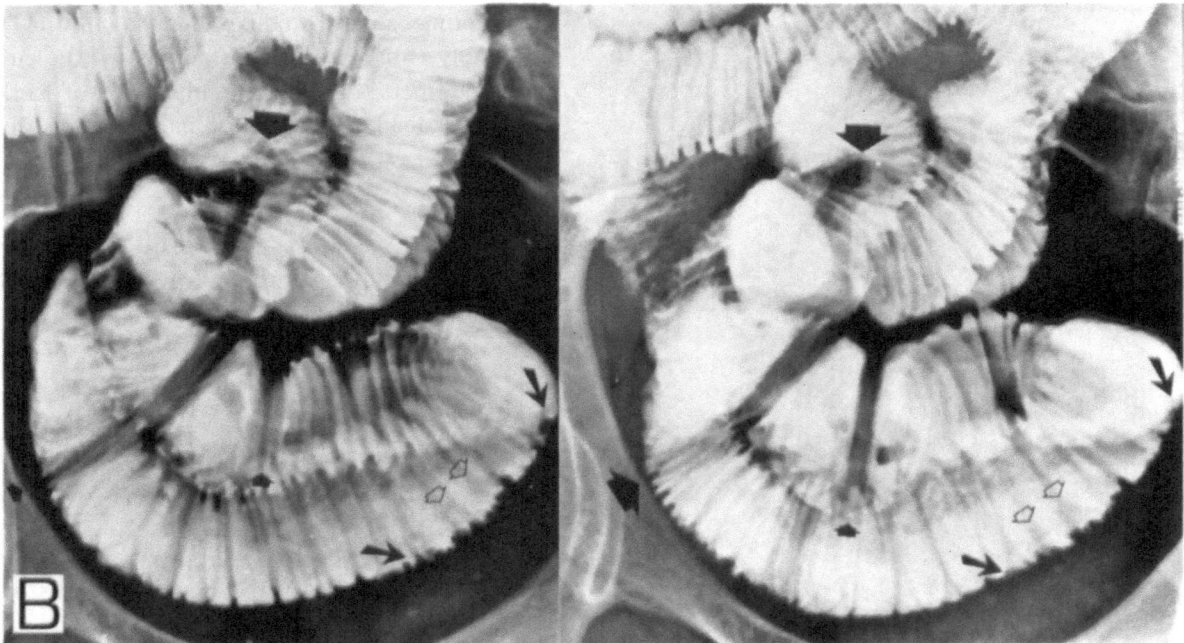

*Fig. 2.6*B. Mild inflammatory-like changes in the wall (between the long arrows) and impressions in the intestinal lumen due to bands (short solid arrows) are only visible because the course of the folds is orderly and the intestine is well filled. The short open arrows show how far these abnormalities extend along the length of the folds.

8

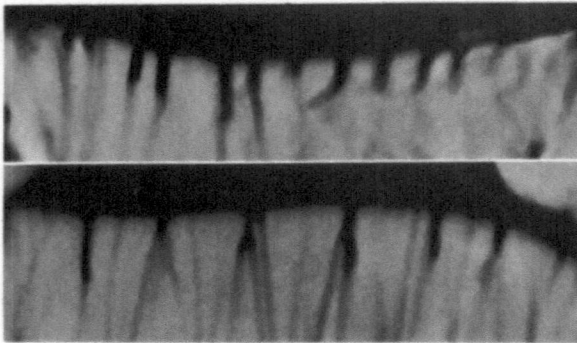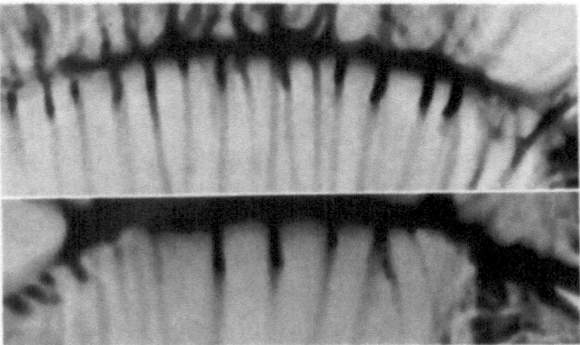

Fig. 2.7. The margins of a fold of Kerkring extend approximately in parallel; the transition from fold to intestinal wall has the shape of a rounded corner.

spiral-shaped. In this region it can be seen that the folds follow a true spiral course in some segments of the intestine while in other segments they resemble more or less a chain of tridents along each wall that mesh together in the center of the lumen (arrow). We have the impression that the latter configuration is more common in the distal jejunum and

that the spiral course occurs predominantly in the proximal ileum.

In the literature it is generally stated that the folds in the distal ileum often follow a longitudinal course. In our opinion, however, this is not true; the configuration of the folds is just as circular as in all other parts of the small intestine. The ileal folds are in fact smaller, thin, and farther apart, and do not contribute significantly to the fold relief – irrespective of the state of contraction of the intestine. The longitudinal folds frequently seen on x-rays of the ileum are obviously wider and higher than the circular ones. Like those on the evacuation films of a colon with few haustra, they must be explained as puckering caused by collapse of the intestinal wall, possibly enhanced by contractions of the circular muscle fibers (fig. 2.9). Circular folds of Kerkring which extend in a longitudinal direction do not exist.

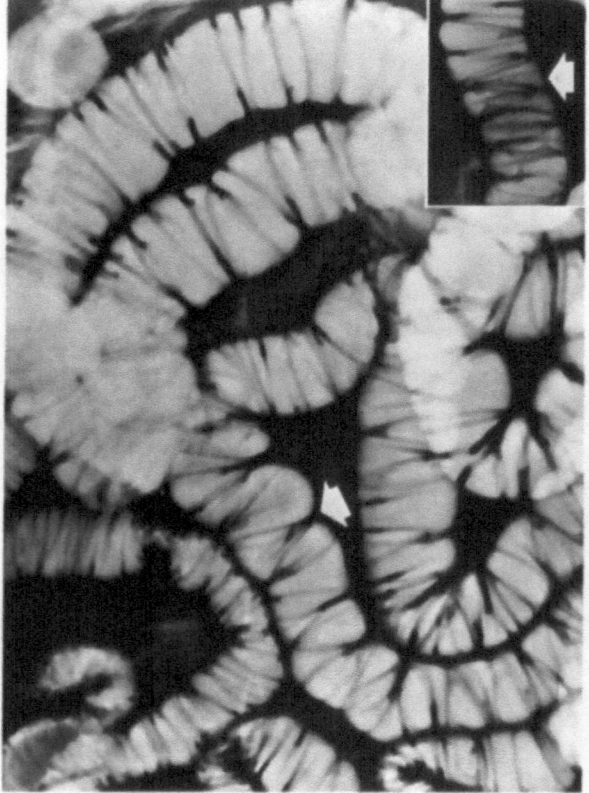

Fig. 2.8. Trident-shaped mucosal folds which mesh together in the region of the jejunoileal transition.

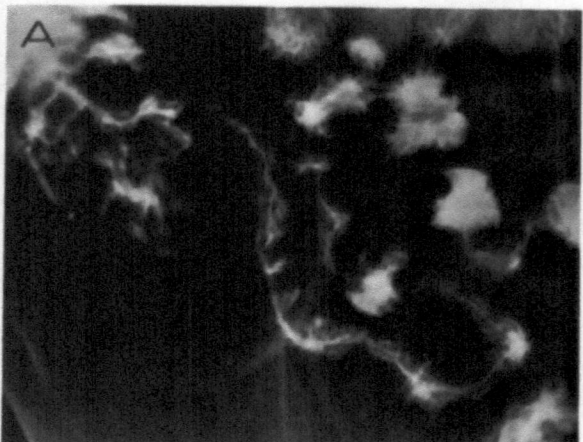

Fig. 2.9A. Longitudinal folds in the ileum in a contracted intestinal loop.

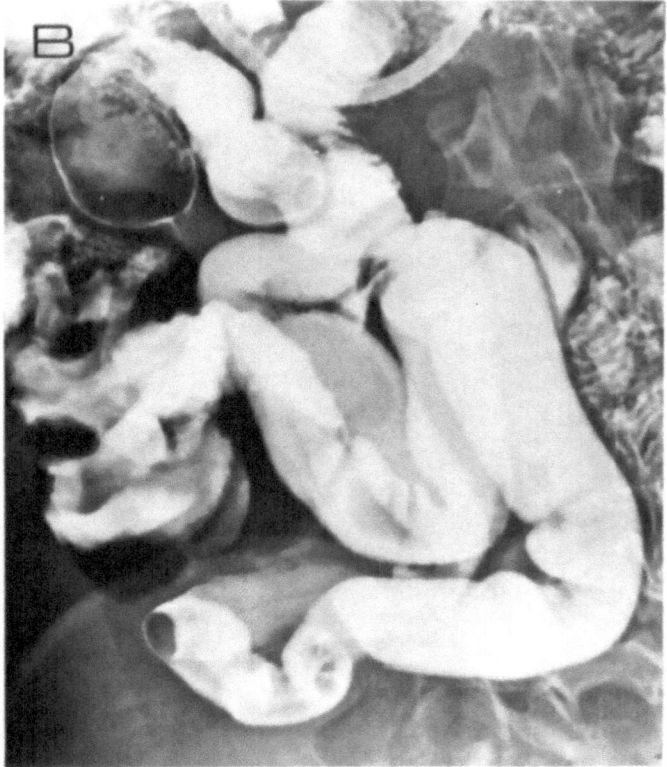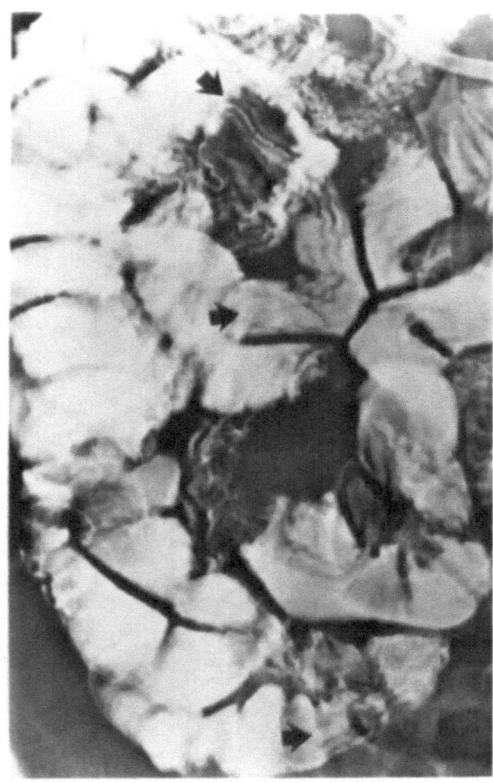

Fig. 2.9B. Case of cured Crohn's disease. When the intestine is well filled, the longitudinal folds disappear entirely (left) so that a completely smooth intestinal wall without mucosal relief is seen. In case of collapse (right), only longitudinal folding is seen. Circular folds have disappeared.

Occasionally in the most distal part of the ileum, an abnormal mucosal pattern is seen: the folds have a longitudinal course on the mesenteric side and a circular course on the other side of the loop (fig. 2.10A). This longitudinal folding can sometimes even resemble an elongated ulcer or a partially filled appendix lying against the distal ileum (fig. 2.10B). The mucosal pattern can, depending upon the state of contraction or dilatation, show very pronounced changes. During contraction, the folds in the jejunum can extend in a more longitudinal direction, as they do in the ileum.

In a resting phase, the folds lie in a very disorderly fashion if the intestine is empty an especially if the muscular tone of the intestinal wall is high. Comparison of the mucosal patterns of one intestinal segment in various stages of contraction (fig. 2.11) illustrates this quite clearly. In this figure it is also obvious that the thickness of the folds is fairly constant and therefore is not influenced by the different phases of contraction.

Whatever the degree of stretching of the intestine, the folds are about 2 mm thick in the jejunum and about 1 mm in the ileum. In the first few decimeters of the jejunum, however, the folds can sometimes be $2\frac{1}{2}$–3 mm thick – although no visible reason can be found. If these folds are normal in shape, they probably have no pathological significance.

Figure 2.12 shows that even if there is marked stretching of the intestinal wall, as in the case of total mechanical obstruction, the folds of Kerkring retain their thickness fairly well. The folds do become somewhat shorter and are smoothed out, which implies that the shorter and thinner ileal folds may be visible only as minute ridges (fig. 2.4).

It can be seen on the x-ray in fig. 2.13 that the thickness of the folds as well as the space between adjacent intestinal loops has clearly increased in addition to the ileal loop dilated as a result of the obstruction. In this case, this is due to Crohn's disease accompanied by lymphedema (see page 127). Only in the proximal part of the jejunum could this fold relief be attributed to dilatation alone; then, however, the intestinal wall would have to be thinner and the distance between the folds less.

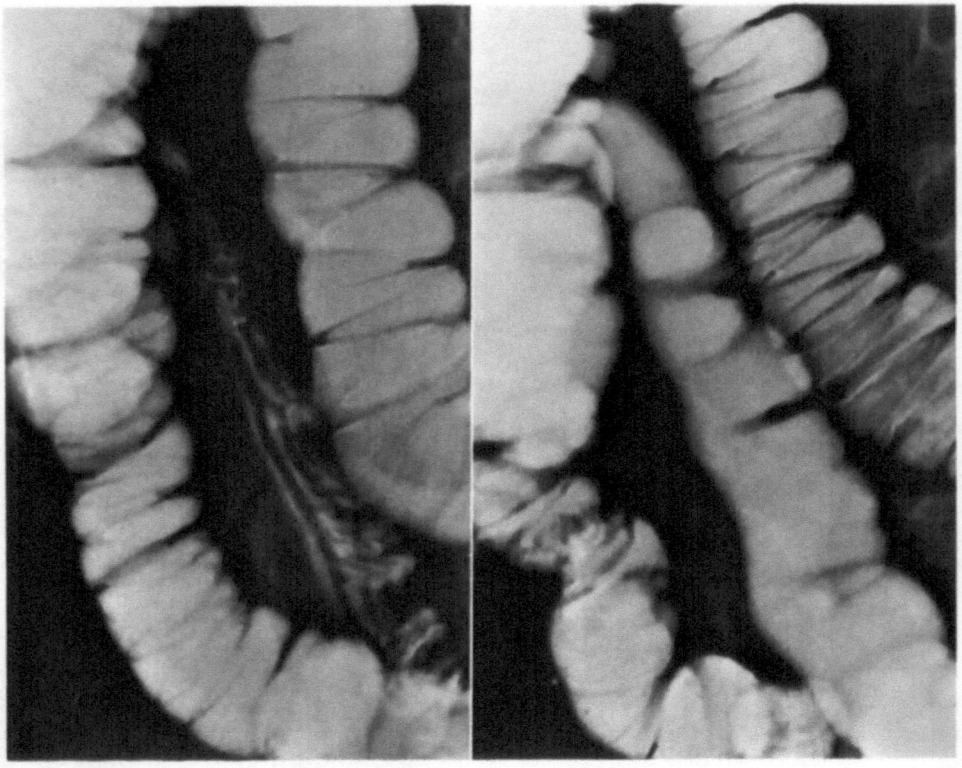

*Fig. 2.10*A. Fold relief occasionally seen in the distal ileum. Longitudinal folds on the mesenteric side of the intestine.

If the jejunum is in a rest phase and there is only moderate filling with contrast medium, then evaluation is difficult. We know this well from conventional examinations. Because the folds intersect one another frequently, particularly in a highly contractile intestine, multiple small round bright spots appear in the mucosal patterns which are highly suggestive of lymph follicles. Since dilatation and a high degree of filling are often impossible to achieve in a contractile intestine, it may be necessary to induce hypotonicity for the purpose of evaluation (fig. 2.14). Because there are fewer folds in the distal ileum, the presence of true lymph follicles is easily demonstrated there. These follicles are frequently encountered in small children under normal circumstances; they disappear when the children are 10–14 years of age. The much larger Peyer's patches can also be seen in the distal ileum in older patients. They are recognized by the cushion-like configurations that occur mainly on the mesenteric side of the intestine (fig. 2.15).

A fine circular sawtooth pattern, like that often seen in the mucosa of a colon influenced by laxatives, may also be found in the distal ileum. This presumably is a result of contractions of the muscularis mucosae (fig. 2.16).

Until the second world war, it was assumed that the intestinal mucosa and the intramural nervous system of infants were still markedly underdeveloped. This was because, for the first 3–6 months, mucosal patterns were never seen on the x-ray films, not even in the duodenum. The appearance of a baby's small intestine on the x-ray films at that time was strikingly similar to that of an adult with a severe malabsorption or 'deficiency state'. This was due to the contrast medium being less stable, and therefore flocculation occurred from mucin and lactic acid. It was assumed that this deficiency state must be ascribed to damaged nerve cells since the pathologist found vacuolar degeneration in these cells. The x-ray films often showed flattening or even disappearance of the relief of the

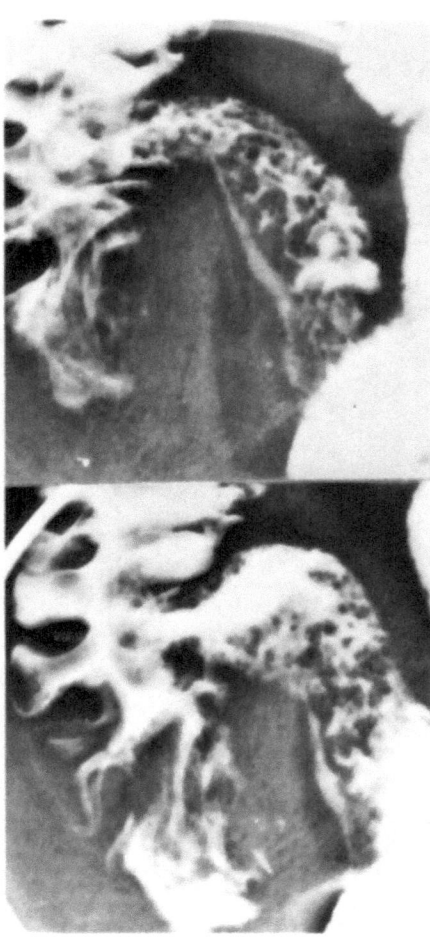

Fig. 2.10B. Misleading pattern of longitudinal ileal fold or fissure-like ulcer, caused by adherence of the appendix in this unusual position.

mucosal folds [76].

Bouslog [22, 23] and Weltz [240] were also not able to observe mucosal patterns on the x-ray films of infants. However, their studies had shown that the mucosal folds are more highly developed both absolutely and relatively than those in an adult and are even present in the third fetal month. The folds are, however, thinner and not as high. Vascularization and cellularity are pronounced in the mucosa. The submucosa is thinner than that in an adult so that the muscularis, the mucosa, and the submucosa of an infant are all of approximately equal thickness. The relative underdevelopment of the muscularis, also in the mucosa, could cause the mucosal folds to be flattened completely by the barium column. All x-ray films published before the second world war show only a pronounced segmen-

tation of the barium column, even in the duodenum. In general therefore one suspects that these examinations were in vain and that the conclusions were probably more often incorrect than correct.

Although the composition of many contrast media has been greatly improved, articles still appear today reporting that mucosal patterns cannot be observed until the infant is several months old. It is also stated, however, that no conclusions may be drawn from this fact.

2. Normal position of the intestine

To be able to understand why a specific configuration of the small intestine is abnormal, as well as how it developed, knowledge of normal development is required. An important phase in this respect is the rotation phase that occurs between the fourth and tenth weeks of fetal development. In the early stages of embryonal development, the digestive tract is a tube-like organ called the archenteron. The superior mesenteric artery already exists; the liver is large and there is little space in the abdominal cavity.

The intestine increases rapidly in length, but the mesentery that attaches it to the abdominal wall does not grow at the same rate, so that loops are formed. This elongation is greatest in the region supplied by the superior mesenteric artery, thus involving the small intestine and the colon. Elongation is much less in the area of the rectosigmoid and especially the esophagus and stomach.

Since the initial enlargement of the fetal abdominal cavity is not sufficient to contain the rapidly lengthening intestine, part of the intestine with the omphalomesenteric duct as midpoint herniates physiologically into the umbilical cord (fig. 2.17A). The steadily growing intestine then rotates 90° with the omphalomesenteric duct and the superior mesenteric artery acting as an axis such that the distal ileum and proximal colon lie on the left side and the jejunum and the proximal ileum on the right (fig. 2.17B). Further growth of the liver is slow so that the space in the abdominal cavity now increases faster than the total volume of the intestinal loops. The latter can then return into the abdominal cavity. During this so-called reduction of the umbilical herniation, the jejunal loops pass behind the

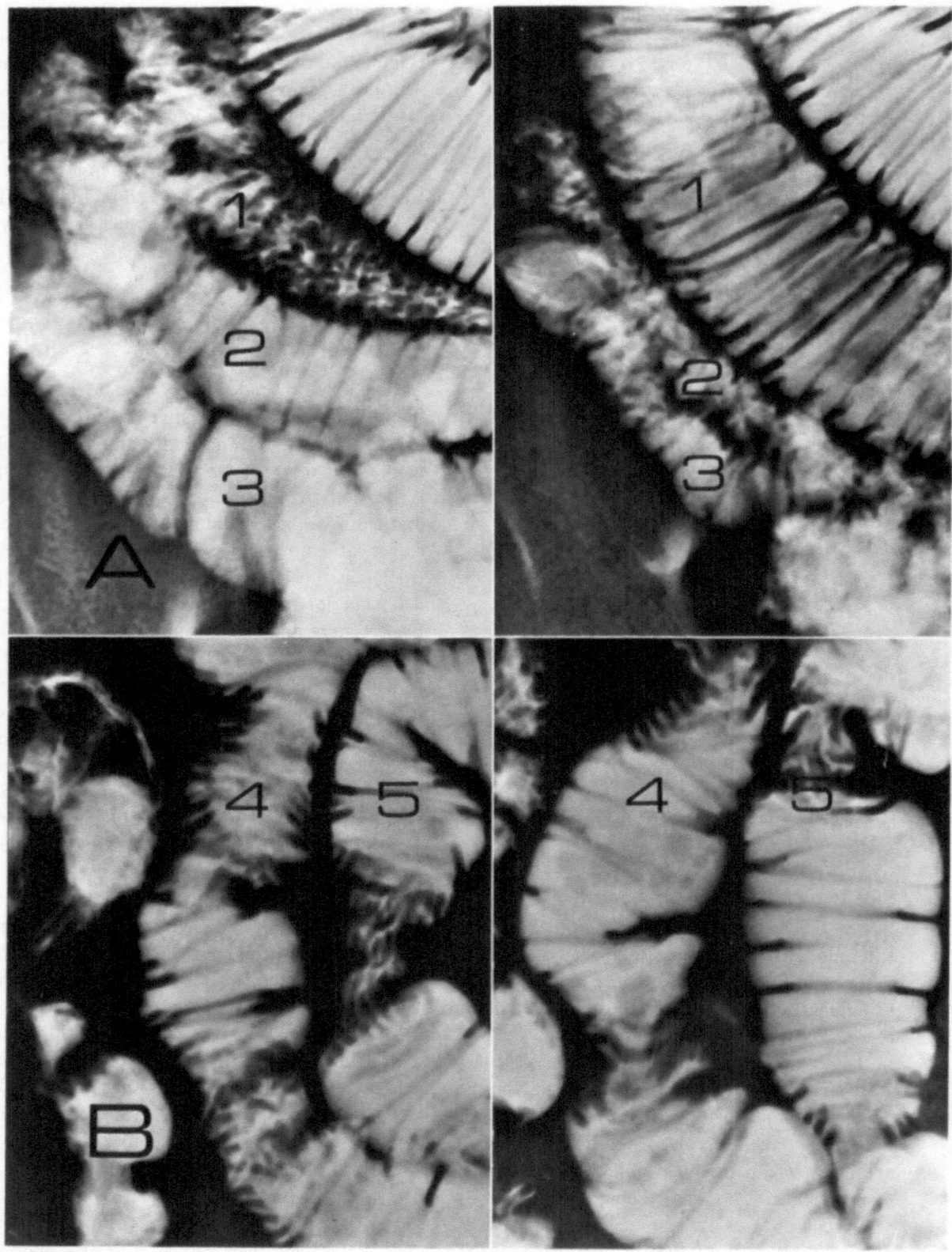

Fig. 2.11. Various phases of contraction of the same intestinal loop. Disorderly arrangement of the folds in the rest or contracted phase, orderly in the dilated phase or when well filled.

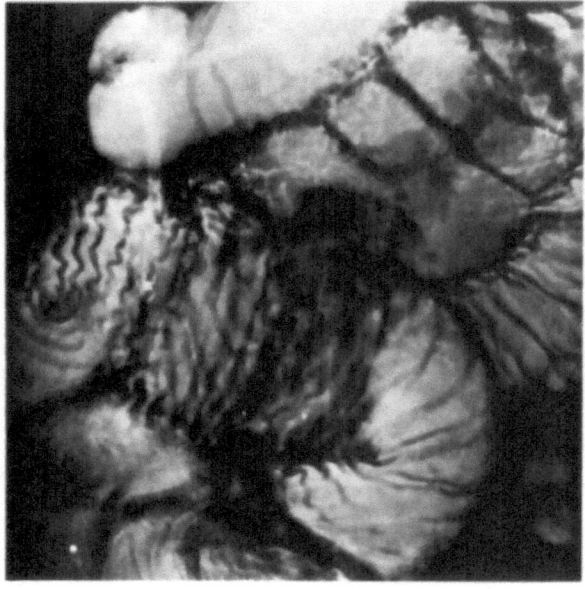

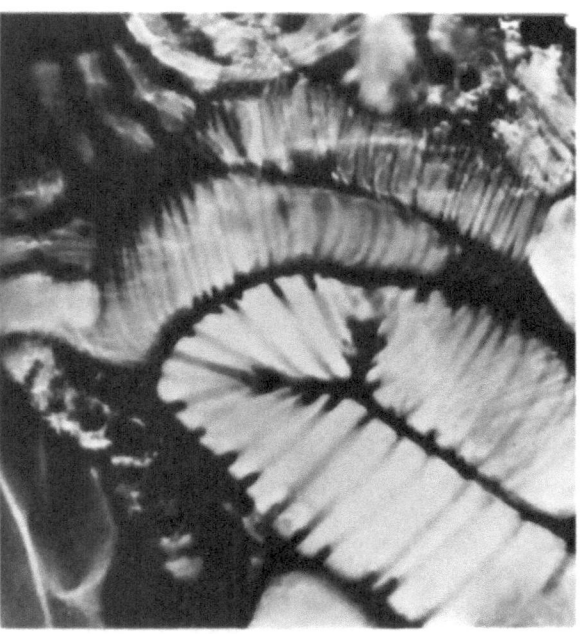

Fig. 2.12. Pronounced stretching of the intestinal wall causes the mucosal folds in the jejunum and ileum to become shorter but barely thinner than normal.

Fig. 2.13. Crohn's disease with obstruction in the ileum. Mucosal folds as well as intestinal wall are thickened.

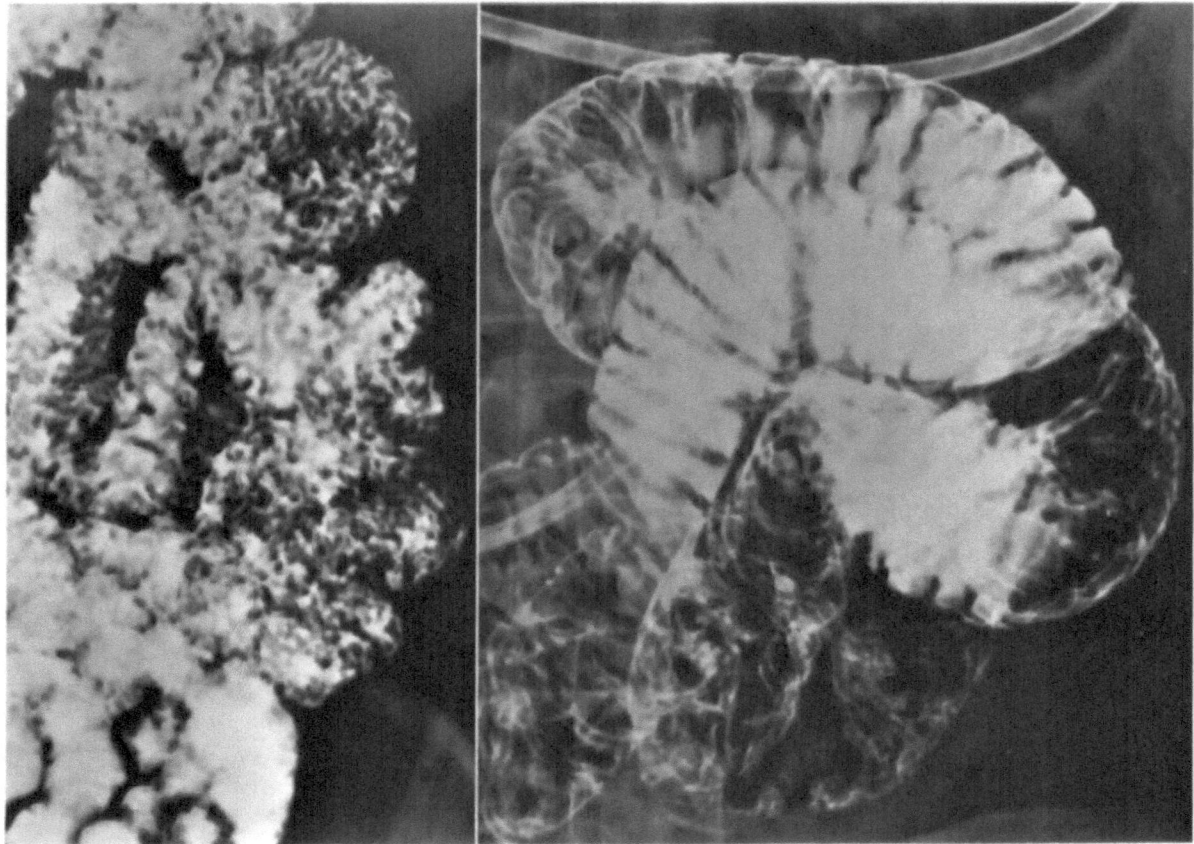

Fig. 2.14. Clear spots in the mucosal pattern that resemble enlarged lymph follicles because the contracted intestinal loops intersect many times. After administration of a hypotonic agent, the illusory pattern disappears completely.

14

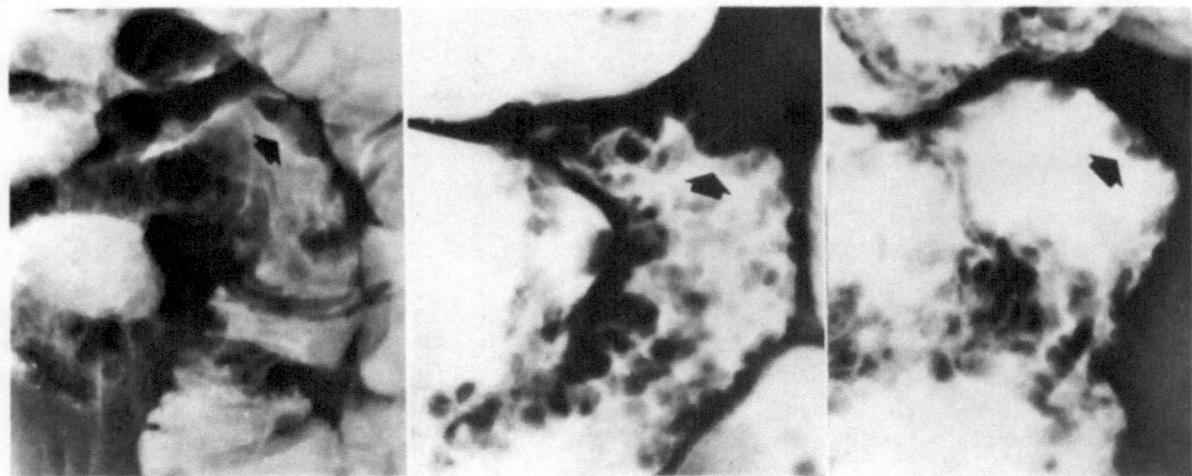

Fig. 2.15. Cushion-like configurations in the mucosal pattern caused by Peyer's patches in the distal ileum.

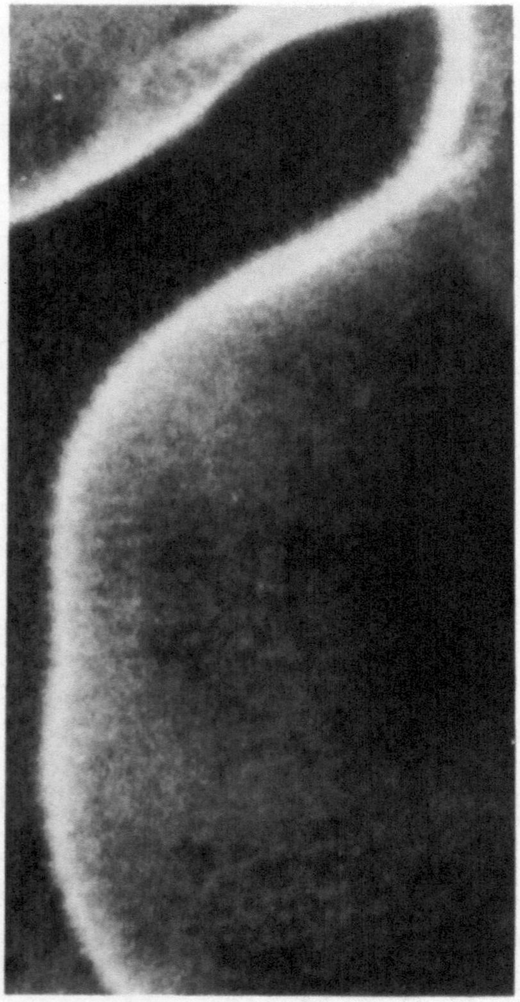

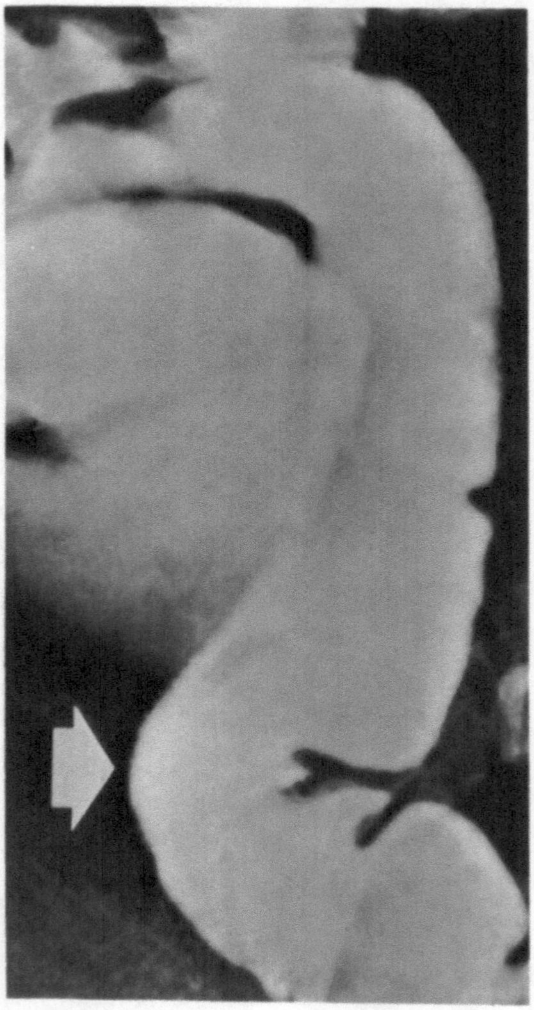

Fig. 2.16. Sawtoothed margins of the wall of the distal ileum due to contractions of the muscularis mucosae (arrow). Similar configurations are also seen in the colon, especially if a laxative is added to the contrast fluid (top left) and in the esophagus and stomach (bottom). (See also page 15.)

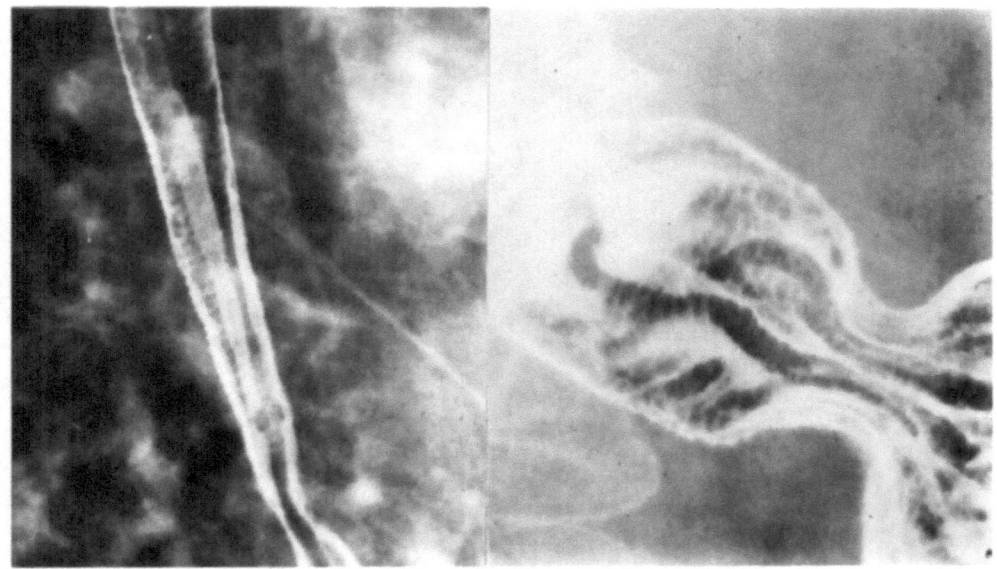

Fig. 2.16.

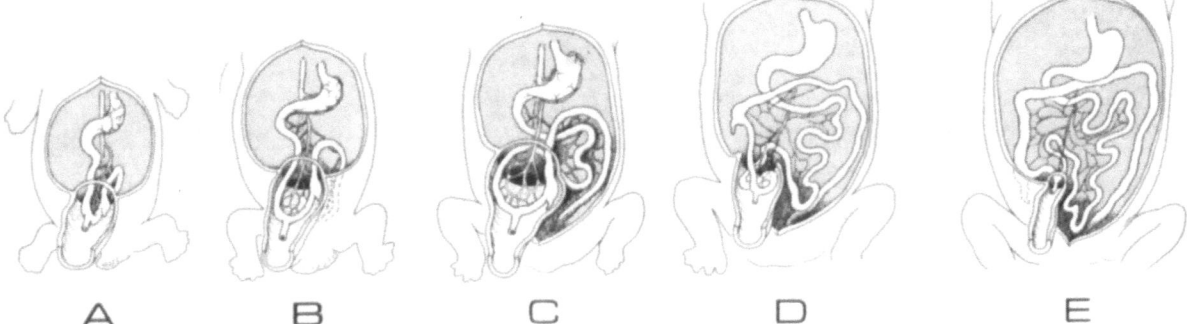

*Fig. 2.17*A–E. Stages of development and rotation of the convolution of intestinal loops in the abdominal cavity.

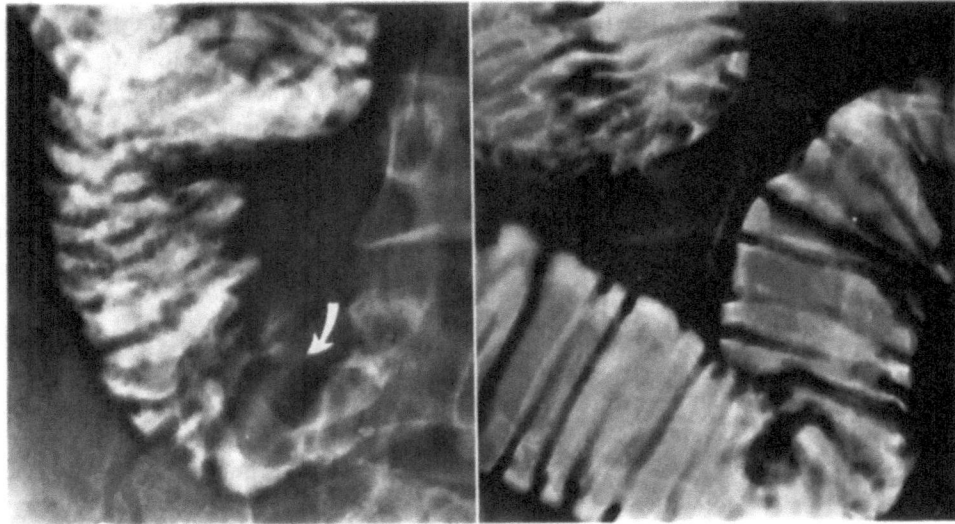

Fig. 2.18. Impression of a jejunal loop on a jejunal loop caused in this case by a sharp curve in the loop.

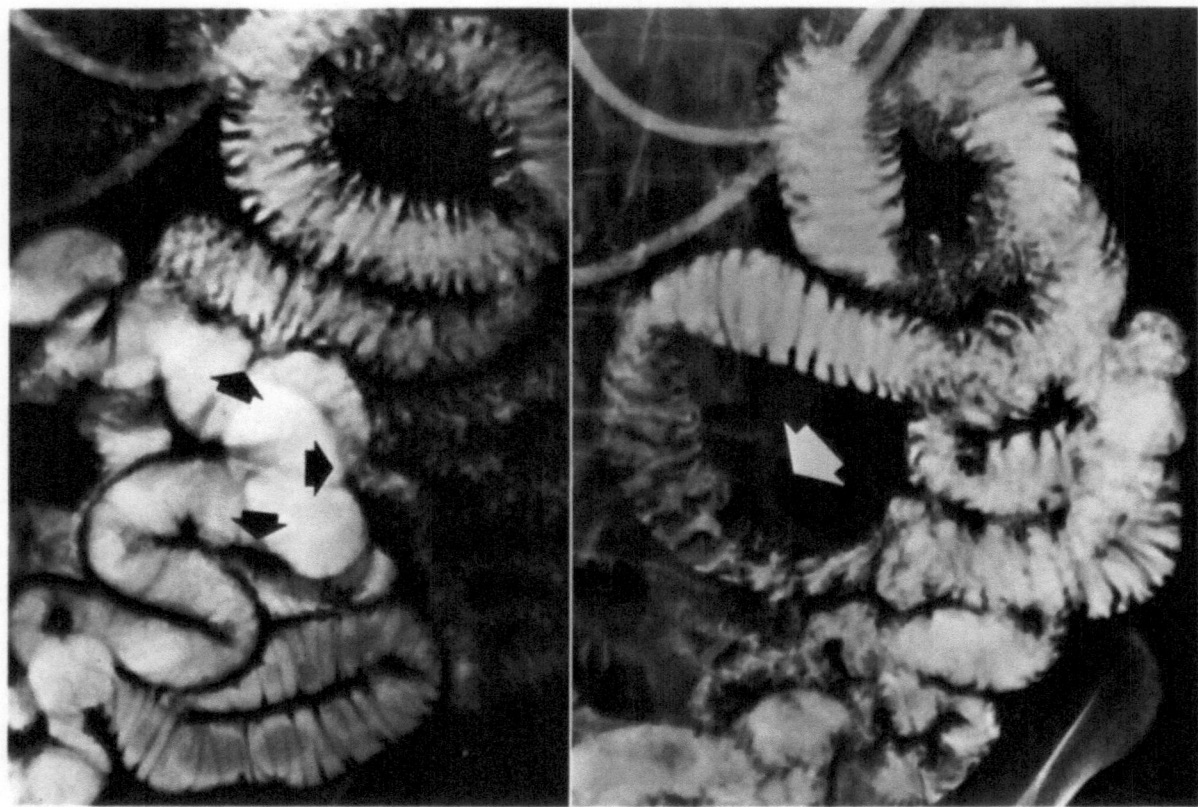

Fig. 2.19A. Impressions on the jejunum caused by ileal loops which were not yet filled with contrast fluid when the x-ray was taken.

superior mesenteric artery to occupy the left posterior abdominal cavity (fig. 2.17C). The left anterior region contains the distal ileum and the ascending colon. The right half of the abdomen contains the still relatively large liver. After the return of the physiological herniation, there is again a rotation around the omphalomesenteric duct and the superior mesenteric artery. As a result of the pressure of the jejunal loops that occupy the left posterior part of the abdominal cavity, the ileocecal section rotates another 180° in the same counterclockwise direction. The cecum is now to be found to the right in the upper abdomen with the ileum, at least the distal half, below it (fig. 2.17D). The loops of the small intestine continue to fold and, as a result of the elongation of the colon, the cecum descends into the lower right abdomen and finally becomes fixed.

When the rotation process is completed, the loops of the small intestine are grouped in the abdominal cavity as seen in fig. 2.17E. The jejunum then lies to the left in the upper abdomen and the ileum to the right and in the middle of the lower abdomen.

According to recent studies, the position of the fully developed intestine is not achieved by rotation; the word 'malrotation' therefore should not be used to indicate an abnormal position of the bowel. Normally, the embryonic intestine is embedded in a mesenchymal mass, which is by no means compatible with the later mesentery, without a coelomic cavity between the intestine and the mesenchyme. As a result of extension of the coelom, segmental growth of the intestine takes place inside the mass in the area surrounded by the coelomic activity. This growth is situated between two parts of the intestine that are still fixed in position within the mass. As the development of the intestine reaches completion, the mesentery develops as a very thin duplicature at the same time.

Welvaart, K.: Etude du développement de l'intestin envisagée parallèlement à la genèse du mésentère. *Bulletin de l'Association des Anatomistes* (March 1965) 921: 926.

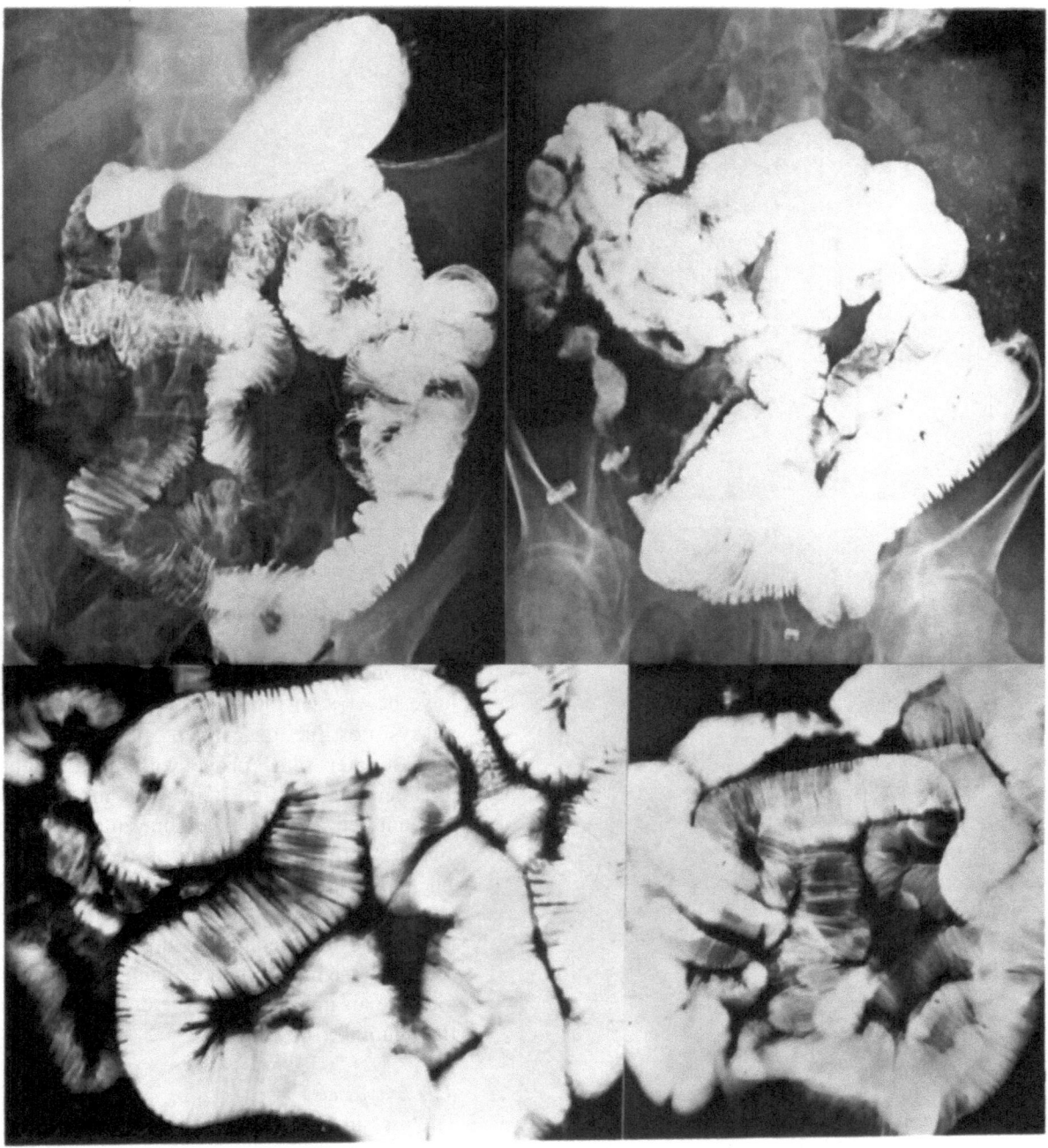

*Fig. 2.19*B. Regular follow-through examination first revealed a large defect between the intestinal loops which was assumed to be a tumor or cyst in the mesentery, even though it was no longer visible in a later stage of the examination (top). A second examination using enteroclysis showed that no abnormalities exist (bottom).

3. Normal impressions on the intestine

Impressions can be caused by other intestinal loops, adjacent organs, vessels, inflammatory infiltrates, tumor tissue and fat. In enteroclysis, the degree of filling of the intestinal loops is greater than in a

conventional follow-through examination so that mutual compression of these loops occurs much more frequently.

3.1. By other intestinal loops
In the jejunum, indentations in the contrast column

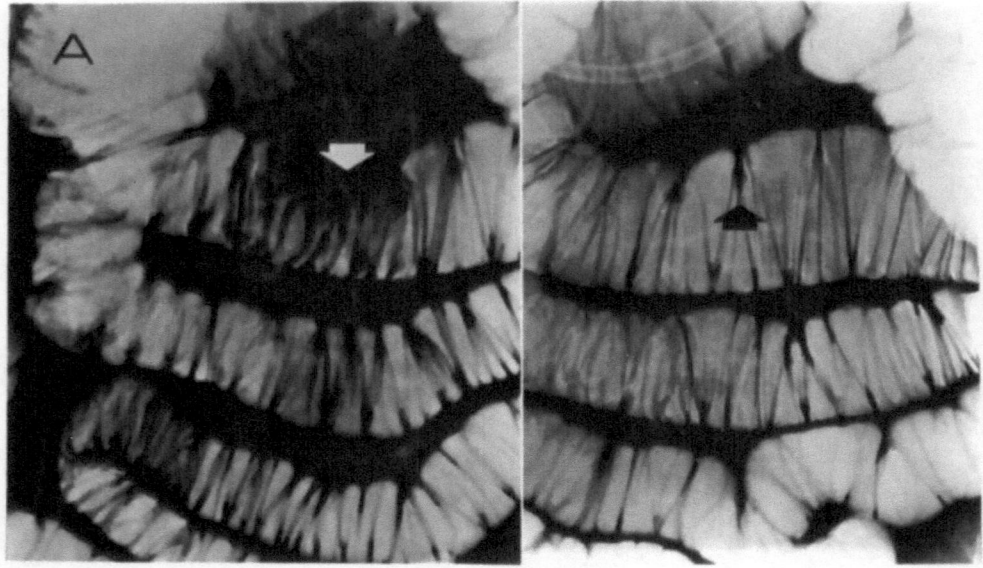

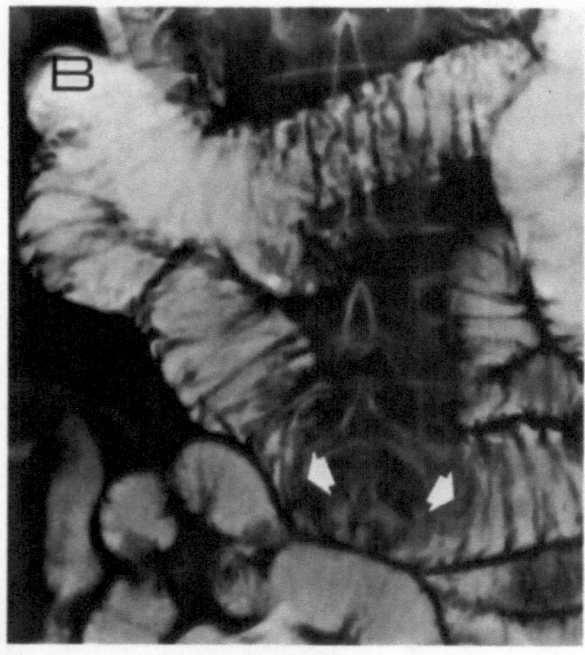

*Fig. 2.20*AB. Temporary impression of unknown origin (abdominal aorta?) on the jejunum.

may be seen, which in later films are shown to be caused by other jejunal loops (fig. 2.18). In general, these impressions are most clearly visible on the largest loops, which usually have the lowest tone or are at that moment in a rest phase. We see fewer impressions on an intestine with active peristalsis, which therefore must have good tone, than on an atonic intestine. Since atony usually affects the proximal intestinal loops sooner than the distal

ones, the most distal loops are more likely to push against the most proximal. An impression of ileal loops on those in the jejunum is therefore likely; we have never seen the opposite (fig. 2.19). It is not always possible to explain an impression even though later films prove without a doubt that it is temporary (fig. 2.20). The most frequently encountered impression of one intestinal loop on another is that of the colon on the small intestine. The most likely explanation for this is the considerable difference in the viscosity of the contents in them. The most common impressions are of the cecum or sigmoid on the ileum; occasionally we may see an impression of the descending colon on the jejunum (fig. 2.21).

3.2. By vessels

The pressure in the veins is so low that indentation by a vein on an intestinal loop is not conceivable. On the other hand, the large arteries frequently cause an impression on the small intestine. Usually we see an indentation in the duodenum due to the aorta where the former passes between the aorta and the superior mesenteric artery (fig. 2.22). The mucosal pattern caused by an aortic indentation can even be so irregular that these indentations mimic tumor growth (fig. 10.7, page 285). An impression of the superior mesenteric artery on the duodenum is rarely visible; it is probably com-

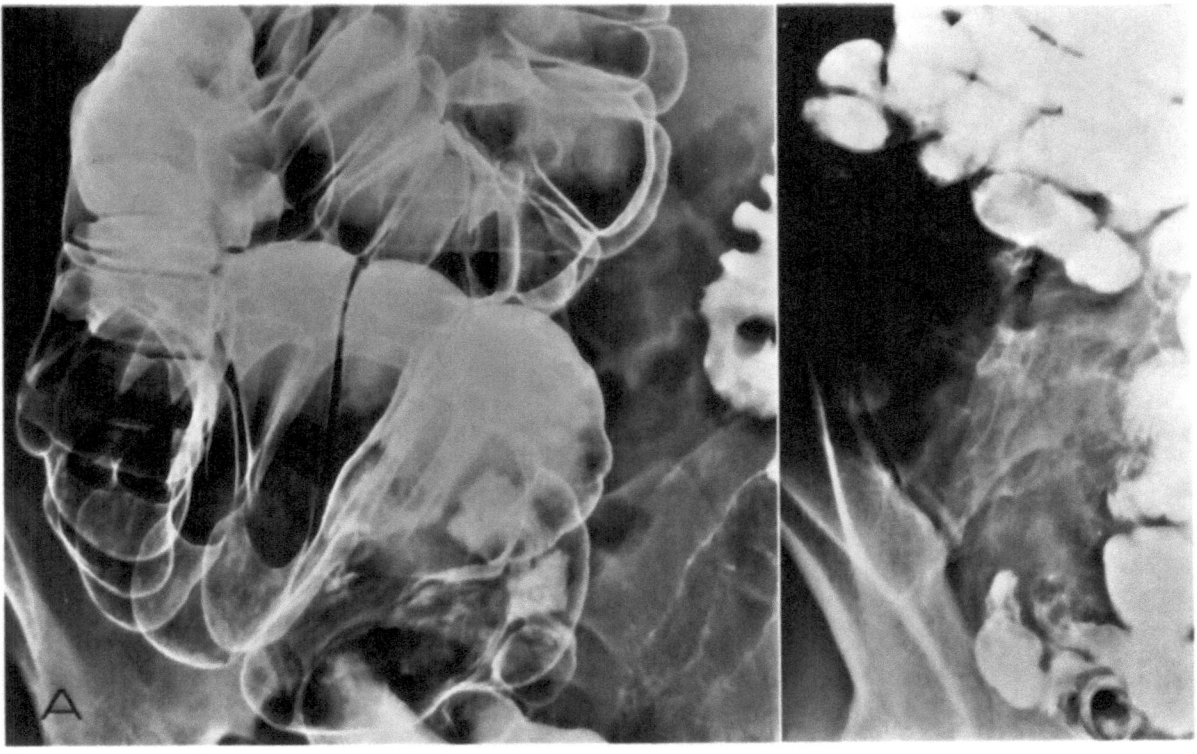

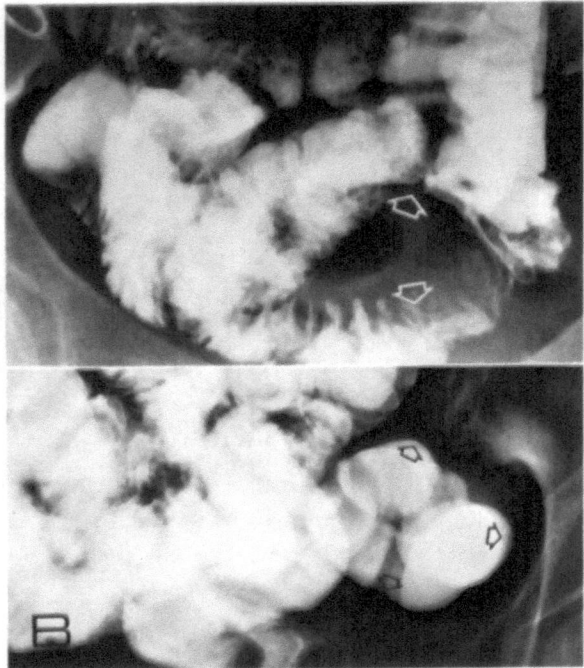

*Fig. 2.21*AB. Several examples of impressions of the colon on the small intestine: (A) the cecum on the ileum; (B) the sigmoid on the ileum.

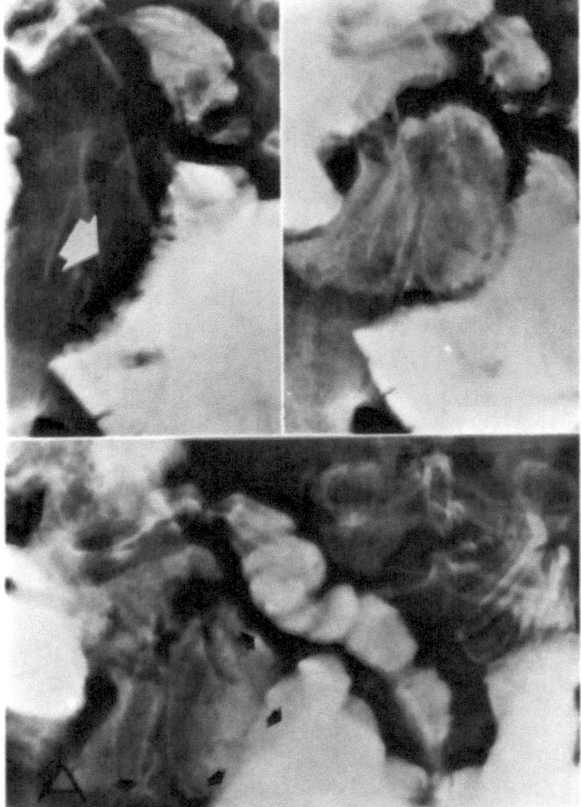

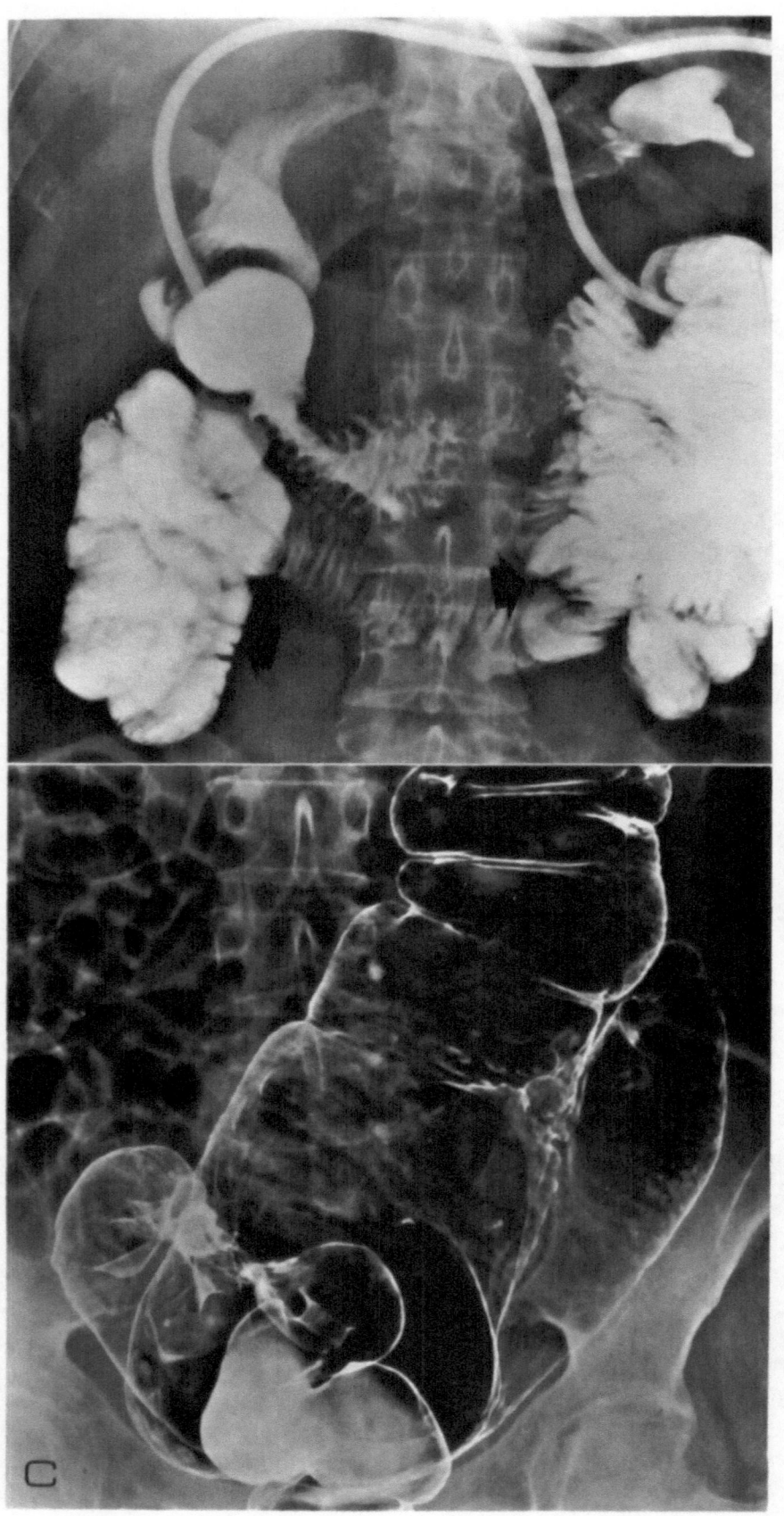

*Fig. 2.21*c. Megasigmoid on the jejunum.

pletely 'overshadowed' by the much larger impression of the aorta.

Another common indentation on an intestinal loop by a large vessel is that of the iliac artery on the ileum at the somewhat narrow pelvic outlet (fig. 2.23). Here too, as in the duodenum and the jejunum, it is striking that such cases involve fairly wide and highly filled intestinal loops, usually as a result of an iatrogenic atony (see chapter 12).

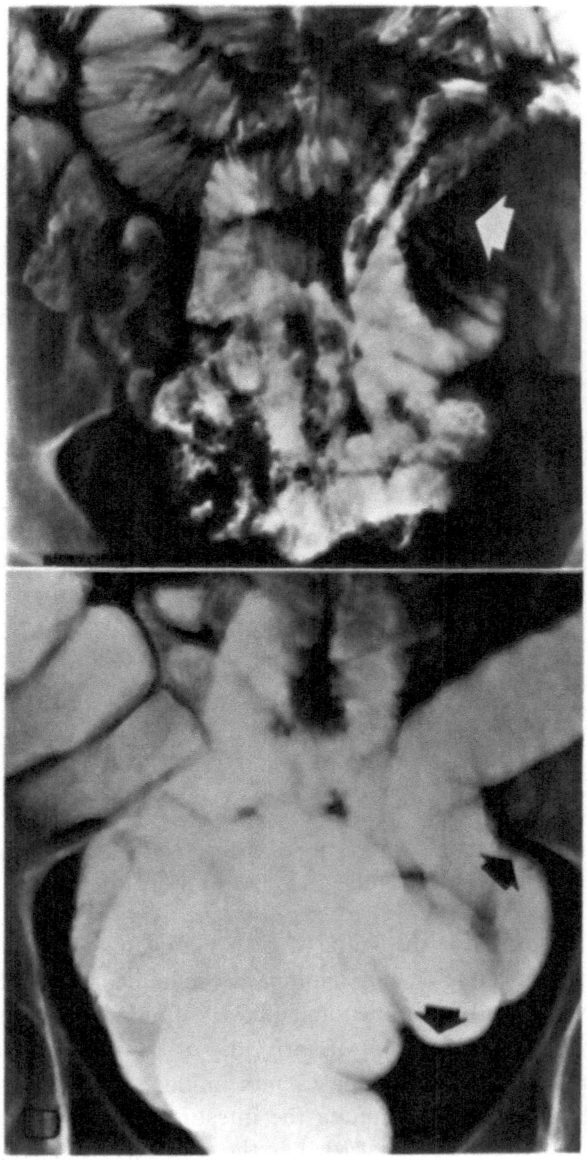

4. Filling defects between the intestinal loops

4.1. Caused by other organs

Exactly in the middle of the abdomen, we sometimes observe an abnormality in the convoluted intestinal loops that is seen only in the prone position; it is because a sagging loop of the transverse colon is filled with feces (fig. 2.24). A fairly recent phenomenon is the appearance of a large abnormality in the convoluted intestinal loops in the lower left or lower right abdomen due to the presence of a heterotopically transplanted kidney (fig. 2.25). Recognition of this abnormality is exceedingly important since the use of compression in this region could cause heavy damage to the transplanted kidney.

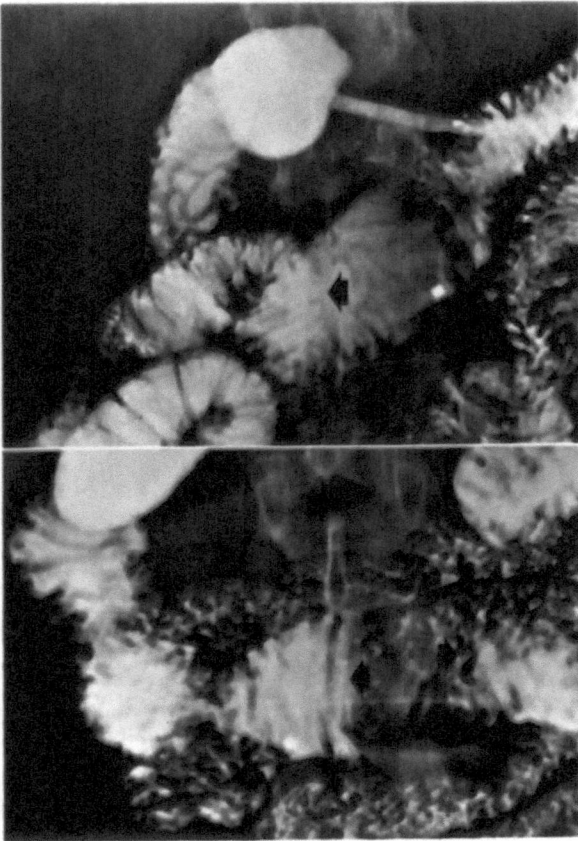

Fig. 2.21D. The descending colon on the jejunum and ileum.

Fig. 2.22. Impression of the abdominal aorta on the duodenum.

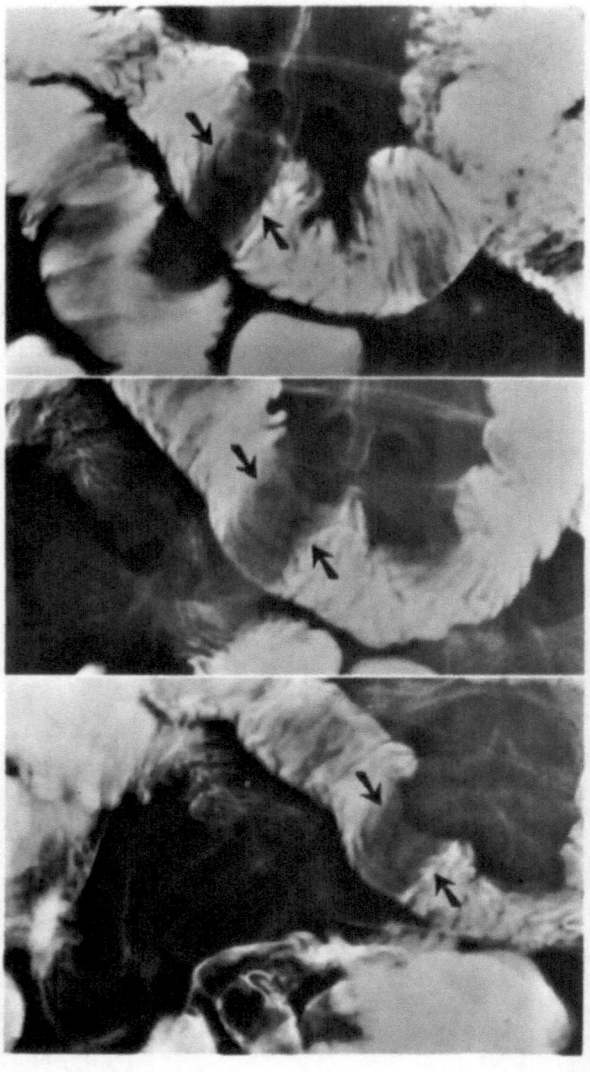

Fig. 2.23. Impression of the iliac artery on the ileum.

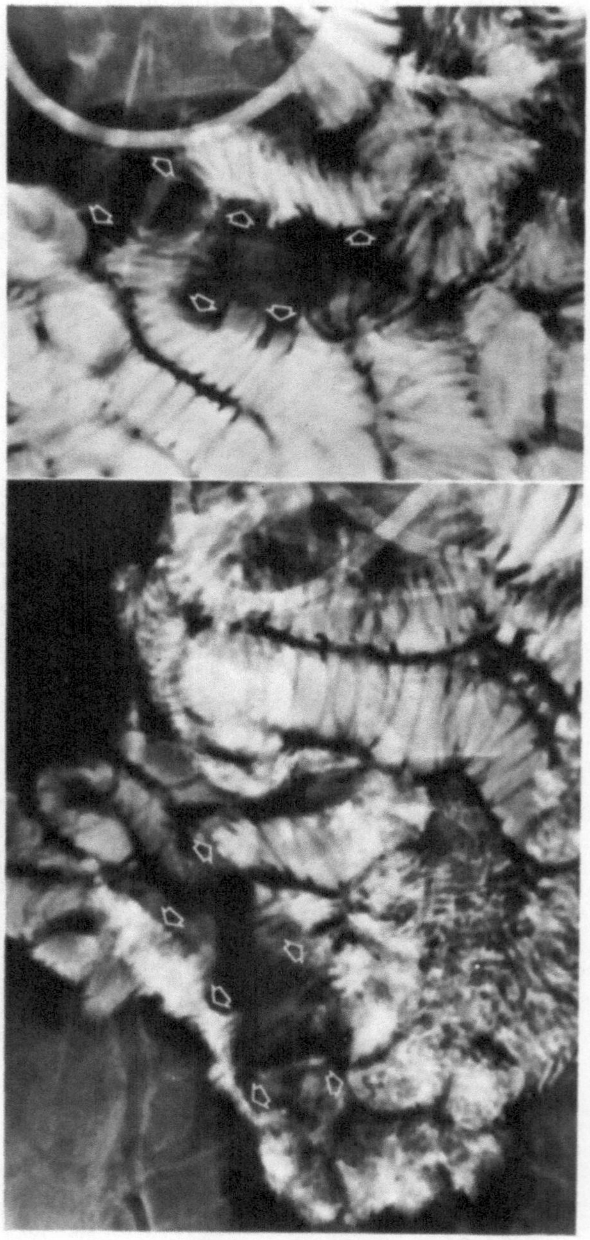

Fig. 2.24. Empty space between the intestinal loops in the mid- and right lower abdomen, caused by the transverse colon.

4.2. *Caused by other tissue structures*

This is not considered a normally occurring phenomenon. For instance, although one would expect to find impressions on the intestinal loops caused by the psoas muscles fairly frequently, they are – for some unknown reason – rarely observed (fig. 2.25B). As far as we have been able to determine so far, marked lordosis of the lumbar spine, hypertrophy of the psoas musculature, a pronounced ptosis of the kidneys, or a clear-cut atony of the intestine do not significantly enhance the development of this phenomenon. A voluminous omentum or degeneration or shriveling of the mesentery can result in empty spaces in the middle of the abdomen or scattered among the intestinal loops; these defects are even larger than those visualized in pyknics (fig. 2.26). In pyknics, there is almost never a convolution of intestinal loops in the minor pelvis

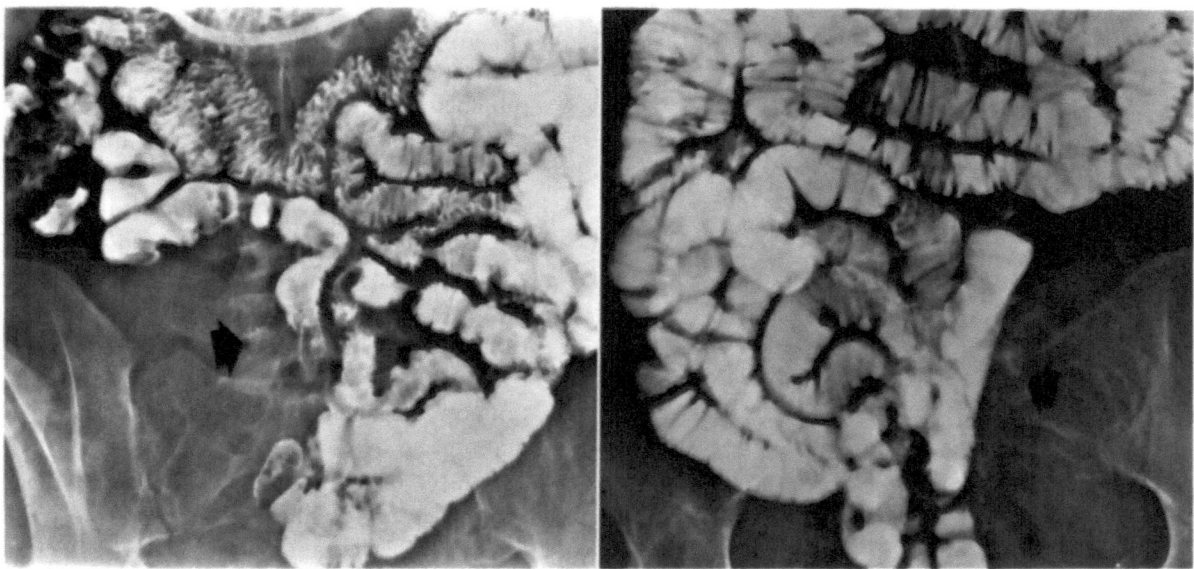

*Fig. 2.25*A. Empty space in the right or left lower abdomen, caused by a heterotopically transplanted kidney.

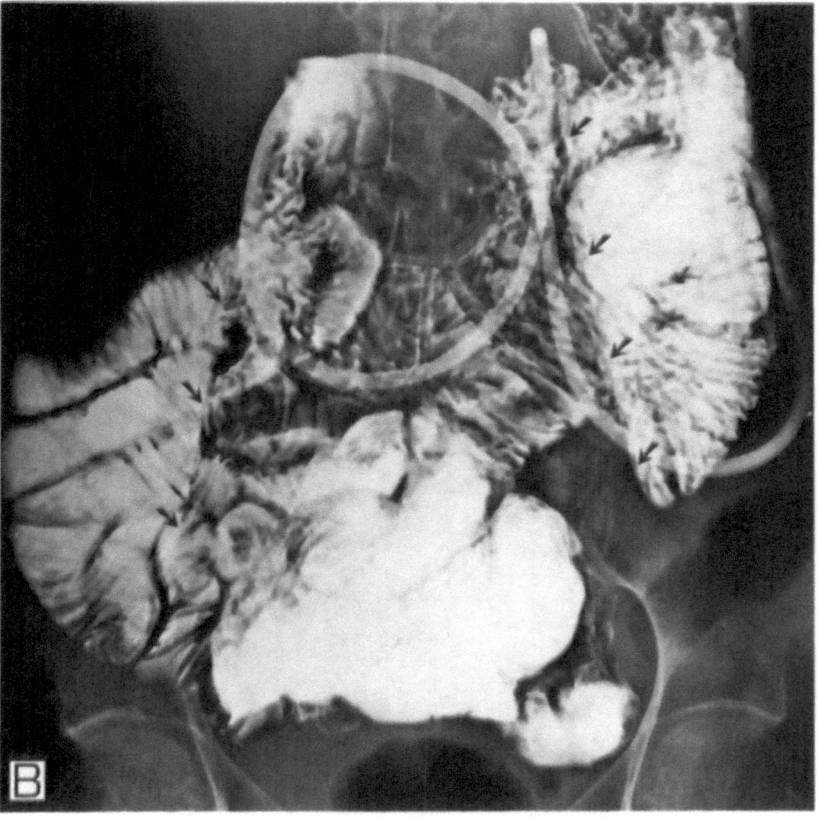

*Fig. 2.25*B. Bilateral sharp lines (arrows) caused by impression of the psoas muscles on the small intestine.

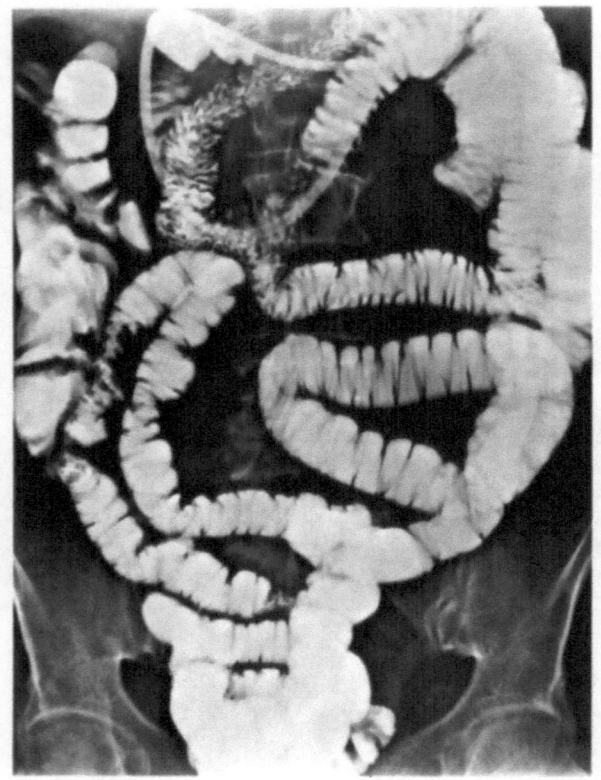

(fig. 2.27). An empty space within the convolution is, however, usually caused by an inflammatory infiltrate, for instance Crohn's disease (fig. 2.28), an inflamed appendix (fig. 2.29A) or an abscess in the abdominal wall (fig. 2.29B). The intestinal loops adjacent to the infiltrate often show deformation and adhesions as well as edematous, irregularly altered or stretched mucosal folds (fig. 2.29B). Approximately the same pattern is seen when the infiltrate is not caused by inflammation but by tumor growth in the intestinal wall or the mesentery (fig. 2.30). A tumor usually causes more pronounced destruction and stenosis than an inflammation.

Tumors or cysts in the wall of the abdomen can sometimes be visualized only when the patient is prone or when compression is used (fig. 2.29B). The opposite may be true for tumors, nodular masses, or cysts located in the mesentery (fig. 2.31).

Fig. 2.26. Unusually large spaces between the intestinal loops in the center of the abdomen, possibly due to mesenteric fat or a copious greater omentum.

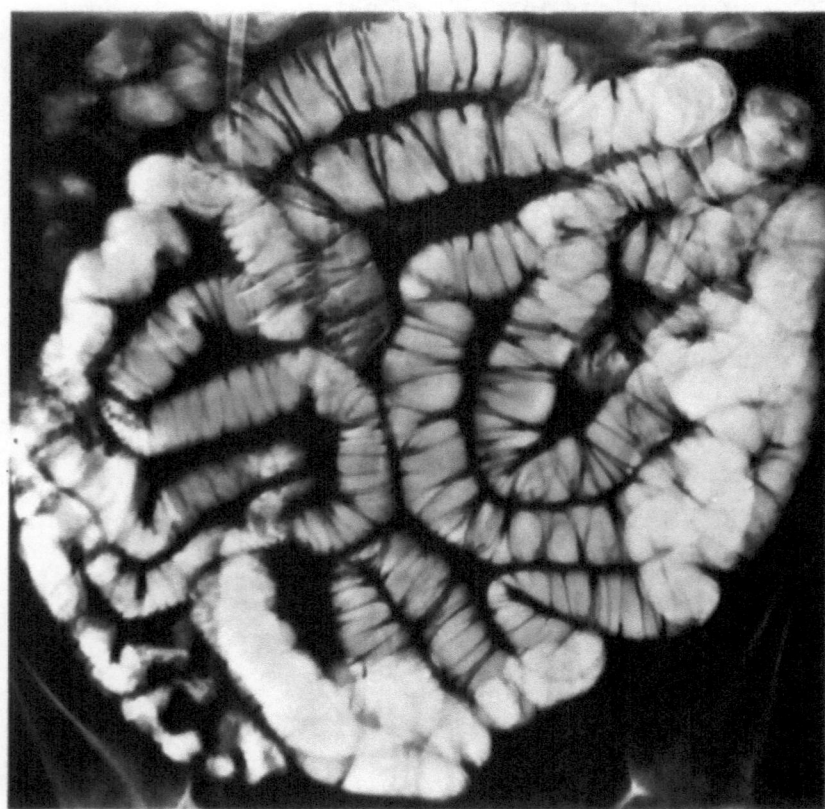

Fig. 2.27. Small intestine of a pyknic, filled with 1200 ml contrast fluid and 600 ml water. No hindrance of superposition.

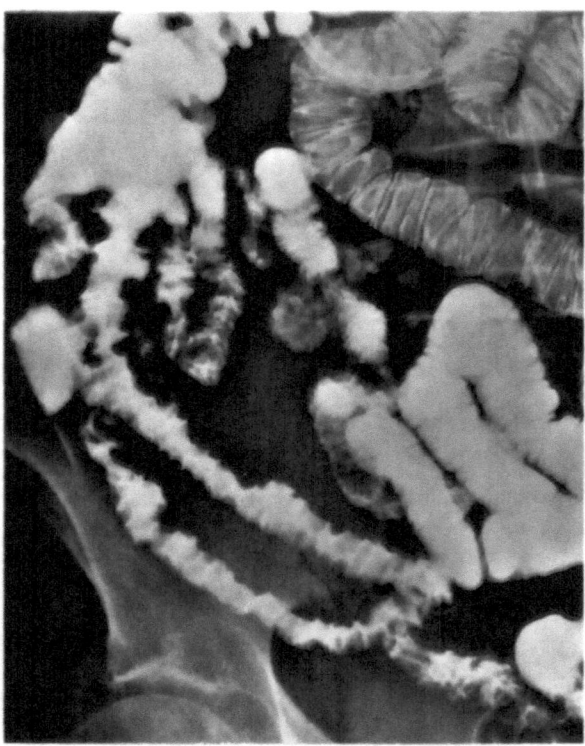

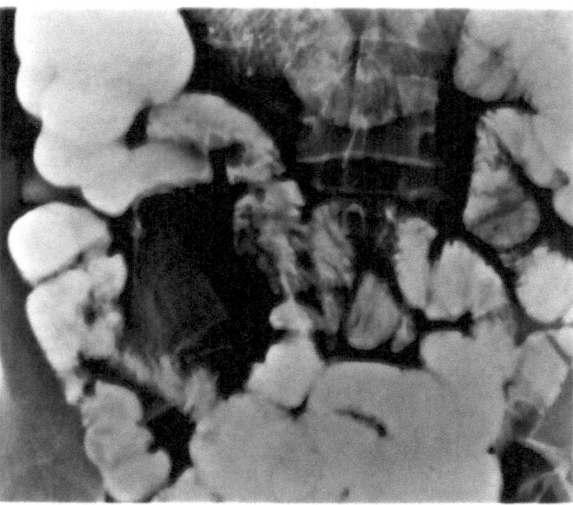

*Fig. 2.29*A. Empty space between the intestinal loops in the right lower abdomen as a result of an appendicular infiltrate.

Fig. 2.28. Greater spaces between intestinal loops as a result of an inflammatory infiltrate or a layer of fat encircling the intestine in Crohn's disease.

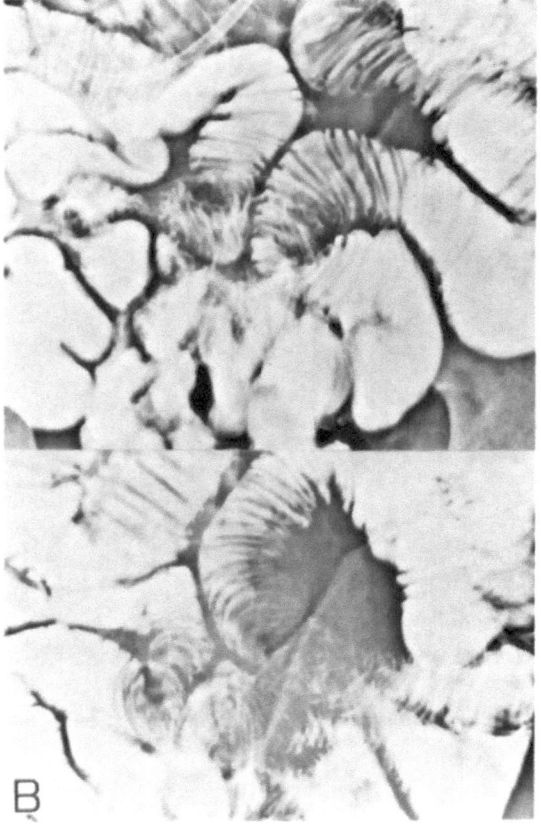

*Fig. 2.29*B. Fusion of intestinal loops to an abscess on the abdominal wall, not or barely visible on the plain film (top). The compression spot film shows that the mucosal folds in the intestinal loops are definitely stretched and that fusion prevents contraction of these loops (bottom).

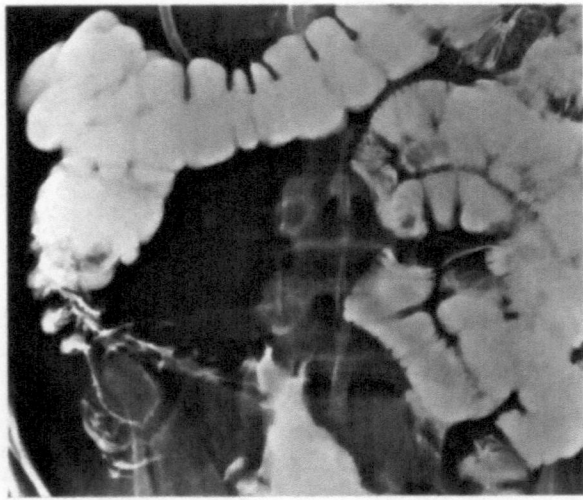

Fig. 2.30. Increased space between intestinal loops caused by tumor growth that has involved the mesentery.

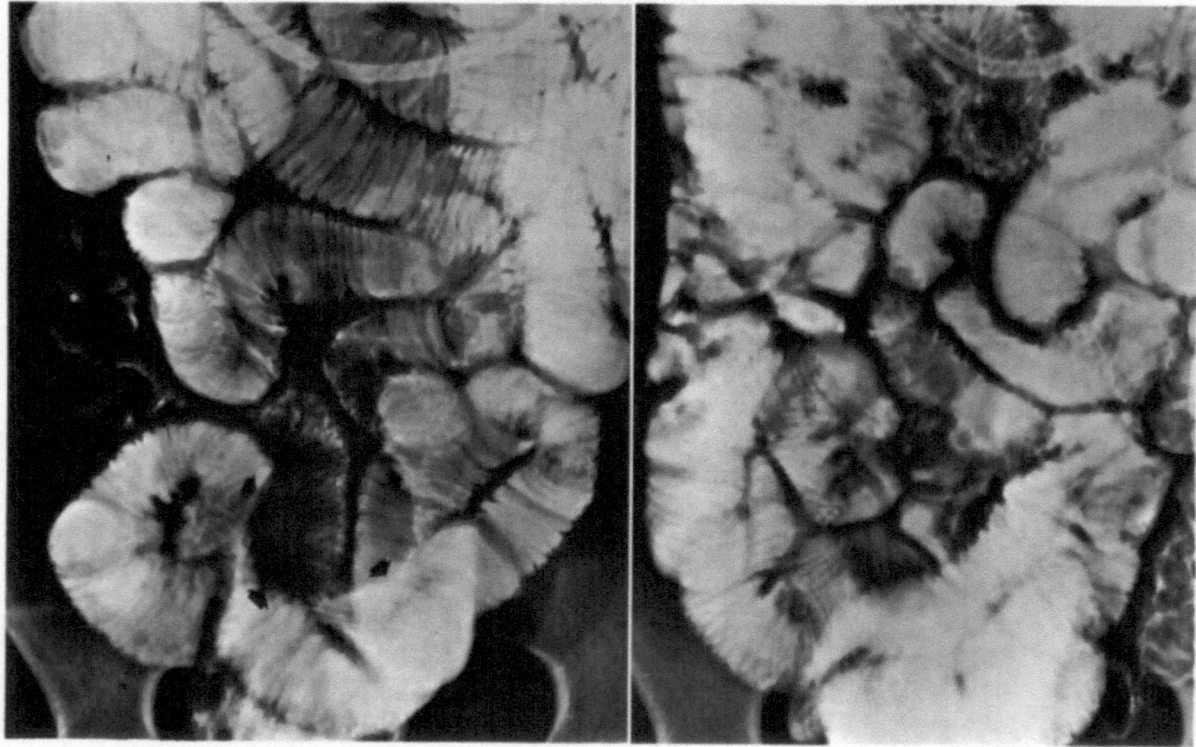

Fig. 2.31. Mesenteric cyst, visible when the patient is in the supine postion (left) and hardly visible in the prone position (right).

3. PHYSIOLOGY

1. Innervation and motility

The parasympathetic innervation of the small intestine occurs via the celiac ganglia by fibers of the right vagus nerve. Cutting the vagus causes a decrease in the motility of the small intestine and therefore a reduced rate of transit. The sympathetic innervation occurs via the splanchnic nerves. The fibers of both systems lie in the mesentery and belong to the central nervous system.

The intramural autonomic nervous system is exceedingly important for the small intestine. It consists of the plexus of Auerbach in the tunica muscularis and the plexus of Meissner in the submucosa (see fig. 2.1).

Loewi (1921) and Dale (1929) showed that when the parasympathetic nerves are stimulated, acetylcholine is produced; in 1933, Cannon demonstrated that stimulation of the sympathetic nerves produces adrenin, which has the same effect as adrenalin. Acetylcholine plays an important role in the transmission of nervous impulses; it is not soluble in fat and cannot pass through the lipoidal membranes of the nerve fibers. Acetylcholine causes contraction of the muscle fibers. Termination of this contraction is caused by the repeated inactivation of acetylcholine by the enzyme acetylcholinesterase. This enzyme can be inactivated by neostigmine; when this occurs, the breakdown of acetylcholine is retarded and the state of contraction or the tone lasts longer. This heightened tone causes an enhancement of the peristalsis, especially in the jejunum.

In 1923, Forssell [57] showed that the movements of the muscularis mucosae are independent and not, as was generally assumed, dependent upon contractions of the tunica muscularis. Using x-ray films and autopsy material, he observed that a given intestinal segment with a lumen of a specific diameter displays highly divergent mucosal patterns. He assumed that the movements of the muscularis mucosae might fulfill an important role in the digestion of food.

In 1922, the physiologists King and Arnold [111] made similar observations but it is not clear whether Forssell was aware of this. They noted that mechanical stimulation of the ends of the villi only caused contractions of the stimulated villi, usually once but occasionally several times in succession. Stimulation at the base of the villi caused contractions of the villi as a group. The mucosa appeared to be stimulated not only locally but also via the splanchnic nerves. The plexus of Meissner probably regulates only the tone. Stimulation of the muscularis mucosae is not possible via the plexus of Auerbach; however, stimulation of the mucosa does cause a relaxation of the tone of the tunica muscularis, followed by a recovery. The rate of this recovery increases as the stimulation is intensified. Physiologically, mechanical stimulation by the food mass is the most important factor causing contractions of the tunica muscularis. The reflex mechanism for these peristaltic waves is regulated via the plexus of Auerbach and it will respond only to stimulation of this plexus [111]. Peristaltic waves of the tunica muscularis are characterized by relaxation before and contraction behind the area stimulated. Although similar in motion to milking, the mechanism involved is not known precisely since it is highly complicated [127]. The longitudinal fibers shorten behind the advancing circular contractions. The frequency of the peristaltic waves is approximately 1 per second. In the case of hypermotility, this frequency increases only slightly, but the contractions clearly become more pronounced. There are fewer peristaltic contractions in the ileum than in the jejunum, and the latent period between stimulation and contraction is the longest in the distal part of the small intestine. In addition, the movements of the villi decrease in the distal direction. This gradual decrease in diverse vital functions from proximal to distal is called the 'metabolic gradient'.

Normally, peristaltic contractions should not occur in the ileum; they are seen, however, when there is an increased irritability of the intestine or a lowered stimulus threshold. The ileum is characterized by segmentation moving in the aboral direction; the intestinal contents are constricted at regular intervals and divided up into the so-called 'segments of Cannon' [128].

Nicotine and stimulation of the vagus influence the tunica muscularis but not the muscularis mucosae [112]. The development of the mucosa appears to be highly dependent upon the blood supply [76, 112]. Abbott and Pendergrass [1] found that when morphine is administered directly into the duodenum, there is a pronounced increase in the tone which decreases in the distal direction; 15–20 min later, the tone decreases – it is once again the greatest in the duodenum and decreases in the distal direction. Using a double balloon to register the change in the pressure in the small intestine, they observed that the motility is highly dependent upon the differences in tone and that the intensity of the peristaltic waves increases with an increase in the tone of the intestinal wall. Lenz and Kreppel [129] studied the influence of Prostigmin, pilocarpine, and arecoline on the motility of the small intestine of a cat, which is structured similar to that of man. The movements of the contrast column were filmed. After Prostigmin was injected, the tone increased and the Cannon constrictions became more pronounced and more frequent; the number of peristaltic contractions also increased. The Prostigmin was ineffective 9 min later and hypotonia occurred.

The intensification of peristalsis produced by neostigmine or Prostigmin is used in intravenous pyelography to remove troublesome small gas bubbles from the small intestine. It is well known that air in the small intestine moves so fast in the distal direction that it takes only several minutes to travel from the stomach to the cecum. Large gas bubbles generally remove themselves from the digestive tract since they cause sufficient stretching of the intestinal wall to induce peristaltic contractions [137].

The effect of Prostigmin is canceled by atropine. Neostigmine has no effect on patients with sprue; it is tentatively assumed that this is due to a disturbed functioning of the nerve cells. In this respect the role of vitamin B deficiencies is still unknown.

The results with pilocarpine and arecoline were similar but more pronounced. In particular, pilocarpine enhanced secretion so that dilution of the contrast medium was greater than with Prostigmin. The mucosal folds were clearly broadened; autopsy showed that this was due to edema. Overdosage of Prostigmin and arecoline caused spasms and dyskinesia; peristaltic waves no longer occurred. An overdosage of pilocarpine did not cause dyskinesia, but there was such heavy secretion and edematous swelling of the mucous membrane that peristaltic waves were no longer possible mechanically.

In 1937, Pansdorf [178] had already observed swelling of the folds of Kerkring caused by pilocarpine in 18 healthy persons. The effect of these three substances, called the muscarine effect, is similar to that of postganglionic sympathetic stimulation and can be neutralized by atropine. Pilocarpine and arecoline act directly on the smooth musculature; Prostigmin acts on cholinesterase.

2. Gastric emptying and transit time

2.1. Peristalsis

The rate of transit of a contrast fluid through the small intestine depends almost entirely on the rate and intensity of the peristaltic movements in the intestine. This motility is in turn dependent on diverse factors that can be utilized by the physician at will, such as caloric value, temperature, and osmosity of the contrast fluid. However, the most important factor, as far as the stimulation of peristalsis is concerned, is the gastric emptying time since this determines the degree of stretching of the duodenum and the proximal jejunum. The latter is essential for the stimulation of good peristaltic movements. If there are no factors inhibiting peristalsis (these are described in detail in chapter 12) and if mechanical passage through the pylorus is unimpeded, then the gastric emptying time depends to a large extent on the degree of filling. These considerations shall now be discussed in more detail.

2.2. Quantity

Henderson [90] studied the gastric emptying time for 110 infants by using specific amounts of contrast medium; he found values of 8–24 h for a newborn child, 4–5 h for a baby two weeks old, and 2–3 h for babies three to four months old. He therefore advised that the fasting period before examination of the baby should be longer than the usual 4 h. He observed that two-thirds of the contrast medium leaves the stomach rather quickly but the remaining one-third takes considerably longer. He also saw that the stomach empties faster when the babies are in the prone or right lateral position and that good mucosal patterns, sometimes even of the proximal ileum, can be obtained only under these conditions. He was not able to find an explanation for this observation.

Even the size of the meal influences the gastric emptying time. Van Liere et al. [132] reported emptying times for 200 ml, 400 ml, and 600 ml in normal individuals. They found that 400 ml of a watery barium suspension took only 16.83% instead of 100% longer to leave the stomach than 200 ml; 600 ml took 38.33% longer. The use of two decimal places suggests an accuracy in conflict with the small number of persons tested. It is also improbable that the second supplementary dosage of 200 ml took $38.33 - 2 \times 16.83 = 4.67\%$ longer to leave the stomach than the first supplementary dosage of 200 ml. However, the inaccuracies caused by these small numbers do not change the importance of their observations. This phenomenon can be explained only by the greater supply that, especially in the beginning, is comparable to a continuous supply in the right lateral position. Henderson observed that the gastric emptying time for a child decreases gradually; this follows in the same line of thought [90].

2.3. Temperature

Gershon-Cohen et al. [71] found that barium test meals cooled to 35°–40° F left the stomach sooner and (therefore) passed through the small intestine more quickly than contrast meals heated up to 140°–145° F. The mechanism of this accelerated gastric emptying and rapid transit after cold meals is not known. The assumption that it is due to insufficient digestion and absorption resulting from decreased secretion is speculative. Gastric secretion decreases markedly when the gastric contents are cold; however, when the gastric contents are warm, secretion increases to only slightly above the norm. For cold gastric contents, secretion returns to normal more rapidly than the increase in the temperature of the gastric contents suggests.

2.4. Nutrients

The influence of nutrients on gastric emptying and transit time through the small intestine can best be studied by using carbohydrates. Glucose was chosen because it mixes easily with the contrast fluid and, with it, the contrast fluid can easily be made hypertonic. Hypertonic gastric contents first become isotonic; during this process, the volume can increase considerably. For example, 215 ml of a 50% glucose solution increases to more than 500 ml after 1 h in the stomach [132]; 100 ml of a 10% glucose solution increases to 128 ml, and 12 min later it is still 122 ml. When a 3.5% glucose solution is administered orally, then 1 h later the glucose concentration in the small intestine is 2.6 mg/100 ml. If a 50% glucose solution is used, this concentration is only 5.3 mg/100 ml, a relatively small difference.

Reynolds et al. [198] compared the gastric emptying time for 33 children by using five different mixtures of the contrast medium. They examined each child five times; their values were:

Contrast medium	Gastric emptying time
1) 60 g Ba + 120 g water	1.9 h
2) 60 g Ba + 120 g milk (2.3% fat)	3.1 h
3) 60 g Ba + 120 g cream (13.3% fat)	4.8 h
4) 60 g Ba + 90 g water + 30 g syrup	3.3 h
5) 40 g Ba + 200 g water + 100 g protein (3.5% fat, 7% protein)	5.0 h

If we consider that the high value of the fifth test is due to the greater amount administered, then we can conclude from the above that fat is the slowest to leave the stomach. This conclusion is in agreement with that of Menville and Ané [155], who carried out similar tests with adults. They found that proteins and carbohydrates retard gastric emptying to the same extent, but fats considerably more. Fat was also the most important factor causing retarded transit through the small intestine. Although the gastric emptying time is shorter after a partial gastrectomy, here too the addition of nutrients to the contrast medium has a delaying effect. Because of the presence of glucose in the proximal part of the small intestine, enterogastrone is produced, a hormone that inhibits the peristalsis of the stomach. Similar mechanisms also exist for fat and possibly protein.

Van Liere et al. [132] introduced 50 ml of an indifferent mixture into the stomach of dogs that had first received an intravenous glucose injection. Autopsy showed that a half-hour later this mixture had moved an average of 141 cm in the small intestine in contrast to 183 cm for the control group. The blood sugar was then 183 mg% versus 99 mg% for the control group. According to their report, the inhibitory influence of a high blood sugar concentration on the peristalsis of stomach and intestine has been known since 1924. A low blood sugar concentration, on the other hand, causes contractions of the stomach and a feeling of hunger.

2.5. Osmosity

In 1907 it was reported that isotonic solutions leave the stomach faster than hypotonic or hypertonic solutions [132]. Gershon-Cohen et al. [70] showed that a hypotonic solution leaves the stomach almost as fast as an isotonic solution. However, when these solutions are introduced directly into the duodenum, then the hypotonic solution causes the pylorus to remain closed until isotonicity is achieved. A solution becomes isotonic much faster in the duodenum than in the stomach although the stomach also attempts to make a hypertonic solution isotonic by fluid secretion.

Using HCl and Na_2CO_3, Shay and Gershon-Cohen demonstrated that the responses of the stomach and the pylorus are the same, whether the hypertonic solution is administered into the stomach or directly into the duodenum by intubation [211]. Johnston and Ravdin [104] administered glucose-barium to dogs after a partial gastrectomy to demonstrate that severe contractions of the small intestine compensate to some extent for the absence of the pylorus. They also observed this in patients.

This peristalsis can vary greatly for the same tone. For a rapid increase in pressure in the intestinal lumen, the stimulus threshold for the development of peristaltic waves is lower than for a slow increase in pressure. The stimulus threshold is also lower for an increased tone than for a decreased tone [40]. If there is a marked increase in pressure or pronounced stretching of the intestinal wall, which physiologically probably does not occur, motility is inhibited after a latent period of 2–3 s. This enterointestinal 'inhibitory reflex' [245] develops more rapidly as the stretching or pressure as well as the length of the intestinal segment involved increases.

2.6. pH

In addition to the caloric value of gastric and duodenal contents and osmosity, the pH also plays an important role [211]. The contents of the duodenum are usually slightly acidic, depending upon the composition of the ingested food. It appears that prolonged closing of the pylorus is not caused by highly acidic contents alone; this occurs also when sodium bicarbonate is introduced via a tube, causing the duodenal contents to become alkaline [37]. This mechanism of duodenal neutralization is the most highly developed in hyperchlorhydria and the least in achlorhydria. The most sensitive reactions to tone and acidity occur in the proximal part of the duodenum and decrease in the distal direction [211].

In an empty stomach, the pyloric ring is relaxed, which explains why the bulb is so often well filled immediately after administration of the first few mouthfuls of barium in a gastric examination. Shortly afterward, the pylorus closes; the latent period for this reaction is several seconds. The tone of the gastric musculature depends upon the conditions in the duodenum and is the stimulus for the development of peristaltic waves. These peristaltic waves are, however, not necessary for gastric emptying; the stomach can also empty if there is sufficient tone and an open pyloric ring. The pylorus is more relaxed in achlorhydria than when there is free acid in the stomach. If the other conditions remain the same, then the stomach empties faster in achlorhydria.

2.7. Emotion

Another well-known fact is that fear and emotion influence the small intestine by causing an increase in tone and an enhancement of the peristalsis. Because there is not enough time for the absorption of fluids, diarrhea develops. The opening and closing of the pylorus is a very complicated mechanism that is only partially understood. Almost everyone who has studied this mechanism has found that a peristaltic wave in the stomach is not necessarily followed by relaxation of the pyloric ring.

4. THE CONTRAST MEDIUM

1. General considerations

During the second world war, barium was the generally accepted contrast medium for examination of the small intestine. The 40-year-old custom of mixing nutrients with the contrast medium was abandoned since this appeared to be the main reason that good mucosal patterns could not be obtained. The importance of fine demonstration of anatomical detail had become paramount since the morphological examination of the small intestine had replaced the functional examination. The omission of nutrients, however, did not improve the characteristics of the contrast medium to an extent such that it could be regarded as ideal and satisfactory for everyone. It was recognized that a good contrast medium suitable for examination of the digestive tract must satisfy many requirements, namely [249]:

1) Sedimentation should not occur after prolonged standing.
2) It must mix easily with all secretions and digestive products found in the stomach and the small intestine without flocculation and segmentation. The contrast medium also had to be insensitive to pH changes.
3) It must adhere readily.
4) The viscosity could vary between that of water and of cream, but no more. In order to prevent the formation of hard masses due to fluid absorption in the colon and the distal ileum, a specific maximum viscosity could not be exceeded.
5) The barium content must be high enough for good contrast.
6) It must have a homogeneous structure.
7) It must have a pleasant taste.
8) It must be nontoxic.

9) It must be inexpensive and easy to prepare without clumping or foam formation. Later these characteristics were expanded to include:
10) It must stimulate peristalsis.

Obviously it is not easy, if at all possible, to find a contrast medium that satisfies all of these requirements. Several of these factors will be discussed separately in more detail.

2. Sedimentation of the contrast medium

A well-known characteristic of barium powder is that it precipitates quickly in aqueous suspensions, as does bismuth. In 1931, Holzknecht wrote in his handbook [97] that the colon mixture must be stirred until just before use. In the same book, Jozef Paluguay wrote that colloidal barium suspensions that gave a better reproduction of relief and that settled less quickly were on the market. He did not see the usefulness of these new media, however, because the same could be achieved by first boiling and then cooling the barium suspension.

The problem of sedimentation had already been studied extensively in 1947 by the pharmacologist Braeckman [24]. He suggested that the formation of clumps of barium particles can be separated into an orthokinetic coagulation. The former pertains to the larger particles and is caused by gravitation; the latter applies to the smaller particles and is caused by Brownian movement. Although an increase in the viscosity of the solution will cause a decrease in both types of clumping, perikinetic coagulation is more effectively combated by adding an electrolyte or peptizing agent to the contrast suspension. In addition, there is of course less coagulation when the particles are smaller: it is also important that the particles be of equal size, other-

34

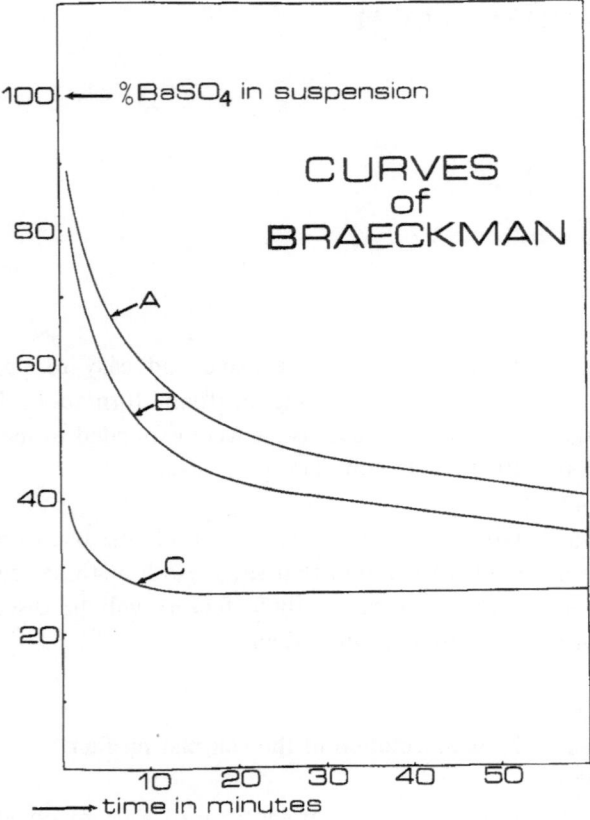

Fig. 4.1. Difference in rate of sedimentation of following mixtures: (A) BaSO$_4$ + 0.01 N sodium citrate + 7.5% arabic gum; (B) BaSO$_4$ + 7.5% arabic gum; (C) BaSO$_4$ + 0.01N sodium citrate.

wise the larger will act as nidus [26]. The latter, however, is physiologically impossible to achieve.

Barium sulfate particles in water have a slight negative charge due to the OH groups on their surface. The agglomeration of these particles is decreased by increasing their negative charge. Brown achieved this by adding a small amount of an electrolyte with many hydroxyl groups, such as sodium carboxymethylcellulose. Braeckman obtained the best results in his experiments with a mixture of 7.5% arabic gum and 0.01 N sodium citrate. On a graph, he showed the differences between the rate of sedimentation of a mixture of BaSO$_4$ and 0.01 N sodium citrate, and the rate of sedimentation of the same mixture with 7.5% arabic gum (fig. 4.1). If too much hydrophilic colloid is added, then the negative charge will become too high and clumping will again occur as a result of the strong mutual repulsion. During this phenomenon,

called 'super settling', a barium mass develops which is so hard and compact that it can no longer be resuspended. A suspension with such a high negative charge has the advantage of being almost insensitive to pH changes in the digestive tract. Therefore, mucus and other substances found in the digestive tract will not cause flocculation. Since in any event 'super settling' must be avoided, some tendency toward flocculation is unfortunately necessary. The rate of sedimentation of many barium sulfate preparations now on the market is so low that this factor no longer plays a role in the examination of patients. The stomach and the intestine are in sufficient continuous motion to prevent pure sedimentation. Letters and Gaul [131] had already reached this conclusion in 1951.

3. Flocculation of the contrast fluid

A phenomenon that perhaps appears quite similar to sedimentation, but must definitely be differentiated from it, is the flocculation of barium particles in the contrast suspension when it comes into contact with specific substances found in the digestive tract, such as hydrochloric acid, gall, and mucin. Mucin is coated with colloidal protein polymers that are usually amphoteric: it is therefore positive in acidic and negative in basic surroundings. Under normal circumstances, therefore, a massive clumping with the negatively charged barium particles will occur in the stomach. We call this phenomenon flocculation. It had already been reported in 1931 by Berg and in 1932 by Frik [65]. Knoefel et al. [114] demonstrated that a 10% solution of barium sulfate flocculates ten times as fast in gastric juice as in water. An increase in the amount of gastric juice causes a further increase in the rate of flocculation until a specific limiting value has been reached, apparently when all the muco-protein has combined. Sedimentation appears to be mainly a physical process, flocculation a chemical process. A contrast medium prepared from barium powder with very tiny particles of approximately the same size, which in addition has a cream-like viscosity and contains a peptizing agent, will produce practically no sedimentation in vitro. Experience with patients has, however, shown that this same medium can, in spite of continuous move-

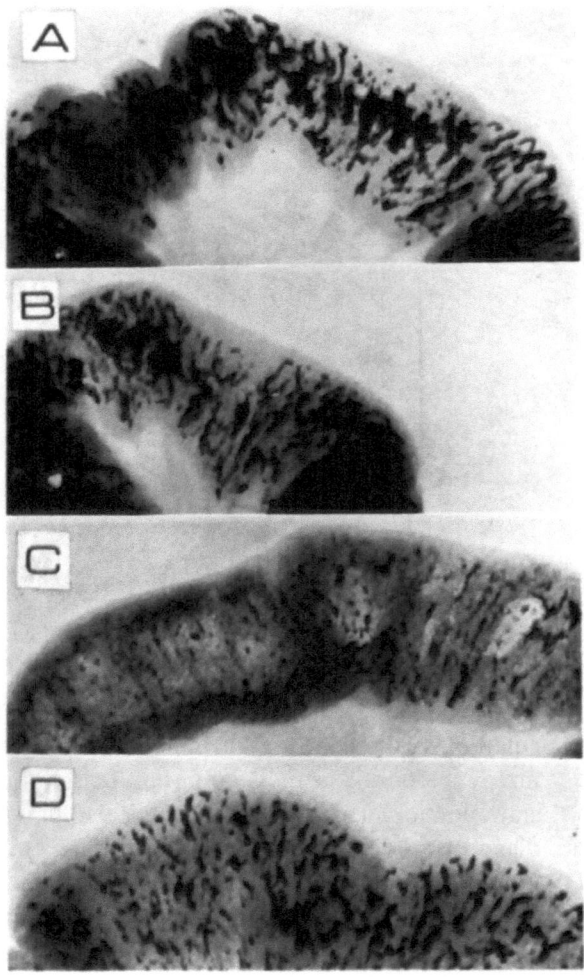

Fig. 4.2. Contrast fluid in isolated intestinal loop during surgery. There is practically no barium left in suspension. Peristalsis induced by injection of Prostigmin. (AB) Beginning of clump formation. (CD) Flocculation (snowflake pattern) (Deucher [43]).

ment, still produce pronounced flocculation when gastric acid or other juices found in the digestive tract are added. The precipitation caused by sedimentation in vitro has a homogeneous structure. Flocculation, on the other hand, produces a precipitation with a coarse, splotchy structure. A complete change in the viscosity of the contrast medium is also possible (fig. 4.3B). Also in vivo, flocculation can be recognized by the coarse, splotchy structure of the contrast medium in the intestinal lumen; this is called the 'snowflake pattern'. The finely spotted pattern, usually left behind after the contrast medium has passed through the jejunum, is also caused by flocculation of the

residual barium. In general it can be stated that these floccules will be smaller when the contrast fluid adheres less readily to the mucosa so that less barium is left behind.

Deucher [43] introduced barium into isolated intestinal loops in surgical patients during the operation and induced peristalsis with an injection of Prostigmin. He then made roentgenograms that showed a finely spotted distribution of the contrast medium in the intestinal loops. In addition, he noted that the outline of the intestinal lumen could not be distinguished clearly (fig. 4.2). Deucher was not able to give a convincing explanation for these phenomena. The retention of contrast fluid between swollen folds that were not able to contract seemed to him the most likely explanation. He assumed that the mucosal swelling was caused by a disturbance in the blood circulation since there were no indications of an infectious process in the intestinal wall. It is now clear that we are confronted here with such a complete flocculation of the contrast fluid that there is no barium left in the suspension at all. The difference between the specific gravity of the suspension fluid and that of the tissue of the intestinal wall has therefore become so small that the outline of the intestinal lumen can no longer be seen.

Deucher showed quite clearly with this experiment that no further morphological information can be obtained once flocculation has occurred. Many radiologists have found that a small dose of contrast medium causes more flocculation than a large dose. It has long been known that flocculation occurs in the foremost part of the contrast column, which disappears as soon as more contrast medium is administered [184]. Patterson even saw flocculation develop with the exceedingly stable Raybar that he introduced directly into the duodenum. For the patients he examined in this way, however, he only used 40 ml of this contrast medium [179].

In a series of in vitro experiments, we studied the occurrence of sedimentation and flocculation. Five barium suspensions of various brands were placed in test tubes, agitated, and then set aside for 30 min. X-rays then made with a horizontal beam showed a very thin and unimportant liquid film on the surface of several brands of contrast medium and some sediment at the bottom of the test tube for

36

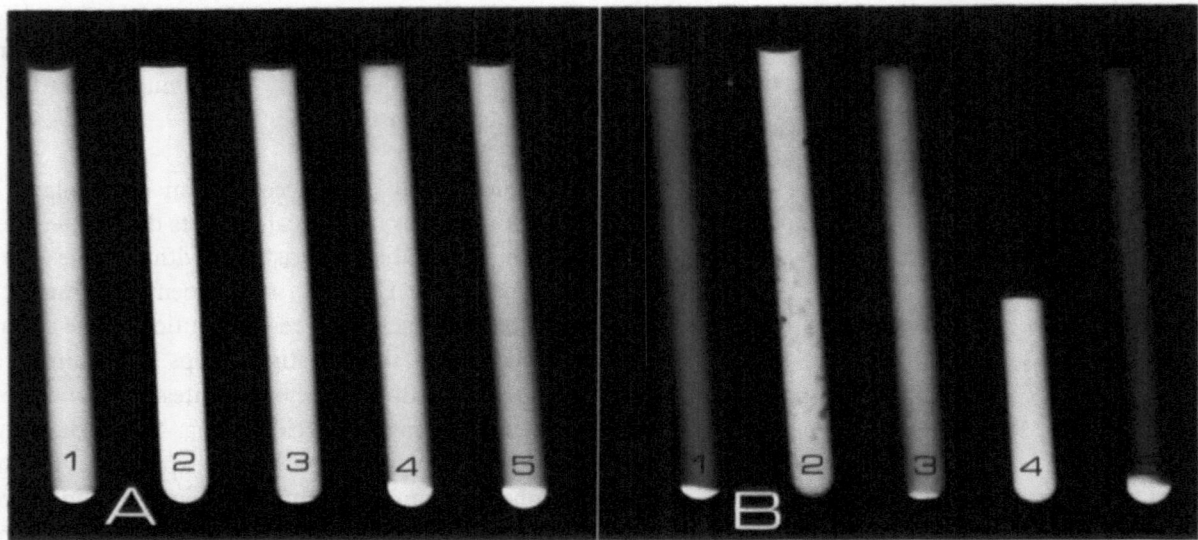

Fig. 4.3. In vitro tests with five current brands of contrast medium, numbered 1–5. (A) After standing for 30 min, only slight sedimentation of barium particles. (B) 15 ml of the same contrast fluids used in A mixed with 5 ml 1/10 N HCl. X-ray after 30 min, brand 2 shows flocculation; for brand 4, there is practically no barium left in suspension.

others (fig. 4.3A). In particular, the structure of brands 2 and 3 appears to remain homogeneous. It is therefore obvious that the annoying effect of sedimentation no longer plays a role, especially in vivo, since the contrast fluid is also in continuous motion. The test was repeated by mixing 15 ml of the same contrast media with 5 ml 0.1 N HCl. A contrast–acid ratio is then created that can occur under physiological circumstances. The films made after 30 min (fig. 4.3B) show that the structure of brand 2 is definitely no longer homogeneous (flocculation). The contrast medium has acquired a gelatinous to pudding-like consistency, and only after energetic shaking could it be removed from the test tube. Brand 3 appeared to be insensitive to the addition of the acid while brand 4 flocculated completely. Although most brands of contrast medium on the market can withstand basic better than acidic substances, tests have shown that their characteristics can change greatly under influence of intestinal juice [60, 250]. It is therefore clear that barium suspensions can completely lose their most valuable characteristics in vivo.

It was exceedingly difficult for the chemical industry to produce a contrast medium that retains its stability in both acidic and basic surroundings. Figure 4.3 shows that not every manufacturer has been successful in this respect.

The fact that the factors responsible for flocculation of the contrast medium were not recognized is certainly the most important reason for the slow development of the radiological differential diagnosis of diseases of the small intestine. Golden assumed that the flocculation and subsequent disintegration into segment clumps of the contrast column resulted from a disturbed motor function of the small intestine, which is a dominant symptom of sprue, and is caused by abnormalities in the intramural nervous system of the intestinal wall [80]. Bouslog [22] agreed with Golden's interpretation because the nervous system in the intestinal wall of babies only a few months old is still underdeveloped. During the examination of the small intestine of these babies, he observed only that the contrast fluid flocculates and finally disintegrates into segment clumps. Caffey supported the assumption of a disordered motor function by reporting that passage through the small intestine lasted 5–6 h for newborn children. In addition, some radiologists, including Golden, Friedman [63], and Goin [75], had found that fear and emotion could cause sudden flocculation of the barium suspension, a phenomenon which is said to have also been observed in animals.

Many other radiologists, including Reynolds et al. [198] in 1940, proved convincingly that floc-

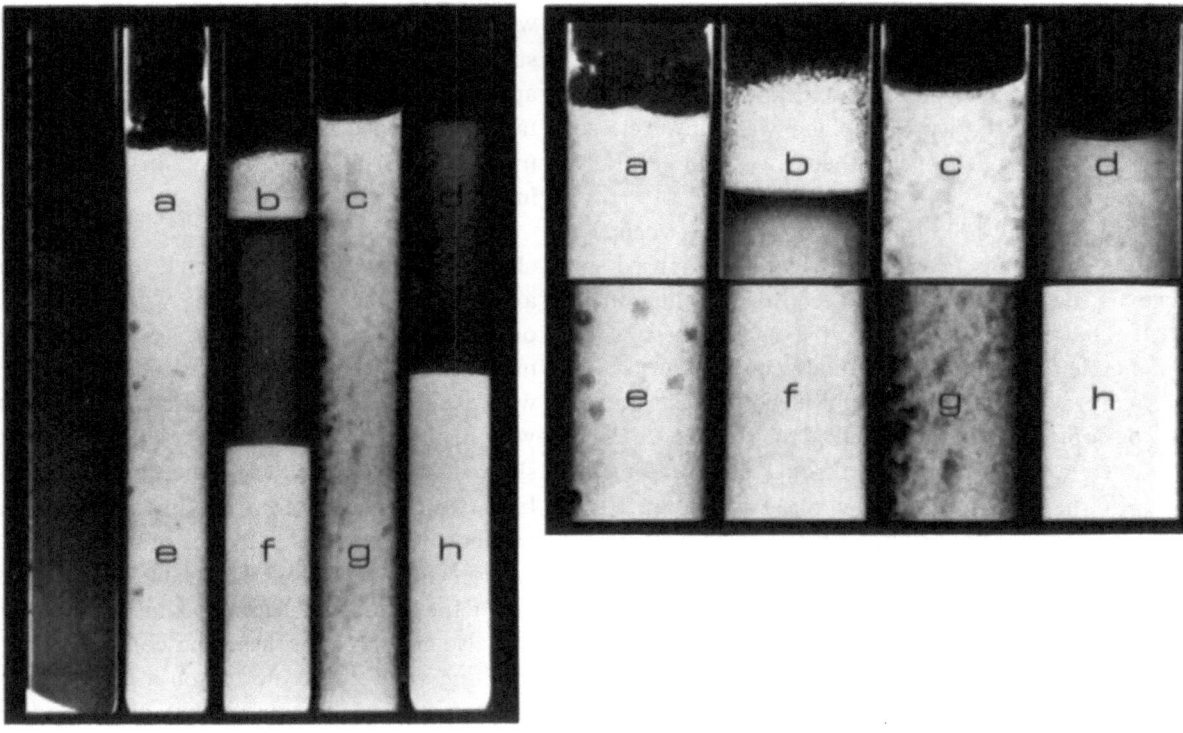

Fig. *4.4*A. X-ray of four barium sulfate suspensions to which artificial gastric juice (pH 1.8–2.0) is added: (*a, e*) pure barium sulfate; (*b, f*) high-quality brand; (*c, g*) low-quality brand; (*d, h*) Alubar 'Wander'. Suspensions *a, e* and *c, g* show flocculation. (*a–d*) Detail exposures of fluid surface. (*e–h*) Detail exposures below fluid surface.

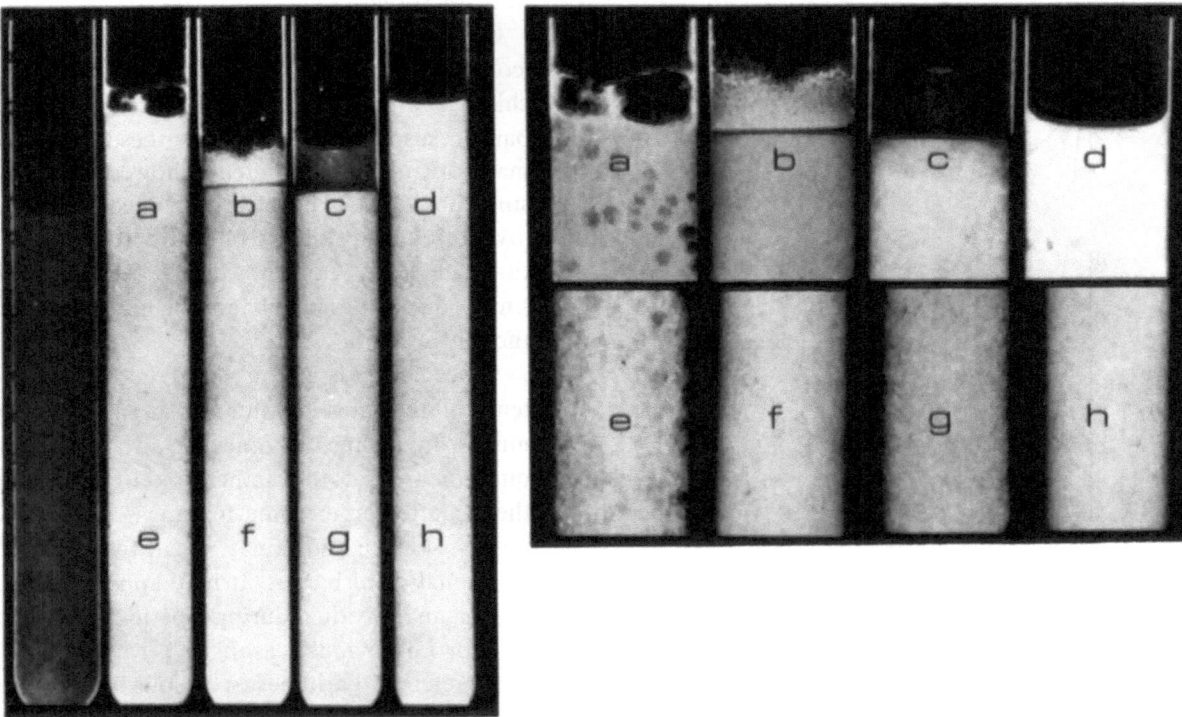

Fig. *4.4*B. Same test as A, but with artificial intestinal juice (pH 8.2–8.4).

culation of the contrast fluid can at least be caused by factors other than those mentioned above, such as gastric acid, hypertonic solutions, proteins, and fats. The authority of Golden was, however, so great that his neurogenic theory was still generally accepted.

Many were not converted until 1949, when the publication by Frazer et al. [60], who used an extensive series of tests, showed that flocculation of the barium suspension in the small intestine of completely normal individuals can be caused by many factors. To avoid the influence of gastric acid, the contrast medium as well as the substances to be tested were administered through a tube directly into the duodenum. They observed flocculation followed by segmentation after adding hypertonic solutions, acetic acid, lactic acid, fatty acids, olive oil, unsaturated fatty acids (sprue patients), and gastric mucus. Gall only caused flocculation in acidic surroundings, not for a pH greater than 6.4. To rebut Golden's theory in a spectacular manner, they demonstrated that the barium suspension also flocculated in the intestines of a deceased person

where a disordered motor function, such as Golden supposed, cannot possibly exist. Furthermore it appeared that flocculation followed by segmentation developed in persons who had consumed a meal rich in fats the evening before the examination.

In the same year, Zimmer [249] compared the characteristics of Alubar, which he considered to be a superior contrast medium, with those of an ordinary barium sulfate suspension and two commercial products by adding artificial gastric juice with a pH of 1.8–2.0 and artificial intestinal juice with a pH of 8.2–8.4. The roentgenograms made showed varying degrees of structural change for at least two of the four contrast fluids and are highly similar to the changes noted for brand 2 during our experiments (fig. 4.4). The rate of flocculation under the influence of gastric and intestinal juices was also measured for these four contrast fluids; the resulting values were plotted on a graph (fig. 4.5). He then studied the homogeneity and the adhesion for these suspensions. Alubar appeared to be better than the ordinary $BaSO_4$ in all respects. In his conclusion, he writes that the use of a pure $BaSO_4$ suspension will often lead to the unjustified diagnosis of sprue.

One year later, Ardran et al. [9] also proved that a 'colloidal' barium suspension does not flocculate in children with celiac disease, but that a normal barium suspension does. After these publications, many others of similar intent followed, but there are still radiologists who have remained more or less loyal to Golden's theory of disordered motor function. In 1959, Golden himself seemed to have similar difficulties in abandoning his original line of thought when he wrote:

'Flocculation is undoubtedly caused by the contents of the intestine and has been attributed to mucus. In as much as mucus is always present the question arises as to whether this effect is related to the quantity or to some unknown quality of the mucus. Flocculation may occur as a result of emotional disturbances. It may appear and disappear in an individual during a period of an hour or two for no obvious reason' [79]. Meanwhile, Golden preferred barium suspensions which did not flocculate but he did not see any advantage in all kinds of special examination techniques.

He administered 240 ml contrast medium orally

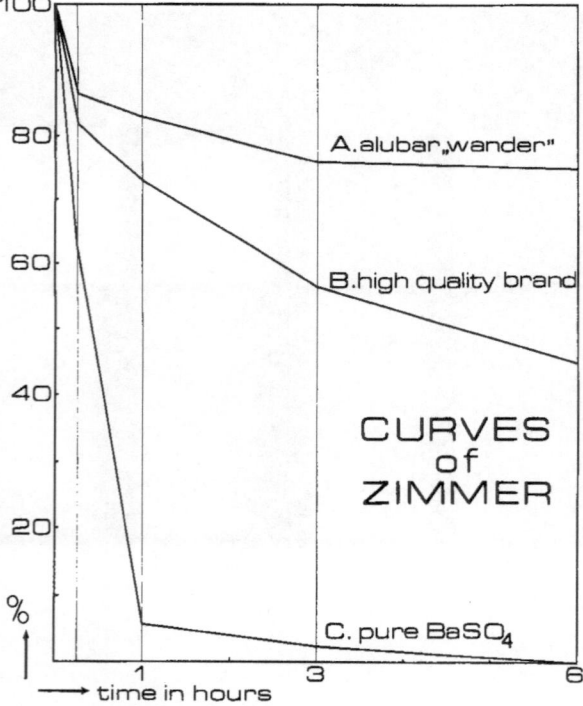

Fig. 4.5. Sedimentation curves of Zimmer [249]. Difference between Alubar 'Wander', a high-quality brand and a barium suspension without additives.

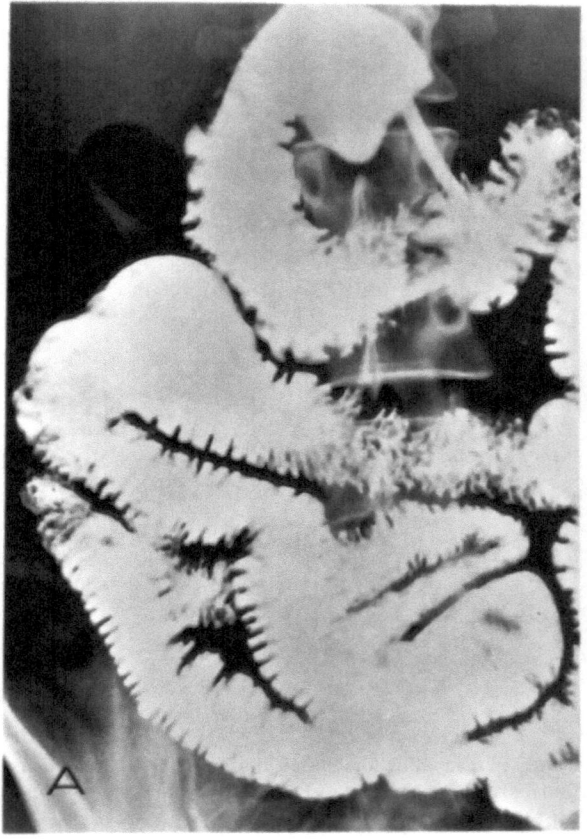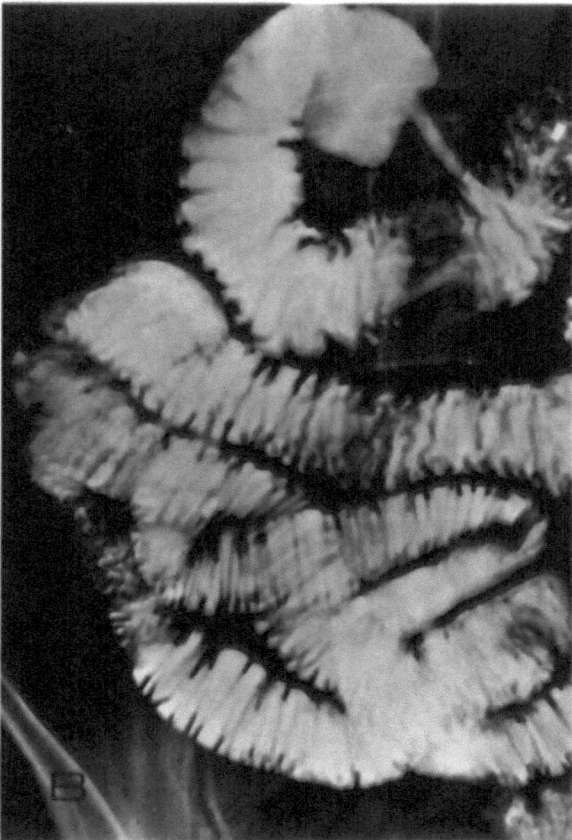

Fig. 4.6. Decrease in contrast and increase in information when a higher voltage is used (A: 80 kV; B: 120 kV). Film density equal for both exposures.

and, if necessary, took spot films. Since Gianturco's article in 1953, he used the 'high voltage' technique because with a low voltage only marginal information was obtained (fig. 4.6).

At a congress in 1960, in reference to a demonstration of the radiological examination of the small intestine where a tumor was not localized, Golden clearly indicated that his opinions had changed in the meantime by stating: 'It would seem that a tumor such as this should easily be detected by a small intestine study (barium follow-through). The segmentation was so great and the distribution so uneven that the tumor could not be demonstrated. It seems possible that this might have been demonstrated by a small bowel enema.'

4. Segmentation of the contrast column

Although the disintegration of the contrast column into segment clumps is usually observed together with flocculation, a separate discussion of this phenomenon is justified for several reasons.

The segmentation picture was known long before that of flocculation. The reason is that flocculation is obtained only when the patient receives a reasonably homogeneous suspension of relatively small particles. When it was still customary to mix nutrients with the contrast medium, this requirement was certainly not satisfied. As mentioned previously, owing to the withdrawal of fluids from the contrast column, segmentation in the colon is a physiological phenomenon: this is also the case in the ileum when transit is very slow. In the fluid-rich duodenum and jejunum, such massive flocculation can also occur that results in increasingly large

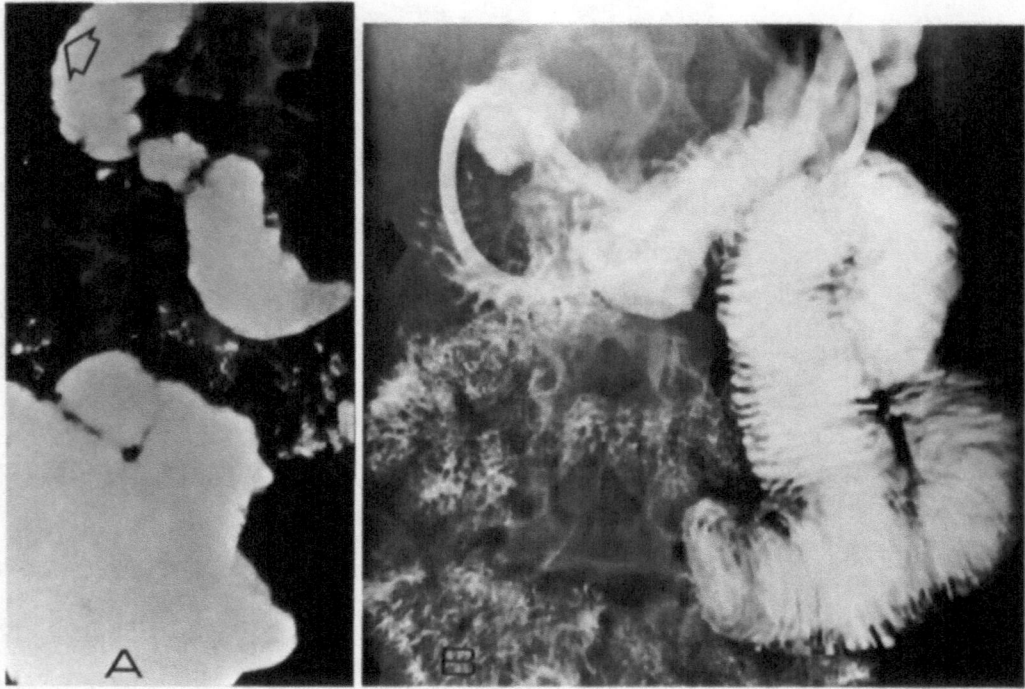

Fig. 4.7. 'Moulage' sign in the duodenum of a patient with celiac disease is caused by total disintegration of the contrast fluid and a pronounced increase in viscosity so that reproduction of the mucosal folds has become impossible (A). A repeat examination using the enteroclysis method showed that the mucosal folds do in fact exist (B).

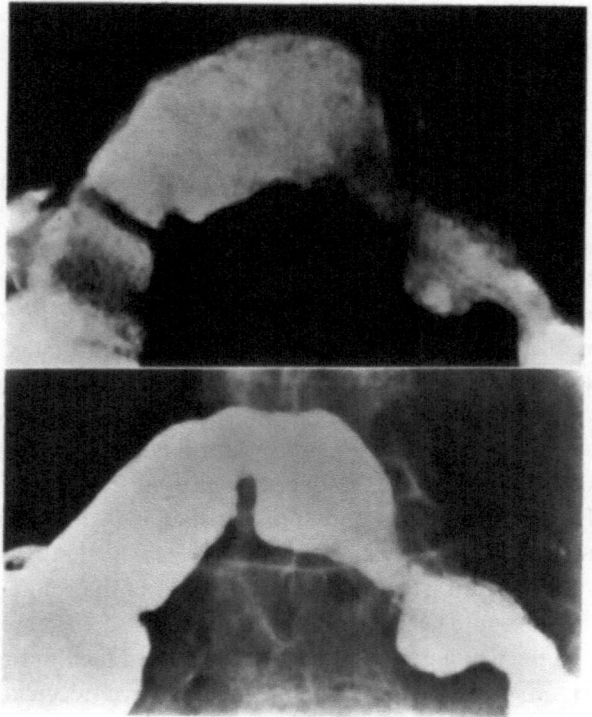

conglomerates and finally segment clumps. In the 1930s this phenomenon was frequently seen in the duodenum and jejunum of infants; a reasonable explanation was unknown [22]. Autopsy material had shown that mucosal folds were definitely present; the fact that Henderson had indeed observed these folds on roentgenological films when the stomach emptied rapidly also could not be explained [90].

In 1934, Snell and Camp [222] described the segmentation of the contrast column in sprue. They saw clumping of the barium and disappearance of the fold relief. They are to be respected, for even then they believed that this was not a specific symptom, but that the same could be observed for other 'diffuse infections'. In 1939, Kantor [108] described the 'moulage sign' that can be seen in the

← *Fig. 4.8.* Only when the exposure dose is high enough can it be seen that the structure of a disintegrating barium suspension has become granular; in other words, underexposure completely masks the fact that a contrast fluid can no longer be used.

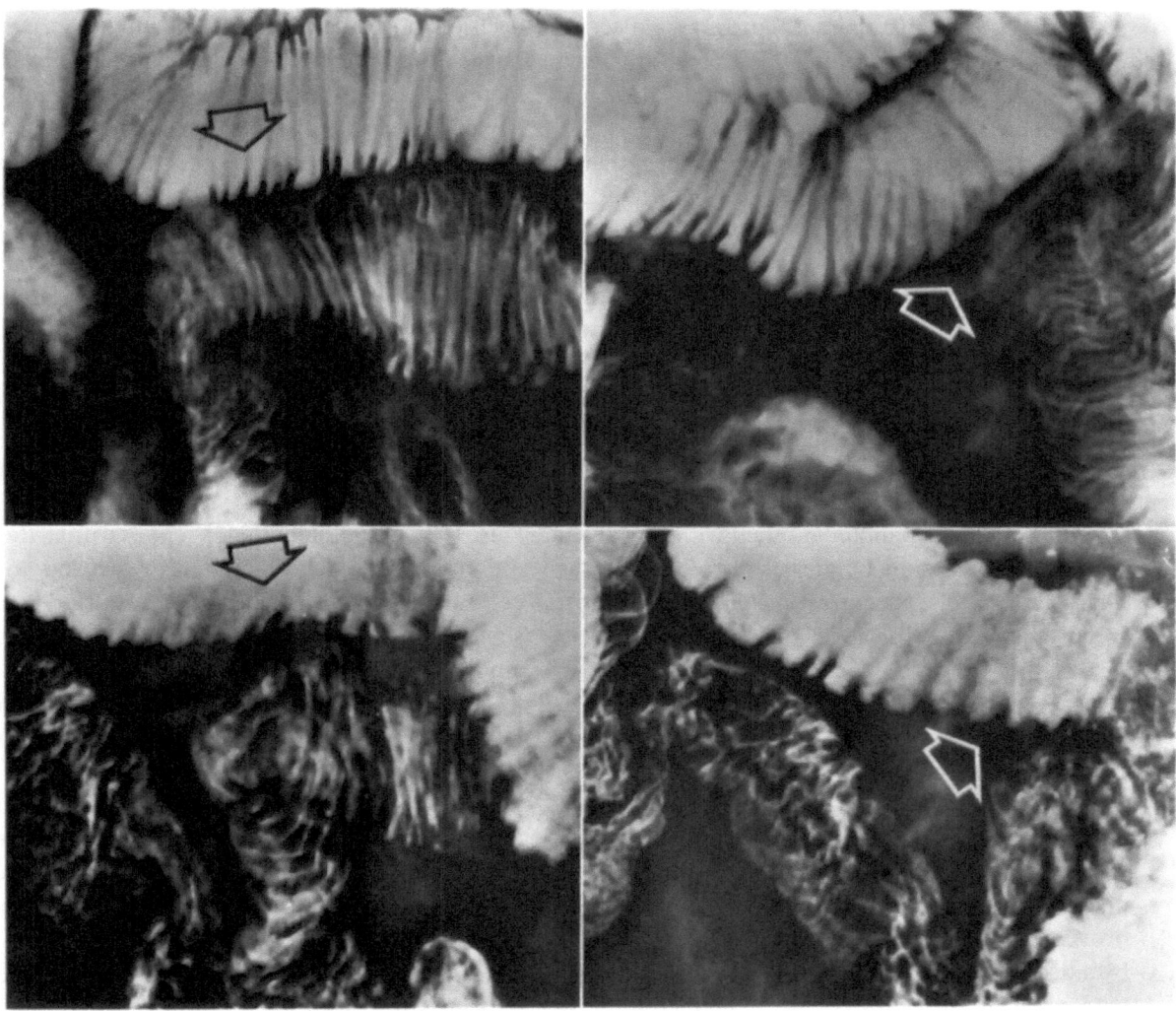

Fig. 4.9. On the two uppermost exposures the mucosal folds appear normal; distintegration of the contrast fluid then developed rapidly with flattening and apparent coarsening of the mucosal folds (two lowermost exposures). The structure of the contrast fluid has become granular.

duodenum or jejunum, where the rigid barium column resembles a wax mold without fold relief (fig. 4.7). He saw this picture in only highly advanced cases of sprue and therefore he thought that in these cases the fold relief was greatly flattened or absent altogether. In fact there will probably always be a heavy and early occurrence of clumping of the barium suspension in such cases. When the roentgenograms are overexposed, the barium column has a grainy appearance (fig. 4.8). In a case of pure mucosal atrophy, without signs of malabsorption, this structure must be homogeneous. Kantor's conclusion that the moulage sign could be considered an indication of the severity of the sprue might still

be correct in spite of the opinion of Snell and Camp; however, this picture has absolutely nothing to do with the condition of the mucous membrane.

In 1961, Marshak [143] was of the opinion that the moulage sign could be the result of hypersecretion and segmentation. In the same article, however, he does mention his surprise at also seeing string sign-like configurations and coarse mucosal folds, which do not seem to agree with the normal autopsy findings. The quality of the published roentgenograms is, however, poor and they are so distorted by flocculation and segmentation that this incongruity between radiological and autopsy findings is not strange. Figure 4.9 shows that flocculation and segment formation of the barium suspension led to an apparent flattening and coarsening of the mucosal folds. Patterns are even possible that do not in the least resemble the actual situation.

From the above, it must be concluded that a radiological examination of the small intestine should be terminated when the contrast fluid shows clear signs of disintegration and apparently is no longer able to provide true images of the intestinal mucosa. It would be ideal if a contrast medium was available that was highly stable, moderately viscous, and adhered readily. In order to prevent the annoying effect of dehydration and thickening of the barium column in the distal ileum during slow transit, it is also desirable that the contrast medium be protected against unlimited fluid withdrawal. Of the numerous attempts undertaken to improve the characteristics of the contrast media, only the most important will be discussed.

5. Additives to the contrast medium for the purpose of improving stability and adhesion

Many radiologists have tried this method to increase the adhesion of the contrast medium to the mucous membrane of the digestive tract. An improvement in adhesion is usually also accompanied by a decrease in the sedimentation and flocculation tendencies of the contrast medium; therefore an attempt aimed specifically at the latter cannot easily be distinguished from the former. Due to the importance of double-contrast exposures for the colon examination, good adhesion is even more important for that examination than for an examination of the small intestine. The reverse holds for sedimentation and flocculation. Adhesion of the barium meal to the intestinal mucosa could be increased by adding tannin since this substance supposedly causes precipitation of proteins on the cellular surfaces and decreases mucin secretion.

For a long time, tannin was used for the colon examination in concentrations of 0.3%–3.0% in the cleansing enema and in the contrast medium. Since it has become known that tannin is absorbed by the mucous membrane [116] and eight fatal cases resulting from necrosis of the liver have been described, use of this substance has been forbidden in the United States [6]. Some do not agree with this decision since they believe that in these cases the possibility of overdosage exists [99]. Tannin is found in tea and, it is said, in red wine. It is not only hepatotoxic but is also believed to be carcinogenic. When perforations occur and the barium mixture containing tannin enters the abdominal cavity, a serious chemical peritonitis develops. To avoid lethal termination, acute surgical intervention and cleansing of the abdominal cavity are absolutely necessary.

As far as we know, tannin has never played a role of any importance in the examination of the small intestine although the influence of a cup of strong tea consumed the evening before the examination has never been studied.

In 1938, Wooldman [242] reported that the addition of colloidal aluminum hydroxide to the contrast medium produced good results. This substance is slightly astringent, does not irritate, and is amphoteric. He had noticed during operations and in autopsy material that a contrast medium containing this substance adheres quite readily to the mucosa.

In 1953, Schufflebarger et al. [215] tried to improve adhesion to the mucous membrane by decreasing the secretion from the intestinal wall in animals and later also in patients. They injected histamine and atropine but were not successful. They did note that the best results were obtained in patients with hypotonic, ptotic stomachs.

Alexander [5] believed that adhesion would be improved if the barium suspension mixed easily with the mucus; he therefore added 1% mucin. He reported improvement for the examination of the small intestine and the colon, but not for esophageal and gastric examinations.

Embring and Mattsson [47] added a wetting agent (Tweens, sodium lauryl sulfate, and saponins) to enhance the mixing of two different water phases, but they were not very enthusiastic about their results.

Many radiologists [26, 47, 114, 183, and others] added carboxymethylcellulose or its sodium salt to the barium suspension and in general reported good results with this combination. Sodium CMC does cause an increase in viscosity, but does not dissolve in gastric juice and does not appear to adhere as readily as the CMC in a 0.5% concentration. Both substances are highly hydrophilic and therefore accelerate transit.

Both the binding of water and the acceleration of transit protect the barium suspension against excessive fluid withdrawal in the ileum. A slight disadvantage of the contrast media containing hydrophilic colloids to restrict dehydration in the ileum is that they cannot be used to diagnose a disaccharidase deficiency [121]. Micropaque does not contain these colloids; for prolonged transit times, however, there is the disadvantage of pronounced dehydration in the distal ileum as a result of fluid withdrawal. Other substances that have occasionally been used to improve the adhesion of the contrast medium are tragacanth and arabic gum [2, 90]. The results described vary widely; this may be a result of the various dosages used. Henderson did not see any improvement when 10 ml 2% arabic gum was added, an observation that we can confirm. We have found that the addition of 10 vol % of the total amount of the contrast medium, thus a considerably higher dosage, does produce satisfactory results. This suspension, however, is rather viscous and becomes thinner and more liquid only in patients with sufficient gastric acid. This decrease in viscosity is not accompanied by flocculation at all; in this case the gastric acid is apparently bound chemically. This chemical combining of the gastric acid must be regarded as specifically preventing flocculation. Substances that bind mucin have the same effect. In addition to the above-mentioned substances, many others have been tested; as a result it has been demonstrated clearly that no single additive has been found that is ideal. Some of these substances are: buttermilk, olive oil, sodium oleate, fecal fat from sprue patients, diverse carbohydrates, lactic acid, citric acid, gelatin, agar, and pectin.

6. Relationship between viscosity, particle size, and adhesion of the barium suspension

Although the adhesive capacity of a suspension can be increased by adding several substances, a minimum viscosity is also a necessary requirement. An increase in the viscosity, however, has the disadvantage of retarding the rate of transit through the pylorus and small intestine. An additional difficulty is that when the viscosity of the contrast medium is too high, the adhesive layer left behind can become annoyingly thick (fig. 4.10). The correct (creamy) viscosity for the suspension, however, does not guarantee that adhesion will be good.

Some radiologists have tried to obtain a clearly visible adhesive layer by preparing solutions with a high specific gravity and a very low viscosity. One example is Brown's mixture [26]. He used sodium carboxymethylcellulose, heparin, and sodium dextran sulfate or sodium cellulose acetate to obtain a thin, liquid suspension containing 75 wt % barium. Embring and Mattsson [48] also obtained a thin, liquid, as well as stable, barium suspension with a specific gravity of approximately 3, as follows: they added 1 g sodium citrate and 9 g sorbitol to a paste-like mixture of 100 g $BaSO_4$ and 40 ml water; a pronounced decrease in viscosity resulted. However, for exposures of the filled, relatively thin ileum, a barium suspension with a specific gravity of 3 is much too high, and therefore not desirable. Only marginal diagnoses can be made with this medium.

For double-contrast exposures, it is in principle a question of personal preference whether a thin liquid suspension with a high specific gravity or a thicker liquid suspension with a lower specific gravity is used. Within certain limits, a clearly visible layer can be obtained with both. At the Academic Hospital in Leiden, experiments were carried out using a segment of stomach stretched over a cylinder and coated with layers of mucus of varying viscosity; it was found that the quality of the radiographs will deteriorate whether the contrast fluid is too thick and also if it is too thin. It should be obvious that good adhesion between the barium suspension and the mucous membrane will not develop until the mucous coating has been flushed off. As already discovered in practice from our double-contrast examinations of the stomach and the colon, the adhesive layer in the phantom improved when the mucus-coated segment was rotated more frequently in the barium suspension. It also appeared that it is more difficult to flush off the mucous coating, and that the visibility of the film of barium covering the mucous membrane decreases, when the viscosity of the contrast fluid is less than that of the mucus. The mucus is easily flushed from the wall of the stomach when the

44

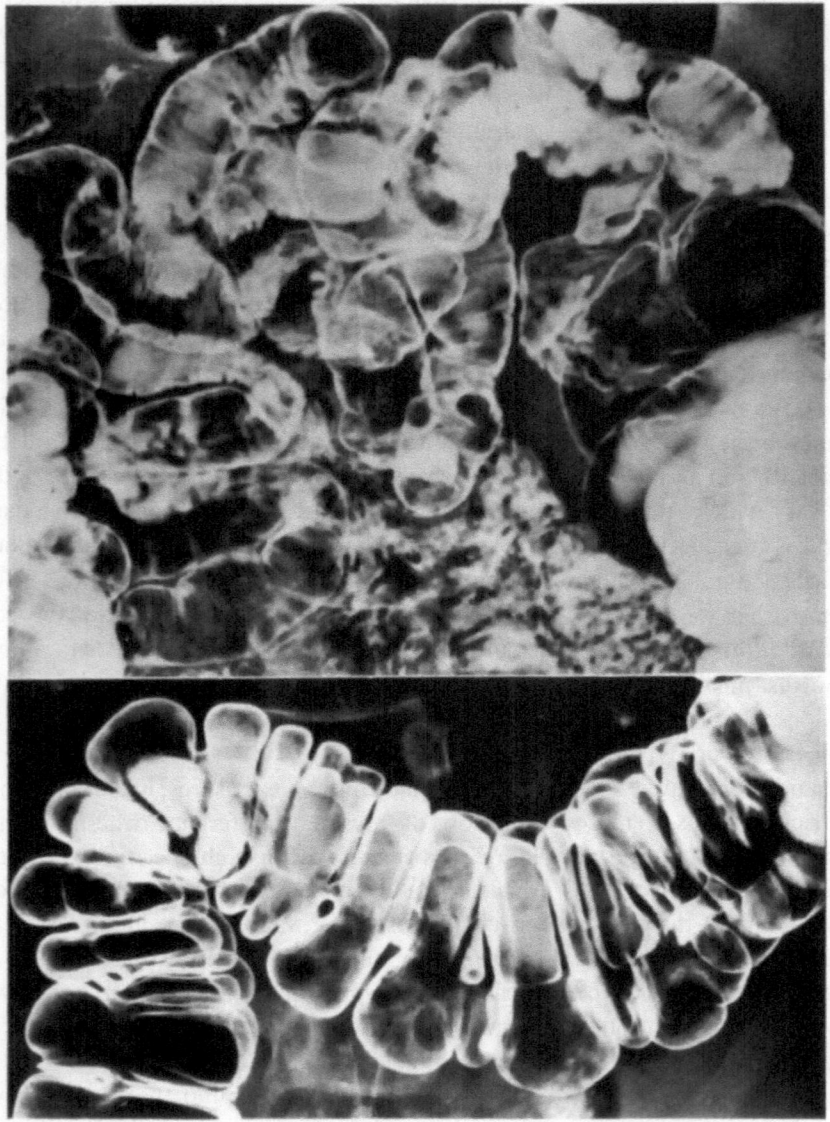

Fig. 4.10. Layer of barium suspension on the intestinal wall is too thick because the viscosity of the contrast fluid is too high. Double-contrast exposure of the colon at the end of the small intestine examination.

viscosity of the contrast fluid is equal to or greater than that of the mucus.

Strangely enough, however, the results are also poor when the viscosity of the contrast medium is much higher than that of the mucus. It was not quite clear whether this should be attributed to inadequate flushing of the mucus or to poor adhesion of the thicker barium suspension to the wall of the stomach. Presumably the latter is the answer since more frequent rotation of the segment in the contrast fluid did not noticeably improve the visi-

bility of the film of barium.

These findings are useful in determining the optimum viscosity of the contrast fluid for the examination of stomach or colon, but not for the small bowel examination since a thick contrast fluid cannot pass through the infusion system fast enough. However, we have found that in rare instances, for example the patient seen in fig. 9.19 (page 210), the mucous coating of the intestinal wall may be so thick that it cannot be flushed off by the much thinner contrast fluid. For the sake of sim-

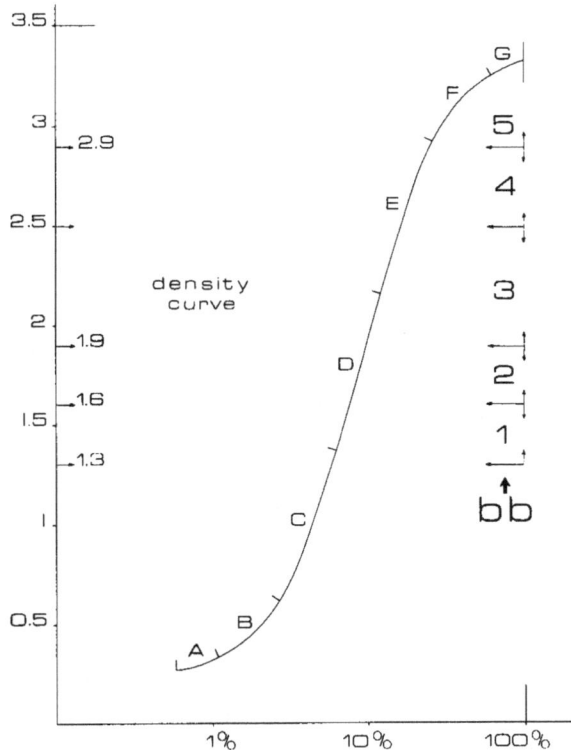

Fig. 4.11. Schematical representation of a film density curve. Background blackenings (bb) 1, 2, 3, 4, and 5 (figs. 4.12–4.18) are indicated on the curve.

plicity, it can be stated that for the examination of the small intestine, the viscosity of the contrast medium is optimal when it is just possible to administer a barium suspension with a specific gravity of 1.3 through the Bilbao tube at a rate of 75 ml/min, with the infusion bag suspended as high as possible above the table.

Various radiologists, including Adam [2] in 1932, have shown that for a good adhesive layer in double-contrast exposures, the 'colloidal' chemical relationships are more important than the particle size. For suspensions with a low viscosity, a particle size of less than 0.4 microns can even be a disadvantage instead of an advantage. Both the specific gravity and the thickness of the adhesive layer are then insufficient for the double-contrast examination. All the factors are present in such a suspension for a barely visible adhesive layer.

Brown pointed out that, for the same weight of barium, the viscosity of a suspension increases as the size of the particles decreases and that the adhesion decreases as soon as the barium content in a suspension becomes greater than 45 wt %. Many

who have prepared barium suspensions themselves for an examination of the esophageal varices will have experienced the truth of this observation.

When requested, the manufacturers of contrast media usually do not supply adequate information about the chemical composition of their product. It was found that often the data supplied were not even correct; this was also true for the particle size given.

Microscopic studies have proven that the grains were usually much larger than indicated, sometimes even significantly larger than prescribed by the American pharmacopeia [159]. In addition, the relative differences in the grain size of the diverse products on the market appeared to be a factor of 4 [48]. Schufflebarger et al. [215] made diagrams of the grain-size distribution of six different brands of barium sulfate and showed that most of the powders also displayed a marked lack of homogeneity. Moreton and Yates [163] compared four commercial preparations and obtained similar results.

7. Specific gravity of the contrast fluid

We have found that generally this exceedingly important factor has not received sufficient attention. Often barium suspensions are used with a specific gravity that is much too high. The choice of the barium content for a suspension is apparently influenced by the spectacular sight of snow-white intestinal loops, preferably against the background of a normally exposed abdominal survey film. As long as there is no annoying superposition, only small abnormalities on the contours of the intestinal loops can be seen clearly on these roentgenograms. In addition, the other organs in the abdomen will also be seen since their blackening falls in the midportion of the density curve (fig. 4.11, section D). Masses in the lumen of the intestine, however, will be easily missed. There is too little difference in contrast with the intense white parts of the intestinal loops. These lie in the lowermost part of the density curve (fig. 4.11, section A). It will be obvious that with this exposure technique, only two very small segments of the contours of these snow-white intestinal loops are visible. The specific gravity of the human body differs only slightly from that of water and can be set at approximately 1. The specific gravity of a concentrated barium suspension, such as undiluted liquid Micropaque, is approximately 1.75. The difference in specific gravity between this contrast fluid and the human body is approximately 0.75; thus it is even less than the difference in specific gravity between the human body and air, which is slightly less than 1.

From this it might be concluded that perhaps air could be an ideal as well as a very inexpensive contrast medium for the examination of the digestive tract. However, the disadvantage of air is that its specific gravity cannot be regulated by means of dilution like the positive contrast media. In addition, air is not capable of adhering to the mucosa and therefore cannot leave traces of its presence. Air is also unable to mix with secreted mucus and therefore cannot penetrate the narrow spaces that are filled with fluid. The greatest disadvantage of air, however, is that disturbing contrast differences are caused by solitary gas bubbles. These are located in approximately the same section of the density curve as contrast differences of the intestinal loops filled with gas. The result is that an isolated gas bubble, for instance, could not be differentiated from a diverticulum of either the anterior or the posterior intestinal wall. Unhindered evaluation of the intestinal loops and the contrast fluctuations caused by diverticula and polypoid tumors can best be made when:

1) The density of these loops differs markedly from that of the (irrelevant) background and its fluctuations.
2) The contrast fluctuations caused by pathological processes of the intestinal wall fall in the steep part of the density curve and can therefore be seen as clearly as possible.
3) The background fluctuations fall in the highest possible section of the density curve, and therefore cause the least possible disturbance.

From the above, it can be seen that theoretically the density of the intestinal loops can best fall in section c and the density for the rest of the abdomen in section G of this curve. The specific gravity of the contrast fluid should then be chosen such that small bulges of the intestinal lumen and narrow fistulous tracts can be seen clearly on the one hand while, on the other hand, mucosal folds and small masses,

even in the lumen of wide loops, do not escape our attention. It is known that a high-voltage exposure technique levels out the contrasts; this has a favorable effect on the density of both the background and the intestinal loops filled with contrast fluid (fig. 4.6). A film blackening such that the background falls in section G of the curve would, however, mean a very high radiation dose for the patient.

Therefore we thought it would be useful to experiment with a phantom to determine how much the background blackening with its fluctuations can be decreased without interfering with the evaluation of the contrast differences in the intestinal loops. It also seemed worthwhile during these experiments to test contrast fluids of different specific gravity in order to determine which specific gravity (s.g.) gives maximum information.

In a 15-cm-thick phantom filled with water that acted as scattering medium, we placed plastic pipes with diameters of 22 and 34 mm. The plastic pipes were filled with barium suspensions with s.g. 1.65, 1.32, and 1.2. In each plastic pipe was a nylon thread holding wooden beads with diameters of 5, 7, 9, and 12 mm. Roentgenograms were made with a voltage of 125 kV and increasing degrees of density of the background (henceforth designated as d.b.), numbered from 1 to 5. These five levels were chosen such that they adequately represented the upper half of the density curve (fig. 4.11). The walls of the plastic pipes could still be seen with d.b. 3; with d.b. 4, they were no longer clearly visible.

The results were as follows:

1) For the contrast medium with s.g. 1.65 in the 22-mm pipe, the largest bead could be seen vaguely with d.b. 2; not until d.b. 4 were four beads visible in this pipe. They could be observed most clearly with d.b. 5 in the 34-mm pipe, the three largest beads were just visible with d.b. 5 (fig. 4.12).
2) For the contrast fluid with s.g. 1.32 in the 22-mm pipe, visibility of all four beads increased as the d.b. increased from 2 to 4. Although clearer with d.b. 4, all four beads in the 34-mm pipe were already visible with d.b. 3; the smallest was very vague. With d.b. 2, no beads were visible in the large pipe (fig. 4.13).
3) For the contrast fluid with s.g. 1.2, the visibility of all four beads in both pipes increased as the

47

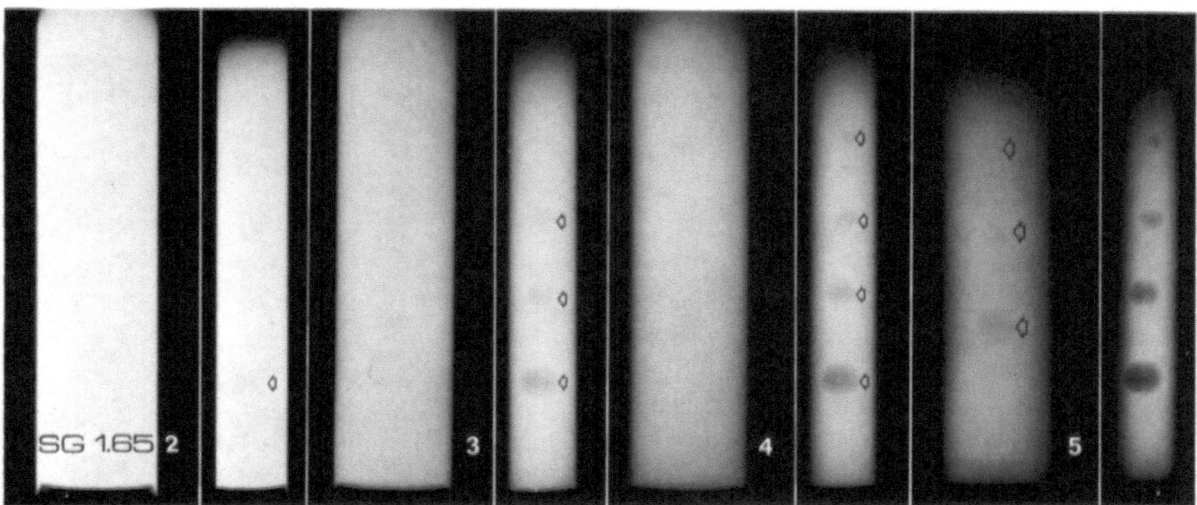

SG 1.65

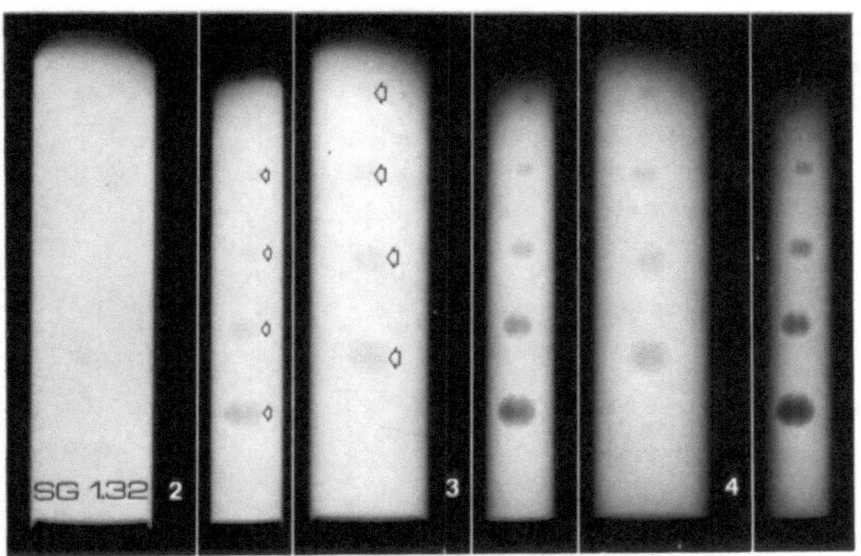

SG 1.32

Fig. 4.12–4.17. Tests on the specific gravity (s.g.) of the contrast fluid. The diameters of the plastic pipes are 14, 22, and 34 mm and of the wooden beads, 5, 7, 9, and 12 mm. The density of the background (d.b.) is shown in white numbers; the values 1 through 5 correspond to the following values on the density curve (fig. 4.11): 1→1.3–1.6, 2→1.6–1.9, 3→1.9–2.5, 4→2.5–2.9, 5→ >2.9. (See also pages 49–50.)

Fig. 4.13

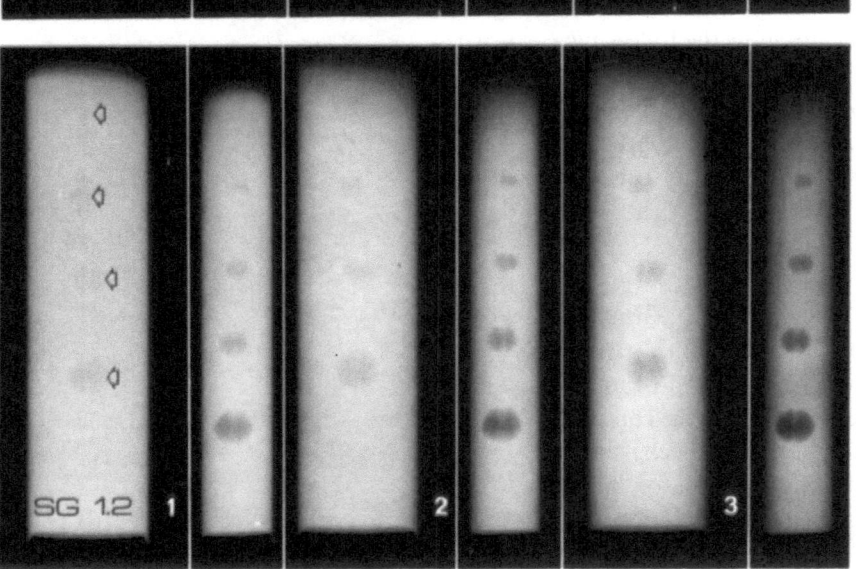

SG 1.2

Fig. 4.14

d.b. increased from 1 to 3 (fig. 4.14).

4) In the small pipe, the beads in the contrast fluid with s.g. 1.32 and a certain d.b. were as clearly visible as the beads in the contrast fluid with s.g. 1.2 and one d.b. lower.

5) When the film density is even higher, the same applies for the large pipe.

The contrast fluid with s.g. 1.2 revealed the beads in the large pipe somewhat more clearly with d.b. 2 than the fluid with s.g. 1.32 with d.b. 3. This difference in visibility of the beads in the large pipe increases as the d.b. decreases to the advantage of the contrast fluid with the lowest specific gravity.

The experiment was repeated, but this time the wooden beads were not located in the middle of the plastic pipes but along the wall. Figure 4.15 shows the results, which are similar to those of the previous experiment. Once again it was apparent that the wooden beads are most clearly visible when the film density is high; in all cases, however, with the same d.b. they are more clearly visible than in the previous experiment. There is again no difference in clearness in the small pipe between s.g. 1.32 with a certain d.b., and s.g. 1.2 with one d.b. less. In the large pipe, however, as the d.b. decreased, the beads were significantly clearer in the contrast fluid with the lowest specific gravity.

The results with s.g. 1.65 were again very disappointing, although somewhat less than in the previous experiment.

For the actual examination of the digestive tract, the results of these experiments show the following:

1) A specific gravity of 1.65 is always much too high for the contrast fluid and density of the background in the lower half of the density curve is always too low. A combination of these two factors is particularly unfavorable, especially for a colon examination.

2) The combination of a relatively high density of the background (approx. 3) and a contrast fluid with a low specific gravity yields the most information. When the specific gravity of the contrast fluid is decreased, the density of the background can also be decreased without a loss of information. This means a lower radiation dose for the patient.

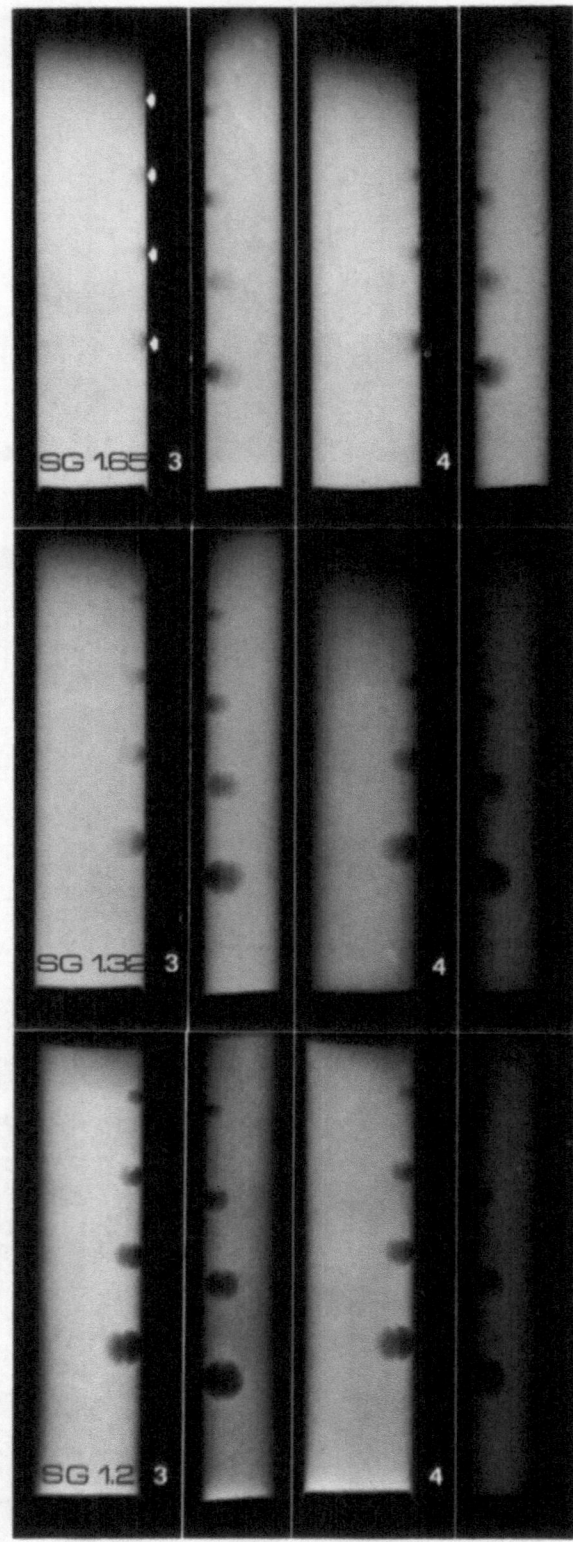

Fig. 4.15

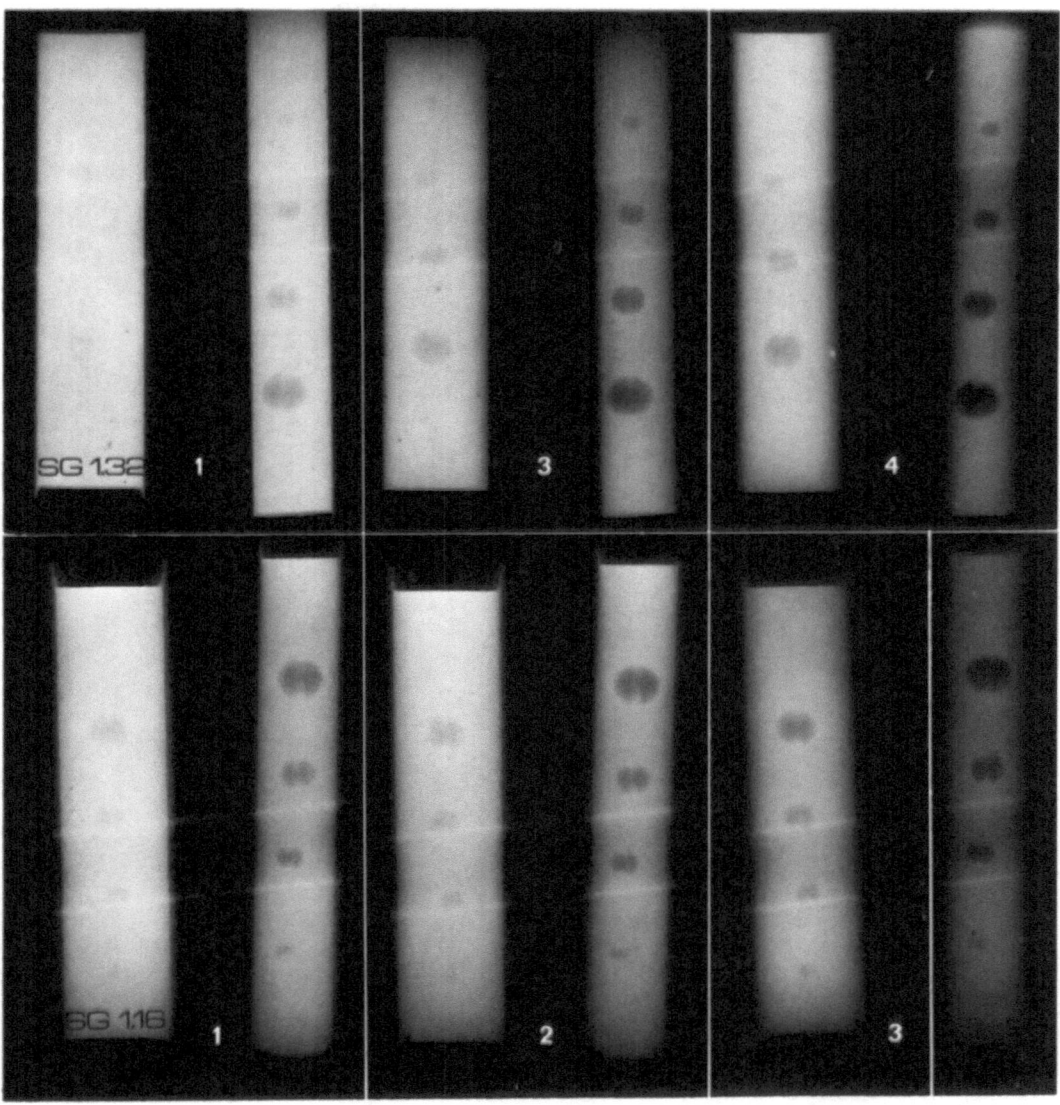

Fig. 4.16

3) For the colon examination, the specific gravity of the contrast fluid must be lower than for a transit examination, and the density of the background must be higher.

4) The loss in information due to underexposure of the x-ray films is less when a contrast fluid with a low specific gravity is used. The loss in information due to a contrast fluid with a high specific gravity can be compensated for by overexposure of the x-ray film.

In order to evaluate the disturbance caused by fluctuations in the density of the background, a new experiment was carried out. A transverse, air-filled plastic pipe, 22 mm in diameter, was introduced into the water phantom. This pipe crossed the two pipes filled with contrast fluid. This time we used barium suspensions with specific gravities of 1.32 and 1.16, and once again exposures with varying d.b. were made.

The results were as follows (fig. 4.16):

1) The disturbing influence of the differences in contrast of the lumen and the wall of the air pipe is the least for the background when the density is high (sections F and G) and for the pipes filled

50

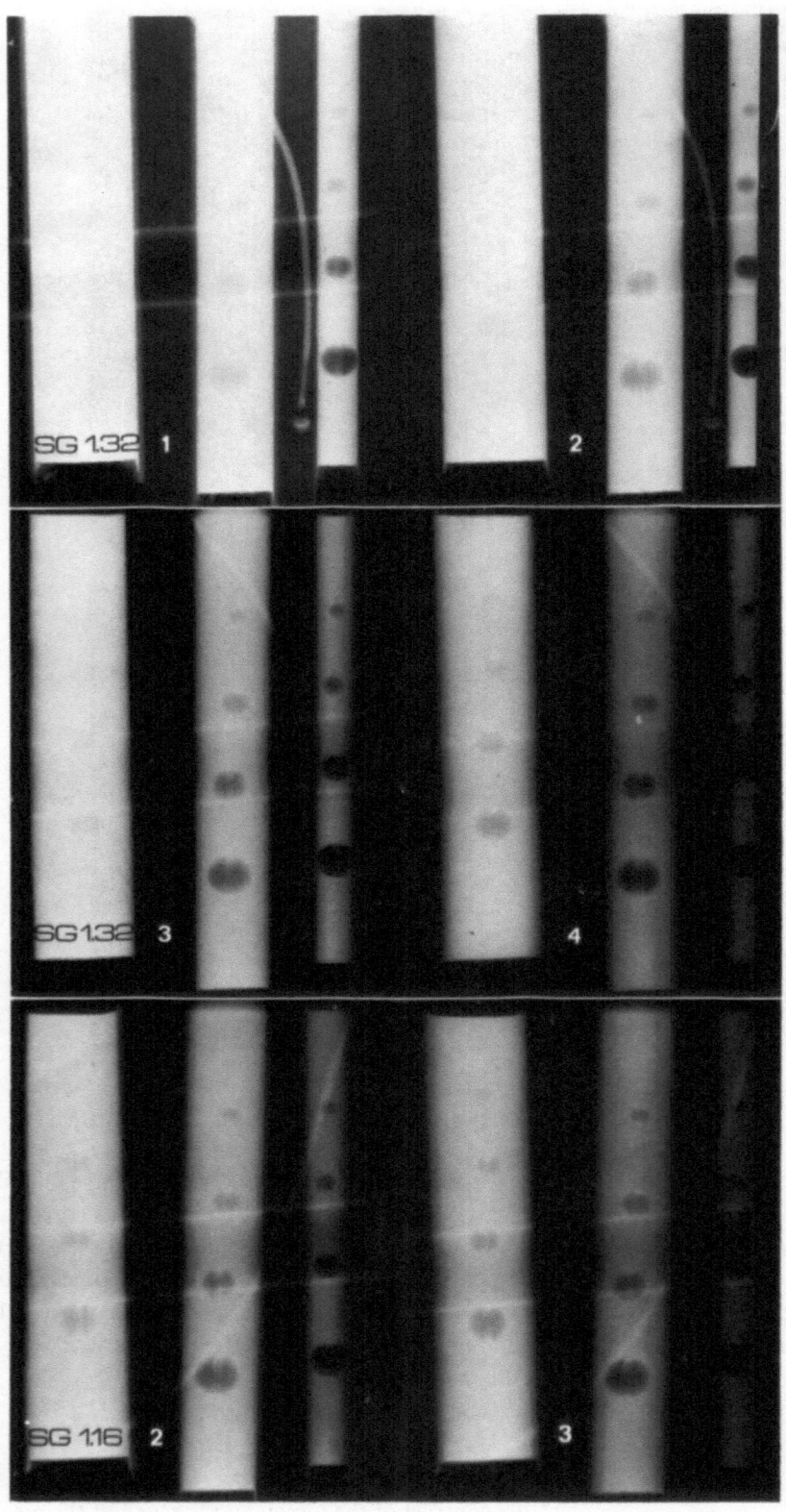

Fig. 4.17

with contrast fluid, when the density is low (sections A and B).

2) The disturbing positive and negative influences of the air pipe are greater for the background as the density decreases and for the contrast column as the specific gravity of the barium suspension decreases.

In spite of the fact that disturbance by background fluctuations is greater for a contrast fluid with s.g. 1.16 and d.b. 3 than for the 1.32–4 combination, s.g. 1.16 is still to be preferred since in the larger pipe the wooden beads are then seen more clearly even with one d.b. less. In practice, the combination of a contrast fluid with s.g. 1.32 or higher and d.b. 1 (normal exposure) is generally used. Figure 4.16 shows that in this way no information on the presence of filling defects is obtained in the large pipe and in the thin pipe only a little. It can also be seen that s.g. 1.16 obviously gives us more information for the same film density.

The practical confirmation of these theoretical considerations was demonstrated nicely with films of the rectum of a patient who visited our department because of rectal blood loss. Figure 4.18A shows that the filling exposures made of the rectum in anterior-posterior, three-quarter, and lateral projections revealed no abnormalities. The specific gravity of the contrast fluid is 1.32; the density of the background is approximately 2.

The difference in contrast between air and tissue is greater than between the contrast fluid and tissue so that we need not be surprised that the double-contrast films made with the same density of the background revealed a large polypoid tumor in the right posterior wall of the rectum (fig. 4.18D).

New films of the rectum were again made using the same contrast fluid, this time, however, with a density of the background of approximately 4 and 5. On these films, the polypoid tumor can be seen (fig. 4.18B).

Finally after thorough evacuation, a third series of filling exposures was made. The specific gravity of the contrast fluid was 1.16 and the density of the background was approximately 2 and 3. These last films show the filling defect in the rectum very clearly. In addition, the contours of the sigmoid loops, which cross each other, can be followed more easily with the contrast medium of lower specific gravity than on the first two series of exposures (fig. 4.18C).

With respect to the examination of the small intestine, if the importance of the specific gravity is neglected, the survey films obtained will inevitably be useless, especially with the enteroclysis technique (fig. 4.19).

The two pipes with the contrast fluid can only be considered representative of a colon that is not too wide and for filling of the duodenum and the jejunum in the manner described in this study (duodenal intubation). The ileum, however, is less wide and mucosal folds only 2 mm thick must also be visible over their entire length without over-exposure of the margins.

Furthermore, small ulcers, diverticula, and fistulous tracts must not escape our attention. The test procedure was therefore expanded to include a 14-mm plastic pipe containing the four wooden beads described previously. This pipe can be considered representative of a loop of the ileum. Finally, a thin plastic tube with a 2-mm lumen was introduced into the phantom such that it crossed several barium columns.

The three pipes and the tube were successively filled with contrast fluids with specific gravities of 1.16 and 1.32. For s.g. 1.16, films were made with d.b. 2 and 3, and for s.g. 1.32, with d.b. 1, 2, 3, and 4 (fig. 4.17).

It is striking that for this series of experiments the greatest amount of information is again obtained with s.g. 1.32 and d.b. 4, or with s.g. 1.16 and d.b. 3. Here the preference for the 1.16–3 combination is greater than in the other experiments because, for the 1.32–4 combination, overexposure almost occurs for the 2-mm tube and the density of the largest bead in the 14-mm pipe is so high that the central hole is no longer clearly visible.

With a contrast fluid with s.g. 1.32, the information in the 'ileum pipe' is greater with d.b. 3 than with d.b. 4; the tube is also more clearly visible with d.b. 3. For the 'colon pipe', the lower specific gravity was usually to be preferred; it is therefore sensible to be guided by this factor so that, for less wide loops, the density can be decreased from 3 to 2 without loss of information, which means a reduction in dosage for the patient. Although the tube is most clearly visible with the 1.32–2 combination, the opacification caused by the two smaller beads in

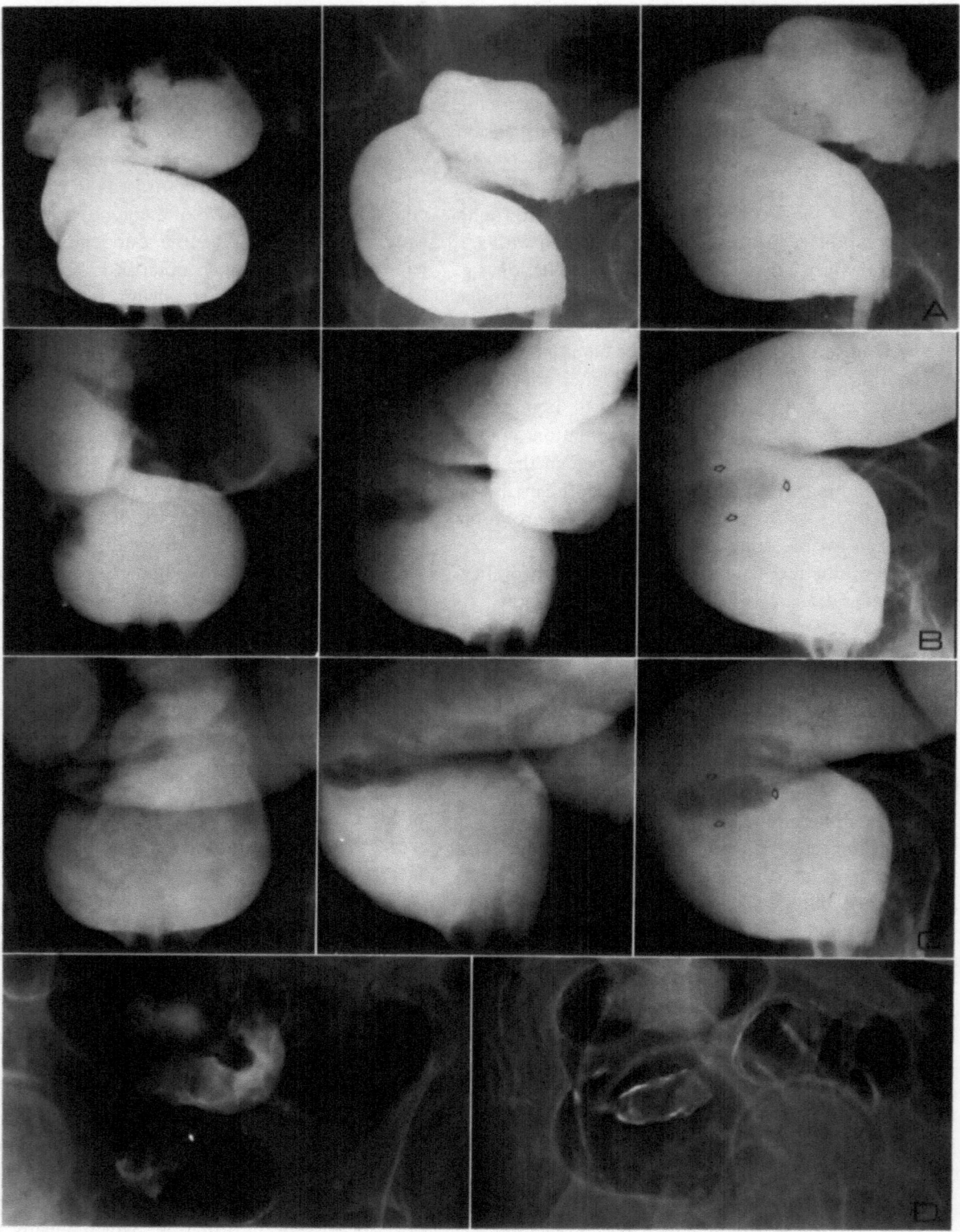

Fig. 4.18. Visibility of polypoid mass in rectum under various exposure conditions. (A) s.g. contrast fluid 1.32, d.b. 2; (B) s.g. contrast fluid 1.32, d.b. 4–5; (C) s.g. contrast fluid 1.16, d.b. 2–3; (D) double-contrast exposures d.b. 2.

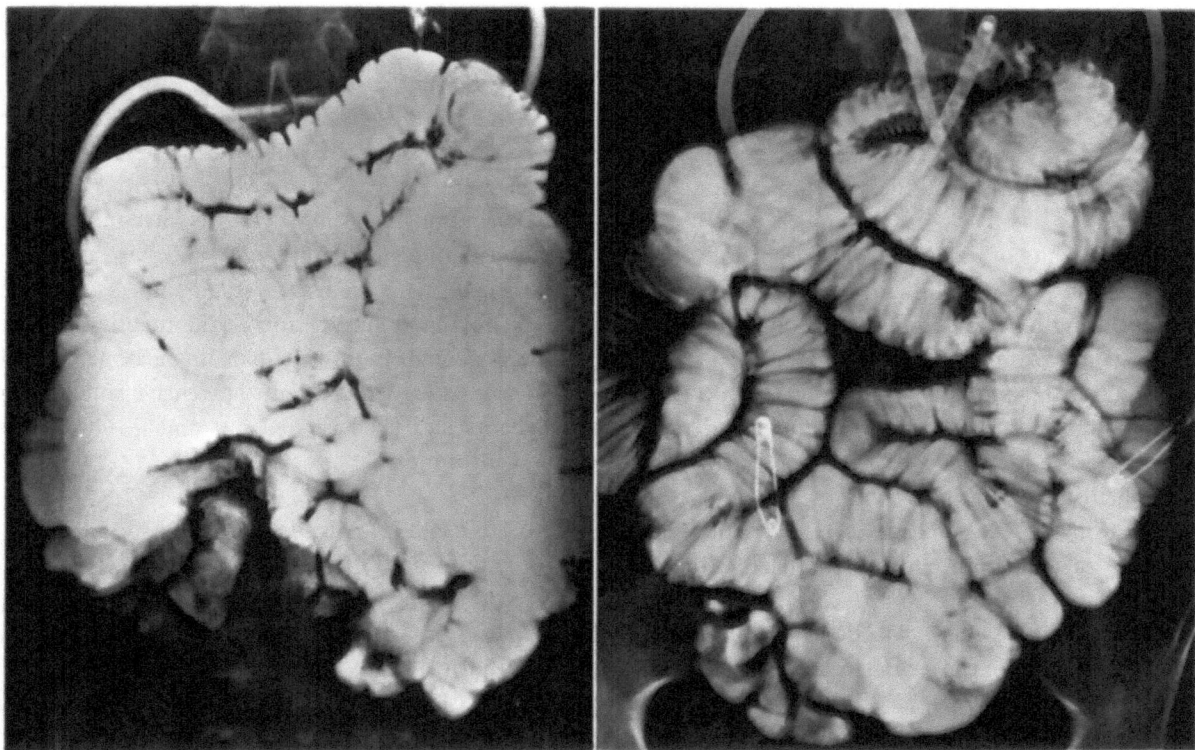

Fig. 4.19. Survey film of an enteroclysis examination executed elsewhere (left). Although the background density is rather high, the information obtained is only marginal. Therefore it must be concluded that the specific gravity of the contrast fluid was much too high. There are no indications that the kilovoltage was low (see fig. 4.6). When the examination was repeated in our department, the results (right) were better because a barium suspension with a lower specific gravity was used so that the density of the background could be lower and therefore the x-ray dosage used was much lower.

Fig. 4.20. Enteroclysis barium concentration (density) and heights of suspension for proper flow rates.

| Abdomen thickness (cm) in prone position | Relationship between weight/volume % and specific gravity | | wt/vol % | s.g. | kV | Flow in ml/min | Height of barium above tabletop (cm) |
	BA Lafayette HD-85 Ratio	H$_2$O (cold tap water) Ratio					
Obese (25/+)	+ 1 (360 ml)	+ 1 (360 ml)	= 42	− 1.32	125	100	200
Normal (20/24)	+ 1 (300 ml)	+ 1½ (450 ml)	= 34	− 1.27	125	100	125
Thin (15/19)	+ 1 (240 ml)	+ 2 (480 ml)	= 28	− 1.23	120	100	90
Child (11/14)	+ 1 (150 ml)	+ 2½ (375 ml)	= 24	− 1.2	100	100	75
Infant (8/10)	+ 1 (100 ml)	+ 3 (300 ml)	= 21	− 1.17	80	75	60
Baby (5/7)	+ 1 (50 ml)	+ 3½ (175 ml)	= 19	− 1.15	60	50	35

Flow rates obey Poiselle's Law. (Miller RE: Faster flow enema equipment. *Radiology* 123: 229–230, 1977.) The above figures apply only to barium Lafayette HD-85, $^3/_8$-inch internal diameter tubing, a plastic (3-ml plastic syringe) connector and 130-cm Sellink type enteroclysis duodenal intubation tube as supplied by Cook, Inc., Bloomington, Indiana. Any other system and any other brand of contrast fluid must be tested to assure flow rates of 100 ml/min for adults, 75 ml/min for infants, and 50 ml/min for babies. BaSO$_4$ should be 10°–15° C; water to be 30° C. Water flows faster than barium and bag must be lower – 40–50 cm. Too fast a flow will cause reflux and vomiting.

54

the 'jejunum pipe' is too vague.

The best results for the examination of the small intestine probably will be obtained with d.b. 2 and a specific gravity for the contrast fluid somewhere between 1.16 and 1.32. Practical experience has confirmed this hypothesis completely.

The results of this series of experiments can best be summarized as follows:

Using only the regular full-column technique for a colon examination, a contrast fluid can best be used with a specific gravity of 1.15 for a thin and at the most 1.2 for an obese patient. The density of the background must lie in the upper fourth of the steep part of the density curve.

For the examination of the small intestine, a contrast medium can best be used with a specific gravity of 1.2 for a thin, 1.25 for a normal, and 1.3 for an obese patient. The density of the background must lie in the third quarter of the steep part of the density curve.

The density for an examination of the digestive tract may therefore never lie in the lower half of the density curve.

If the conditions described here are satisfied, then the density of the intestinal loops filled with contrast fluid will fall in the lower fourth of the steep part of the density curve.

Although the specific gravity is the easiest to work with scientifically, and the most suitable parameter for comparing the various densities of the barium solution, this parameter is never used. In order to be able to compare the specific gravity with the most common parameter, the weight volume percentage, the Radiology Department of the Indiana Medical School worked together with a company in Lafayette, Indiana, which produces contrast media, to prepare the table shown in fig. 4.20. For the benefit of those concerned, this table also indicates the ratios necessary for dilution to the required density for the various groups of patients as well as the correct level of the bag of contrast medium above the examination table to obtain the proper rate of flow of the contrast fluid (see also pages 53, 95, and 466).

8. Contrast media other than barium sulfate

8.1. Barium carbonate

In 1959, the gastric examination of a number of patients was carried out by using barium carbonate. In eight patients there were severe symptoms of poisoning, including cyanosis, irregular heart activity, intestinal complaints, and paresis. In the six patients who died as a result, autopsy revealed a hemorrhagic infiltration of the meninges and cerebral edema. Before the barium carbonate had been administered to patients, extensive animal experiments had been carried out and no ill-effects had been found [139].

8.2. Disadvantages of barium suspensions

In addition to the great difficulties still encountered in producing a sufficiently stable barium suspension that is at the same time protected against fluid withdrawal, several other disadvantages of this contrast medium are mentioned in the literature.

1) Owing to the higher viscosity of a barium suspension in the ileum, it cannot deeply penetrate narrow fistulous tracts in this area.
2) As a result of leakage from perforations or fistulas, the formation of barium granulomas can occur.
3) As a result of aspiration, a necrotizing bronchopneumonia can develop.

Some radiologists have therefore tried to find a contrast medium that does not have these disadvantages. They have considered organic iodine compounds. The thin liquid aqueous iodine solutions are just as unsatisfactory. This will be discussed in more detail in this chapter.

8.3. Suspensions of an organic iodine compound

Jones et al. [106] studied tetraiodophtalimido-ethanol; they were able to produce a very homogeneous suspension with a particle size of 1–2 microns. This fluid contains 73% iodine, barely precipitates, and adheres more readily to the mucosa than barium suspensions. By adding gelatin, the characteristics of the suspension were further improved. From animal experiments it appeared that the toxicity of this contrast medium is as low as that of barium sulfate; for the latter it has been shown that particles varying from 0.04 to 0.1 micron in size can be absorbed by the intestinal mucous membrane. These particles, which do not end up in the bloodstream but in the lymphatic channels, form less than one ten-thousandth of the normal barium suspension [4]. The organic iodine compounds were tested in several experiments with dogs; it appeared that much smaller mucosal lesions could be localized with this contrast medium than with barium.

In 18 patients and a number of students, a total of 56 follow-through studies and four colon examinations were carried out. The resulting roentgenograms were very clear. One objection was that fluid absorption in the distal ileum and the colon caused even greater dehydration of the contrast fluid than barium. Unfortunately the preparation of this contrast medium was so time-consuming and expensive that the experiments had to be terminated.

8.4. Aqueous iodine solutions

In 1958, the first publications appeared on the use of Urokon, Hypaque, and Renografin as contrast media for examination of the digestive tract. Shortly thereafter, similar articles were also published in England and Germany. A true avalanche of reports from enthusiastic users broke loose after the introduction of Gastrografin about 1960. After Gastrografin, which consists of 76% Urografine mixed with a wetting agent, a sweetener, and a flavoring, several other brands were introduced, but they have never been generally accepted. Most radiologists believe that Gastrografin is ideal for use when barium fails due to flocculation or when barium is contraindicated. The following examples of the latter are mentioned:

1) Atresia or fistulas in the tracheo-esophageal area (danger of aspiration).
2) Special cases of pre- and postoperative diagnosis of the digestive tract, such as bleeding ulcers, suture leakage, or perforations.
3) Partial obstructions that cannot be passed by barium or where dehydration and thickening of the barium suspension might occur.

There were also publications reporting the use of Gastrografin for all patients and for the colon examination as well as the examinations of the

stomach and the small intestine. Shehadi even reports a series of 1500 patients [213]. Robinson and Levene [202] prefer Renografin over barium for the gastrointestinal examination. In 1959, Lessman and Lilienfeld [130] had already studied and compared the experiences of various radiologists. It appeared that the amount of Gastrografin used per examination varied widely. Some used only 25–50 ml of a 76% concentration and others used ten times as much. There was general satisfaction with the reproduction of the gastric mucosal relief and the greater ease with which a pyloric stenosis could be diagnosed or a fistulous tract filled. However, they all discovered that dilution of the contrast medium in the small intestine was so great that morphological evaluation of this area was absolutely impossible. In addition, no one succeeded in making acceptable double-contrast exposures. Some authors reported that more than 50 ml can cause abdominal cramps, vomiting, and diarrhea. Reasonably satisfactory colon films can be made because absorption of fluid causes an increasing contrast in this area [213]. In this way it was sometimes possible to obtain good filling of the colon on the proximal side of a stenosis, which could not be passed by the barium from the distal side. It remained impossible to localize tumors in the small intestine, although the diagnosis of 'obstruction' could often be made on the basis of the presence of wide dilated intestinal loops. Some radiologists believe that when Gastrografin has not yet reached the colon 4 h after oral administration, a postoperative ileus is due to an obstruction and not a paralysis [236].

Rubin et al. [204] were not able to confirm this opinion. Berger, of Philadelphia, agrees with Rubin, and at a conference he showed slides of four patients. In these cases the Gastrografin was visible in the colon within 15 min although a definite obstruction did exist in the small intestine, which apparently could easily be passed by the thin liquid Gastrografin. In approximately 2% of the patients, some of the iodine contrast medium is excreted into the urine [92]. This is believed by some to indicate an obstruction, perforation, or other pathological condition in the digestive tract [164]. Although surgical confirmation has often supported this line of thought and Tosch has shown with radioactive Gastrografin that this can indeed occur [232], disap-

56

pointment [246] and false positive results have also been reported in this respect [203]. On the other hand, we once saw an accumulation of an aqueous iodine solution in the distal ileum after an angiography in a patient without any evidence of bleeding in the digestive tract (fig. 4.21). In 1959, Lessman and Lilienfeld pointed out the strong hyperosmotic characteristics of Gastrografin and the dangers this can cause in case of intestinal obstructions [130]. Since the osmotic value of 50 ml 70% Urokon is equal to that of 15 g magnesium sulfate, a dose of 6 ml/kg body weight can cause such excessive fluid withdrawal that the circulating plasma volume can decrease 15%–30%. Harris et al. have described lethal complications in children due to the hypovolemia. They also showed that the osmotic force of Gastrografin in isolated intestinal loops can be so great that blood circulation in the intestinal wall can be seriously disturbed [87]. In addition, the vomiting and diarrhea caused by Gastrografin can further disturb an already critical electrolyte balance [173]. It has therefore become

clear that, for cases of suspected obstruction in the small intestine, it is far from certain that Gastrografin is the most suitable contrast medium. If considered desirable, then it must in any event be handled with extreme caution and used only when the clinical condition of the patient permits it. Furthermore, when Gastrografin is used, it must be realized that this contrast medium does not adhere easily, and therefore reliable morphological information can be obtained only when filling is complete. In addition, Gastrografin is such a thin liquid that fistulous tracts or perforations may not be discovered because the contrast medium passes so rapidly that there is not enough time for penetration of these small defects.

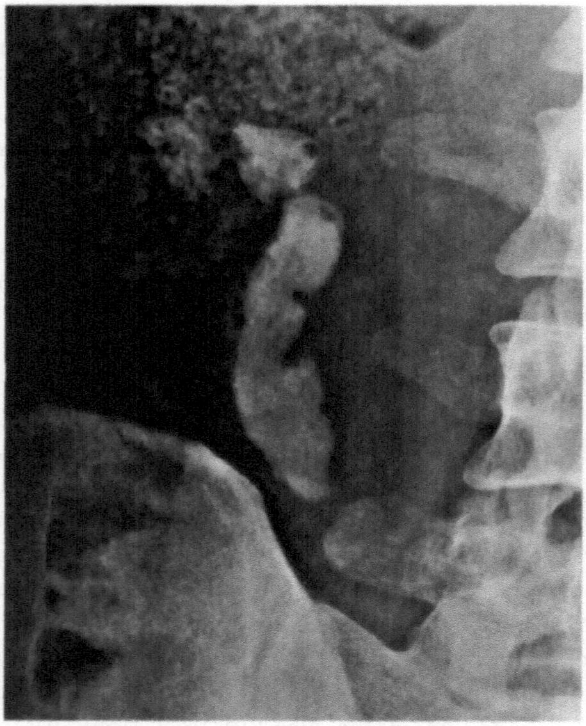

Shehadi wrote in 1960 that the introduction of the aqueous iodine contrast medium could be considered a milestone in the diagnosis of the digestive tract [212]. Fortunately since then the use of Gastrografin has lost some of the ground it had taken by storm. However, a new landmark in the diagnosis of the digestive tract will be reached when use of this medium is a rare exception.

8.5. Gastrografin–barium mixtures

A number of radiologists did not simply stop using Gastrografin, but have attempted to obtain better results by mixing it with barium [74, 226]. They expected the mixture to have the better adhesive characteristics of a barium suspension on the one hand, and the transit acceleration and the ability to mix with gastric and intestinal juices without flocculation of Gastrografin on the other. The combination of these two entirely different contrast fluids was tested in every possible ratio, especially in Japan where it is still used for gastric and duodenal examinations. During these tests it appeared that the tendency of barium to flocculate does not decrease; it even increases as the amount of barium in the mixture decreases. The transit acceleration of the Gastrografin–barium mixture does not depend particularly on the ratio, but is almost directly dependent upon the absolute quantity of Gastrografin.

Shehadi [213] and Stecken et al. [226] report the strange phenomenon of separation of barium and Gastrografin already occurring in the jejunum. The Gastrografin produces less contrast as a result of the absorption of fluid, and it travels rapidly to the

Fig. 4.21. Aqueous iodine solution in the distal ileum after an angiography.

cecum while the barium remains in the jejunum. Furthermore, Stecken et al. observed that not only stenosis and hypotonia but also meteorism clearly delays the rate of transit. Various radiologists believe that 150 ml barium suspension and approximately 30 ml Gastrografin is still the most satisfactory ratio. This is probably because there is so little Gastrografin in this mixture that it barely affects the barium suspension. Furthermore, it is possible that the 30 ml Gastrografin does not visibly separate from the barium in the duodenum and the jejunum, but absorbs sufficient fluid to cause transit acceleration. Due to the faster transit, a larger portion of the intestine can be radiographed with the still usable barium suspension than would otherwise have been the case.

5. METHODS OF EXAMINATION

1. 'Physiological' examination of the small intestine

In chapter 3, it was noted that addition of nutrients to the contrast medium was abandoned during the second world war. The problems involved in the functional examination were found to be considerably greater than those for the morphological examination. Furthermore, it was recognized that a functional examination must also be evaluated morphologically. It is therefore necessary that the morphological examination of the small intestine first attain a much higher degree of perfection. In the 1960s, only Mattsson et al. [47, 153] advocated a return to this method; however, their published photographs of the ileum were very poor. The nutritional composition of the 300 ml contrast meal administered by Mattson et al. is approximately the same as Borgström's and is as follows:

153 g BaSO$_4$
12½ g protein
15 g fat
12½ g lactose
25 g dextrose
200 ml water

In one of their articles, they report that their examination technique gave very constant transit time, in contrast to the highly variable data from the literature. The authors thereby showed that they had little insight into the reasons for these variations.

It is customary for many radiologists to give their patients something to eat or drink whenever a standstill of the contrast column has occurred in the ileum. This has, of course, nothing to do with a physiological examination. This additional food is usually given to renew stimulation of peristalsis.

Sometimes, however, it is done only to decrease the patient's feeling of hunger.

Some radiologists have set rules; Pirk and Vulterinova [185], for instance, give a small meal after 3 h if the stomach is empty and the cecum has not yet been reached. Patients who have undergone gastrectomy receive this food after 2 h.

If this is done, it must be realized that a large, liquid meal will induce more active peristalsis and faster transit than a small, more viscous meal. In the first case, the additional food is more likely to ruin the roentgenograms of the ileum, if this has not already occurred as a result of the long transit time.

2. Single administration of the contrast medium

2.1. Normal amount

For examination of the small intestine, most radiologists, including Golden, have the patient drink approximately 250 ml of the contrast fluid. Usually this is preceded by a gastric examination whereby the mucosa is studied by using approximately 50 ml contrast fluid. The number of exposures subsequently made of the small intestine is highly dependent upon the rate of transit but probably even more upon the attitude of the radiologist. Many are in the habit of making films at equal time intervals even when the rate of transit continues to decrease. This is not correct, because the patient receives an unnecessarily high radiation dose. It also means a waste of film.

There is no waste of film for those who believe that an examination of the many meters of small intestine can be carried out with only three [247] or even two [164] exposures. This method is very poor for good diagnosis and should be abandoned, even when each of these exposures clearly shows practically the entire small intestine.

2.2. Small amounts

Some radiologists use small quantities of contrast fluid; for example, Laws et al. administer only 100 ml undiluted Micropaque, even for sprue patients [123]. This is probably done to avoid the annoying effect of superposition, but this exaggerated fear is paid for with flocculation and segmentation. Morton, who used only 70 g Micropaque powder mixed with 200 ml of an ice-cold physiological salt solution [167], also obtained poor results. He made only two exposures, but probably the information would not be increased much by an increase in the number of films.

2.3. Large amounts

For many years, an increasing number of radiologists have switched to the use of large quantities of the contrast medium for examination of the small intestine.

Although there was no general acceptance, Weltz in 1937 had already pointed out that the quality of the x-ray films of the small intestine is highly dependent upon the degree of filling [240]. He also reported that this requires rapid gastric emptying and that stretching of the small intestine is the main stimulus for the induction of good peristaltic waves. Furthermore, he believed that a large amount of contrast medium offers the best buffer action against the detrimental effects of secretion and absorption in the intestinal canal. He noted that the contrast intensity in the ileum is greater than in the jejunum, but that this phenomenon is less pronounced for a rapid transit because there is apparently not enough time for fluid absorption.

In view of the time in which he worked, his insights can be regarded as brilliant. If he had had a better 'sales technique', the development of the radiological examination of the small intestine would certainly have advanced much faster.

According to published articles, Marshak had similar views but did not reason them as well as Weltz. In any event, Marshak's great contribution was that these improvements in technique were widely published in his numerous articles after 1954 [143–149]. He routinely used 480 ml contrast fluid and, when the small intestine was dilated, sometimes 600 ml or more [147].

In 1963, Caldwell and Floch examined 32 patients twice and thereby showed that the transit time is significantly shorter when the amount of contrast medium is chosen according to Marshak (480 ml) rather than Golden (240 ml). For the former, the average transit time was 2.25 h and for the latter, 3.25 h [33].

Many authors believe that it is desirable to make compression exposures of the ileum, whereby the loops that cover one another are forced apart [143, 225].

Numerous radiologists also find that diagnosis is considerably improved when several exposures are made, one immediately after the other. The same intestinal loops are then seen more often in approximately the same stage of filling [244, 247]. Caldwell et al. [34] pointed out that delayed gastric emptying can still cause flocculation and segmentation even when 500 ml stable barium is administered.

It is striking that none of the radiologists who use large quantities of contrast medium feel that either the use of ice water or drugs to accelerate passage is necessary.

3. Fractional administration of the contrast medium

3.1. Method of Pansdorf

In 1927, Pansdorf [178] introduced this method based on the entirely reasonable assumption that the best technique for administering the contrast medium must be extreme fractionation. He gave his patients one tablespoon to drink every 5 min and thought that only in this way could distribution of the contrast medium throughout the small intestinal loops be guaranteed. Furthermore, the annoying effect of superposition would be very slight at the most. He reasoned that each roentgenogram would then show as many loops as possible.

Pansdorf was probably not sufficiently aware of the numerous factors that can completely disturb this theoretically uniform supply. Ideal fractionation exists only when administration of the contrast medium is matched by gastric emptying through the pyloric canal (fig. 5.1). In addition, the stability of the contrast medium is too low to withstand such an unfavorable ratio with respect to the intestinal fluids. It is, however, possible that at

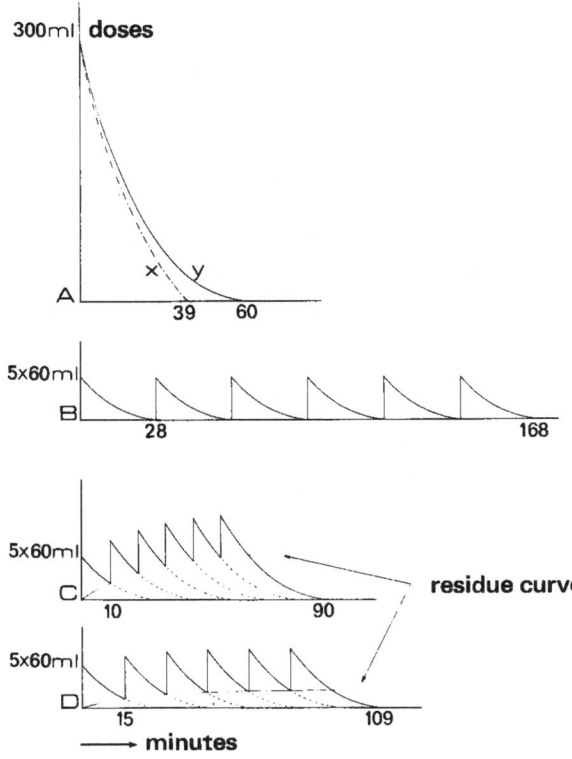

Fig. 5.1. (A) Gastric emptying curve: *y*, sitting or standing position ——; *x*, right lateral position –·–·–; (B) Ideal fractionation: rate of supply equals rate of emptying. (CD) Fractionation: rate of supply is greater than rate of emptying so that an increasing amount of residue is found in the stomach.

the time of Pansdorf this technique of fractional administration of the contrast medium was not as unfavorable as it is now. After all, the contrast medium used then was highly unstable, even without the addition of food, and disintegration occurred anyway in the proximal part of the intestine. Possibly a distribution of flocculation or segmentation was to be preferred over large segment clumps. In the future should there ever be a completely stable contrast media, then it is conceivable that the principle of fractional administration might regain favor.

3.2. Modification of Weltz
In 1937, Weltz [240] introduced important changes in the method of Pansdorf by first giving a single dose of 200 ml contrast medium for the gastric examination. For the subsequent follow-through study, the patient drank approximately 30 ml every 5 min. As mentioned previously, Weltz believed in a large dosage of contrast medium. Although his method appears to resemble fractionation, this is in fact not true. The stomach is continuously filled to a large extent and fractionation is probably only meant to keep the patient from feeling that his stomach is much too full.

3.3. Modification of Naumann
Naumann [171] administered two doses of 200 ml a half-hour apart. Again this method cannot be regarded as true fractionation; it is used to administer a slightly larger amount of contrast medium without discomfort to the patient.

3.4. Fractionation by the pyloric muscle
It is useful to realize that every quantity of contrast medium administered orally is passed to the small intestine in fractions by the pylorus. The size of these fractions differs for every patient and is partly dependent upon:

Pyloric function	Right lateral position
Peptic ulcer or tumor	Drugs to enhance peristalsis
Gastric acid concentration	Temperature, osmosity, and caloric value of the contrast fluid

4. Administration of cold fluids with the contrast medium

4.1. Method of Weintraub and Williams
In 1941, Weintraub [239] noted that drinking ice water after a meal enhanced peristalsis and caused diarrhea. Using this observation, he gave ice water after a barium meal and found that in about 50% of the cases, the cecum was reached within a half-hour. The quality of the pictures, however, was not very good although it improved when he replaced the ice water with cold physiological salt solution. It was remarkable that passage of the contrast medium through the small intestine proceeded even more rapidly. After some experimentation, he finally settled on the following technique:

1) Gastroduodenal examination with a mixture of 120 g barium and 120 g isotonic salt solution at room temperature.

2) After this examination, 240 g ice-cold physiological salt solution is administered and after 5 min, a new roentgenogram is made.

3) Immediately after this x-ray film, another 240 g ice-cold physiological salt solution is administered and again a new roentgenogram is made after 10 min.

4) Still another film is made 15 min later, and if necessary, every 30 min afterward.

As a result of the large amount of fluid given in total (700 ml), transit is rapid and the barium does not thicken in the ileum. He even reports that when the transit time is short, the quality of the films is good and it is poor when the transit time is longer. It is understandable that this method of examination is not very pleasant for the patients.

4.2. Simplified variations

Golden found the method of Weintraub too arduous and in addition believed that the great haste involved was not opportune since precise following and evaluation of the transit films already cost too much time. Many other authors also found this method of examination too laborious, but they did want to profit from the passage acceleration caused by a cold liquid. The simplifications introduced are so similar that they will not be discussed as separate modifications.

Ettinger [50] gave a glass of ice water after first examining the stomach with a mixture of 120 g barium and 120 ml water. Hudak [99] gave a glass of ice-cold physiological salt solution 10 min after a small barium meal and, 10 min later, 1 mg Prostigmin.

Bendick [16] gave 200 ml ice-cold soda water after the contrast meal. He had noted that the gas formation induced peristalsis. This gas travels rapidly and completely independently to the cecum and therefore does not accelerate passage of the contrast medium. Apparently Brown's experiences were similar [25]. In spite of the fact that he gave three glasses of ice-cold soda water, in only 60% of his patients had the cecum been reached within 2 h. He tried to prevent the pronounced flocculation and segmentation of the contrast fluid that then occurred by using Raybar, the most stable contrast medium then known. Morton [167] gave the patient a mixture of 200 ml ice-cold salt solution and only

70 g Micropaque powder. Like those of Hudak, his photographs show only flocculation and segmentation of the contrast fluid and demonstrate quite clearly how unsuitable this technique is.

All the authors in this group report a transit time to the cecum of 1.5–2.0 h, considerably longer than the method of Weintraub. No one apparently recognized the importance of the large quantities; they all used 200 ml instead of 700 ml like Weintraub. In this connection it is most interesting to note the technique of Brown, who did give approximately 600 ml fluid. The passage acceleration that this large dose should have produced was completely neutralized by the retardation caused by the release of gas from the soda water.

5. Administration of the contrast medium through a tube directly into the small intestine (enteroclysis)

Publications between 1920 and 1925 by Einhorn, who introduced the contrast fluid into the duodenum through a tube and obtained outstanding films, gave Pesquera the idea in 1929 of using this method for filling the entire small intestine [184]. He administered a mixture of barium and water, which also contained a small amount of gum acacia. Although no quantities are reported, the article indicates that he let the infusion run slowly and as long as necessary to reach the cecum, usually no longer than half an hour. He reports that he was able to diagnose a lymphosarcoma in the distal ileum in this manner. This certainly can be regarded as a success in radiological diagnosis at that time.

Ten years later, Gershon-Cohen and Shay [69] did some experiments on the function of the pylorus and noted that the closing mechanism was very good. After the duodenum had been filled by using a tube, the entire contents quickly disappeared into the jejunum; reflux into the stomach occurred only when the pressure of the infusion was too high. They used this method to administer 800–1200 ml contrast fluid and they were surprised by the rapid rate of transit through the small intestine. The cecum was reached in 8–15 min. This interval would probably have been even shorter if the pressure of the infusion had been higher; their level of difference was only 25 cm.

In 1943, a publication by Schatzki [206] appeared, reporting on 75 patients examined in this manner. He intubated a supple Rehfuss tube with an olive-shaped metal end into the duodenum and let 500–1000 ml barium suspension with a lower specific gravity than he normally used for a gastric examination run through this tube. In half of his patients the cecum was reached in 15 min. For four patients, reflux into the stomach occurred; in these cases the average transit time was more than 40 min – considerably longer. The rather low percentage of reflux and the relatively long transit time for such an examination with large amounts of contrast fluid probably indicate that his infusion was given under low pressure.

Once reflux into the stomach had occurred, Schatzki tried to end it by sliding the tube further into the duodenum, decreasing the pressure of the infusion, or acidifying the barium mixture. He was not successful with any of these methods, so he concluded that these factors do not influence the development of reflux. The correctness of this conclusion is, however, very doubtful since it is obvious that once reflux has occurred, the pylorus will continue to open to allow the gastric contents to pass on to the duodenum. While the infusion is flowing, the pressure in the duodenum will probably be higher than in the stomach and opening of the pylorus will therefore have a reverse effect.

Schatzki's great contribution is that he pointed out the importance of administering large quantities of the contrast medium in the right lateral position. He had found that interruption of the contrast column lengthens the transit time considerably, thus allowing more time for dehydration in the ileum.

In 1951, Lura [136] reported on a series of 300 patients; he examined the small intestine of these patients by using the infusion technique and found an average transit time of 15 min. It had been difficult to pass the tube through the pylorus in 5%–10% of the cases.

In 1960, Scott-Harden et al. [119, 208] and Pygott et al. [193] described an improvement in the technique for duodenal intubation. They passed two catheters, one inside the other, into the pars media of the stomach, which can be felt as well as seen by fluoroscopy since the outer end of both catheters is marked by a metal ring. The outer more rigid catheter has an outer diameter of 5.8 mm and the inner more pliable catheter has a lumen 1.5 mm in diameter. The inner catheter is then slid through the outer into the pyloric canal. It appeared that curling of the catheter could often be prevented by placing the patient in the right lateral position.

In spite of this simplification of the technique, they were still not able to get the catheter into the duodenum in 7% of the patients, which must be considered a high percentage. We have found that beginning this procedure with the more rigid catheter was probably the reason for their failure.

Both catheters remain in place; only the end of the inner catheter with the narrow lumen lies in the duodenum. Pygott et al. then used a syringe to administer 50 ml contrast fluid into the duodenum as often as necessary. It is possible that, as a result, continuity of the contrast column is occasionally interrupted. Also, the outflow through this narrow lumen is probably too low to cause sufficient stretching of the duodenal wall to induce good peristalsis.

Scott-Harden administered only 80 ml of a thin Microtrast solution, directly followed by a $MgSO_4$ solution. This method will certainly not lead to good results since both the hyperosmotic $MgSO_4$ solution and the low dose of contrast medium induce marked flocculation.

In 1965, Patterson et al. [179] reported that they had injected 40 ml Raybar in 15 sprue patients through a duodenal tube; 15 min later they administered 500 ml ice water as well as a $MgSO_4$ solution. They obtained flocculation in this manner even with this exceedingly stable contrast medium. Here we are confronted not only with an abuse of a good examination technique, but also with an entirely misplaced conclusion drawn from their experiments: 'for sprue, an examination technique of duodenal intubation offers no advantages over oral administration of the contrast medium.' It is noteworthy that orally they did not give 40 ml Raybar with ice water and $MgSO_4$, as would be expected, but 120 g undiluted Micropaque solution!

The only techniques that might be regarded as a variation of the preceding are those of Greenspon and Lentino [82] and Friedman and Rigler [64]. In 1960, they reported that they introduced a double-lumen Miller-Abbott tube (fig. 5.2) into the small intestine just beyond the area they wished to examine.

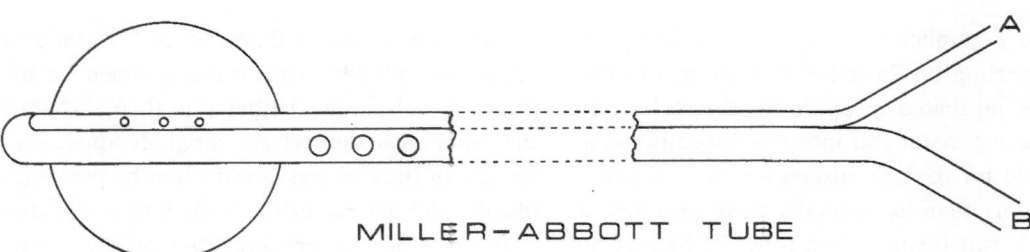

Fig. 5.2. (A) Air inflow. (B) Contrast fluid.

It can take several days for the end of the tube to reach the desired location. The balloon is filled with 50–60 ml air through tube A so that passage beyond this location is not possible. Contrast fluid is then administered through tube B. In this way, according to the authors, one-fourth of the small intestine can be examined without the annoying effect of super-position. Because the intestine is suddenly occluded, the patients cannot easily tolerate more than 600 ml contrast medium. Abdominal cramps can also be caused when the contrast fluid is injected too quickly or its temperature is too low. It is clear that this method of examination is not suitable for routine use and is probably also seldom necessary.

6. Retrograde administration of the contrast fluid

In the 1920s and 1930s some authors believed (correctly) that it is better to examine the distal ileum by using the colon enema technique rather than the small intestine transit examination.

Although the situation had changed somewhat in 1964, Figiel and Figiel [52] pointed out that retro-grade filling of the ileum could still mean a welcome supplement to the transit examination for the diagnosis of strictures, adhesions, ulcerations, fistulas, and diverticula. They demonstrated this with the x-rays of a number of patients examined in this manner. They found abnormalities that were confirmed surgically while the normal transit examination had revealed nothing.

Miller [160, 162] found that the appearance of the ileum in particular is determined by peristalsis and tone to such a large extent that constricting lesions in an early stage and smaller mucosal lesions are definitely missed during a transit examination. The functioning of the pylorus causes intermittent, irregular, and incomplete filling so that the elasticity of the intestine cannot be determined. Furthermore, flocculation and segmentation often completely distort the evaluation. At that time, Miller was of the opinion that enteroclysis is a good method of examination but the duodenal intubation before-hand too troublesome. He therefore propagated retrograde filling of the entire small intestine. Although it is possible to reach the stomach in nine out of ten patients (fig. 5.3C), he advises terminating the filling of the small intestine as the duodenum is approached. It is obvious that this filling must occur under fluoroscopic control and that one must be careful that the contrast fluid does not enter the lungs by way of the stomach and esophagus. In many patients it is possible to pass Bauhin's valve easily (fig. 5.3AB) but sometimes it is difficult or impossible. This can be overcome in most cases by oral administration of 1 mg atropine before the examination; this may also cause a decrease in the secretion of intestinal juices and in forward peri-stalsis, which would greatly facilitate retrograde filling. He now uses 0.5–1.0 mg glucagon i.v.

The amount of contrast medium needed to fill the colon and small intestine is sometimes less than 2 liters, sometimes considerably more. More than 4.5 liters are never given, even if the duodenum has not yet been reached.

Miller later changed this method slightly by replacing the barium suspension with a physiological salt solution as soon as the ileum begins to fill. When the infusion of the contrast medium is terminated, the colon is emptied by first lowering

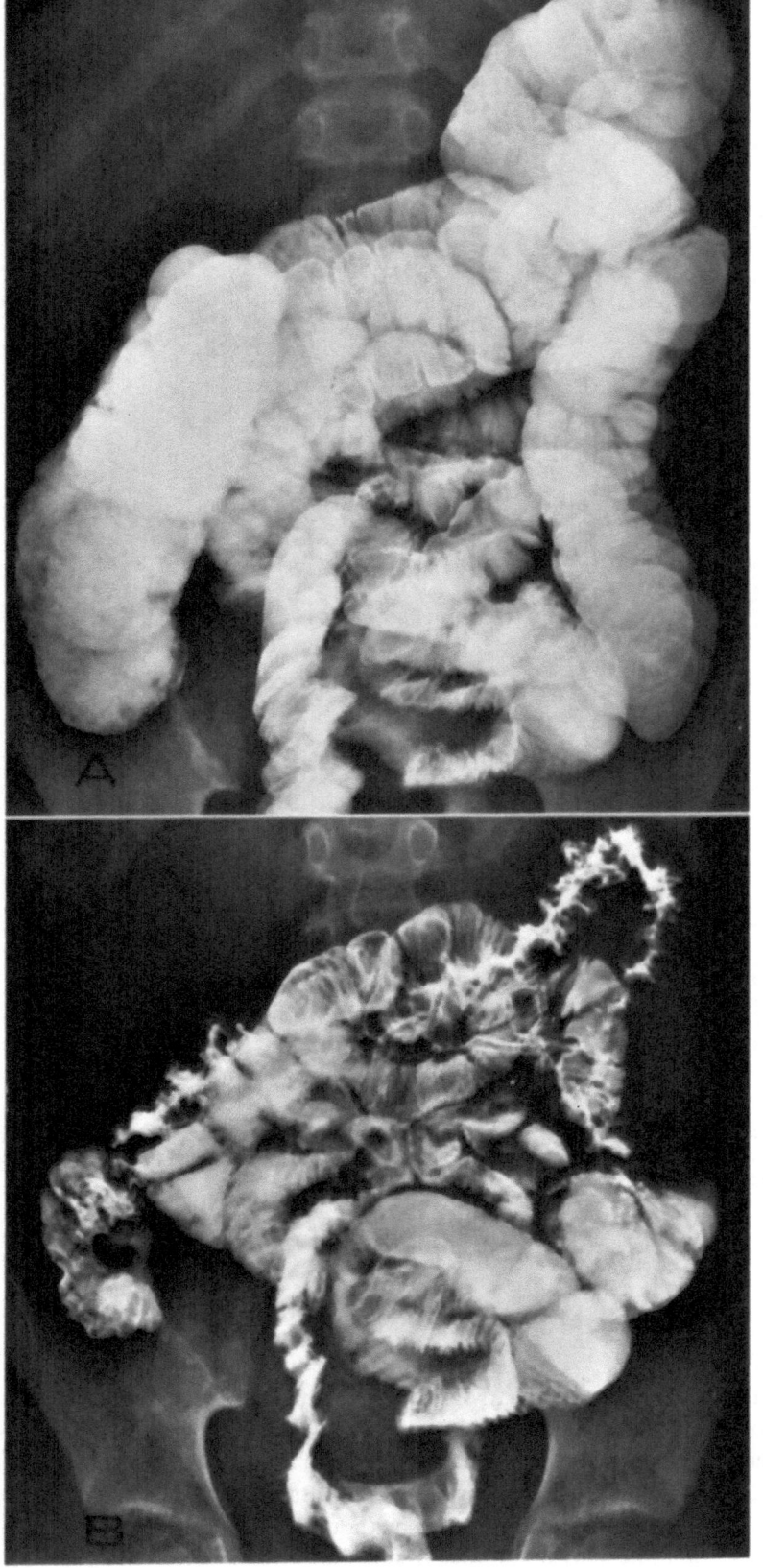

*Fig. 5.3*AB. Roentgenogram of retrograde filling of the small intestine. (A) Survey exposure after filling of the colon and ileum; a hypotonic agent was not administered. (B) Survey film after evacuation; the colon is now empty.

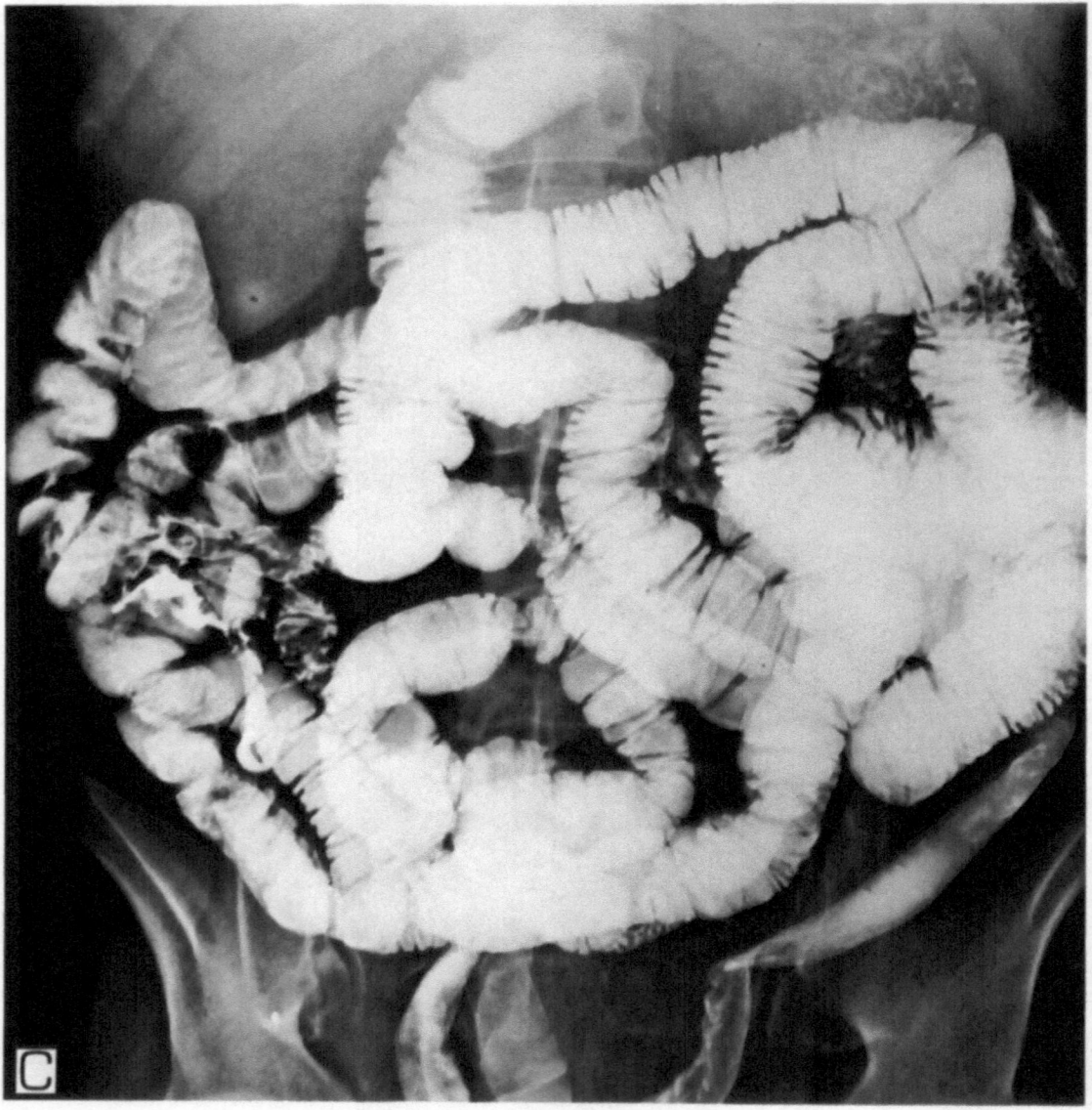

Fig. 5.3c. Retrograde small bowel enema with complete filling of the small intestine. To pass the ileocecal valve, 1 mg atropine was used. After complete filling of the colon with contrast fluid, water was used to push this into the small intestine. The roentgenogram still shows the diluted barium suspension left in the rectosigmoid after evacuation.

the plastic infusion bag below the level of the table and then sending the patient to the toilet. Films of the small intestine are subsequently made; if desired of course, films of the colon can be made at the beginning of the infusion period. In our hospital this later modification of Miller's technique is used

to our complete satisfaction. The contrast fluid is of course not that for a colon enema but the same barium suspension used for oral enteroclysis. If it is possible to pass Bauhin's valve and fill the small intestine without giving a drug to induce hypotonicity, the time available for making roentgen

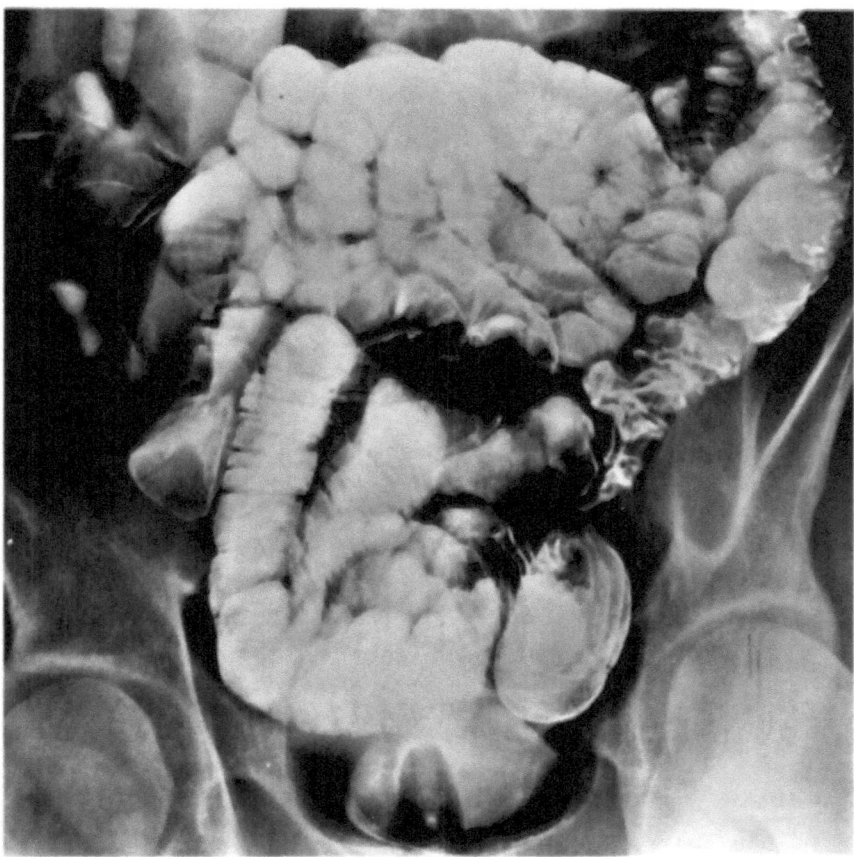

Fig. 5.4. Survey exposure after evacuation; in this case the ileum could be filled only after a hypotonic drug was administered. Evacuation of the colon was of course fairly difficult.

films is quite short since the small intestine will empty quickly. The patient must be permitted frequent but short periods for evacuation, which can easily be done by lowering the bag under the level of the table.

If retrograde filling of the small intestine is not possible without atropine or Buscopan, then the patient must be allowed to evacuate for much longer periods (fig. 5.4). We have found that the small intestine films are best made as soon as peristalsis resumes.

An enormous advantage of this method is that stenotic processes in the small intestine can be approached very quickly from the distal direction (fig. 5.5). Proximal approach in these cases costs more time and, moreover, an annoying dilution of the contrast medium can occur in the dilated loops.

Figure 5.6AB shows a series of films taken when enteroclysis turned out to be impossible because of a stenotic obstruction in the pars antralis due to

Crohn's disease. Retrograde filling of the small intestine revealed multiple abnormalities in the region of the duodenum and the jejunum; the ileum, however, was free of abnormalities.

In the case of fig. 5.6C, it was impossible to fill the fistulous tracts via the proximal way.

7. Combined methods of examination

Without a doubt, many radiologists use methods that are not described here or that are made up of elements or variations of specific methods of examination.

An example of such a combination is the approach of Bugyi [29], who first examines the gallbladder and stomach according to the method of Gianturco [72], then the small intestine by using a variation of the method of Weintraub, and finally takes pictures of the orally filled colon.

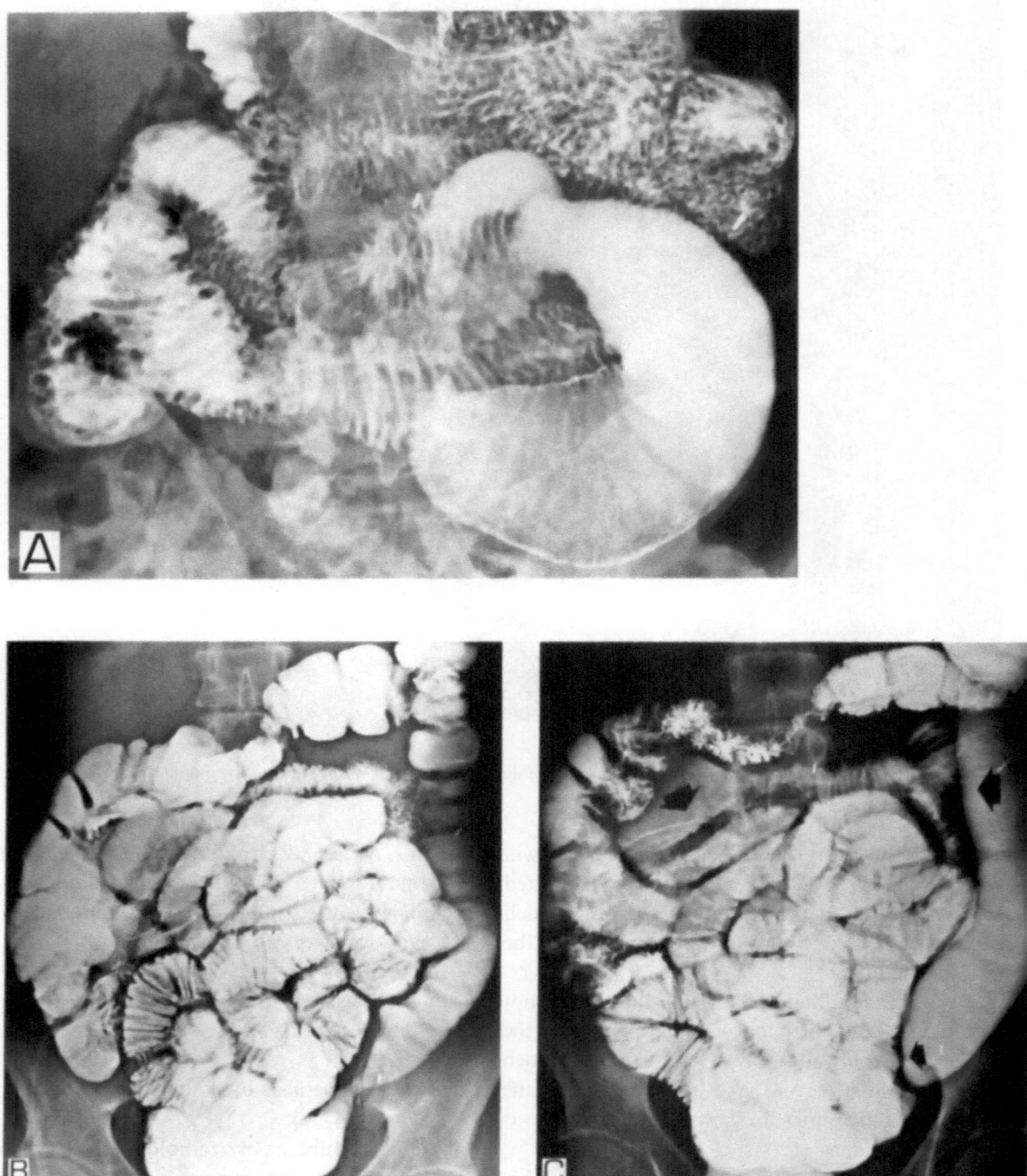

*Fig. 5.5*A–E. (A) As a result of a stenosis in the jejunum due to radiation enteritis, it was not possible to obtain adequate filling of the ileum. (B) Filling of the ileum via the colon appeared to be possible without administration of a hypotonic agent. (C) The exposure after defecation showed edematous mucosal folds in the left upper quadrant, extensive fusion and obliteration of the mucosa in the right upper quadrant, and a stenosis in the sigmoid. (D) The mass of ileal loops in the minor pelvis became accessible for compression after filling the rectosigmoid with air. (E) Spot films using compression reveal a skip lesion in the right lower quadrant.

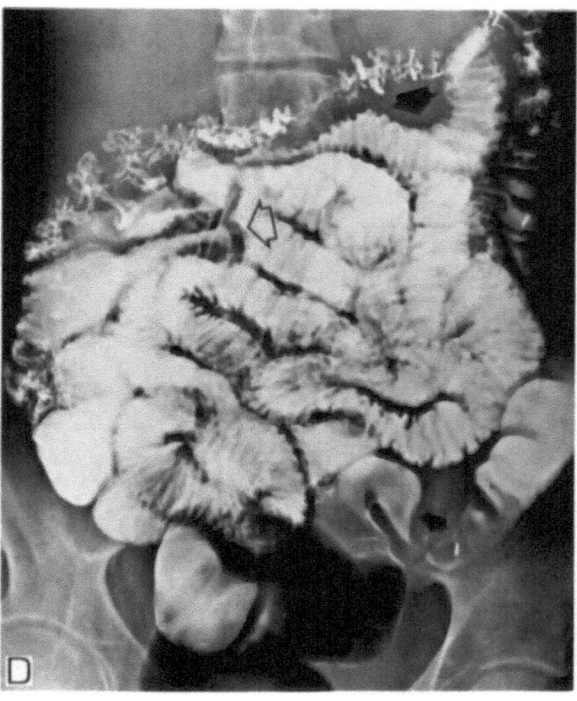

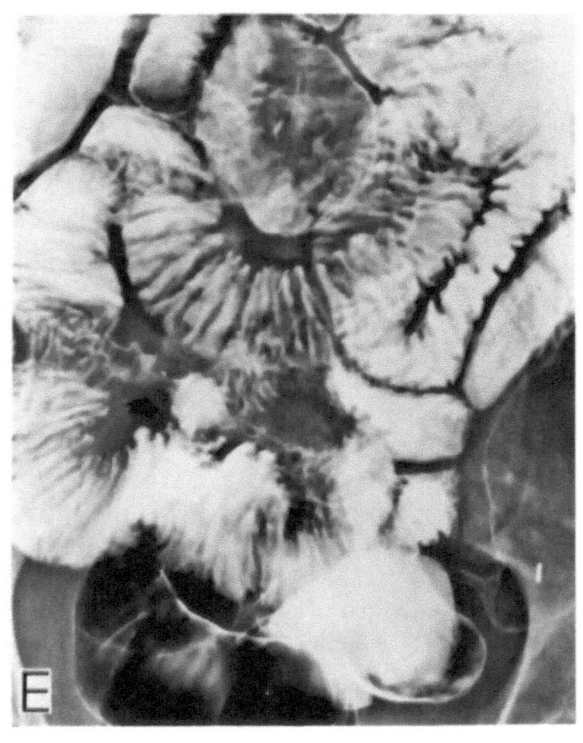

*Fig. 5.5*D E. See legend on page 68.

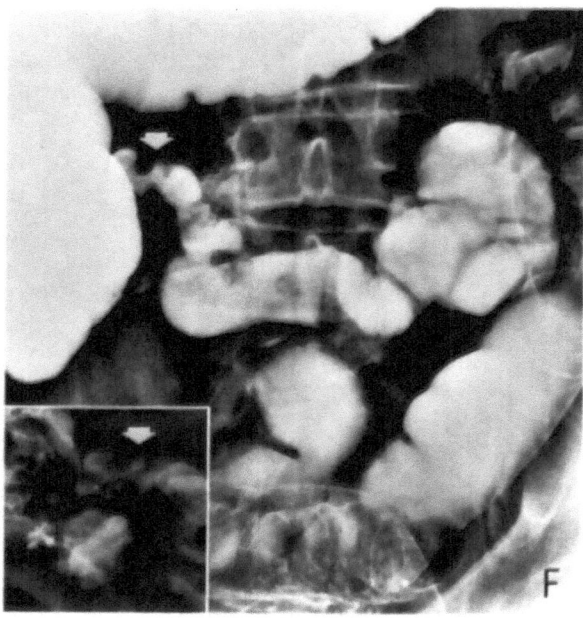

*Fig. 5.5*F. With the enteroclysis technique, this small tumor in the distal ileum was not reached although 2500 ml contrast fluid and water were administered and the examination was continued for 1 h. The tumor was quickly visualized via filling of the colon. The patient had been hospitalized five times elsewhere because of rectal bleeding.

The following procedures occur in the following order:

1) On the morning of the examination, gallbladder films are taken first. On the afternoon of the previous day the patient swallowed the necessary tablets.
2) After the gallbladder films are taken, the colon is cleansed by means of an enema.
3) The next step is the gastric examination; no details are given.
4) After the gastric examination, the patient receives 100–200 g paraffin oil, which is a laxative and also induces contraction of the gallbladder.
5) A half-hour later, films of the contracted gallbladder are taken.
6) The patient is given a glass of ice-cold salt solution.
7) Films of the small intestine are now made every 10 min.
8) Films are made of the orally filled colon 4–6 h after the beginning of the examination.

Unfortunately the article contains no films of his

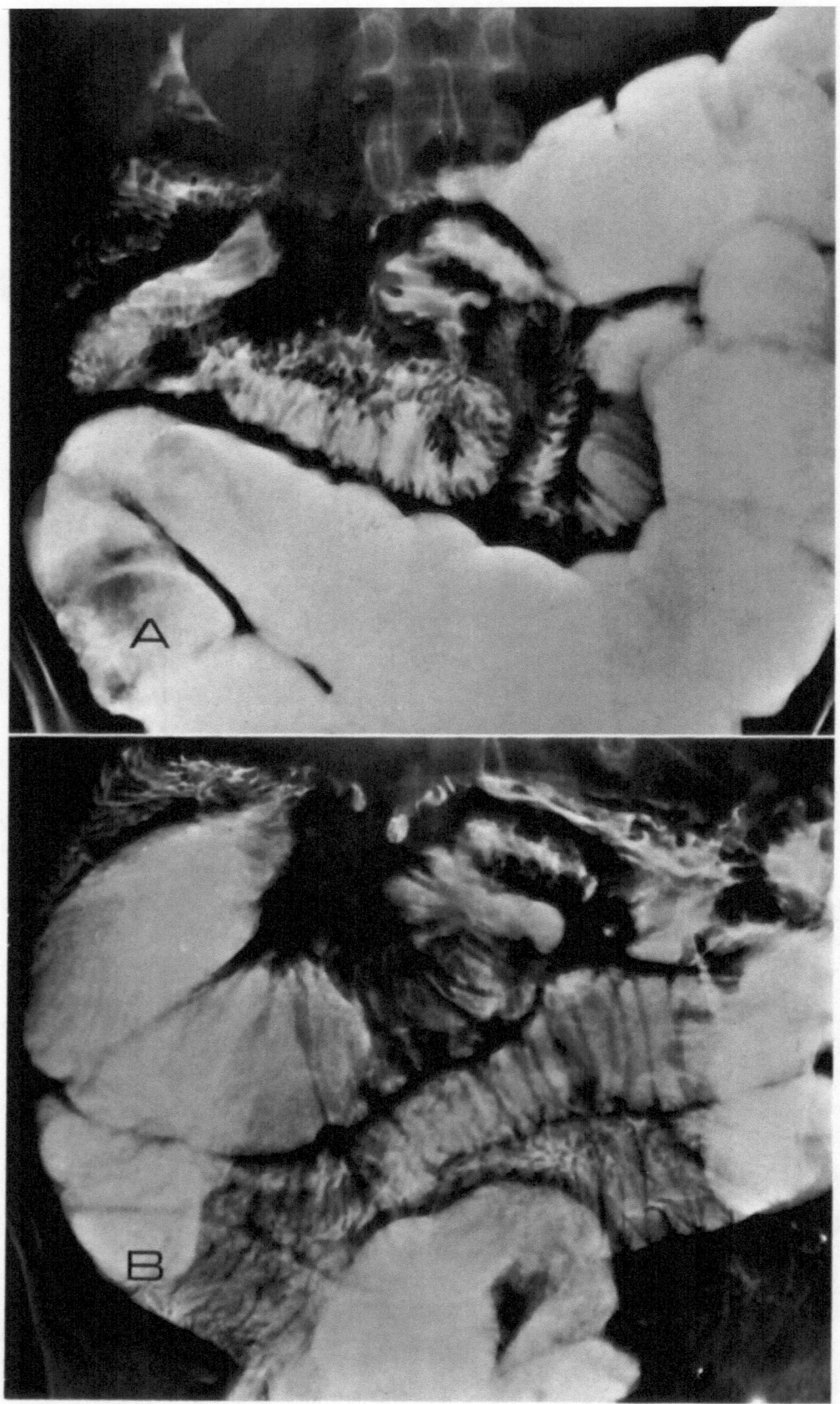

*Fig. 5.6*AB. Retrograde filling of the colon and the entire small intestine (A). Because of a highly obstructive abnormality in the pars antralis of the stomach resulting from Crohn's disease, an enteroclysis examination for evaluation of the small intestine appeared to be impossible. After evacuation (B), only the loops of the small intestine were filled. Several skip lesions were found in the duodenum and the jejunum as well as a fistula to the stomach.

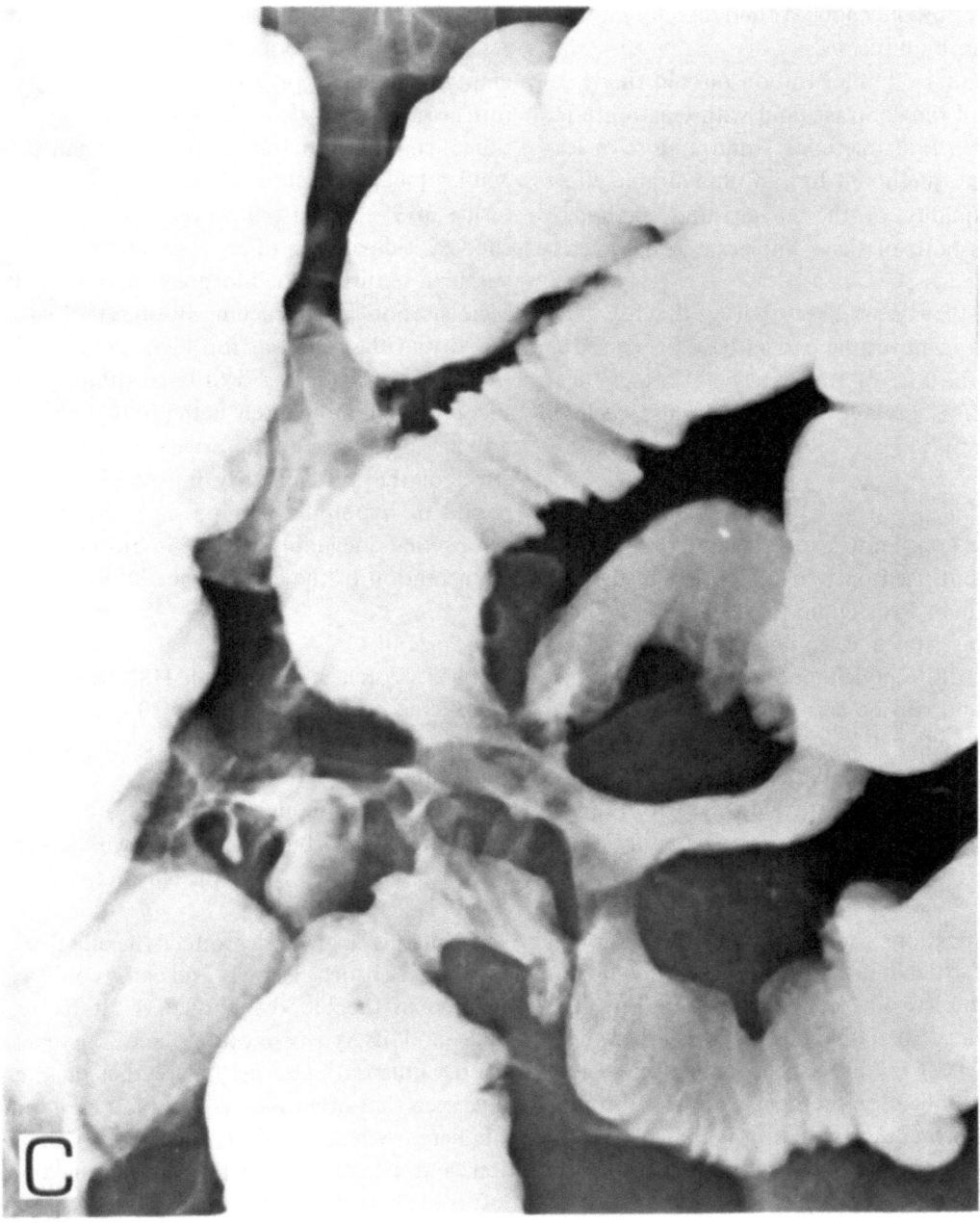

Fig. 5.6c. Retrograde filling of an area of extensive fistulization in the ileum. Filling via the proximal route turned out to be impossible because the contrast fluid flowed via another fistula into the colon instead of the ileum.

results. Bugyi suffices with the statement that he is highly satisfied with this method and that a colon enema examination occurs only upon strict indications.

8. Use of drugs to accelerate transit

The radiologists' increasing lack of time and the high demands on the patience and endurance of the patient are the reasons why shortening the length of the examination has been an objective for so many years. This can be accomplished by:

1) Drinking very large quantities of contrast fluid.
2) Administering the contrast fluid directly into the duodenum by infusion.
3) Supplementary administration of cold fluids.
4) Mixture of the contrast fluid with Gastrografin. The patient finds methods 1 and 2 more or less unpleasant, method 4 has an unfavorable effect on the quality of the image, and method 3 combines both of these unpleasant characteristics.
5) In the past few years, several drugs that are in no way unpleasant for the patient have been used to increase the rate of transit. The effect of these drugs differs greatly; we shall discuss each of them briefly.

8.1. Prostigmin

A substance long known for its accelerating effect on transit, but used only seldomly, is neostigmine methylsulfate or Prostigmin. In chapter 3, we have seen that this substance inhibits acetylcholinesterase so that the acetylcholine is protected against hydrolysis and can be active longer. The effective dosage for adults is 0.75–1.0 mg, and for children, 0.25–0.5 mg. It can be administered subcutaneously, intramuscularly, or intravenously; with the latter, the effect is the strongest but lasts only a few minutes. The effect of Prostigmin can be neutralized by atropine.

Contraindications for the use of Prostigmin are: recent myocardial infarction, volvulus, intussusception, and complete obstruction or perforation of the small intestine. Prostigmin has no effect when there is dysfunction of the nerve cells, as in sprue.

An older publication on the use of this substance in a follow-through examination is that of Hudak [99] in 1951. As a result of a combination of factors, however, the photographs published are very poor. Hudak used only a small amount of contrast fluid (not specifically reported) and afterward he even gave a glass of ice-cold physiological salt solution. This had to result in complete flocculation and segmentation of the contrast medium.

In 1962, Friedenberg et al. [62] also found that, in a series of almost 500 patients, 400 ml ice-cold salt solution had the same effect of transit acceleration as 400 ml water with 0.5 mg Prostigmin. The quality of the mucosal patterns was better with the latter.

Margulis has used Prostigmin for examination of the stomach and small intestine of many thousands of patients to his complete satisfaction [140, 142]. As a result of the more active peristalsis, the gastric emptying time is approximately half as long. Therefore he saw a decrease in the percentage of examination of children with flocculation and segmentation. Müller [168] published his experiences with neoserine in 97 patients; however, 10% of the cases showed side-effects of a respiratory or cardiovascular nature. Like Margulis, he also still saw segmentation in the ileum. Both radiologists believed that the tone was too high, presumably still reverting to Golden's 'disordered motor function' theory. Much more likely is the following explanation based on personal observations: after the short effect of the intravenously injected Prostigmin, a period of hypotonia and passage retardation develops that inevitably results in flocculation and segmentation of the contrast medium.

8.2. Sorbitol

In 1957, Porcher and Caroli [188] described the passage acceleration caused by 30 g sorbitol without the development of hypersecretion and segmentation. The latter, however, is contested by many authors although it must be noted that an overdosage of sorbitol or mixing with other substances often appears to be the reason for their poor results [138, 139].

Sorbitol is a glucose product (hexahydric alcohol) that is absorbed slowly and causes only a slight increase in the blood-sugar curve. It has caloric value and is hyperosmotic, which can cause indistinct mucosal patterns. In previous chapters we have seen that other factors can play an important role here, such as quantity, method of administration, and composition of the contrast medium.

It is likely that the lowest effective dosage will be the best because a higher dosage will cause a linear increase in fluid absorption but a gradual decrease in transit acceleration. It is therefore probably correct to use 10–20 g as advised by the manufacturer and not to increase to 30 g as some do [223]. Manecke and Schmidt [138] found the same; they obtained poor results with 20–30 ml Karion F (variation of sorbitol) and only 20 ml barium suspension. With 5–10 ml Karion F, the mucosal patterns were good, but there was only a slight acceleration of transit. As a compromise they gave their patients 10 ml Karion F at the beginning of the examination; 1 h later, the patient received another supplementary dose of 20 ml after films of the ileum had been made. Furthermore, sorbitol is both cholecystokinetic and cholagogic; these two characteristics again have a favorable and an unfavorable aspect. The transit acceleration caused by these substances is favorable, the flocculation is unfavorable.

For Sack [205], the transit acceleration caused by gall was the reason for enhancing contraction of the gallbladder for follow-through examinations. He gave his patients Diabenol, a mixture of 10 g sorbitol and 4 g powdered egg, but not before the stomach was almost half-empty. Diabenol does accelerate transit but also retards gastric emptying. In 20% of the patients, the substance was not successful, usually because of insufficient contraction or absence of the gallbladder. The evening before the examination, Sack prescribed a liquid diet and a laxative to cleanse the colon. The mucosal patterns of ileum and colon on the films published are of good quality: it is quite clear that the barium suspension has retained the proper viscosity because of the rapid transit time (30 min!). Unfortunately Sack does not provide any further data; it seems likely that the quantities and characteristics of the contrast medium administered contributed more to his good results than did Diabenol.

8.3. Metoclopramide (Primperan)

Since about 1966, metoclopramide has been used increasingly for transit acceleration. Because of its effect on the brain stem, this substance is supposed to activate and regulate the tone and peristalsis of the small intestine and stomach without influencing secretion. This substance can be administered both orally and by injection; the effective dose is 10–20 mg for an adult (1 ampule of 2 ml = 10 mg). Intravenous injection produces the quickest effect; within 5 min, enhancement of peristalsis can be seen clearly as both the number and intensity of the peristaltic waves increase. We have found that the effect lasts only 15–20 min; however, most radiologists report a slightly longer effective period [98, 101].

Diverse authors report that with Primperan (trade name) transit is accelerated to such a degree that the cecum is usually reached in 1–2 h [101]. In these publications it is striking that the contrast medium dose is usually not mentioned although this factor is at least equally important for the transit time [34].

Some authors are justifiably of the opinion that accelerated gastric emptying is an important factor for the transit acceleration caused by metoclopramide. Howarth et al. [98] report that the gastric emptying time is halved by Primperan.

Many also believe that the improvement in the mucosal patterns of the ileum can be ascribed to a decrease in dehydration of the contrast medium as a result of the acceleration of transit. It is strange that the dilatation of duodenum and proximal jejunum frequently seen by accelerated gastric emptying is often believed to be due to a decrease in tone.

The more active peristalsis of the stomach is a time-saving factor for the gastric-duodenal examination and in addition can be useful for duodenal intubation and for cinematographic examination of fixed and immobile sections of the gastric wall.

If it seems necessary to use a transit-accelerating drug, metoclopramide (Primperan) appears to be the best choice at present. This preparation is not hydrophilic and, as a result of the accelerated gastric emptying, causes stretching of the duodenum and thus transit acceleration.

6. GENERAL CONSIDERATIONS

For the examination of the small intestine, it should be realized that this organ is several meters long and lies convoluted in a small space. Owing to tone and peristalsis, the mucosal patterns of each intestinal section vary greatly in different phases.

The objective of the radiological examination is to discover restrictions in the mobility of the mucosa and anatomical abnormalities of the intestinal wall in an early stage. When the contact between the contrast medium and the mucosa is good, abnormalities can easily be observed. One condition is that each intestinal section be shown on at least two exposures without superposition. It is often difficult to locate the related intestinal segments on various films so that it is wise to make two exposures in succession. In the case of hypertonic, contracted loops, the highly folded mucosa lies even more loosely over the innermost layers of the intestinal wall so that deeper abnormalities in this wall can be concealed completely. In general, in a hypotonic or dilated intestine, abnormalities located outside the mucosa are seen more easily since the mucosa then lies against this abnormality smoothly and with few folds (fig. 2.6A). We have less difficulty also when an abnormality is seen in the narrow space between two loops that are in a more or less hypotonic phase. This combination of favorable factors seldom occurs.

In certain cases, if we should find it desirable, dilatation of the small intestine can be enhanced by an injection of atropine or TEAB (tetraethylammonium bromide). With atropine, the movements of the muscularis mucosa still exist, not with TEAB; the paralyzing effect of this substance is so strong that there is no motion at all [96]. The same is true of glucagon.

After these preparations are injected, passage comes to a standstill. As a result, superposition increases due to dilatation and possibly also length-ening of the small intestinal loops. Intervention with these drugs is therefore to be considered only in the last phase of the examination after sufficient normal exposures have been made.

Theoretically, it appears sensible to restrict superposition by fractional administration of the contrast medium. The most even distribution of the contrast fluid in the small intestine is obtained by dividing the total amount into as many fractions as possible, which are then administered so slowly that the continuity of the contrast column is just maintained. The contrast medium could also be administered until the cecum is reached and then a number of exposures of the entire small intestine are made. In this way, with a restricted number of photographs, the greatest amount of information could be obtained.

Just as sensible, theoretically, is the method of following a small amount of contrast medium to the cecum without the slightest problem of superposition. With this method, of course, exposures must be made within short time intervals, which means prolonged radiation exposure for the patient. With oral administration of the contrast medium, we must realize that we can regulate the supply to the stomach easily but that the passage from stomach to duodenum can be regulated only by influencing the pyloric mechanism.

Orally administered contrast medium does not leave the stomach at a constant rate, but at a gradually decreasing rate. When Henderson's [90] results are plotted on a graph, the resulting curve will resemble curve A in fig. 5.1. It shows clearly that greater gastric filling lengthens the gastric emptying time only slightly while the average rate of gastric emptying increases. The decrease in the tone of the gastric wall and the gradual decrease in the supply of contrast medium to the pylorus cause the curve to become increasingly horizontal as the stomach becomes almost empty. We have seen that the rate of gastric emptying increases in the right lateral position. When the stomach is full, the effect is insignificant; when it is nearly empty, however, there is an obvious gain as a result of the considerably improved supply of contrast medium to the pylorus.

In the left lateral position, gastric emptying will be the slowest. Some mothers learn to lay a baby on this side after a feeding and to alternate between the right and left sides. It is possible that this factor plays an important role in the high average gastric emptying time determined for babies [22].

With fractional administration of the contrast medium, the stomach is only partially filled; in the ideal case, emptying will occur according to curve B of fig. 5.1. For equal fractions administered too rapidly, the stomach will empty approximately as shown on curves C and D of fig. 5.1.

Mixing proteins and carbohydrates through the contrast fluid inhibits peristalsis and keeps the pylorus closed for longer periods. For fats, this effect is even more pronounced; 8 h after a meal rich in fats, peristalsis of the stomach is still retarded. In addition it appeared that in healthy individuals flocculation and segmentation of the contrast medium occurred only when they had consumed a meal rich in fats the evening before [59, 198]. Experiments with dogs also showed that a high or low blood-sugar curve can markedly influence gastric peristalsis and the rate of transit [132]. Hunger contractions when the blood sugar is low also occur in humans.

The pylorus remains closed when the contents of the stomach or duodenum are highly acidic or basic. For patients with achlorhydria this closing mechanism does not function as well; the pyloric ring is more relaxed and the stomach therefore empties quickly.

We also saw that isotonic solutions leave the stomach the fastest and that hypotonic solutions do not take much longer. However, when a hypotonic solution is introduced directly into the duodenum, the pylorus will remain closed until a condition of isotonicity is achieved [70]. Hypertonic solutions retard gastric emptying considerably, even when they are administered directly into the duodenum. In the stomach, a hypertonic solution gradually becomes isotonic as a result of heavy fluid secretion

of the gastric wall. This can be accompanied by a considerable increase in volume.

Cold fluids leave the stomach much faster and warm fluids only slightly slower than a solution at body temperature [71]. The rapid transit of a cold fluid through the small intestine can certainly be ascribed in part to the accelerated gastric emptying. The reaction of gastric peristalsis and the pylorus to the direct administration of cold or warm fluids into the duodenum has unfortunately not yet been studied. The mechanism for this temperature sensitivity is also unknown. Furthermore it is important to know that the activation of the neutralization mechanism in the duodenum, a reaction to milieu disturbances of all kinds, does not begin until after the bulb and then decreases in the distal direction [1, 13, 70, 111, 127, 197, 211].

The contrast medium has a very difficult time during a gastrointestinal examination; it must successively endure the influence of gastric acid, intestinal juice, and fluid withdrawal without losing its proper characteristics. In some cases, there is also the detrimental effect of fatty acids, gall, or lactic acid, which practically no contrast medium can tolerate.

Diverse brands can withstand the effect of gastric acid and mucin reasonably well, but only a few contrast media can endure dehydration without becoming practically useless. The viscosity then becomes so high that the soft mucosal folds cause few impressions, or none at all. The specific gravity of the contrast mass increases; it retains, however, its homogeneous structure.

We can see that any contrast medium is about to lose the battle when flocculation develops; if, in addition, segmentation has already developed, then it has definitely lost. The structure of these segment clumps is not homogeneous as in the case of dehydration; the genesis is also different. If a highly thickened contrast medium is no longer able to produce true mucosal patterns, it must then be obvious for a splotchy segment clump (fig. 6.1). In 1942, Bouslog had already seen moulage-like patterns in small children that were not in agreement with the normal mucosal patterns seen at autopsy. The reason for this incongruity was then not understood.

If we study the curves of Braeckman and Zimmer, we learn that disintegration of the contrast

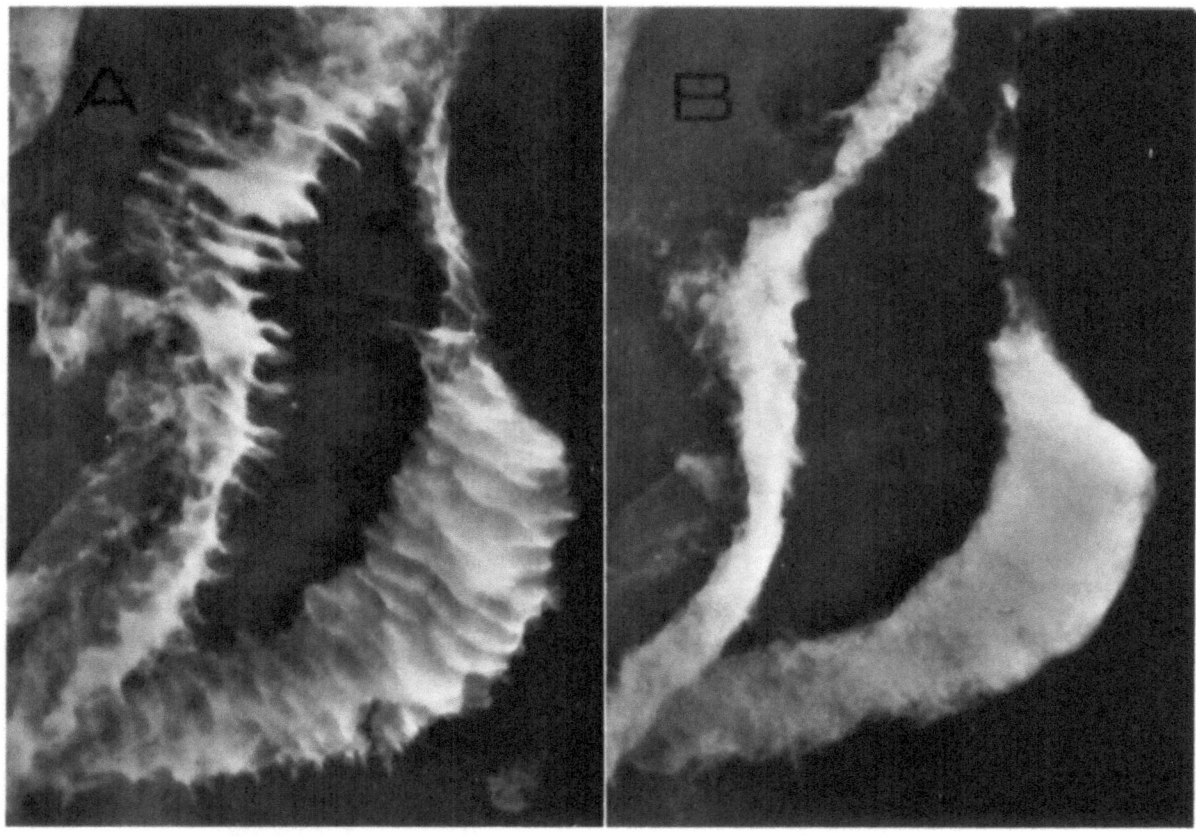

Fig. 6.1. Liposarcoma of the mesentery invading the wall of the jejunum. (A) Coarse irregular mucosal folds. (B) 30 min later, the contrast fluid has disintegrated (granular structure) and can no longer reproduce the mucosal patterns.

medium is a physicochemical process that proceeds gradually, and that even in the most unfavorable circumstances we can still make a number of useful roentgenograms (fig. 6.2).

From the preceding, it is quite sensible to give large amounts of contrast medium; the influence of harmful substances on the contrast medium is then less. Furthermore it is obvious that this dosage must pass through the small intestine as rapidly as possible; reaction with the harmful substances is then short-lived and the detrimental effect is as small as possible.

Another important advantage of an extremely rapid passage is the lack of time for dehydration of the contrast medium in the distal ileum and the colon. Because a low viscosity is maintained, mucosal patterns with a maximum reproduction of detail can also be obtained for these sections of the intestine. It is not easy to choose among the large number of brands of contrast medium on the market. There are some that are reasonably satis-

factory, but no single brand can be called ideal.

In 1932, Adam [2] reported that the characteristics of the contrast medium suspension are determined predominantly by chemical additives and not by the particle size, as is so often suggested by the manufacturers. The requirements for a contrast medium used for a gastrointestinal examination are much higher than for a colon examination. For the latter, good adhesion to the mucosa is of decisive importance; for the former, sufficient stability to prevent flocculation is of even greater importance. Furthermore the viscosity may not be too high and must be maintained as far as possible under the influence of fluid withdrawal in the ileum.

Supplementary administration of cooled fluids and fluid-attracting or secretion-enhancing substances is strongly discouraged. Mixtures of glucose, Gastrografin, or sorbitol, with the contrast fluid has an unfavorable effect in this respect. It is difficult to determine with certainty whether or not Prostigmin and metoclopramide are completely free

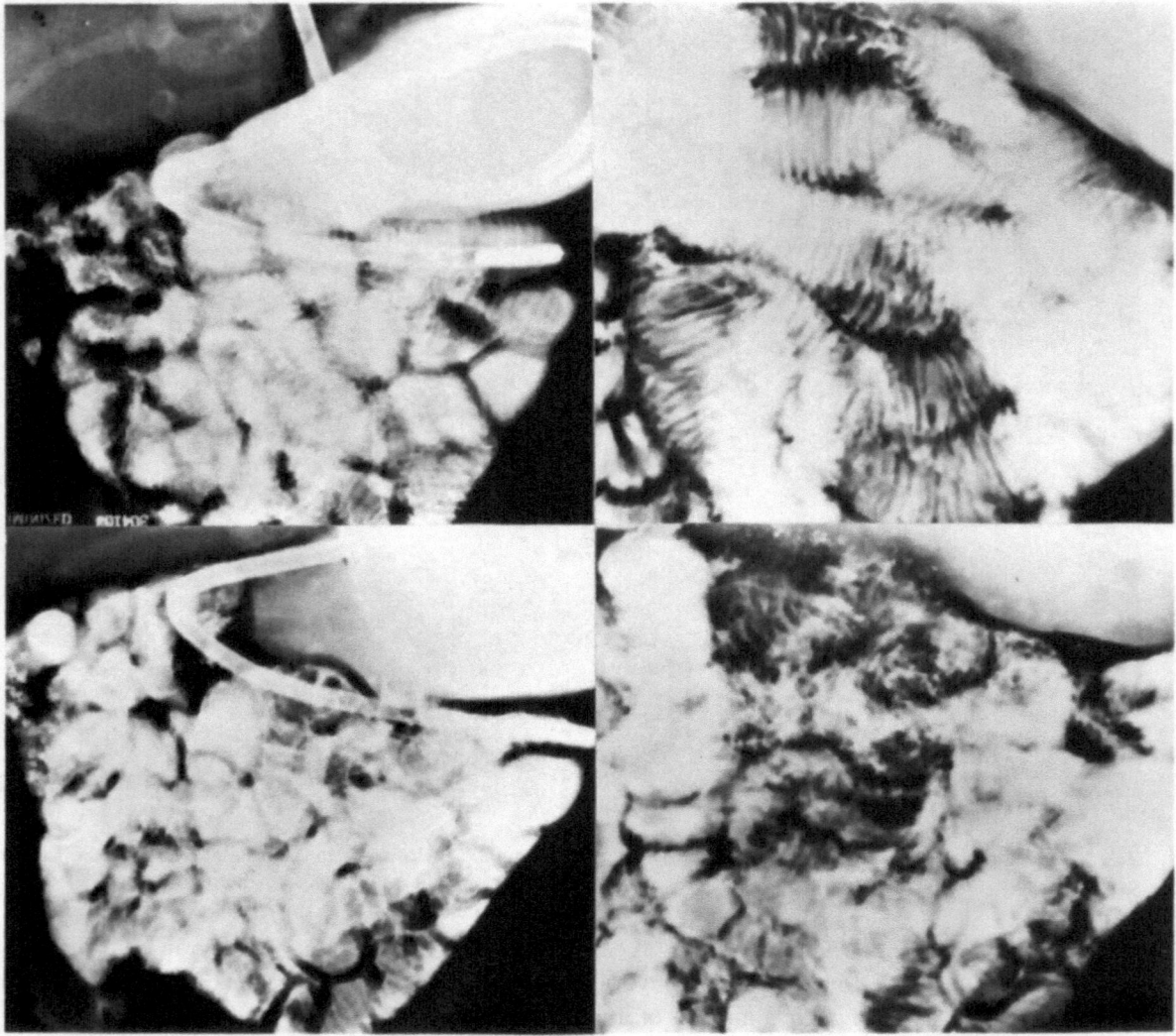

Fig. 6.2. Enteroclysis examinations of a 3-month-old baby (left) and an 8-month-old baby (right). Good reproduction of jejunal folds during contrast medium infusion (top). After the tube had been pulled back into the stomach, the rate of flow to the small intestine decreased and within several minutes severe flocculation developed so that the examination had to be terminated (bottom).

of a secretion-enhancing effect.

When Rieder [200] introduced his standard 'meal' at the beginning of the century, this meal was in general use and recording the transit time was probably useful. This harmony, however, did not last very long because the methods of examination and the use of contrast media became highly diversified. It is therefore not surprising that the average transit time reported between 1930 and 1950 by prominent radiologists varied between 2 and 5 h, with extreme values of 1 and 8 h [134]. From the above, it is obvious that including these values on x-ray films and in reports is totally unimportant today. It is better to omit them since they can lead to incorrect conclusions.

Summarizing, it must be concluded that a large quantity of contrast medium should be administered by infusion directly into the duodenum. It should be administered so quickly that stretching of the duodenum induces maximum peristalsis, but not so quickly that peristalsis is inhibited by the enterointestinal reflex mechanism or so quickly that the patient will vomit. The amount of contrast medium must be as large as possible, but then again not so large that the problem of superposition develops.

The contrast fluid must be hypotonic; hypertonia

stimulates fluid attraction and therefore dilution of the contrast fluid; isotonia does not stimulate contraction of the pyloric muscle and enhances the development of reflux into the stomach.

Other advantages of bypassing the stomach are that the detrimental effect of gastric acid on the contrast fluid is eliminated and the rate of supply to the duodenum is no longer dependent upon the pyloric function.

Since most brands are reasonably stable in alkaline surroundings, we are less restricted in the choice of contrast medium; the adhesive quality and the viscosity can be the decisive factors. The unrealized ideal of standardization of the contrast medium, desired by so many radiologists, has outlived itself as a result of this method. A continuous supply of contrast fluid without the annoying influence of air bubbles, which possibly also retard transit, is guaranteed only in the right lateral position. The patient may possibly also lie on his back or on his abdomen but, in any event, the left lateral position is incorrect.

The question of the most favorable temperature for the contrast medium requires further investigation. It is true that an ice-cold contrast fluid does enhance gastric emptying and intestinal peristalsis. When administered into the duodenum, however, there is also relaxation of the pylorus so that reflux into the stomach can occur. A warm contrast fluid keeps the pylorus closed longer but can even work as a transit decelerator when administered directly into the duodenum. For our examinations therefore a relatively neutral standpoint is taken: all patients received the contrast medium at room temperature or slightly cooler ($\pm 15°$ C). Also unanswered is the question of the most favorable location for the end of the tube in the duodenum. It is probable that

reflux into the stomach is more likely when the end of the tube lies proximal; then when the contrast fluid is administered, maximum stretching of the duodenum occurs quite close to the pylorus, which then may not close as completely.

Another factor is the pyloric ring that is usually relaxed; it takes several seconds before contraction occurs. At least some reflux of contrast fluid into the stomach will occur when the end of the tube lies close to the open pyloric canal.

Thirdly, a tube located in the proximal part of the duodenum can easily slip back into the stomach as a result of regurgitation.

On the basis of these somewhat speculative considerations, in our patients the end of the tube is placed in the duodenojejunal area, although it must be assumed that the peristalsis induced by stretching of the intestinal wall is less here than close to the bulb. In practice this has been proved true.

It is possible that in achlorhydria reflux of the contrast fluid into the stomach will occur sooner. This question cannot be answered and requires further study. As mentioned previously, reflux cannot be terminated once it has occurred. The best thing to do is a supplementary dosage of contrast medium administered at once as well as stimulation of gastric emptying with Primperan. Obviously the patient must lie on the right lateral side between exposures.

In all cases we must concentrate on 'forcing' the contrast medium to the cecum as quickly as possible. Especially in patients with a possible malabsorption syndrome, the disintegration of the contrast medium can occur so quickly that examination of the small intestine must be considered a 'case of great haste'.

7. THE ENTERAL CONTRAST INFUSION

1. Preparation of patients

Even more important than for a conventional follow-through study is the thorough cleansing of the patient. It is desirable that the stomach be entirely empty and thus contain no fasting gastric residuum. Should there be gastric fluid in the stomach, the pyloric ring will not close properly since it is a natural reaction of the stomach to dispel its contents through the pylorus. When an infusion is running, the pressure in the duodenum is probably greater than the pressure in the stomach so that an open pyloric ring will have a reverse effect on gastric emptying and reflux of contrast fluid into the stomach from the duodenum will occur. Since the presence of feces in the cecum will tend to retard the rate of passage through the ileum, the patient must follow a low-residue diet and the colon should be thoroughly cleansed. It is also preferable that the last meal on the day before the examination be free of fats.

Comparison of the results of examinations when the patients did and did not receive a laxative beforehand has shown that less contrast fluid is required to reach the cecum when it is cleansed than when it is contaminated. It is easier to project the separate ileal loops in the lower abdomen with a low dose of contrast fluid than with a high dose that causes greater intestinal filling. An additional advantage of a well-cleansed cecum is that, although the x-rays then obtained of this part of the intestine are inferior to the films from a routine colon examination, they are still usable.

It is exceedingly important that castor oil, or any other purgative given for laxation of the colon, be administered orally. It is not advisable to cleanse the colon by means of a rectal-cleansing enema. We have found that a cleansing enema can sometimes cause extensive reflux of the clyster fluid into the ileum. Some of this clyster fluid is often retained in the ileum and proximal colon and will mix with the contrast fluid flowing in from the proximal direction. As a result, the mucosal patterns in this important part of the intestine can be evaluated only with great difficulty or not at all. It is true that the disadvantages of a rectal enema can be overcome entirely or to a large extent by waiting 1–2 h before beginning enteroclysis, but then one can no longer speak of a short examination.

Very good results for cleansing the large bowel are obtained if the day before the examination the following diet is used:

7 a.m. –	30 g magn. sulf. in 300 ml water; 2 Dulcolax tablets.
9 a.m. –	600 ml tea or lemonade; 2 boiled eggs. 30 g (1 slice) of white bread with 30 g (1 slice) of cheese.
11 a.m. –	600 ml coffee, tea, lemonade, or water.
1 p.m. –	60 g of white bread and 2 slices of cheese (no butter!). 600 ml tea or water.
3 p.m. –	600 ml coffee, tea, lemonade, or water.
5 p.m. –	skinless cooked chicken or cooked fish. 200 ml beef-tea. No potatoes, vegetables, or fruits!
7 p.m. –	30 g magn. sulf. in 300 ml water; 2 Dulcolax tablets.
9 p.m. –	600 ml coffee, tea, beer, lemonade, or water.

Whenever possible, preparation of the patient should also include discontinuation of drugs that inhibit peristalsis in the intestine. In general it can be stated that such a drug should be discontinued for a period that depends upon the length of time the patient has been taking the drug (see also chapter 12).

82

If the patient has received antispasmodics, sedatives, or tranquilizers for many months or even years, then discontinuation just before the radiological examination will serve little purpose since these drugs must be discontinued for many months before any improvement is noted in the peristaltic movement in the intestine. In addition, just prior to or during the examination, no drug should be given that enhances the production of bile or contraction of the gallbladder. Bile pigments do in fact stimulate peristaltic action in the intestine, but on the other hand also tend to promote disintegration of the contrast fluid. An initial advantage can therefore become a disadvantage if the examination has to be prolonged.

Finally, the patient must be told that large amounts of fluid will be administered during the examination. As a result, he may have to micturate frequently and there may be some diarrhea for several hours afterward. This should be taken into account when planning the trip home; it might even be wise to remain in the waiting room of the radiology department for 15 min or more. He should also be made to empty his bladder and bowels just prior to the examination. Otherwise he might do so on the examination table!

2. Duodenal intubation

Fear of the time-consuming intubation procedure is often the main reason that enteroclysis has not been introduced as a routine procedure in some departments of radiology. If, however, the trouble is taken to practice this technique several times, and if the directions described below are followed, then experience will show that this fear is without foundation. After some practice, duodenal intubation of most patients only takes several minutes and fluoroscopy requires 10–30 s at the most. In only a few patients out of every hundred will intubation prove to be difficult for various reasons. It may then take 10 min, sometimes slightly longer. These difficulties are, however, insignificant in comparison to the improved results and the much shorter examination (15–30 min). Only in cases of obstruction or drug-induced atony of the small intestine can the examination last 1 or 2 h, depending upon the dose of contrast medium. This is still very short

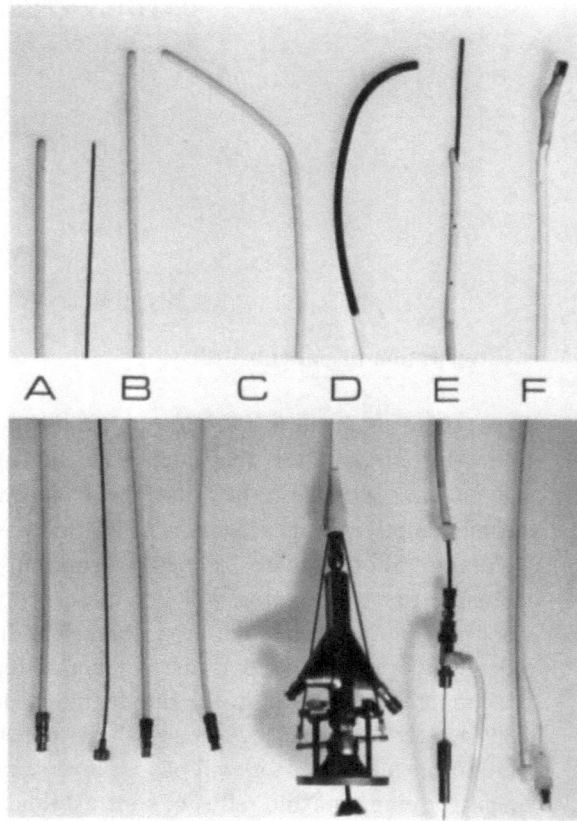

Fig. 7.1. Tubes sold by Cook and Söborg in Denmark.
(A) Bilbao-Dotter: guide wire and tube of equal length. (B) So-called Sellink modification: tube 6 cm longer than guide wire. (C) Acute angle of 20° in the distal end of the guide wire and the tube. (D) Tube which can be guided. (E) Tube which is also suited for taking blind biopsies. (F) Very long tube with inflatable cuff at the tip, used for selective fillings.

when compared with the conventional follow-through studies that can last all day in such cases, in spite of the administration of large amounts of contrast fluid and drugs to accelerate transit. Furthermore, the roentgenograms of a conventional examination will become useless much sooner because of disintegration, pronounced dilution, or thickening of the contrast fluid.

Of the tubes on the market today, the best choice is the extended Bilbao-Dotter tube (fig. 7.1B), which was designed especially for enteroclysis. The guide wire of this tube has the correct degree of rigidity; those used for angiography are too flexible.

In comparison with the original Bilbao tube (fig. 7.1A) designed for hypotonic duodenography, the tube in the new model is not shorter than the guide wire but is instead several centimeters longer. This offers the following advantages:

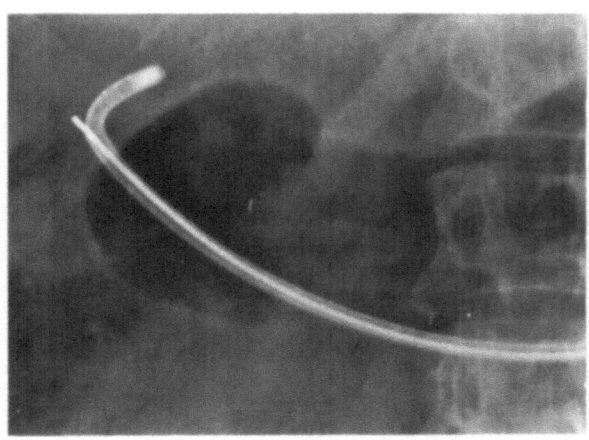

Fig. 7.2. With the original Bilbao-Dotter tube, it was possible that the guide wire would extend through one of the side openings, thus perforating the wall of the stomach or damaging the mucous membrane.

1) Perforation of the wall of the stomach is eliminated since the tip of the guide wire can no longer extend through the side openings in the tube (fig. 7.2).
2) For large atonic stomachs, the old tube was too short and the tip could not reach the distal part of the duodenum.
3) The end of the tube automatically remains flexible, which makes it easier to pass through the pylorus.

To prevent introduction of the tube into the trachea, the patient must keep his neck straight. Furthermore, the patient should sit or even stand. The stomach is then in a lower part of the abdomen than when the patient is in a supine position. In this way troublesome coiling of the tube in the fundus is often prevented.

Sometimes however this is not enough. Then it may help to have the patient breathe in or out as deeply as possible as the tube is pushed into the fundus. The gag reflex causes the least trouble if the tube is pushed in as quickly as possible until it is past the glottis. Some radiographers are so proficient in this respect that local anesthesia is completely superfluous. Furthermore we do not advocate anesthetization of the pharyngeal region because we would rather be sure that the patient will not choke after the examination. Another undesirable possibility is that the absorbed anesthetic could relax the smooth musculature of the

intestinal wall during the examination.

If desired, the tube can also be inserted through one of the nostrils instead of the mouth; this port of entry is better in infants since it is easier to secure the tube with tape after it has been positioned. It should, however, be remembered that it can be a little more difficult to manipulate the guide wire through the fixed curve of the nasopharynx than through the open mouth when the head is tilted backward. The physician or radiographer quickly slides the tube in until the tip is approximately in the pars antralis of the stomach; this is verified under fluoroscopy. The guide wire is now introduced; it is inserted to within 5 or 6 cm of the tip of the tube, which therefore remains quite flexible. For low atonic stomachs, the flexible part of the tube must be even longer, for instance 10 or 12 cm; it is then easier to pass through the pylorus. The patient himself, now lying on his back or right side, pushes the combination of guide wire and tube further; progress is checked by intermittent fluoroscopy. As soon as the flexible tip of the tube approaches the pylorus, it will begin to flap from side to side. If at that instant it is not possible to pass through the pylorus quickly, we recommend applying light pressure with the tip of the tube and then waiting until the spasm of the pyloric ring subsides. Sometimes it is useful to pull the guide wire back several centimeters. If too much pressure is applied against the pyloric ring, the tube will curl back in the direction of the fundus. If the guide wire is inserted into the outermost tip of the tube, curling of the tube would in fact be prevented but instead of passing through the pylorus more easily, the tube will cause a prepyloric sack-like bulge in the wall of the stomach on the side of greater curvature.

As soon as the tip of the tube has passed the pyloric ring, the guide wire must be pulled back to within 5 or 6 cm of the pyloric ring on the prepyloric side. Take care that the guide wire does not enter the duodenum, where it must follow a curved path and therefore is much more difficult to pull back. In cases of doubt, the patient must lie on his right side. Only in this position can it be determined with absolute certainty under fluoroscopy whether or not the tube has passed the pyloric ring. It will then be seen that the tip of the tube first extends posterior and perpendicular to the spinal column and then, in the retroperitoneal region,

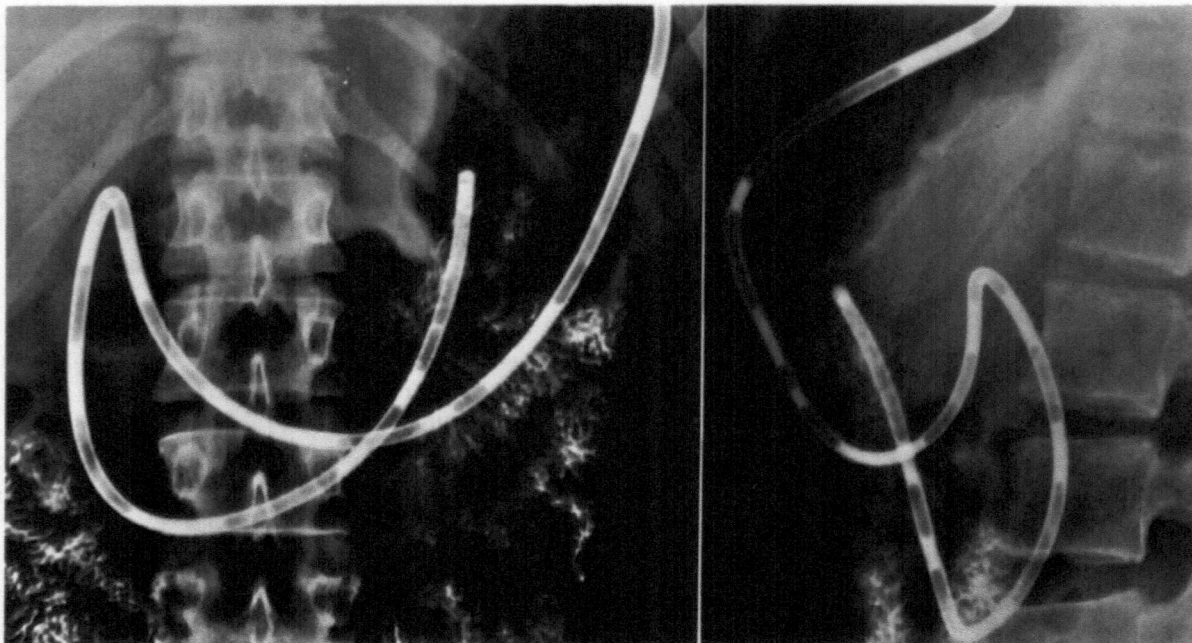

Fig. 7.3. Normal position of the tube after intubation; α-configuration in AP projection, reversed α in right lateral projection.

downward (fig. 7.3). A rare exception to this rule is seen in fig. 7.4; it is of course also obvious that in the case of a duodenum en guirlande, the descending path of the tube will also be abnormal (fig. 7.5). In the case of seriously ill or highly rheumatic patients as well as accident victims with multiple fractures of the extremities, the patient may have to remain on his back for the introduction of the tube as well as the actual examination. Then it is not possible to have the patient lie on his side in order to check on the position of the tube. When a supine position is mandatory, the following criteria will be helpful (fig. 7.6):

1) The tube with guide wire always lies more or less taut along the greater curvature side of the stomach. If the tip of the tube moves back along this same line in the direction of the pars media, then it is likely that it has coiled in the stomach. It is, however, possible that the tube is in fact located in the duodenum (fig. 7.4). This can be determined by administration of a very small test dosage of contrast medium, 20 ml at the most. As it arrives in the duodenum, the contrast fluid is immediately expelled in the distal direction; if it ends up in the stomach, the mucosal folds typical of this organ will be seen.

2) If the tip of the tube moves back above the level of the greater curvature of the stomach, then it is probably in the duodenum.

3) The tube is almost certainly in the duodenum when it extends toward the median plane below the level of the greater curvature. This is already fairly certain when it is seen under fluoroscopy that the tip of the tube crosses more or less perpendicular to the part of the tube lying along the greater curvature of the stomach.

4/5) Curling of the tube in the pars antralis of the stomach is almost always directed toward the median plane. Passage through the pylorus can be directed toward either the median or the lateral plane. If the tube curves downward in the direction of the lateral plane, the pyloric ring has almost certainly been passed even if the tube happens to extend back toward the median plane at the level of the greater curvature side of the stomach.

Once in the duodenum, further positioning of the tube seldom causes problems. This phase can also be executed by the patient himself while the physician checks under intermittent fluoroscopy that the guide wire is pulled back 5–8 cm each time it approaches the pyloric ring. When Treitz's ligament is reached, the guide wire can be removed entirely.

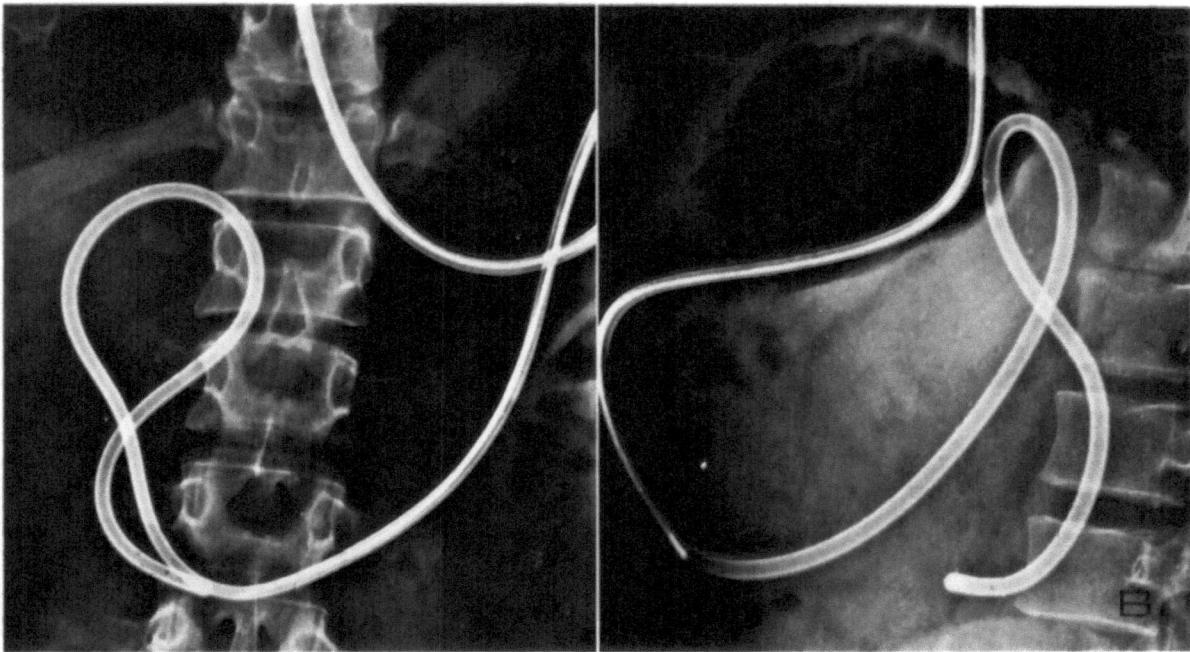

Fig. 7.4AB. Rare variation of a correct positioning of the tube. (A) In the AP projection, the tube passes through the pylorus in the medial direction and then extends back along the side of greater curvature but outside the stomach; it appears, however, as if the tube did not pass through the pylorus but has coiled in the stomach. (B) In the right lateral projection, the tube does not move perpendicular to the spinal column but first extends in the opposite direction and then drops down into the retroperitoneal space.

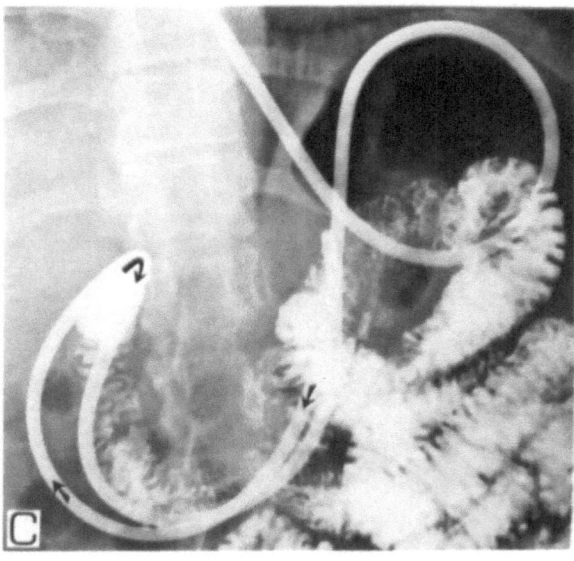

Fig. 7.4C. In this case the position of the tube is the same as in case 1 in fig. 7.6. Here, however, the tube was correctly positioned; this can only be verified by turning the patient on his side or by a test injection of barium.

In a normal stomach, the tube now appears on the screen to lie in an α-configuration in the AP as well as lateral projection (fig. 7.3); this is of course not true in the event of a steerhorn stomach.

In some rotational anomalies (common mesentery), the ligament of Treitz is located to the right of the spinal column (fig. 7.7B). In a flabby atonic stomach, a misleading pattern may be seen in the anteroposterior projection because the side of greater curvature of the stomach may appear to lie on the lateral side of the pyloric canal (fig. 7.7C).

When the tube coils above the diaphragm and thus is projected somewhere on the heart shadow, it is possible that it has turned above the cardia in the distal esophagus, which may or may not be dilated, or that it has ended up beyond the cardia in a diaphragmatic hernia (fig. 7.7D). Also an intrathoracic position of the stomach after removal of the esophagus may be the cause of a strange position of the tube and may lead to intubation problems (fig. 7.7E).

It is important that the tube does not curl in the

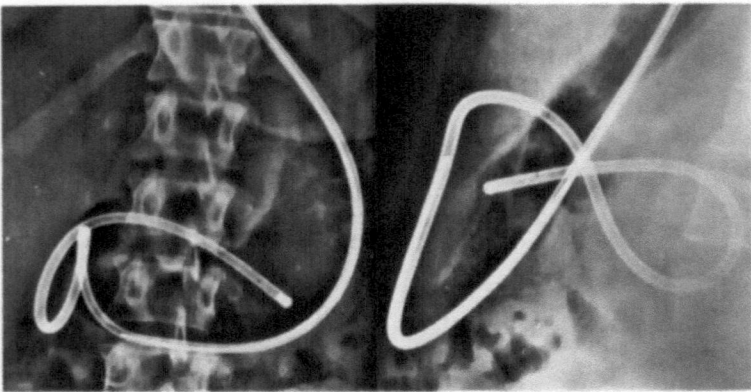

Fig. 7.5. Duodenum en guirlande: after passing through the pylorus, the tube first moves downward slightly and then upward again.

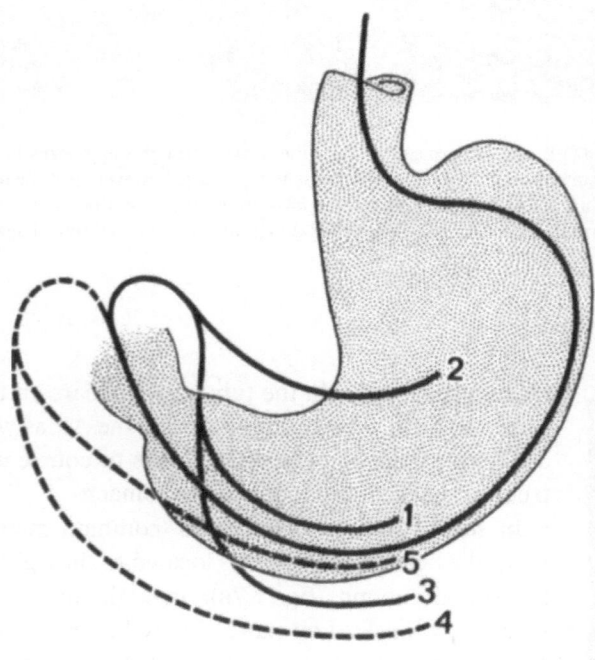

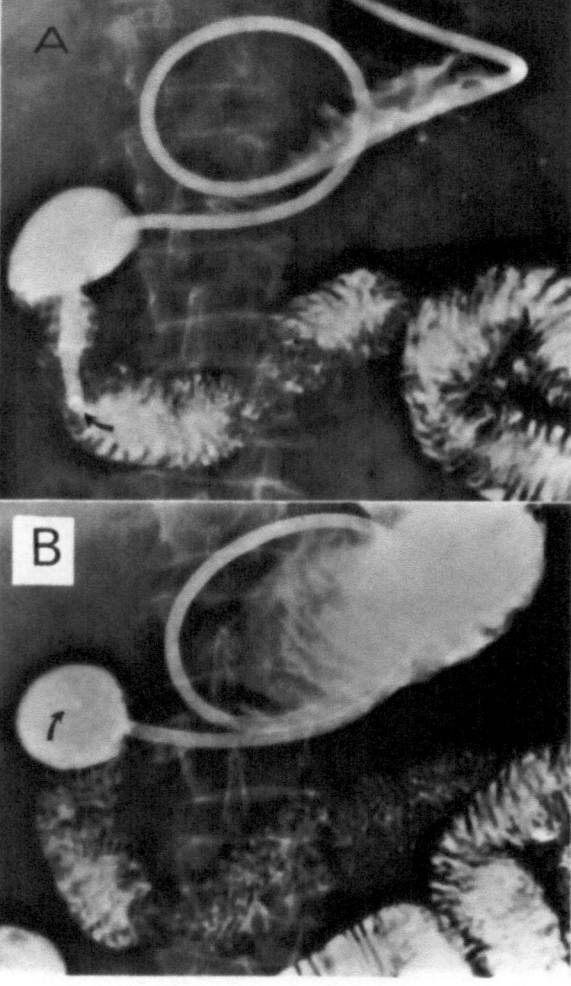

Fig. 7.6. Possible positions of the tube when the patient is in supine position. (1) The tube is usually not correct because it passes through the pylorus in the medial direction and turns back along the side of greater curvature in the stomach. (2) The tube is probably correct because it turns back in a plane above the level of the side of greater curvature of the stomach. (3) The tube is almost certainly correctly positioned because it crosses the side of greater curvature and then turns back at a lower level. (4/5) The tube passes through the pylorus in the lateral direction; the tube is then correct even if it turns back at the same level as the side of greater curvature.

Fig. 7.7A. Loop of the tube in the stomach (A). 1 or 2 retroperistaltic movements are enough to jerk the tube out of the duodenum by the loop (B).

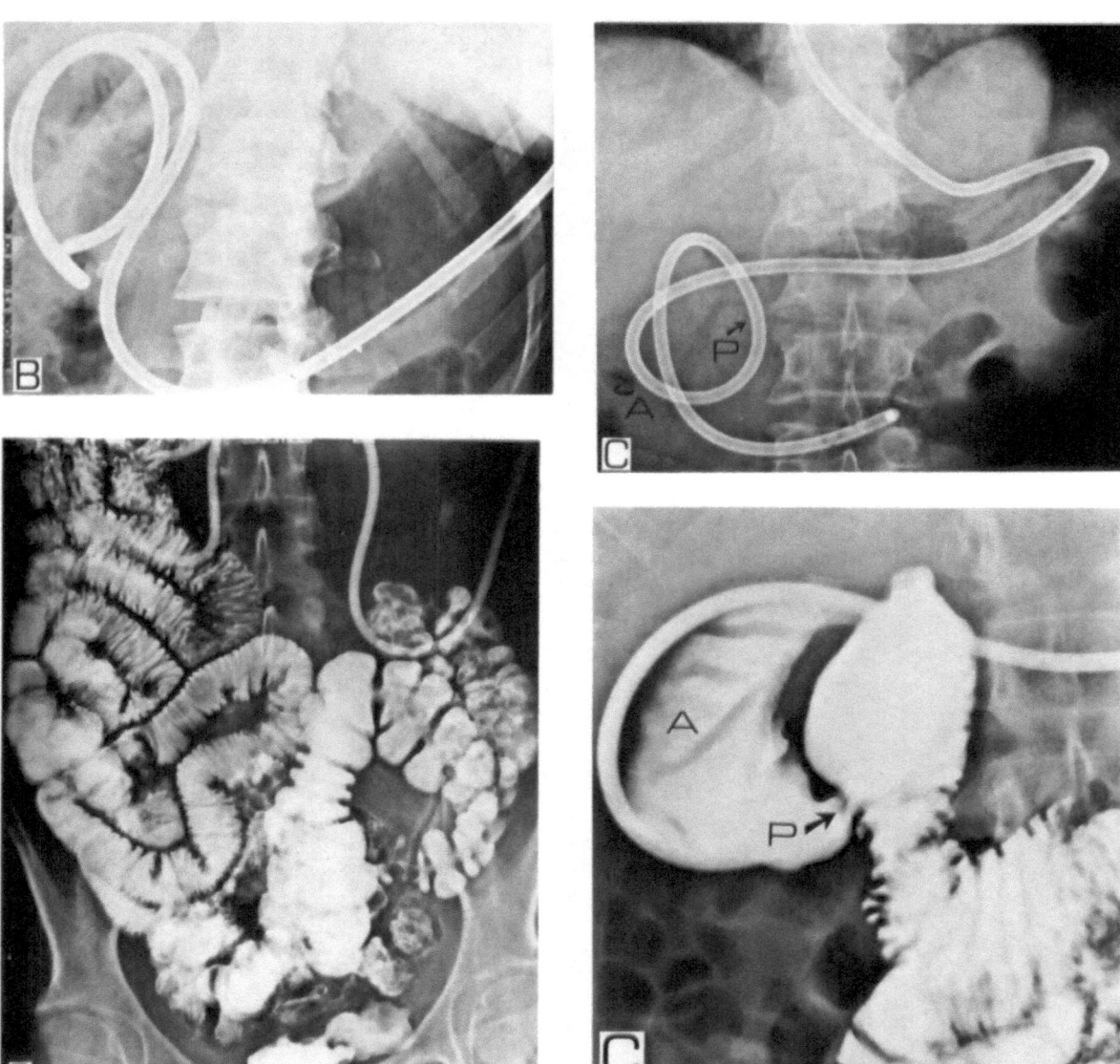

*Fig. 7.7*B. Rotational anomaly with ligament of Treitz as well as jejunal loops on the right side of the vertebral column.

*Fig. 7.7*C. In an atonic stomach, the antrum (*A*) is sometimes clearly situated lateral to the pyloric canal (*P*); the tube then appears to lie in a very strange position on the AP projection.

stomach; otherwise if the patient should become nauseated, one or two pronounced retroperistaltic movements along the loop in the tube will cause the tube to be jerked out of the duodenum (fig. 7.7A). When the duodenum is atonic and dilated as a result of the use of certain drugs or in cases of scleroderma (see chapter 12), a functional stenosis may develop where the duodenum passes between the aorta and the superior mesenteric artery (mesenterial root syndrome). In the prestenotic sac-

culation, the tube tends to curl back in the direction of the pylorus. In these cases, inadequate closing of the pyloric ring enhances the chance of reflux of the contrast fluid into the stomach (fig. 7.8). Therefore it is better not to push the tube beyond the point where it tends to curl. When the tube has become stiff due to frequent sterilization, it often slides into the duodenum easily without the help of a guide wire. It is also possible, however, that the tube will become too stiff and can no longer pass along the

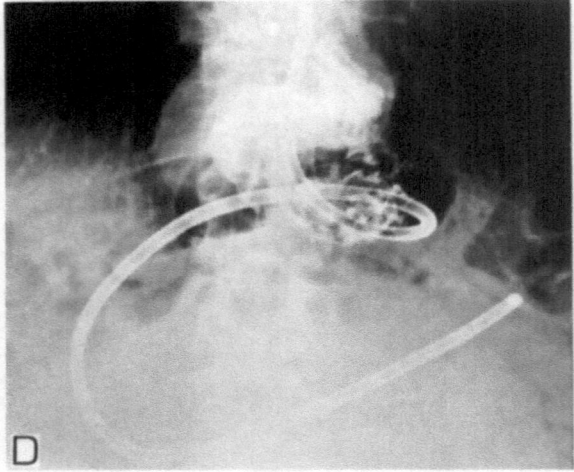

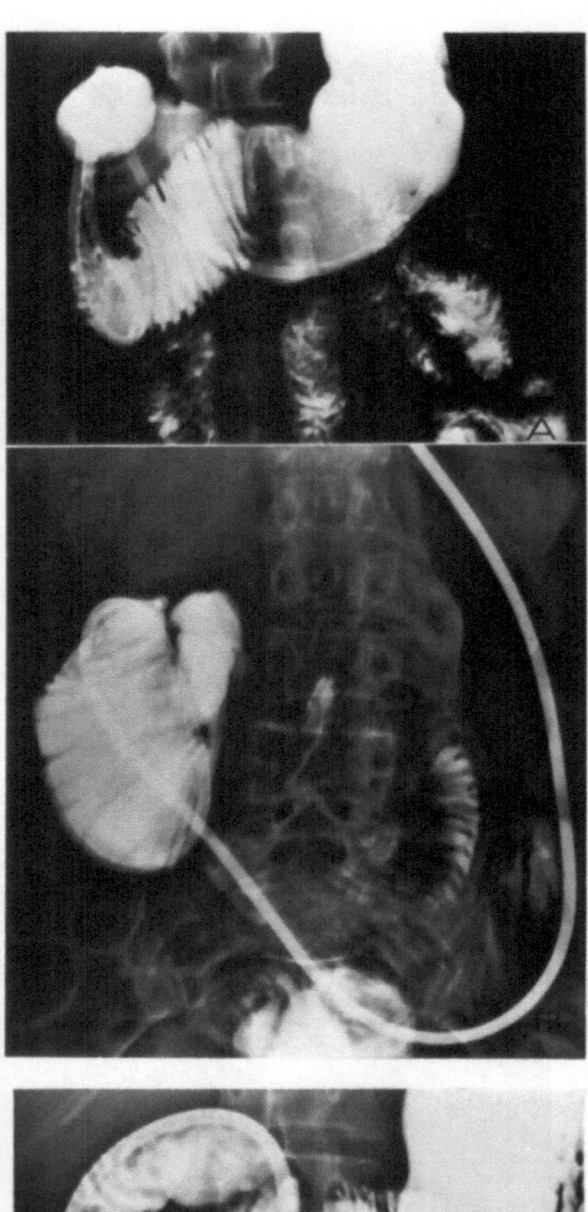

Fig. 7.7D. Loop in the tube above the level of the diaphragm in a fairly large diaphragmatic sliding hernia. It was difficult to get the tube past this hernia. Administration of a small amount of contrast medium through the tube revealed the nature of the problem.

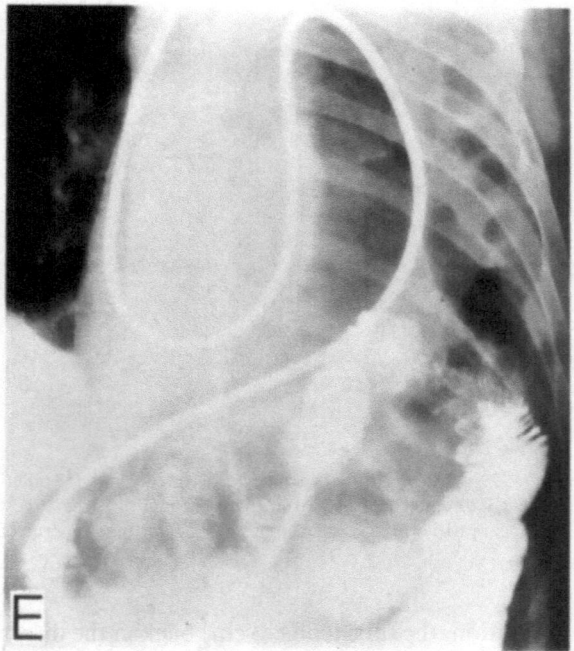

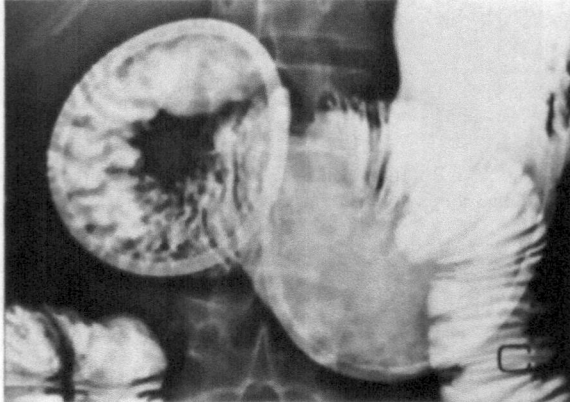

Fig. 7.7E. Strange position of the tube, caused by intrathoracic stomach after esophagectomy.

Fig. 7.8. (A) The tube turns back in a prestenotic sacculation in the duodenum that has developed as a result of a mesenteric artery. syndrome. The tip of the tube is in the duodenal bulb and is therefore close to the pylorus so that a large quantity of contrast fluid flows back into the stomach. (B) The tube coils in the descending limb of the duodenum, which is greatly dilated as a result of scleroderma. (C) It is not always possible, especially in those patients who use drugs for atony, to pass the spinal column or the aorta with the tube. The chance of reflux to the stomach is then considerably greater and we recommend decreasing the rate of flow of the contrast fluid to 50 ml/min and to administer metoclopramide to the contrast fluid.

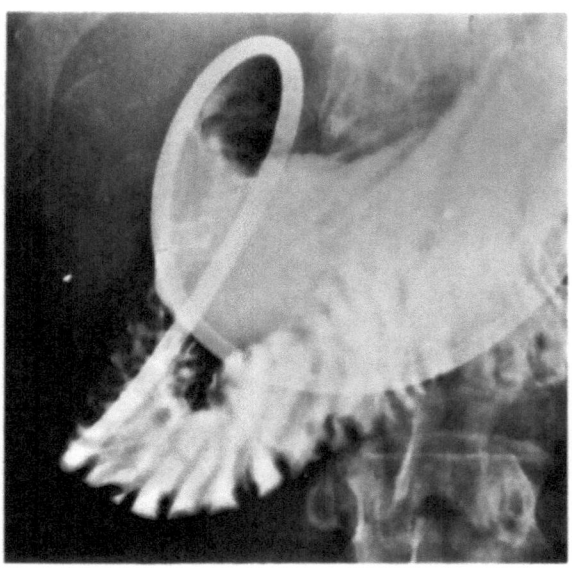

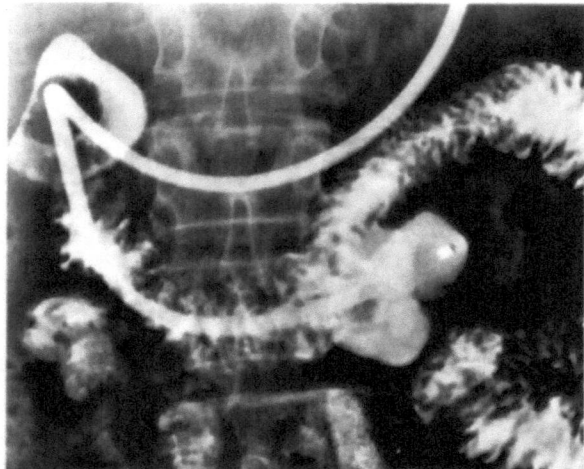

Fig. 7.9. It is no longer possible to pass through the junction between the descending limb and the horizontal portion of the duodenum when the tube has become too stiff as a result of frequent sterilization.

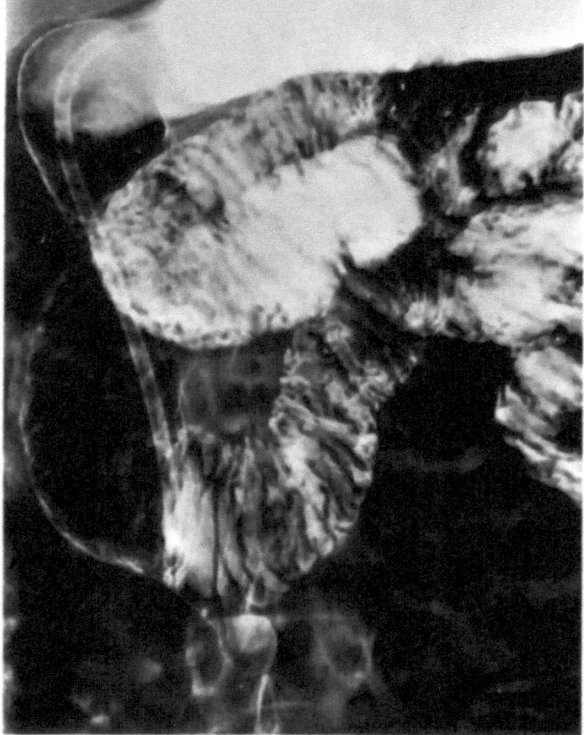

curve in the duodenum to Treitz's ligament (fig. 7.9). If the tube should remain lodged in the descending limb of the duodenum or is seen to plunge downward, then the tube may have ended up in a diverticulum located in the outer curve of the duodenum (fig. 7.10), or it may have even unexpectedly perforated the wall of the diverticulum; this is, however, a rare phenomenon. When the Bilbao-Dotter tube curls in the fundus of the stomach, as can sometimes occur when the stomach lies high up in the abdominal cavity as in pyknic patients, the following can be attempted:

1) It certainly is worthwhile to buy an extra guide wire and bend the tip to form a gentle curve of 60°–90°. After this guide wire is pushed into the extended Bilbao-Dotter tube as far as possible, the unit is introduced until the rounded part of the guide wire is located in the fundus of the stomach and the flexible tip of the tube just touches the wall of the stomach on the side of greater curvature. By

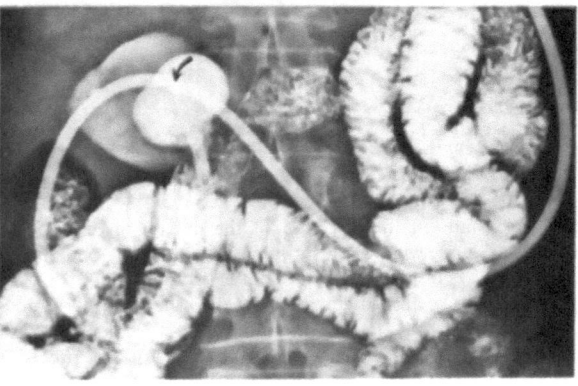

Fig. 7.10. If the tube becomes lodged in the duodenum or if it drops down too far into the descending duodenum, this can be due to diverticula in the outer curve of the duodenum. Beware of perforation!

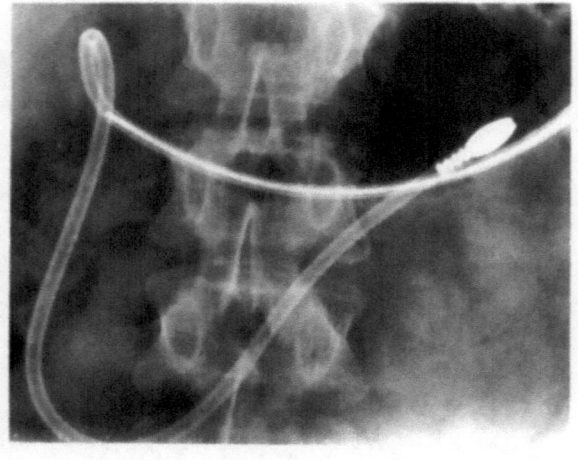

Fig. 7.11A. Flexible tube with metal olive on the distal end.

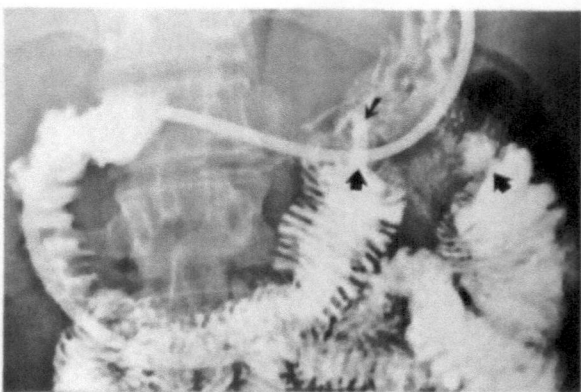

Fig. 7.11C. Spasm of the intestinal wall (→ ←), caused by too much pressure of the tip of the tube.

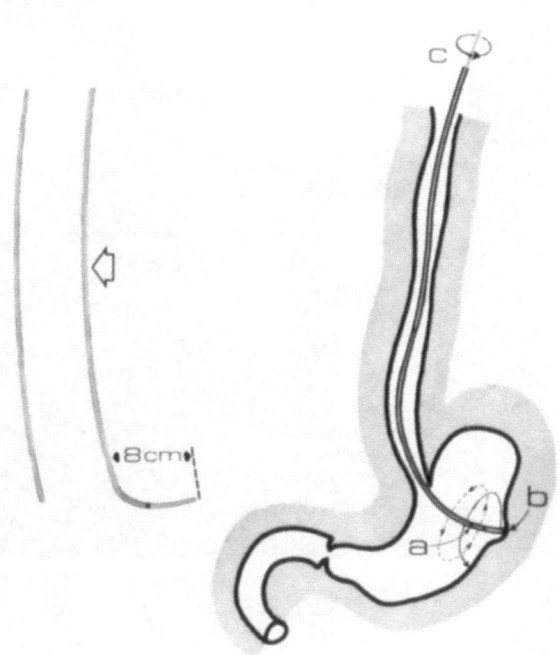

Fig. 7.11B. Procedure in the event of coiling in the cardia. Insert the bent guide wire (arrows) until the tube slightly nudges the wall of the stomach (b) and then rotate at c until the end of the guide wire points in the direction of the antrum. Now replace the curved guide wire with a straight one. Note: if the end of the tube with the bent guide wire does not touch the wall of the stomach (a), it will keep springing back into the incorrect position. Slow rotation of the guide wire and tube together will usually avoid this problem. An upright position for this procedure is recommended.

rotating the guide wire slowly by its knob, it is now easier to push the unit in the direction of the pars antralis without coiling. As soon as this maneuver has been completed, the curved guide wire is replaced by a straight one. For this procedure, which must be carried out under fluoroscopic control, the physician must stand at the head of the patient, who lies in a supine position on the table (fig. 7.11B).

2) If there is only a single loop, one can still try to slide the tube into the required position in the duodenum. The tube should be long enough for this procedure since the stomach is never very long in pyknic patients. As soon as the tube is in position, then it may be possible to uncoil the loop in the fundus; this should be done very carefully, although a sudden tug may sometimes also be successful.

3) Have the patient lie on his stomach and push the tube back and forth quickly several times. To prevent coiling in the esophagus as a result of this maneuver, it is recommended that the guide wire be pulled back so that the last 10 cm of the tube remain flexible. Success is more likely if the same maneuver is carried out with the patient standing instead of in the prone position.

4) Remove the Bilbao-Dotter tube and use a soft radiopaque tube with a metal olive on the distal end (fig. 7.11A). If the patient assumes a prone position and subsequently the right lateral position, then because of the weight of the metal olive, the tube will almost always fall in the direction of the pylorus without coiling. If it is difficult to introduce the guide wire into this tube, which is often rather

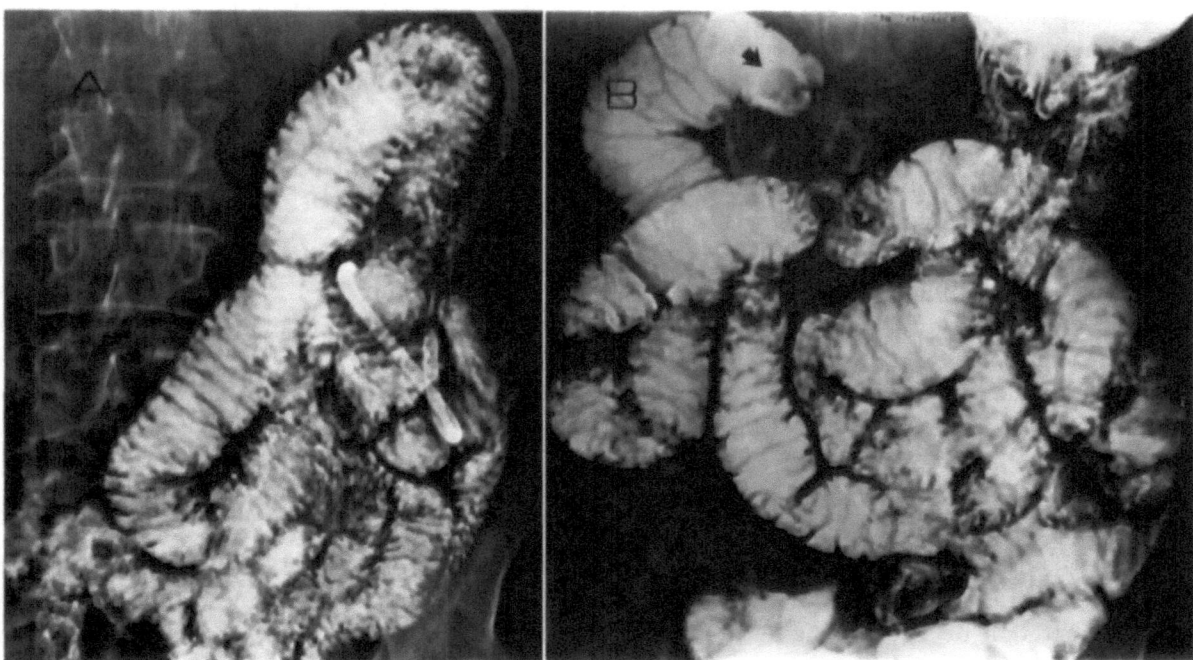

Fig. 7.12. Example of the positioning of the tube after a partial gastrectomy of the BII type. If the tip of the tube extends far enough into the jejunum, there will be no reflux of the contrast fluid into the resected stomach in spite of the absence of a pyloric ring. Many of the loops of the small intestine are in a state of contraction and there is no contrast fluid in the afferent loop (A). It was, however, possible in this particular case to fill the afferent loop after a hypotonic agent had been administered (B). At the end of the duodenal stump is a polypoid lesion resulting from the introverted line of suture (arrow).

thin, then the guide wire should be greased with oil, vaseline, or catheter lubricant. Only in very rare cases is it not possible to pass the metal olive through the pyloric ring within several minutes. In such cases, if the history or a previous follow-through examination does not indicate an organic reason for this failure, we sometimes give a metoclopramide injection and have the patient rest quietly on his right side for several minutes. We have found that this approach is always successful. When metoclopramide is administered intravenously, the rest of the examination must be carried out very efficiently; it should be completed before the peristaltic movements begin to decrease (see page 73). The duration of the examination can be shortened somewhat by slightly increasing the rate of flow of the contrast fluid and by decreasing the dose. An increased flow is obtained by administering the barium suspension under high pressure by using a pneumocolon apparatus, or by greater dilution of the suspension. If the reduced contrast becomes too troublesome, it can, if necessary, be compensated for by lowering the kilovoltage. As soon as the

contrast fluid runs in, we may see a persistent spasm at the duodenojejunal junction. The reason for this phenomenon is that the tip of the tube exerts too much pressure on the intestinal wall; this can be eliminated by pulling the tube back slightly (fig. 7.11c).

3. Partial gastrectomy

It is a mistake to assume that enteroclysis is not worthwhile in a patient who has undergone a partial gastrectomy. With the exception of the abnormal positioning of the tube (fig. 7.12), these examinations cannot be differentiated from those performed in patients with a normal stomach. Introduction of the tube is never difficult after a BI type operation; after a BII type, the tube may sometimes end up in the afferent loop.

Spontaneous gastric emptying is often markedly reduced after partial gastrectomy of the BI type; on the other hand after a BII type operation, the gastric capacity is exceedingly low. Both groups of patients find it extremely difficult to drink large amounts of contrast fluid whereas one or more liters can be administered without problem via the duodenal tube. Although the absence of pyloric musculature frequently causes reflux of the contrast fluid in a proximal direction, this need not always occur – not even after a BII type operation. Reflux of course becomes less likely as the length of the tube in the jejunum increases. After a partial gastrectomy of the BII type, whether accompanied by a clinical malabsorption or not, transit through the small intestine can sometimes be so rapid that the rate of flow of the contrast fluid must be increased in order to obtain sufficient filling of the loops of the small intestine. It is therefore not surprising that the afferent loop usually cannot be filled. If visualization of this loop is considered essential, for example because of bleeding, then the administration of a hypotonic agent is indicated (fig. 7.12B).

4. Special types of tubes

(William Cook – Söborg – Denmark; Bloomington – Indiana – USA)

Because the tube does coil in the fundus of the stomach in some patients, we asked the manufacturer (William Cook) to design a new unit: the tube and guide wire are almost equal in length and are bent at a 20° angle ± 5 cm from the distal end (fig. 7.1C).

Although we have used this tube successfully many times when the Bilbao tube failed, we have in fact had more favorable results with a guide wire that we bent in the shape of a curve (see page 90); in spite of this, however, we still sometimes have to use the olive tube in order to reach our goal. It is possible that a guide wire with a slightly curved tip will eventually appear to be a more universal guide than the normal straight guide wire of the Bilbao-Dotter tube.

The above-mentioned manufacturer also made another intubation unit that is rather costly because of its limited lifespan; it is the so-called guided unit. In the wall of this tube are four wires that are connected to a revolver-shaped handle; this enables the tip of the tube to be moved in any direction

desired (fig. 7.1D). The tube, which is available in any length desired, is not only useful for intubating the efferent loop after a partial gastrectomy of the BII type, but can also be valuable when postoperative leakage along the suture line must be bypassed to provide proper nourishment to the patient.

A third modification, also by the same manufacturer, is a tube that can be used to take blind biopsies in the duodenum and proximal jejunum (fig. 7.1E). This last tube, like all the preceding ones, has an outer diameter of only 5 mm.

5. Administration of contrast fluid

By means of a series of tests with a phantom (chapter 4.6), it was established that the optimum specific gravity of the contrast fluid for a normal patient is 1.25, for an obese patient 1.3, for an extremely slender patient or a child ± 1.2, and for a baby 1.15. Moreover, the contrast fluid must be hypotonic and fairly cool (± 15° C) (chapter 3); however, administration of a fluid that is too cold causes a vomiting reflex.

Addition of sorbitol and other glucose products to the barium suspension must be avoided since these substances are markedly hyperosmotic and therefore absorb considerable amounts of fluid. As a result, the quality of the mucosal patterns becomes quite inferior (fig. 7.13A) and disintegration of the contrast fluid is promoted. Furthermore the barium suspension must not foam; the popular brands Micropaque and Microbar, for instance, do not satisfy this requirement at all (fig. 7.13B).

Tiny gas bubbles can be very troublesome and are exceedingly difficult to differentiate from multiple lymph follicles or a candidiasis (fig. 7.13C).

A comparative study of extensive patient material has shown that when the rate of flow of the contrast medium averages 50, 75, 100, and 125 ml/min, the amount of contrast fluid required to reach the cecum is 655, 695, 745, and 835 ml, respectively (M. Oudkerk, PhD dissertation, 'Infusion rate in enteroclysis examination', Leiden University, 1981). Furthermore it appeared that:

1) When the rate of flow is 50 ml/min or less, filling of the intestine is so inadequate that the possi-

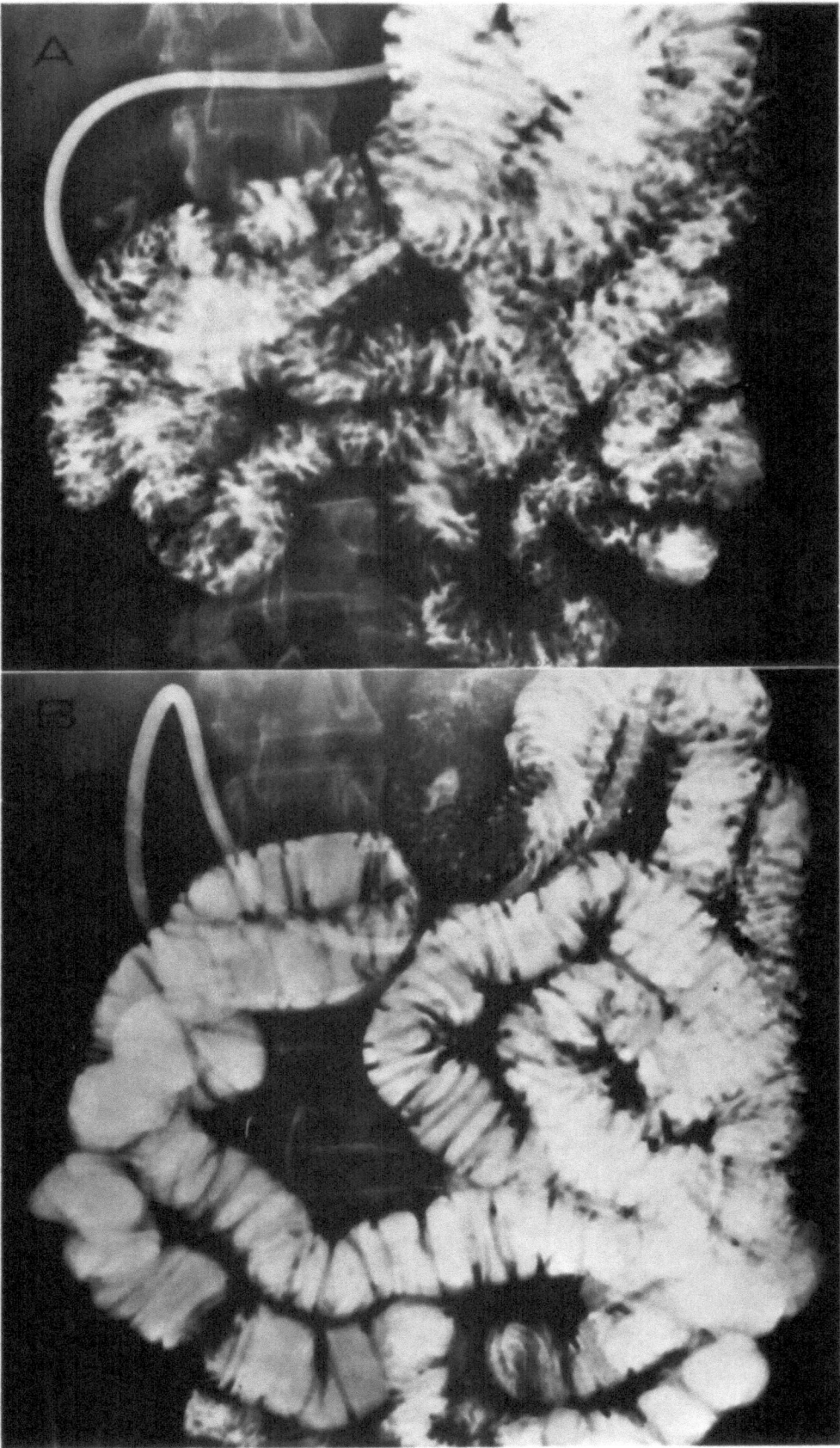

Fig. 7.13A. (A) Dilution of the contrast fluid and vague margins in the jejunum when 40 g glucose was added to the contrast fluid. (B) Enteroclysis was repeated five days later by using exactly the same procedure but without the glucose. The greater contrast intensity and sharp mucosal patterns are obvious.

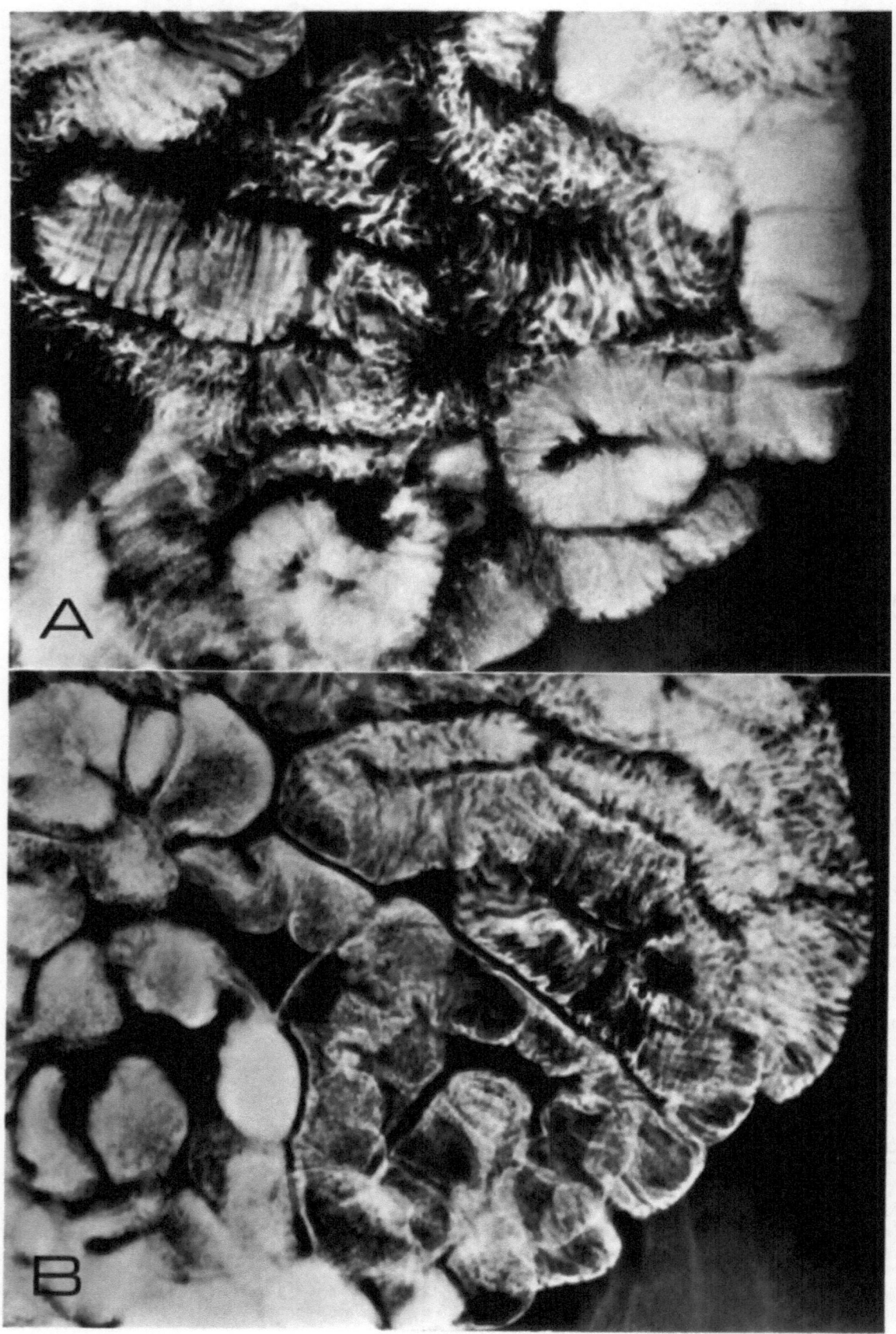

Fig. 7.13B. (A) Antifoaming characteristics of the contrast fluid in this convolution of intestinal loops are insufficient. (B) An extremely troublesome foam develops after air insufflation.

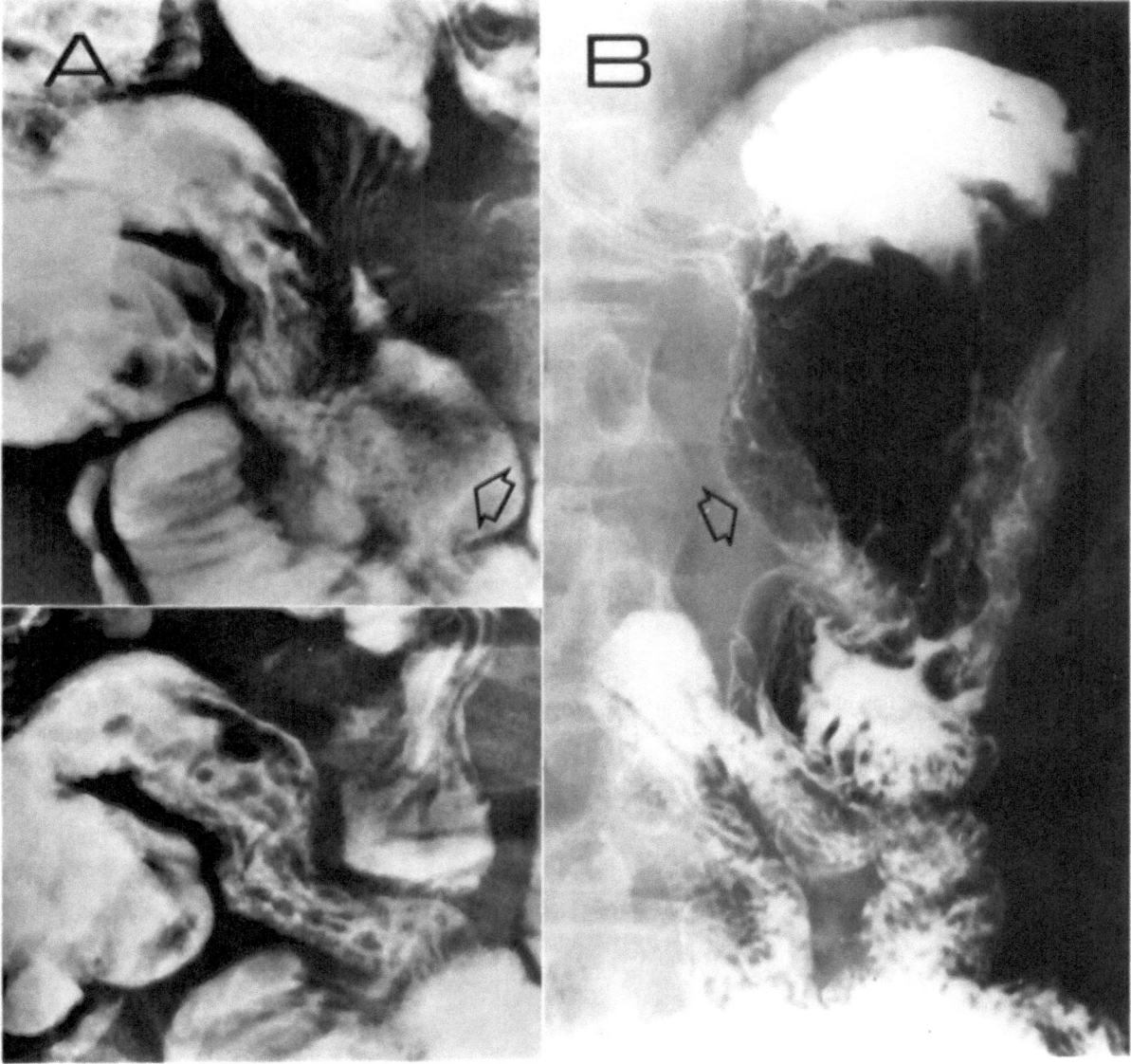

*Fig. 7.13*C. (A) Filling defects of approximately the same size as in fig. 7.13B, caused by lymph follicles. (B) Similar filling defects due to colonies of *Candida albicans* in a patient who has undergone a BII partial gastrectomy.

bilities for evaluation are as limited as those of the conventional transit examination. Disturbed motility, moderate obstructions, mucosal atrophy, and small mucosal lesions can no longer be demonstrated.

2) When the rate of flow is 100 ml/min or more, paralysis of the intestine develops sooner as the rate increases and ever-increasing amounts of contrast medium are needed to reach the cecum. The examination takes longer, reflux to the stomach develops earlier, and evaluation of disturbed motility becomes practically impossible. It

becomes increasingly difficult to take good spot films by using compression, especially in the lower abdomen.

3) Changes in the viscosity and temperature as well as the degree of dilution of the contrast medium needed to obtain the desired specific gravity appear in practice to have such an influence on the rate of flow that totally unacceptable deviations were measured during the enteroclysis examination. For our experiments therefore it was necessary to administer the contrast medium via a specially designed high-precision pump.

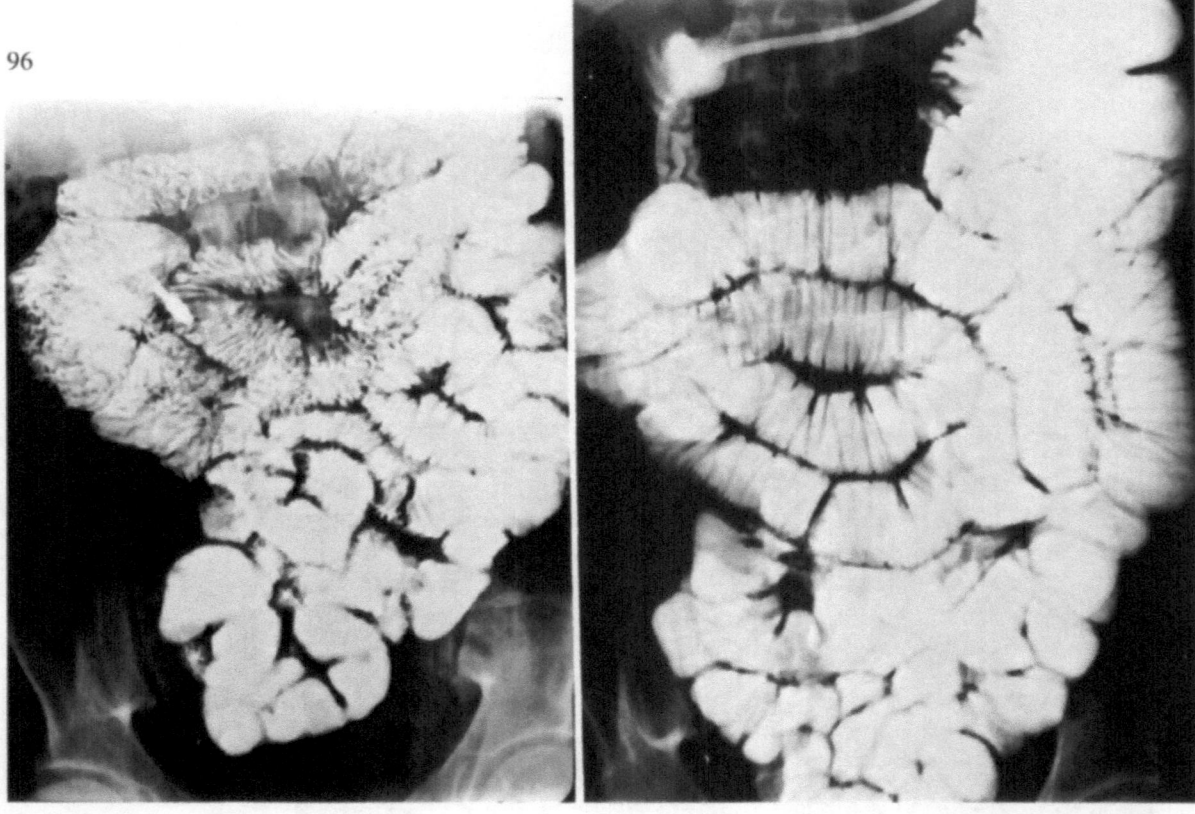

*Fig. 7.14*A. The rate of flow of the contrast medium for the examination of this patient was 50 ml/min (left side) and 100 ml/min (right side), respectively. The hypotonia and reduced peristalsis due to the excessive use of sedatives are not apparent on the left hand film: they are however clearly visible on the right.

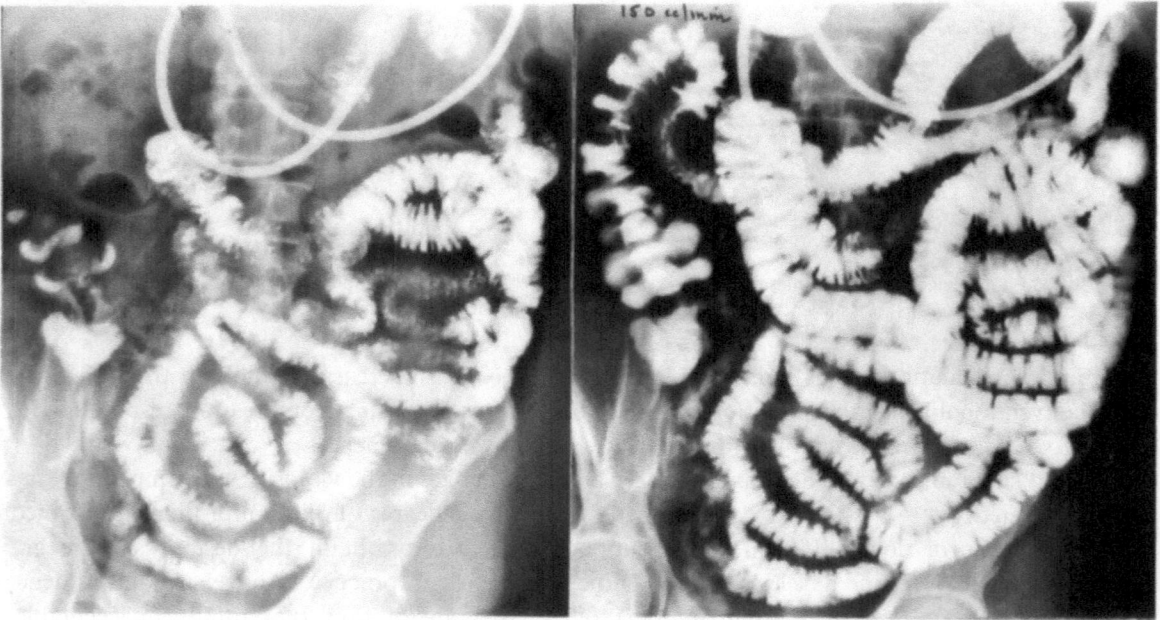

*Fig. 7.14*B. Patient with hypermotility as a result of collagenosis. This is clearly visible on the left-hand x-ray; only 200 ml of contrast medium administered at a rate of 75 ml/min were required to reach the cecum. Because the intestinal loops were not sufficiently full for anatomical evaluation, the rate of flow was subsequently increased to 150 ml/min and additional films were taken (right side).

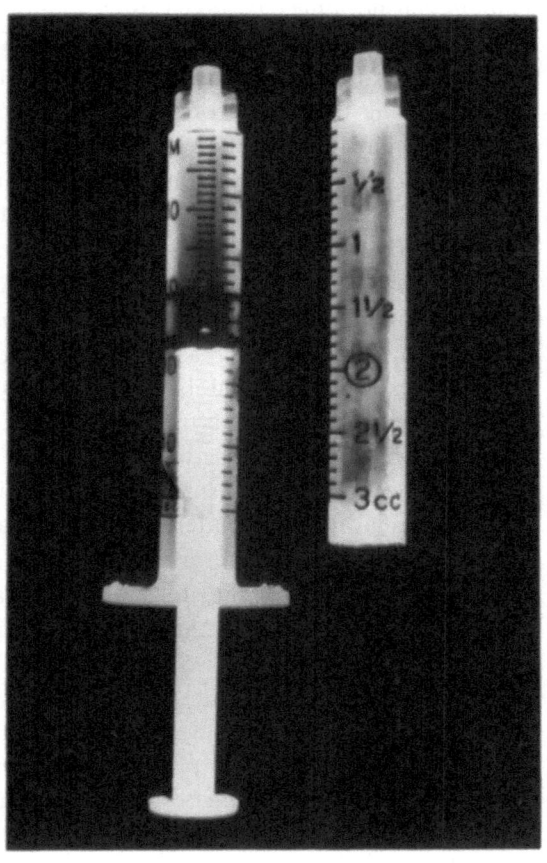

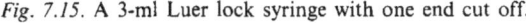

Fig. 7.15. A 3-ml Luer lock syringe with one end cut off.

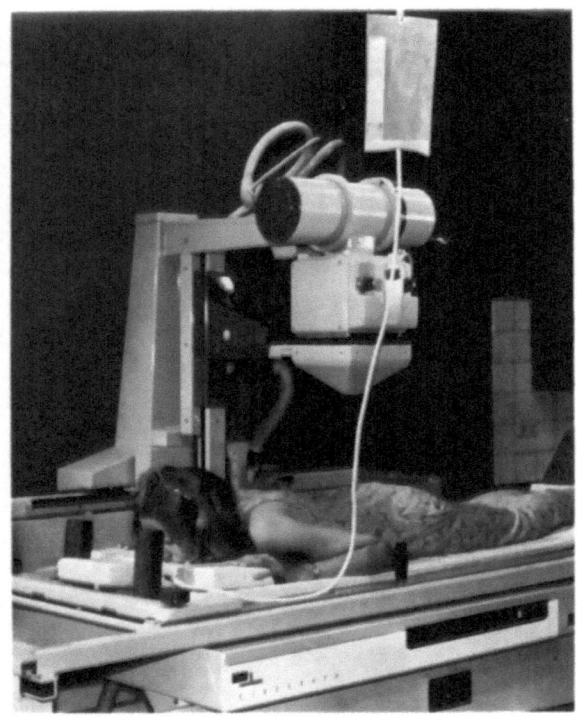

Fig. 7.16. Our infusion system used for enteroclysis. (1) Extended Bilbao-Dotter tube. (2) Plastic connecting piece (available in various sizes and models). (3) Bag and tube 2 m long, also plastic and available in diverse models. (4) Hook that can be adjusted in height via a rope and a pulley mounted on the ceiling.

4) It could be established with certainty that 75 ml/min is the most favorable rate of flow for an enteroclysis examination and that a deviation of more than 15% is not permissible. The effects of variations in the rate of flow are clearly illustrated in fig. 7.14.

Since the routine use of a pump causes insurmountable problems, the influence of the viscosity and the temperature must be limited as much as possible. This can be achieved by using a contrast medium with the lowest possible viscosity, for example a high-density barium suspension diluted to the required specific gravity. It should be obvious that such a contrast fluid will not produce useful double-contrast films; consequently, if this type of examination is indicated, a separate examination with a contrast fluid of higher specific gravity and better adhesiveness must be performed.

The results of a double-contrast examination of the ileum are far better when the examination is planned beforehand and can thus be carried out properly. It is recommended that no more than 300–400 ml of a contrast fluid with a relatively high specific gravity ($\pm$ 1.6) be administered; once the contrast fluid has reached the cecum, if necessary with the aid of a metoclopramide injection, air insufflation is started – both rectally and via the tube.

The best connection between the Bilbao tube and the plastic tube of the infusion bag is a 3-ml plastic Luer lock syringe with the proximal end sliced off (see fig. 7.15). To obtain the correct rate of flow with the dilutions specified for barium Lafayette HD-85, see the table shown in fig. 4.20 (page 53). Our infusion system is shown in fig. 7.16.

The easiest method is to administer the contrast fluid while the patient is in a prone position. In this

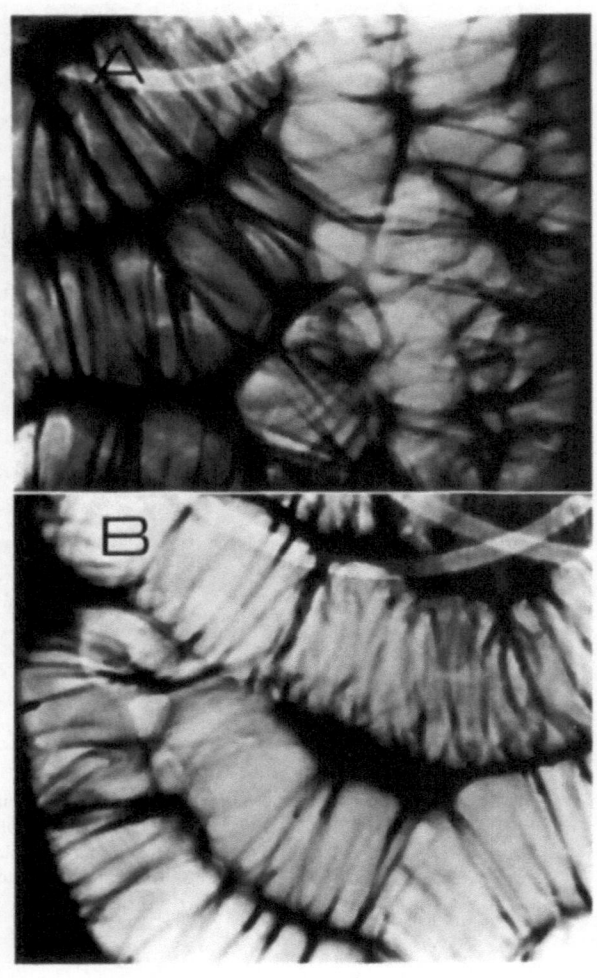

Fig. 7.17. Filling of the proximal jejunal loops with a contrast fluid of lower specific gravity (A). The contrast fluid in the more distal loops still has a high specific gravity (B).

position the intestinal loops remain in a well-ordered group longer, and geometric projection with both the common Bucky table and the tele-command apparatus is better. If the patient is slightly nauseated, it is wise not to move the table any more than absolutely necessary. We also recommended that the rate of flow of the contrast fluid be increased gradually to the maximum value during the first minute. This is very true when the tip of the tube is not in the most distal part of the duodenum. If the tip of the tube lies in the proximal half of the duodenum, it is better for the patient to lie on his right side during administration of the contrast fluid since otherwise reflux into the stomach is quite likely to occur. A disadvantage of the right lateral position is of course that x-rays of the

jejunum can no longer be taken after administration of the first 200–300 ml contrast medium. Loss of these early films is, however, less objectionable than increasing the chance of reflux into the stomach by turning the patient on his stomach or back for these photographs. Once reflux occurs, it can as a rule no longer be averted and will gradually increase during the rest of the examination. Approximately half of the fluid not yet administered will end up in the small intestine and the rest in the stomach. Gastric emptying as well as intestinal peristalsis can be improved by giving 20–30 ml metoclopramide through the tube and placing the patient on his right side between exposures. To facilitate interpretation of suspicious configurations in the intestinal mucosal patterns, we customarily take our survey exposures in pairs – the second x-ray being 10–30 s after the first. A considerable advantage of this method is that the diverse intestinal loops on the various exposures retain their mutual relationships and are therefore easy to recognize and compare. However, the mucosal folds on the two exposures will appear quite different since they fall in different phases of contraction. If after an initial dose of 600 ml the cecum is not yet reached, a second dose is administered immediately or at the most several minutes later. If the cecum has almost been reached or a confusing clump of ileal loops has developed in the minor pelvis, it is better to give only 300 ml. If the contrast medium still has a long way to go to reach the cecum and superposition of the intestinal loops is not too pronounced, then the second dose should be 600 ml. As a rule we dilute the second dose of barium suspension somewhat, mainly because it is easier to see through two or three superimposed loops when the specific gravity is lower (fig. 7.17). Dilution of course means that the viscosity of the barium solution is reduced. As a result the bag of contrast fluid must be placed closer to the table. Otherwise the rate of flow will become too high and reflux to the stomach may occur, followed by nausea and vomiting.

If during the first infusion of 600 ml contrast medium, it is noted that peristalsis in the intestine is particularly slow, then, depending upon the weight of the patient, 20 or 30 ml metoclopramide should be added to the second dose of 600 ml. It is not wise to administer this drug intravenously since the

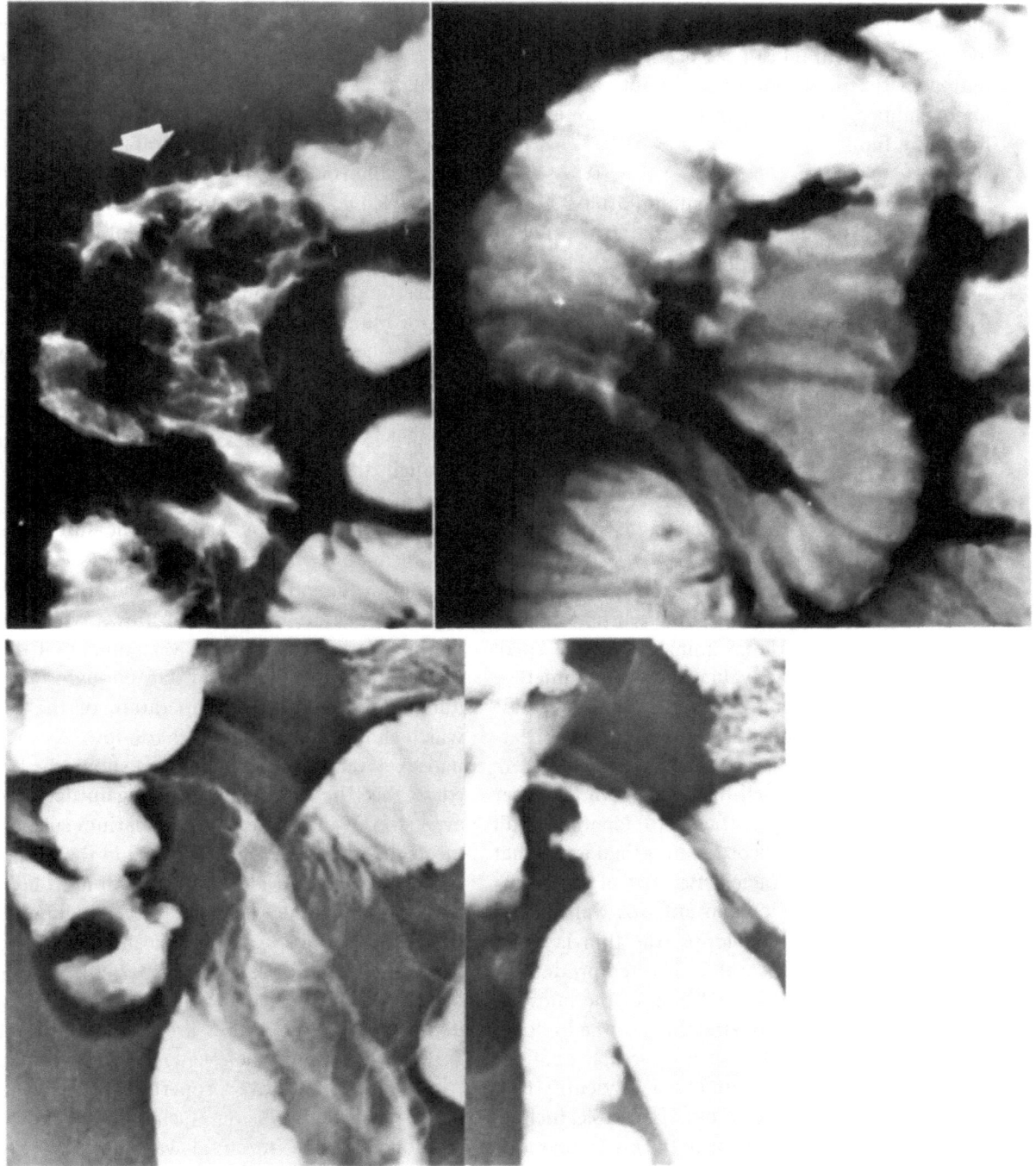

Fig. 7.18. Recurrence of Crohn's disease after an ileocecal resection (top). The swollen mucosal folds are clearly visible when the intestinal loops are only moderately filled, but are difficult to see when the loops are well filled. This is also the case with the shriveled mucosal pattern opposite to a longitudinal ulcer in the second patient (bottom).

period of action is then much shorter. Furthermore, there can be a subsequent fairly long period, lasting 30–60 min, of greatly reduced peristalsis due to fatigue of the overloaded and probably already atrophied smooth musculature. Only when the cecum has almost been reached can a dose of 2 ml metoclopramide be administered intravenously without objection. In this case the period of action (about 10 min) is sufficient to complete the examination before atony develops. The entire examination is carried out under intermittent fluoroscopy and spot films are taken by using compression. If a telecommand apparatus is not available and the Bucky table is used, it is better to wait until the cecum has been reached, as seen on the survey exposures, before making spot films – not only of the last ileal loops but of course of all the other loops of the small intestine. For a standard examination of the small intestine without conspicuous abnormalities, our routine procedure is to take the following films:

2 × 24/30 of the proximal jejunum after 300 ml;
2 × 35/35 of the entire abdomen after 600 ml;
2 × 35/35 of the entire abdomen after the cecum has been reached;
4–12 spot films (2–3 × 24/30).

If the case is without complications, the total length of the examination is 15–30 min, including duodenal intubation; the total exposure time is 3–5 min.

6. Administration of water after the barium suspension

As in the colon examination, mucosal patterns are an essential part of the examination of the small intestine, especially for evaluation of inflammatory diseases. The shriveling process and swollen folds (fig. 7.18) give the mucosa a conspicuous appearance that could easily have been overlooked if there were only x-rays in a well-filled state. On the other hand it is often very difficult to identify small abnormalities of the mucosa in intestinal loops that coincide or have contracted. Because of the superposition of the posterior and anterior walls of the usually twisted intestinal loops, the thin layer of barium coating the mucosal folds often produces a maze of curved lines. Better filling of the intestine causes a greater degree of stretching of the folds; as a result they lie in a more or less circular configuration and abnormalities are easier to identify (fig. 7.19). Each examination should, if possible, include at least a few roentgenograms of the intestinal loops in a well-filled state. However, a high degree of filling of the intestinal loops also means that it is more difficult to project them freely by means of compression. Greater filling should therefore be carried out toward the end of the examination and after a number of films have been made of the partially filled loops in order to avoid the problem of superposition. In the proximal part of the small intestine, the degree of filling of the loops is regulated fairly easily by adjusting the rate of flow

of the contrast fluid. In the distal part of the ileum, however, this no longer applies. Instead, the degree of filling is determined mainly by the ease with which the contrast fluid passes through Bauhin's valve to the cecum. Since the distal ileum is often the site of abnormalities, it is not acceptable to simply acknowledge these disrupting factors. In most cases a very reasonable degree of filling of the important last part of the small intestine can still be obtained by exerting pressure on the region of Bauhin's valve with a blunt compressor, and also by forcing the contrast column in a distal direction as quickly as possible.

The best way to force the contrast column onward is to administer 600 ml or more of water through the tube. Since water has a very low viscosity, a rate of flow of 150–200 ml/min can easily be achieved by hanging the infusion bag 40–50 cm above the level of the table (see page 53). It is, however, possible that the patient, not being able to tolerate this rate of flow, will become nauseated. This can happen very quickly if the tip of the tube is not placed far enough into the duodenum, and if the temperature of the water, which should be 30°–37° C, is too low. As soon as nausea develops, the infusion bag should be lowered so that the rate of flow will again decrease or even stop. If the viscosity of the barium suspension meets the requirements established in the preceding sections, then this water infusion will not only give better x-rays of the well-filled distal small intestinal loops, but will also produce excellent double-contrast films of the jejunum (fig. 7.20). The troublesome large differences in density seen when double-contrast exposures are taken with air (fig. 7.21) do not occur when water is used. Depending partly on the adhesive properties of the contrast fluid, the water infusion flushes the barium suspension from the intestinal wall fairly quickly so that in general these roentgenograms must be taken within about 1 min. In addition, after administration of the water infusion, disintegration of the barium suspension develops rapidly in the zone where water and contrast medium mix so that one is forced to discontinue the examination (fig. 7.22).

6.1. Water-push indications
Several common indications for administration of water after the barium suspension are:

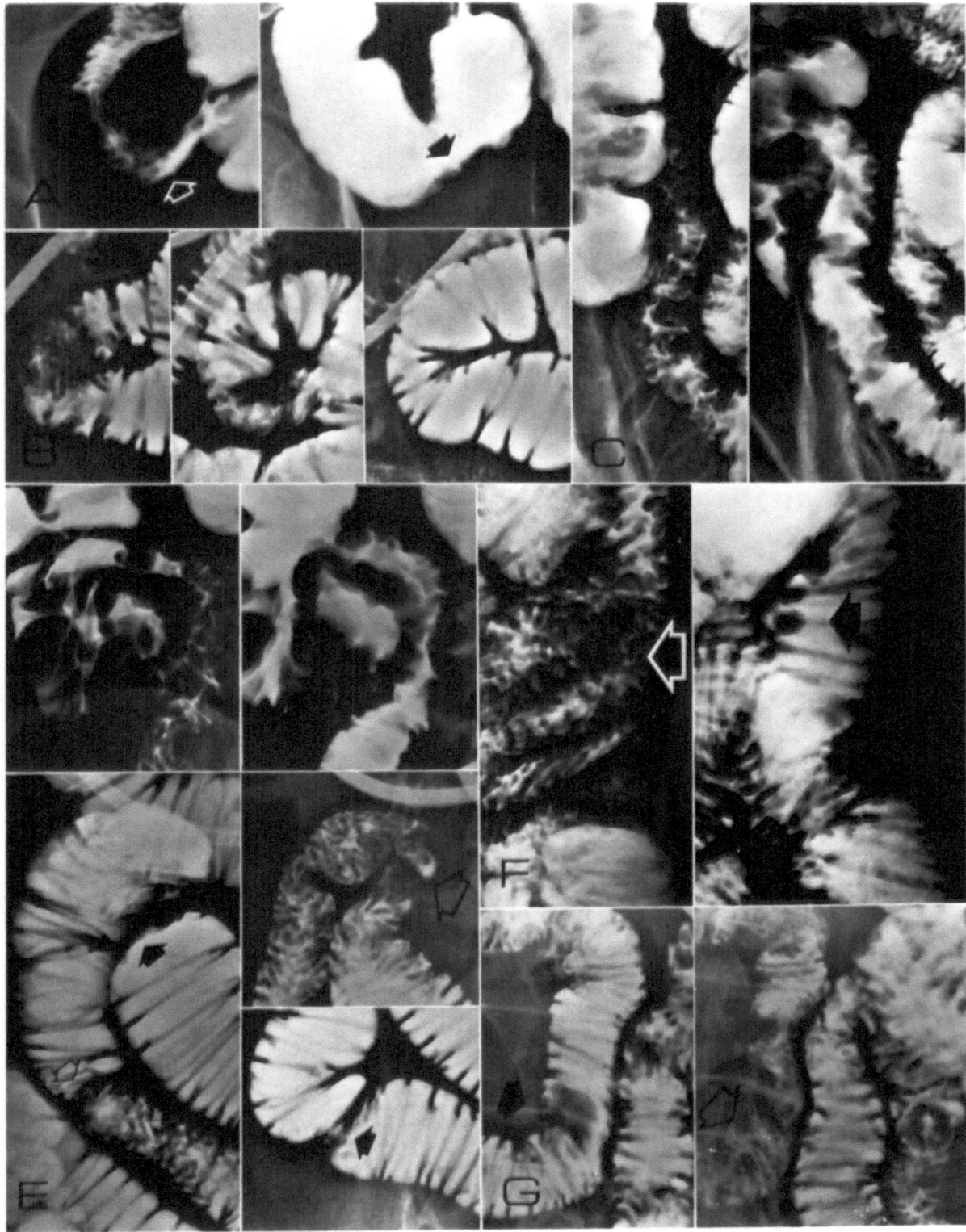

Fig. 7.19. Several examples of abnormalities in the small intestine that are seen most clearly when the loops are well filled. (A) Local ulceration in Crohn's disease. (B) Atrophy of the mucosa as a result of celiac disease. (C) *Yersinia EC* infection. (D) Appendicular infiltration. (E) Aspecific ulceration. (FG) Metastasis of melanoma.

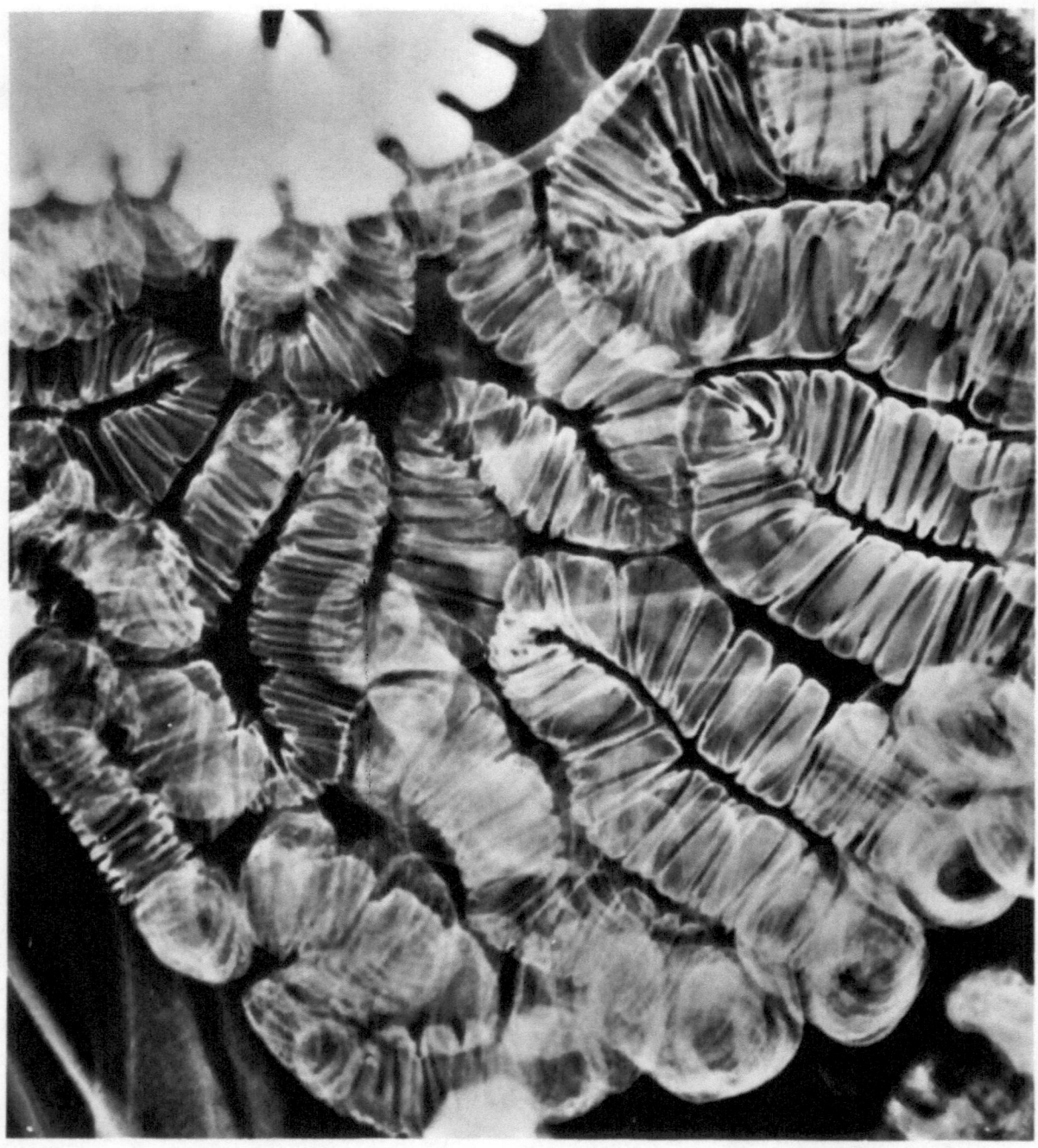

Fig. 7.20. Double-contrast exposures of a jejunum after water is administered. A thin film of contrast fluid remains on the mucosa for 15–30 s.

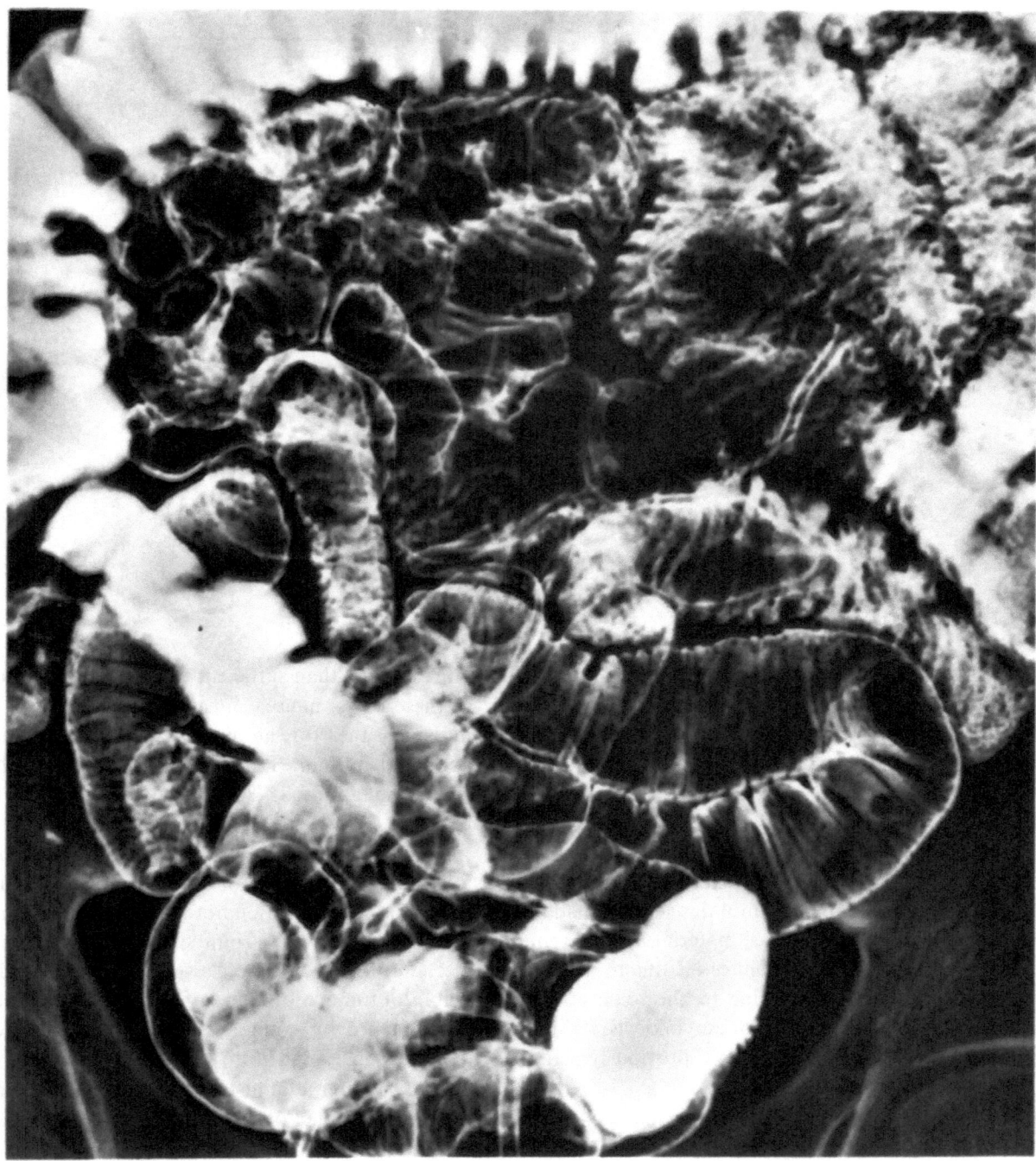

Fig. 7.21. The contrast differences are considerably greater and therefore very troublesome on double-contrast exposures taken after air is administered instead of water. The time available for taking the x-rays, however, is much longer.

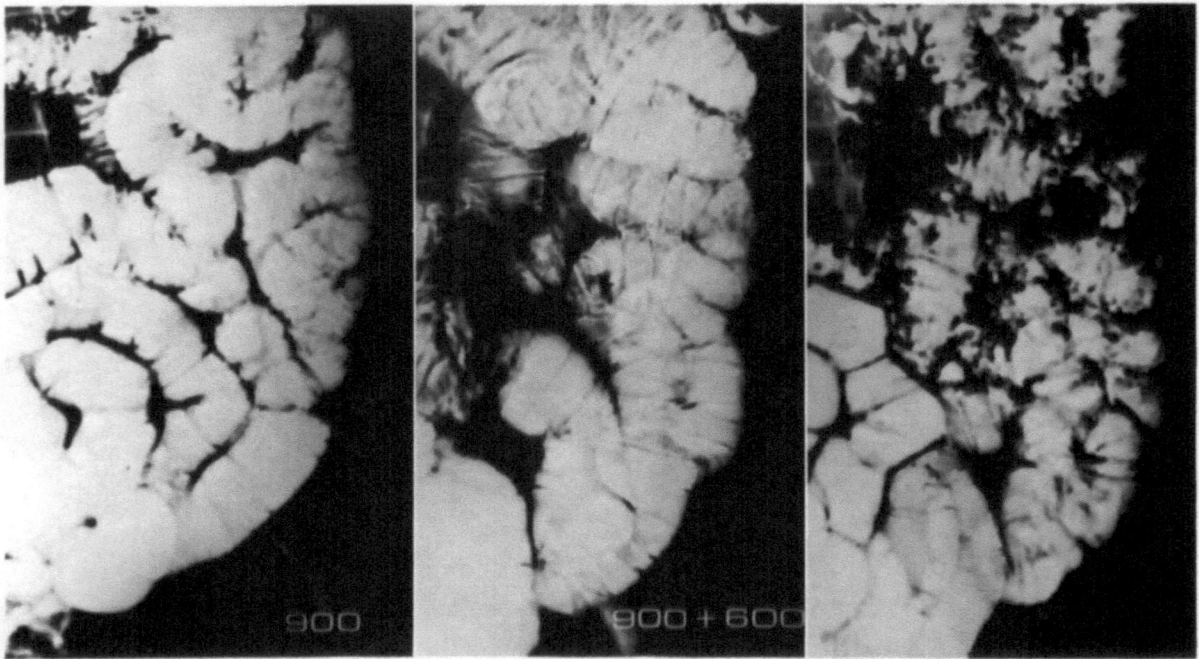

Fig. 7.22. Disintegration of contrast fluid by mixing with an excess of water (flocculation).

In colitis, the contents of the colon mix with secretions induced by infectious diseases and are found in large quantities in the distal ileum as a result of reflux from the cecum through an inadequate Bauhin's valve. In the past this contamination often led to the incorrect diagnosis: 'reflux ileitis' (fig. 7.23.)

In fig. 7.24, the cobblestones in the distal ileum did not become obvious until this segment had been flushed clean with contrast material. In the event of disturbed motility in the intestine due to neurological disorders, damage due to the toxic effect of some drugs, scleroderma, or amyloidosis, residue of food consumed several days previously can be found in the distal ileum (fig. 7.25).

Useful films of the ileum can be made only when the contamination in this part of the intestine has been removed. Quite often if the ileum is not empty, the cecum is not reached even after administration of 1200 ml barium suspension. Administration of even more barium might lead to a persistent obstipation from dehydration in the colon in diseases accompanied by disturbed motility. As a rule we avoid giving more than 1200 ml barium suspension; a supplementary infusion of 600, sometimes 1200 ml water can then be quite effective. Since there is already more than sufficient dilatation of the loops in these cases, nausea must be prevented and the infusion is therefore administered slowly at a rate of about 50 ml/min. To achieve this, the waterbag should hang only 25–30 cm above the level of the table.

In addition to disturbed motility or a contaminated ileum as a result of an inadequate Bauhin's valve, the cecum is often not reached after administration of 1200 ml barium suspension in cases of mechanical obstruction caused by shriveled skip lesions or tumors. In such cases too, which are often accompanied by a manifest or incipient ileus, enteroclysis is extended to include slow water infusions. If, after administration of a total fluid dose of $2\frac{1}{2}$ liters, the obstruction has not yet been reached, which sometimes does occur, no further fluid is administered and further developments are awaited as in a conventional examination. Our experience has shown that free projection of the intestinal loops by means of the compression technique can cause insurmountable problems when the dose exceeds $2\frac{1}{2}$ liters, and sometimes even sooner. A worthwhile contribution to anatomical diagnostics is then no longer possible. In some cases, the maximum permissible fluid dosage for enteroclysis

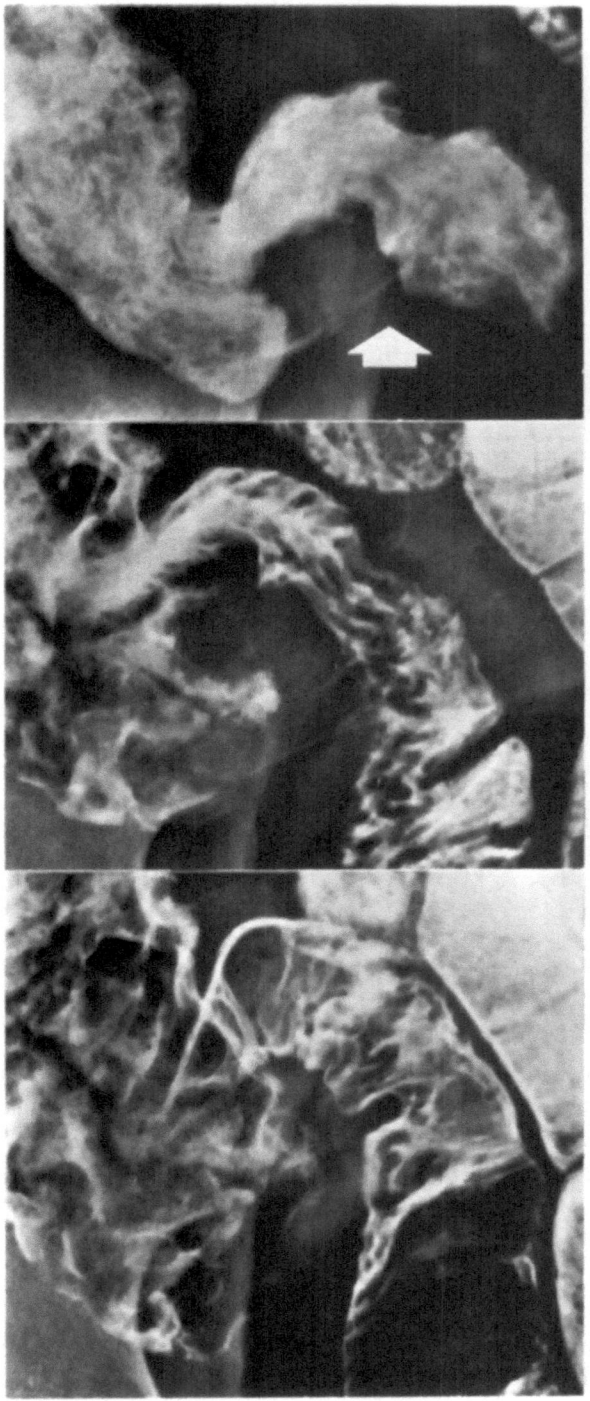

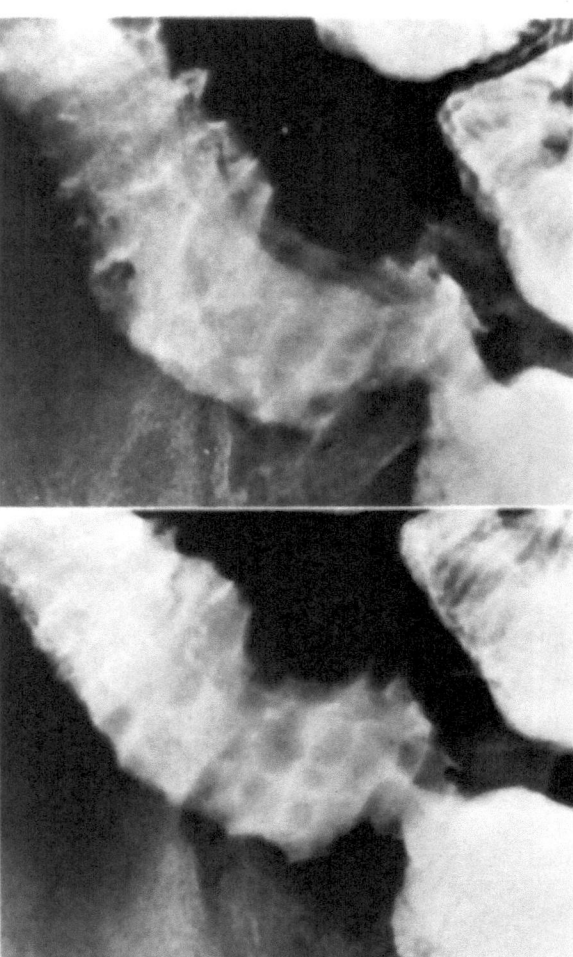

Fig. 7.24. Swollen mucosal folds and cobblestones in Crohn's disease that were clearly visible only after the contamination in this loop was flushed away.

depends partly on what the patient's heart and kidneys can tolerate. This should be determined in consultation with the attending physician.

For various reasons, rectal filling of the colon with contrast medium is not always possible. By means of the method described above, enteroclysis can give very worthwhile roentgenograms of the colon. This can be supplemented, if necessary, with air double-contrast exposures via rectal insufflation or through the tube or both. The procedure for such an examination of the colon is as follows: after 900–1200 ml barium suspension has been introduced into the small intestine through the duodenal tube and x-rays have been taken, the entire contrast dosage is forced into the colon by means of an equally large water infusion. The small intestine can

Fig. 7.23. Misleading pattern of a so-called 'reflux ileitis' in ulcerative colitis (arrow) that disappears after the distal ileum is flushed clean with a large dose of contrast medium.

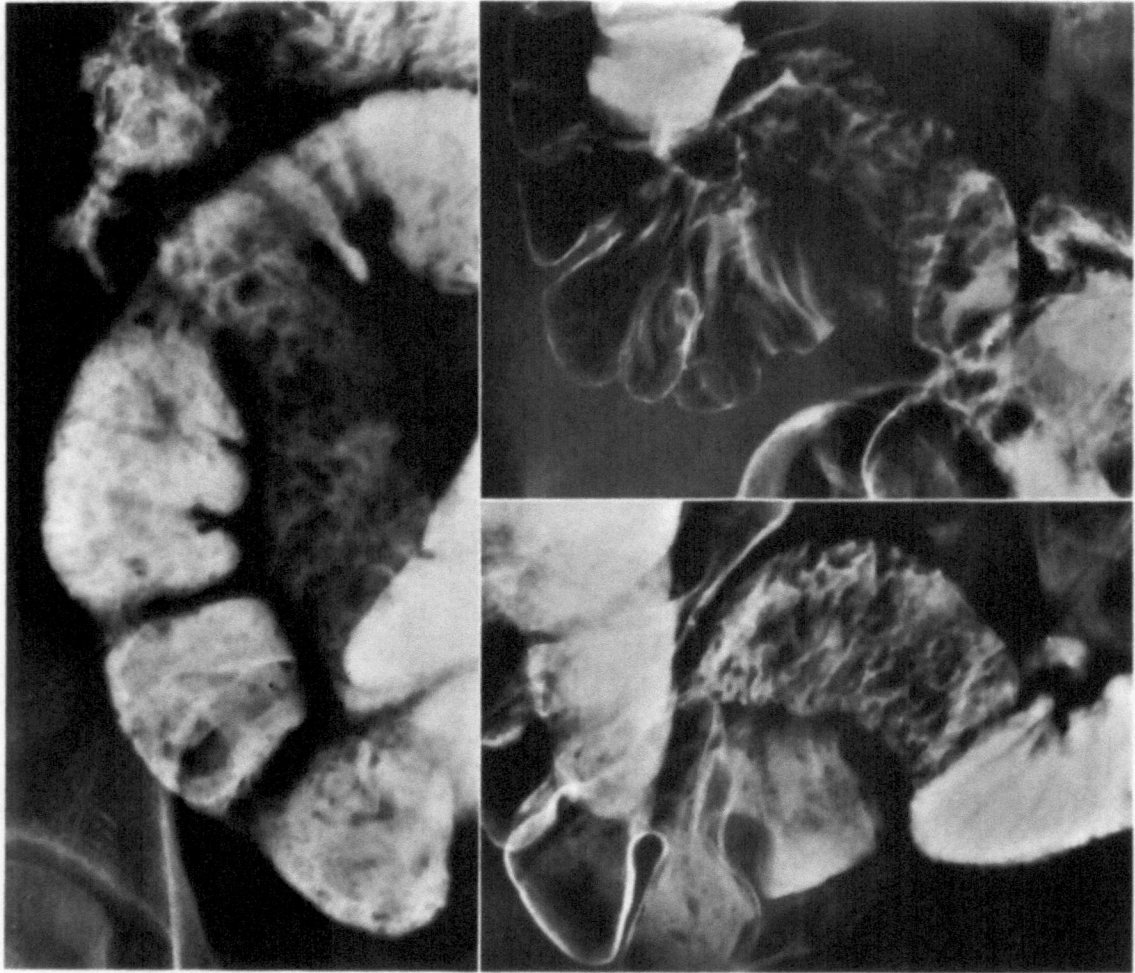

Fig. 7.25. Evaluation of the mucosa in the ileum in a patient with drug-induced atony of the bowel is possible only after the food residue has been forced out of the colon.

in this way be flushed clean in several minutes so that residual barium in the jejunum or ileum will not interfere with the colon films (fig. 7.26). Because many patients feel a strong tendency to evacuate their colon during the examination, it is better to bring in a rectal cannula beforehand.

A relatively rare indication for administration of water after the contrast medium infusion is when the cecum and the distal ileum are difficult to find. By filling the small intestine with water, the colon and distal ileum become more clearly visible against this background (fig. 7.27).

In summary, administration of water after the barium suspension is indicated in the following cases:

1) To obtain a better degree of filling of the distal ileum after the cecum has been reached.

2) To obtain filling of the distal ileal loops when the contrast column has almost reached the cecum. One could in this case also give an additional 300 ml contrast fluid, but water is cheaper!

3) Flushing of the distal ileum when it is contaminated with food residue or by reflux from the colon as a result of an inadequate Bauhin's valve.

4) Filling of the rest of the small intestine after 1200 ml barium suspension has already been administered and the cecum is not yet reached. In general this occurs in the event of a functional or mechanical obstruction.

5) For double-contrast films of the jejunum, filling with water is greatly preferred over filling with air. One disadvantage, however, is that there is very little time available to take the films.

6) If it is necessary to examine the colon with contrast medium administered orally, the entire

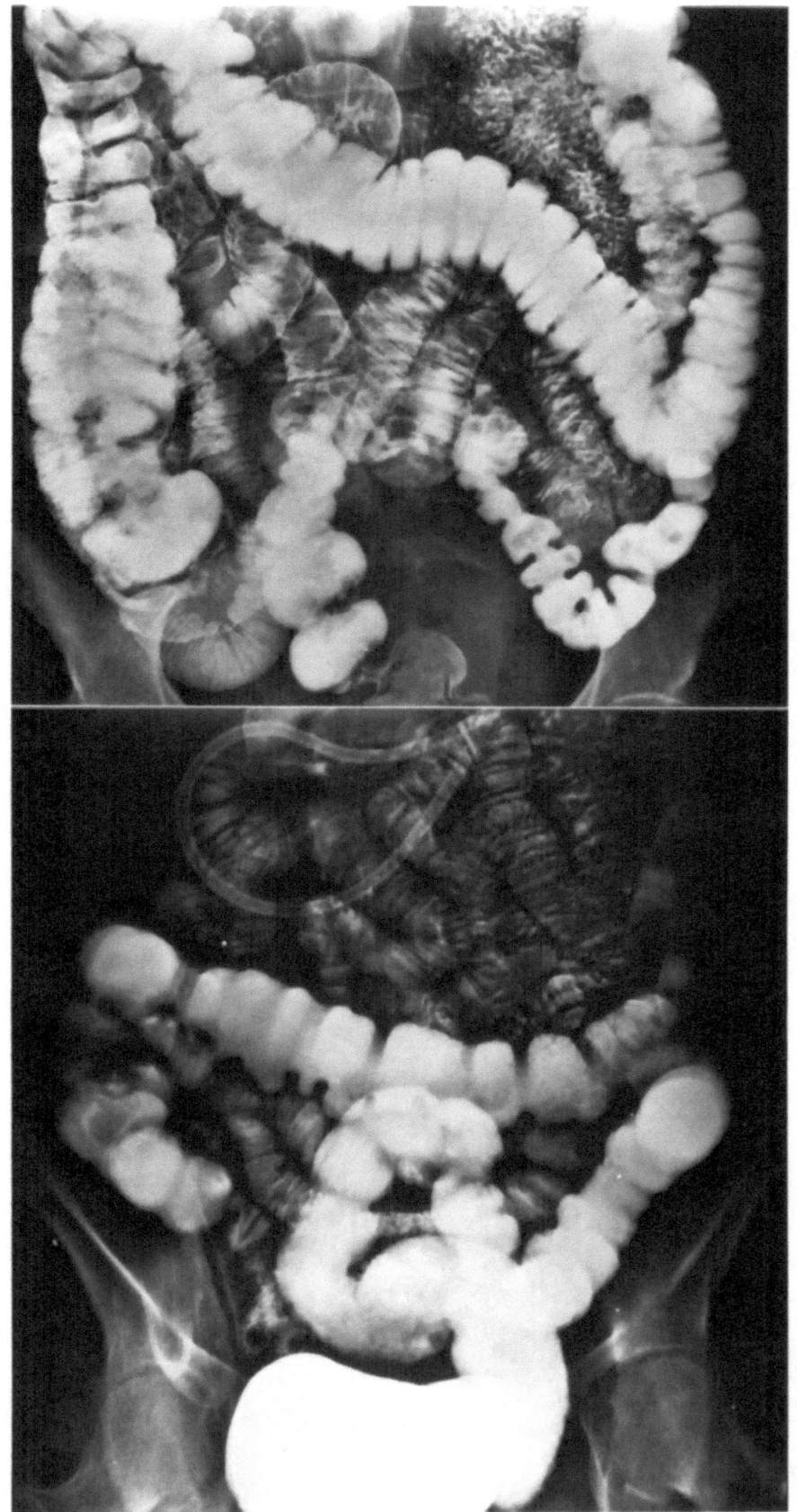

Fig. 7.26. Examples of the survey exposures of the colon after the jejunum is flushed clean with water. Useful reproduction of the mucosa in the colon is then generally no problem at all. (See also page 108.)

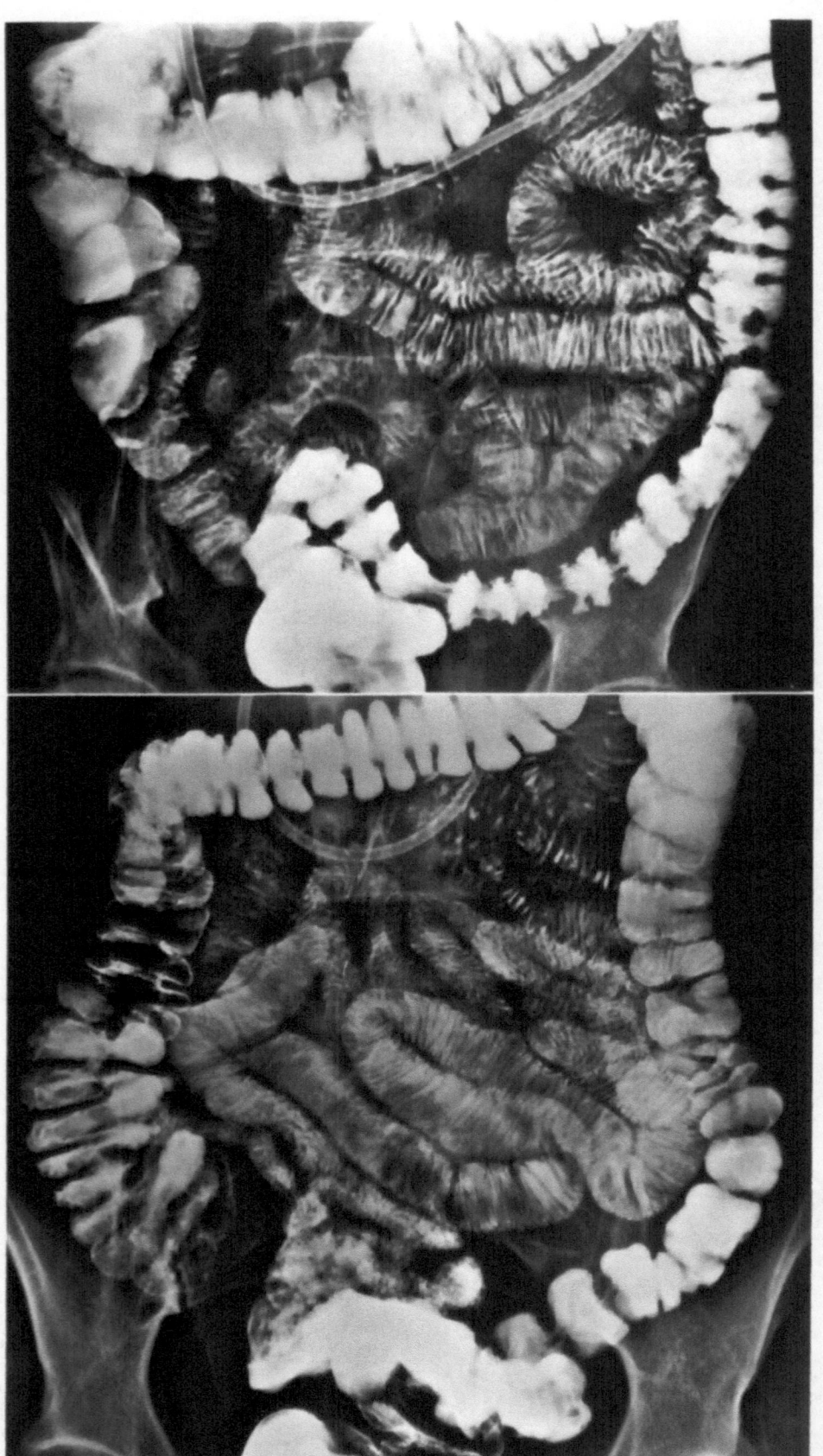

Fig. 7.26. See legend on page 107.

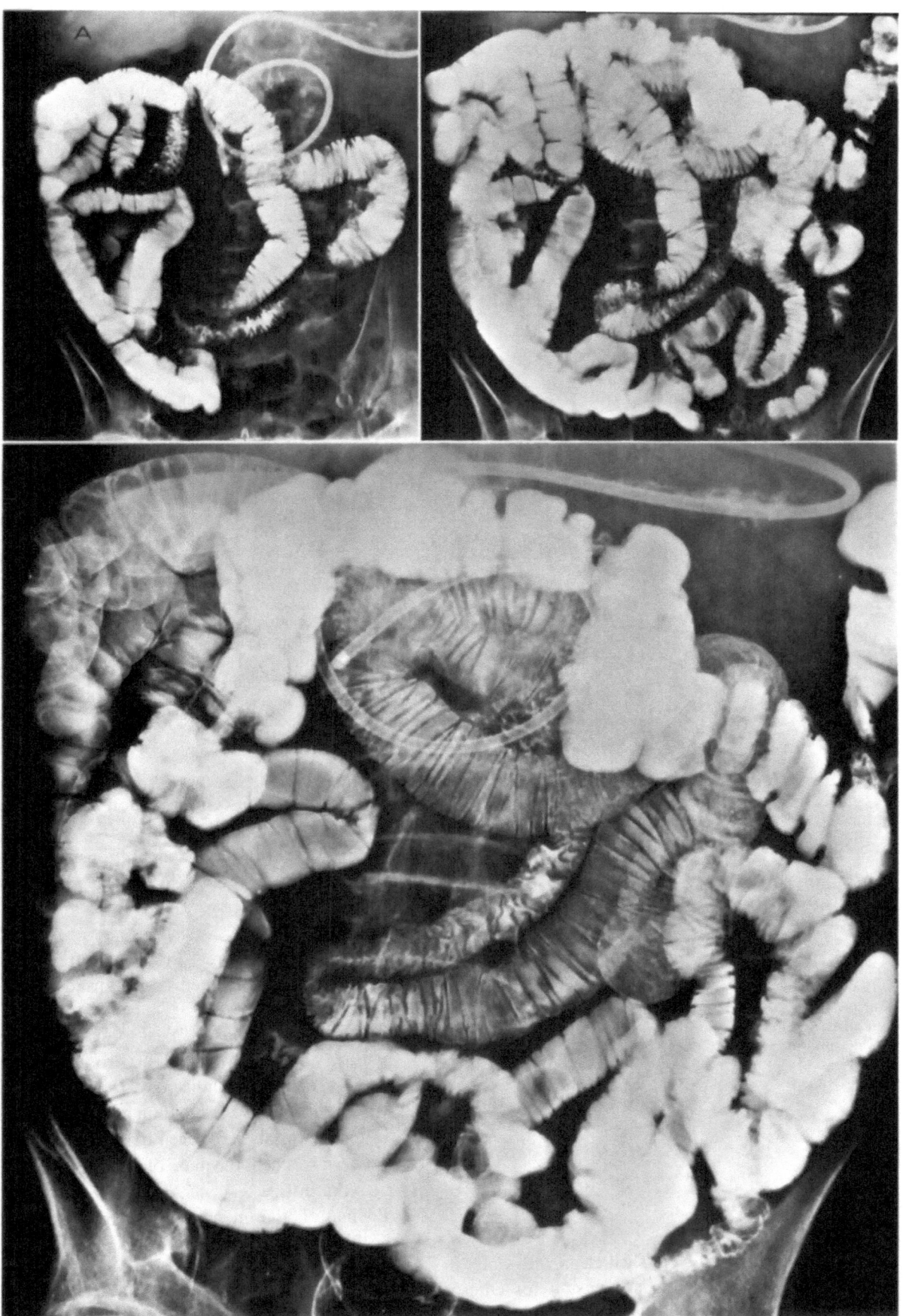

*Fig. 7.27*A. Positional anomaly of the small intestine: the ascending colon is difficult to find. Filling of the jejunal loops in the right half of the abdomen (top left). Now the ileal loops are also filled and parts of the colon are visible in the upper left quadrant. The cecum, usually located either in the lower right quadrant or high up under the liver, is not visible here (top right). After the jejunum is filled

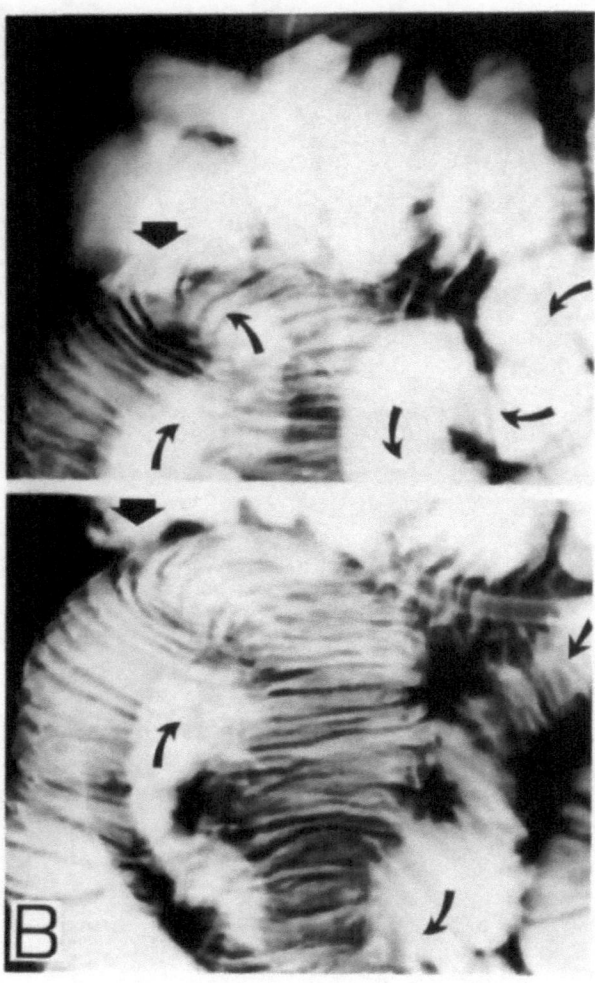

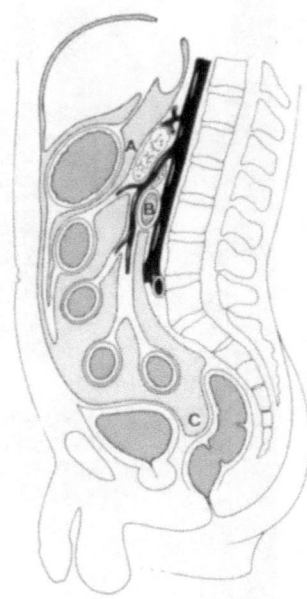

Fig. 7.28. Lateral cross section of the abdominal cavity. (A) Via the foramen of Winslow or an opening in the transverse mesocolon, the jejunal loops may end up behind the stomach in the bursa omentalis. (B) The duodenum can be pinched between the aorta and the superior mesenteric artery. (C) By filling the bladder and the rectum, the ileal loops are forced out of the minor pelvis.

7) Position of the ascending colon and the distal ileum cannot be identified (fig. 7.27).
8) To provoke prestenotic dilatations, useful for the easy and early detection of strictures caused by tumors or ulcers.

There are a number of reasons why a water infusion should *not* be administered or has disadvantages:

1) When there is a mass of ileal loops in the pelvis minor, it is always necessary to use the air-contrast technique and to try to reach the cecum with as little contrast medium as possible. When water is administered, even if the cecum has not yet been reached, the mass of ileal loops will only increase in size.
2) Edema of the mucous membrane is usually visible only when the intestine is moderately filled. Administration of water before the cecum has been reached and all loops have been visualized in this phase greatly increases the chance of overlooking this important finding.

*Fig. 7.27*B. Ileocolic anastomosis (thick arrow) that was not visualized until water was administered so that the overlying jejunal loops became transparent. In the distal ileum (thin curved arrows), the mucosal folds were clearly thickened due to a recurrent Crohn's disease; this was totally invisible before the water infusion.

small intestine can be flushed clean with water in 5–10 min. The barium suspension for enteroclysis is then used again for the colon examination.

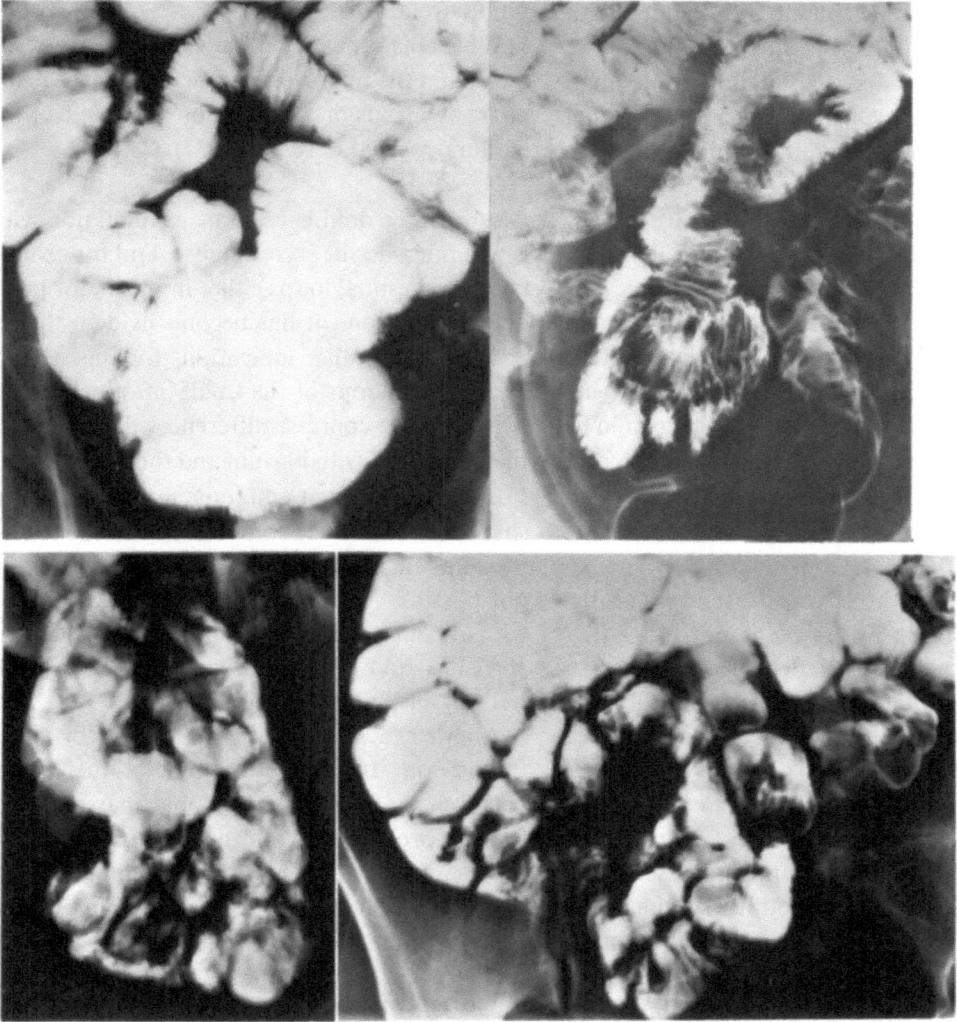

Fig. 7.29. Rectal air insufflation with the patients in the prone position is often sufficient for free projection of the ileal loops in the minor pelvis.

3) If water is administered too soon, the segment of intestine that is stretched will be too long and motility will be paralyzed. Disturbed motility, at least in the distal half of the intestine, can then no longer be seen.
4) Administration of water causes rapid flocculation of the contrast medium so that the presence of malabsorption cannot be determined.
5) As a result of the greater degree of filling of the entire small intestine, it will be much more difficult to take compression spot films.
6) The administration of too much fluid in patients with cardiac insufficiency can be dangerous.

7. Administration of air after contrast fluid

Often in slender individuals the ileal loops may already have clumped together in the minor pelvis after administration of 600 ml contrast fluid or even less. Since this part of the abdominal cavity is not accessible for compression, special measures must be taken to force the mass of ileal loops out of the minor pelvis. The drawing in fig. 7.28 shows that if the patient lies on his stomach in a slight Trendelenburg position, the heavy barium-filled ileal loops are most likely to drop spontaneously in the direction of the navel and the posterior abdominal wal. The result is, however, often disappointing. The next step is to try filling the bladder with water, the rectosigmoid with air, or both. For hygienic reasons, we believe that filling the bladder with water through a catheter is not very desirable. Moreover, this procedure costs more time than rectal air insufflation. One might consider asking leptosome patients to hold their morning urine. We feel, however, that this causes the patient considerable discomfort; in addition it could have an adverse effect on the motility of the small intestine via the autonomous nervous system. Furthermore, for the reasons discussed previously, the patient should evacuate just before the examination to be sure that the colon is as empty as possible. Selective emptying of the colon without emptying the bladder would be difficult and we object to this approach for that reason. Filling only the rectosigmoid with air often turns out to be sufficient to project the deep-lying ileum freely (fig. 7.29).

In general this method is also useful when the cecum is located deep within the minor pelvis (fig. 7.30). In these cases it is better to administer so much air rectally, that the cecum is also filled.

The lowest part of the cecum can also be filled with air and even, via reflux through Bauhin's valve, the distal ileal loops. Rectal air insufflation of the distal ileal loops can be helpful when oral air insufflation takes too long as in diseases accompanied by greatly reduced motility of the small intestine. If peristalsis is normal, oral air insufflation of the tangle of ileal loops is certainly the best and quickest way to increase the chance of evaluating the mucosal patterns in this section. Air is administered intermittently through the duodenal tube with the insufflation balloon; at the same time the expression on the patient's face must be observed closely. When the air is administered too rapidly, sensations of pain due to cramps are immediately visible on the face. Therefore a better method is to let the patient perform this air insufflation himself. The total amount of air to be administered can be estimated at about 1 liter. The air causes pronounced local stretching of the small intestine resulting in such an active peristalsis that the cecum is often reached within 1 min. Each and every time it is an experience to watch the rush of air through the meters of small intestine and to note at the same time that this active peristalsis does not influence the rate of flow of the barium suspension in the small intestine. In fact it even appears that, as a result of the passage of air, the flow of contrast

fluid is retarded.

When the air reaches the segment of the ileum located in the minor pelvis, the loops can be forced apart by means of compression and can be projected almost separately (fig. 7.31).

Although the double-contrast examination with air is without a doubt exceedingly useful for examining tangled intestinal loops either in the minor pelvis or due to adhesions, it has become evident that there are not many other indications for this technique. Because the loops of the small intestine are greatly twisted, large contrast differences develop between the parts filled with barium and those filled with air. Furthermore, the numerous more or less ring-shaped shadows are often very troublesome, especially when separation of the air-filled loops is not possible. Therefore we are of the opinion that with the air-contrast technique only, Meckel's diverticula, and strictures, whatever the cause may be, will easily be overlooked.

Another, although rare, indication for air insufflation via the duodenal tube is the suspected occurrence of very tiny polypoid masses or lymph follicles protruding from the intestinal mucosa. On the survey x-rays these polyps, sometimes only 1 mm long, are visible only along the margin of the contrast column. On air double-contrast films, they can be seen throughout the entire intestinal loop (fig. 7.32). To examine a patient for the presence of such subtle abnormalities it is particularly important that the contrast fluid does not foam; otherwise differentiation from gas bubbles in the intestine can become exceedingly difficult or even impossible.

The exposure time for the x-ray must be short because of the large quantity of air in the exposed area. Quite often double-contrast films are mistakenly taken with a low tube voltage. We have found that this is admissible only when a solitary freely projected loop is involved. Evaluation of double-contrast films with air is easiest when the intestinal loops contain only a little barium and when air insufflation is carried out during the last stage of the examination. If during enteroclysis it appears that a mass of intestinal loops has formed in the minor pelvis, or if it is known or becomes clear that adhesion has occurred, it is not wise to decide too quickly to give a second dose of contrast fluid; it is better to wait or to give metoclopramide.

113

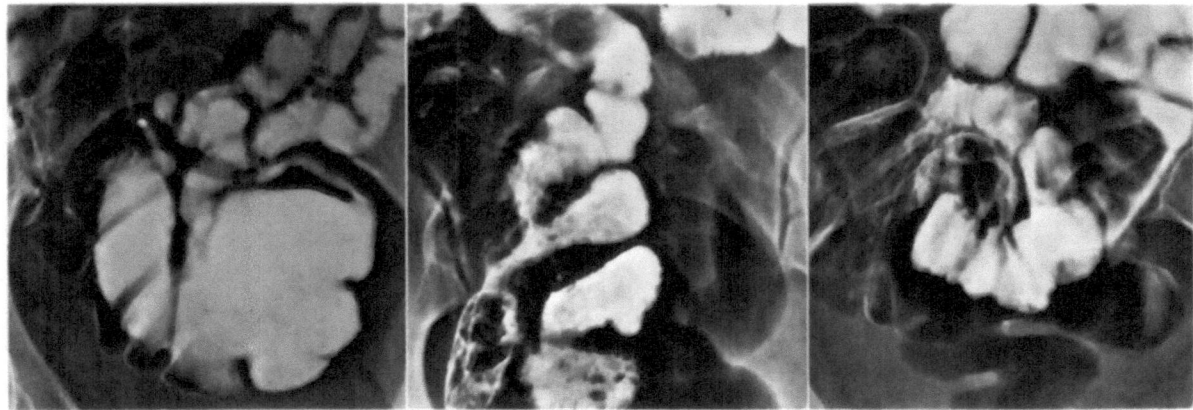

Fig. 7.30. Filling the rectosigmoid with air, and if necessary continuing insufflation until the cecum is also filled with air, is a good method for forcing the deep-seated ileocecal segment out of the minor pelvis.

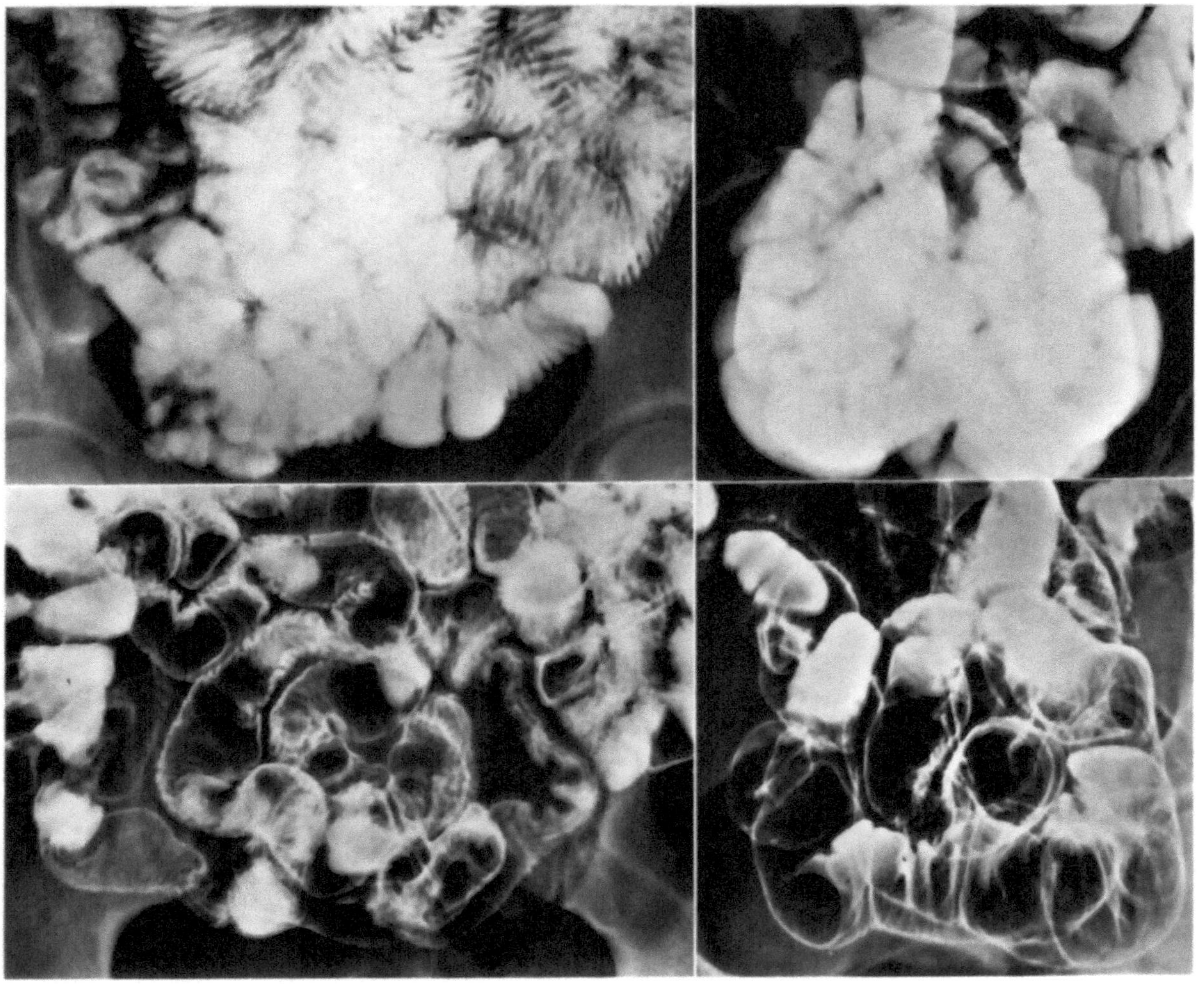

Fig. 7.31. Two examples of free projection of the ileal loops in the lower abdomen and the minor pelvis by using air insufflation through the duodenal tube. The patient is in the prone position.

114

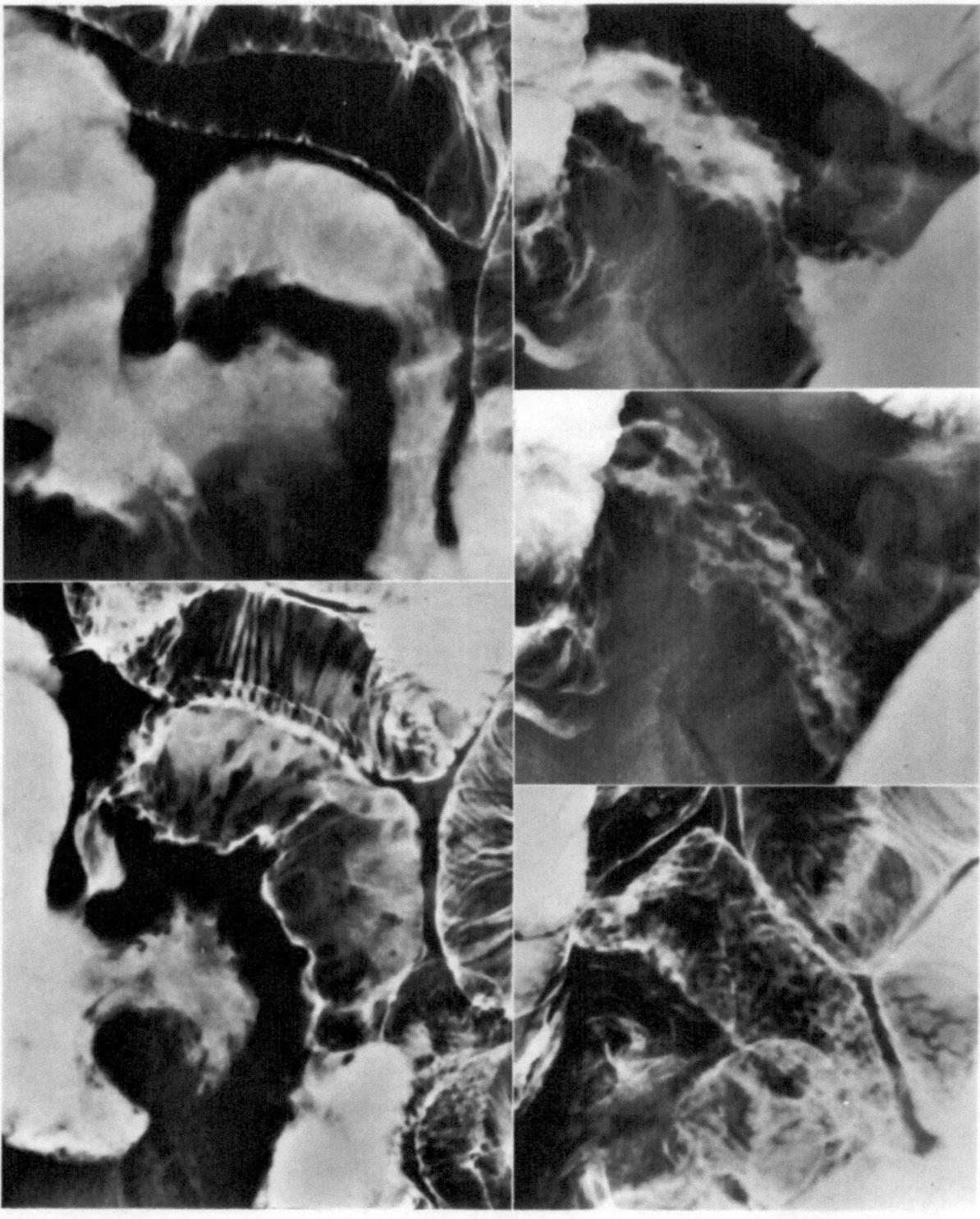

Fig. 7.32. Two examples of lymph follicles in the distal ileum that are clearly visible on the double-contrast exposures but could not or barely be seen when the loop was filled with barium only.

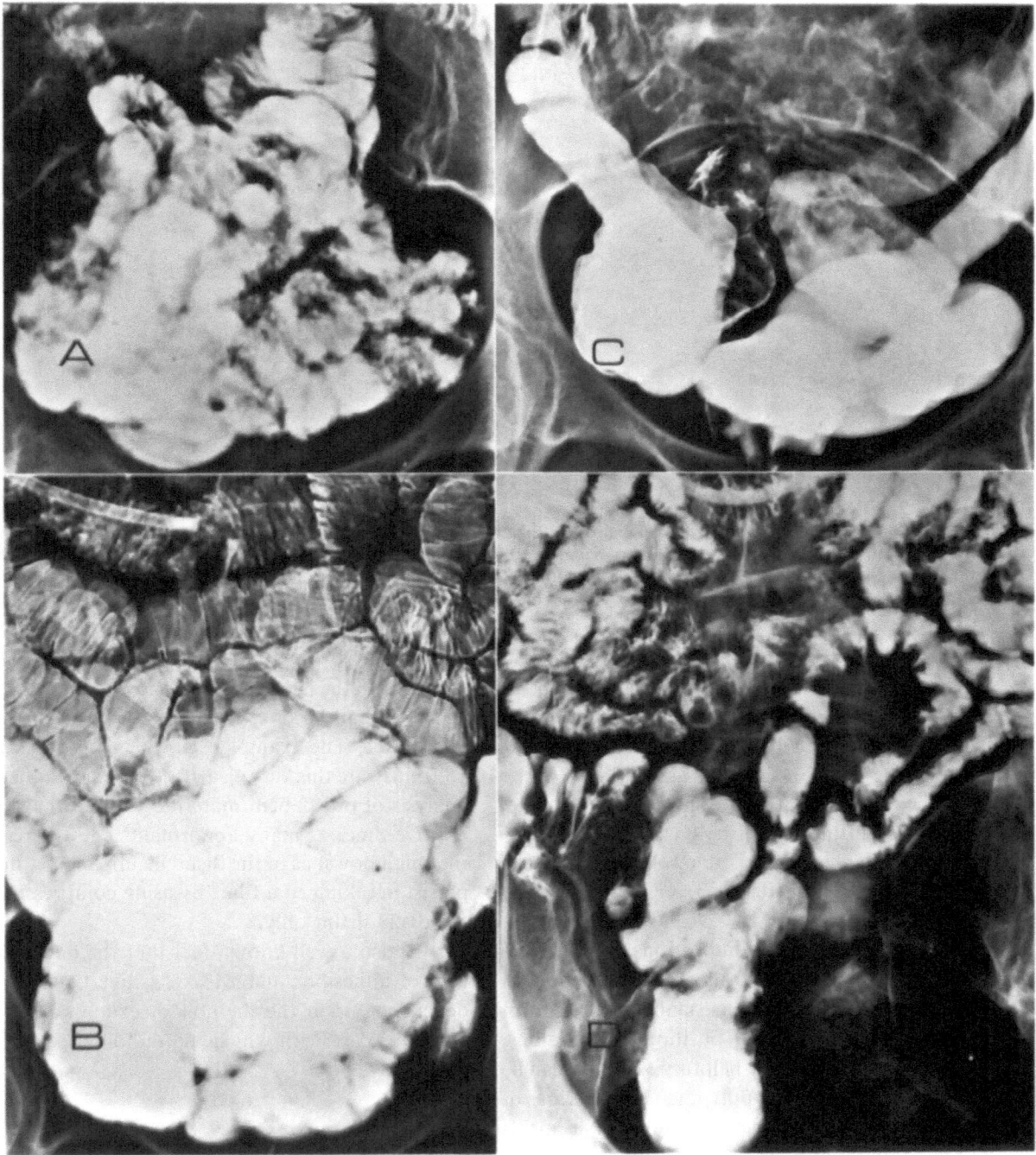

Fig. 7.33. The results of an incorrect decision as to procedure during the course of the examination. There is a clump of ileal loops in the minor pelvis. (A) Because the cecum had not yet been reached, water was administered. (B) The results of this decision. Although the reasoning was in principle correct, this step was apparently undertaken without consideration of the problems that could be expected during free projection of the distal ileum since a previous colon examination (C) had already indicated that the ileocecal segment was deep-seated. (D) The survey exposures obtained after 2 ml metoclopramide was administered intravenously, on the basis of the original situation seen in A, and air was insufflated rectally. Air insufflation via the duodenal tube would serve no purpose.

HOW TO SEPARATE ILEUM LOOPS IN SMALL PELVIS

USE AIR AND COMPRESSION

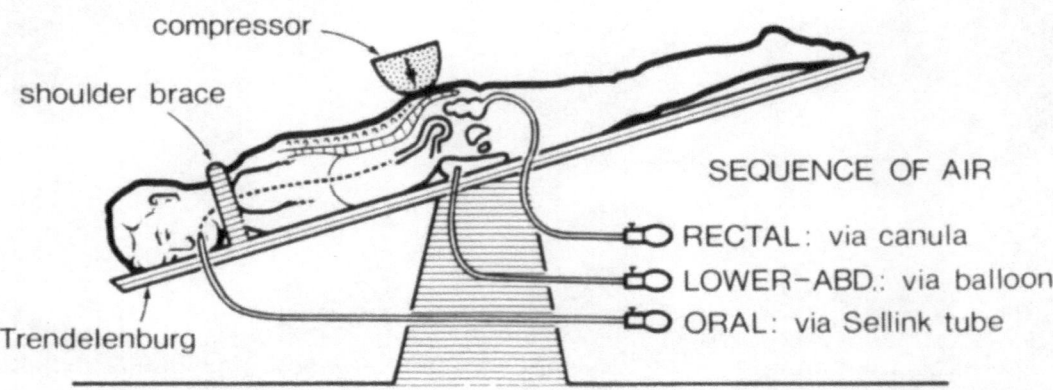

Fig. 7.34. Position of the patient during the combined insufflation and special compression technique. The sequence of steps is usually as follows: (1) Place the balloon under the lower abdomen. (2) Rectal air insufflation. (3) Air insufflation via the duodenal tube. (4) Fill the balloon between the patient and the table with air. (5) Compression on the dorsal side of the patient. (6) If necessary, direct roentgen rays along craniocaudal axis.

When a mass of ileal loops is discovered in the minor pelvis, the decision to give a supplementary dosage of water can be disastrous. The mass will only become larger as a result and usually can no longer be untangled at all – even a belated attempt to use air insufflation will be unsuccessful. A new examination is the only possible solution after such an incorrect decision (fig. 7.33).

In summary therefore, the indications for a double-contrast examination with air are fairly limited in enteroclysis. If loops of the small intestine form clumps as a result of their position or adhesions, this technique can be very helpful; it should also be considered if follicular or polypoid abnormalities of the mucosa are a distinct possibility. Air insufflation should never be carried out before the contrast fluid has reached the cecum. Time and a little patience are sometimes required.

We have found that carefully executed compression, also before air insufflation, and spot films of the entire small intestine, not just the distal ileum, are absolutely essential – a fact that certainly has not yet become apparent to all radiologists. We have seen many cases in which distinct abnormal-ities in both the jejunum and the lower abdomen are poorly visualized or even impossible to find on the plain films. The examples shown in figs. 16.4 and 16.5 illustrate this very clearly. Moreover, statistical analysis of our patient material revealed that there are five times as many abnormalities in the rest of the small bowel as in the distal ileum, and yet many persist in taking spot films by using compression of the distal ileum only.

It is also a well-known fact that the demonstration of adhesions and Meckel's diverticula is not dependent upon the method of examination, but upon the care with which the radiologist works.

8. Compression technique

When it appears that neither rectal nor oral air insufflation is enough to force the distal ileum out of the minor pelvis for adequate projection, a combination of these two methods can be attempted. This combined air insufflation, as well as the subsequent application of compression, can be divided into a number of steps as follows (fig. 7.34):

1) The patient lies on his stomach in a slight Trendelenburg position. Between the lower abdomen and the table, just above the symphysis, is an empty inner tube of a soccer ball or balloon from a compression paddle, which is connected by a long tube to an insufflation bulb. In this way, in spite of the prone position, compression can be exerted on the intestinal loops from the abdominal side. However, the balloon is not blown up until air has been administered rectally at least (see 2) and often also orally (see 3).

2) A cannula in the rectum is connected by a long tube to a second insufflation bulb. One almost always begins with rectal air insufflation since it takes less time than 'oral' insufflation and causes the patient the least discomfort.

3) Air is administered orally through the Bilbao-Dotter tube, which is connected to a third insufflation bulb.

4) Pressure can be exerted on the dorsal side of the patient by means of an electric or manually operated compressor or a tourniquet as used in intravenous pyelography.

Careful execution of this technique, which after some practice only requires a few minutes, gives the results seen in fig. 7.35.

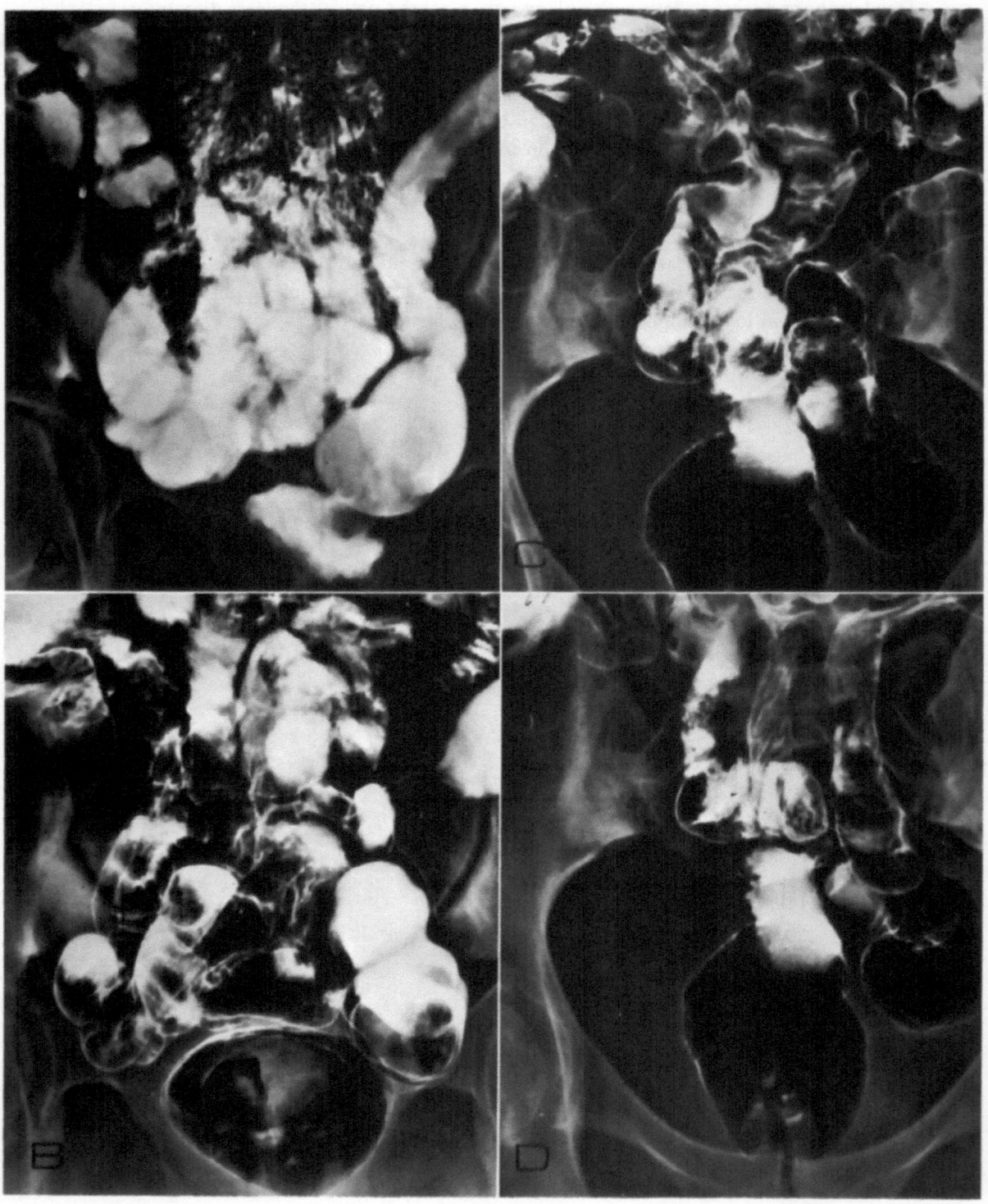

Fig. 7.35. Two examples of the results obtained with the special compression technique and combined air insufflation: (A–D) Patient 1; (EF) Patient 2.

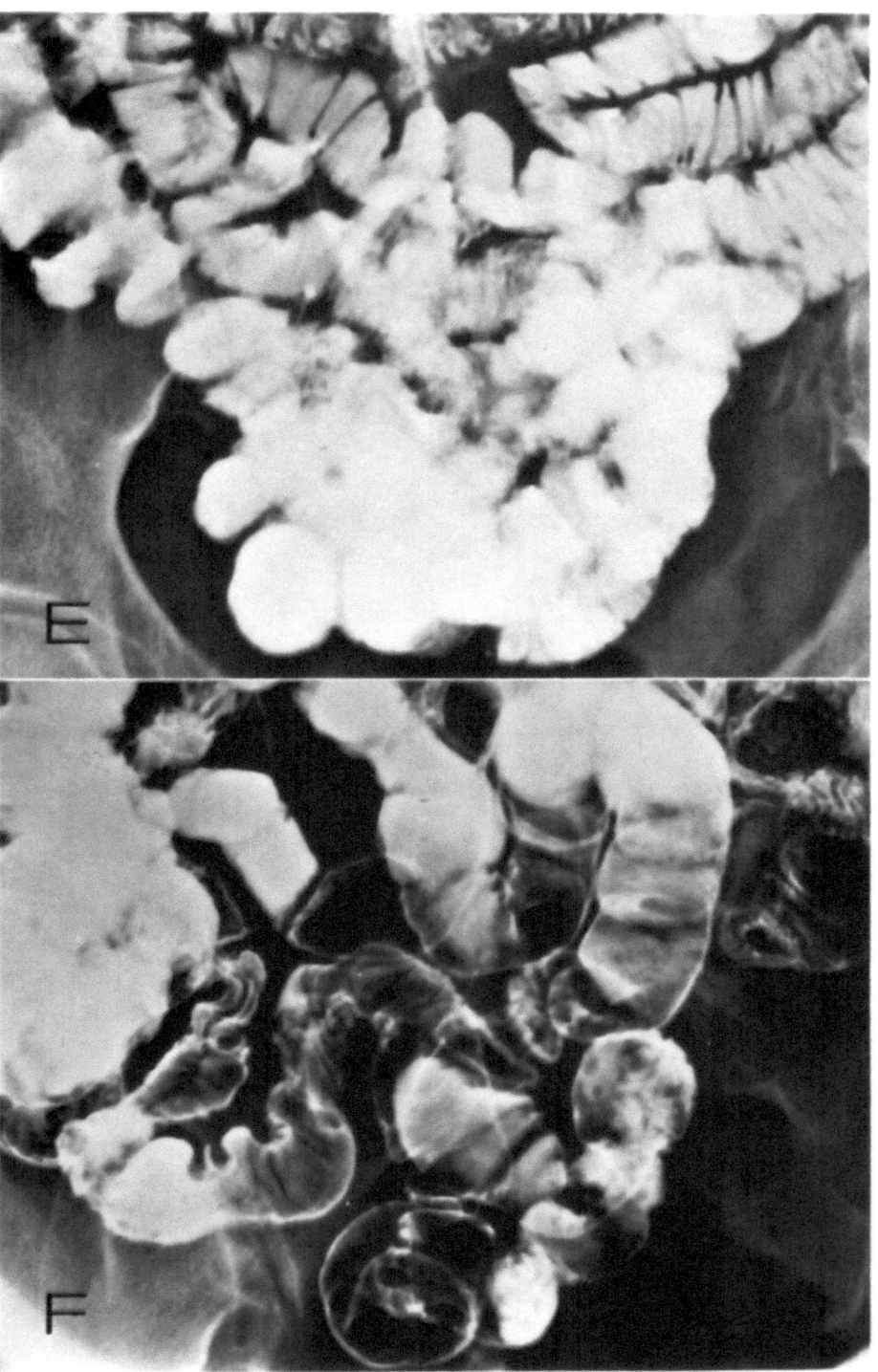

8. BASIC SIGNS OF ABNORMALITY

In order to establish a diagnosis on the basis of the roentgenograms and fluoroscopic examination, it is above all essential that the physician be thoroughly familiar with the normal roentgenological patterns and their variations. Only then can the abnormalities seen on the x-rays be identified as such. In some cases, the patient's history and the clinical data can be quite useful for the determination of the correct diagnosis; in fact they are sometimes indispensable since the mucosa shows only a limited number of reaction patterns. Moreover, several radiological signs are not specific and can be encountered in various, sometimes quite different, diseases.

1. Changes in the mucosal pattern

Changes in the shape of the folds of Kerkring can be subdivided into three main categories:

1) the original shape of the fold is still easily recognized,
2) the original shape cannot be recognized, and
3) there is evidence of destruction.

1.1. Swelling and edema

The most common abnormality although certainly not the most easily recognized, at least when only moderate, is edema or mucosal swelling. On the other hand, this diagnosis is also quite often established incorrectly when the coarse folds are a consequence of a misleading pattern (see chapter 8.7).

Edematous swollen folds are found in diseases that are associated with protein deficiency and hypoalbuminemia, as in inflammatory processes and disturbed protein synthesis, among others. The margins of each fold then do not always lie parallel – instead the folds can assume a somewhat biconvex omega-like (Ω) shape whereby the base of the fold does not change. The thickness of the intestinal wall increases only slightly or not at all (fig. 8.1K–N). In Whipple's disease and lambliasis, the surface of these folds can be covered with tiny nodular swellings that bulge out into the intestinal lumen (see page 245).

In the distal ileum, where the mucosal folding can appear to be longitudinal, the swollen folds become more numerous and begin to follow a twisting course. The mucosal relief appears somewhat disordered, although the continuity of the folds can still be followed, for instance in *Yersinia EC* infections (fig. 8.2). In Crohn's disease, ulcerations develop at the bottom of deep longitudinal grooves in the swollen mucous membrane of the ileum and the jejunum. The continuity of these grooves is broken by numerous deep ulcerations that lie perpendicular to the longitudinal folds, causing a cushion-like relief – the so-called cobblestone pattern (fig. 8.3). This cobblestone relief, a result of a markedly swollen mucosal surface, is, however, not specific to Crohn's disease but is also encountered in many other disorders such as periarteritis nodosa (fig. 8.4), lymphoreticular infiltration in the mucosa (fig. 8.5), and even after repositioning of an intussusception (fig. 8.6B).

Cobblestones will develop only when pronounced edema and clearly visible circular mucosal folds occur together. Because of the pronounced edema, the mucosa and submucosa – and possibly also the underlying muscular layer – become much thicker and the inner diameter of the intestinal lumen becomes much smaller. The excess mucosal surface must then, of necessity, form longitudinal folds. If the mucosal folds of the involved segment are very small or even absent, then the x-ray will show only longitudinal grooves. If there are pro-

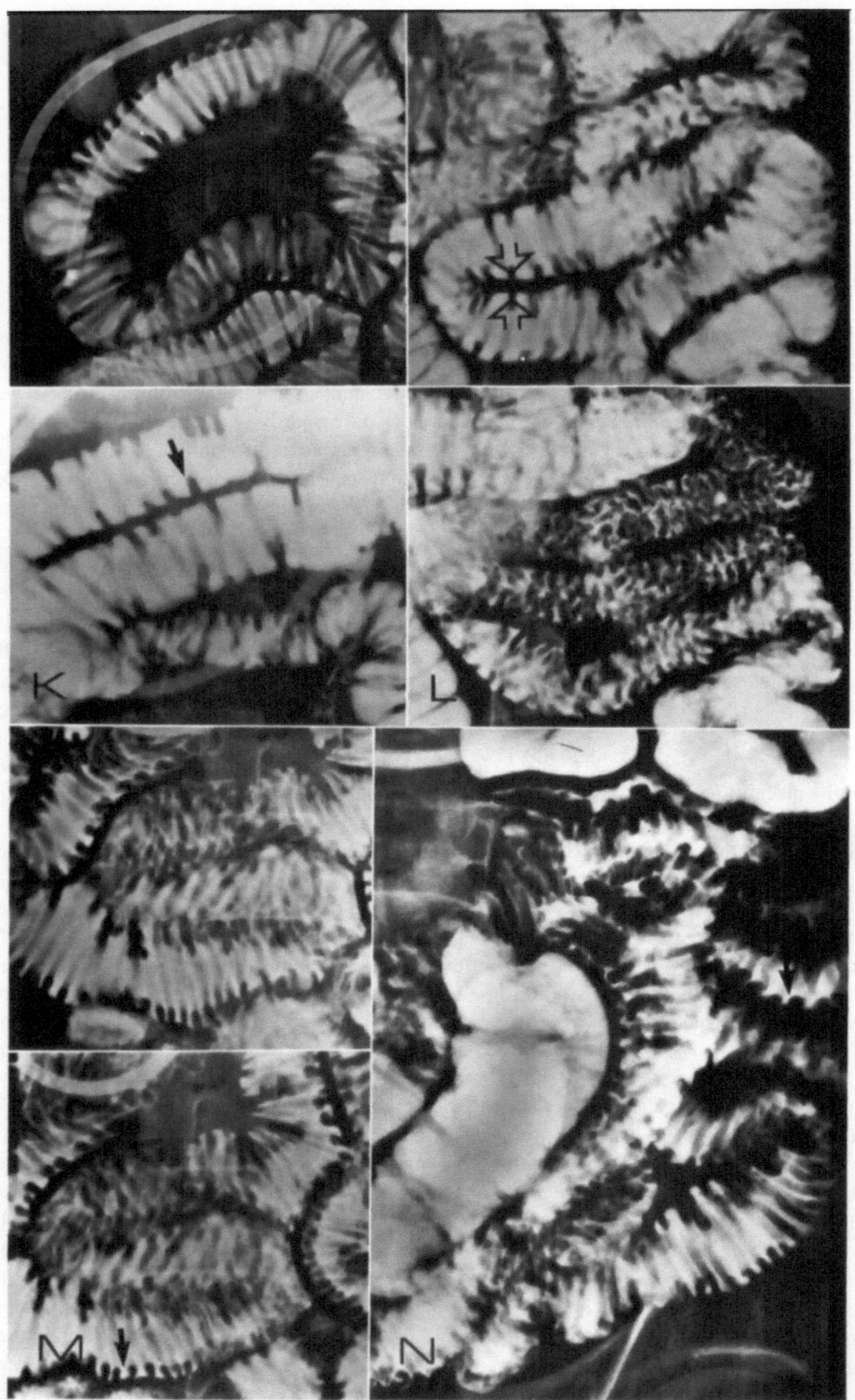

Fig. 8.1. Four patients with edematous swollen folds due to hypoalbuminemia. (ᴋ) Only swollen folds, no thickening of the intestinal wall. (ʟ) Swollen folds and thickening of the intestinal wall. (ᴍ) Biconvex or omega-shaped folds but no thickening of the intestinal wall. The patient has Crohn's disease of the colon. (ɴ) Omega-shaped folds and thickened wall in the bowel of a patient with celiac disease.

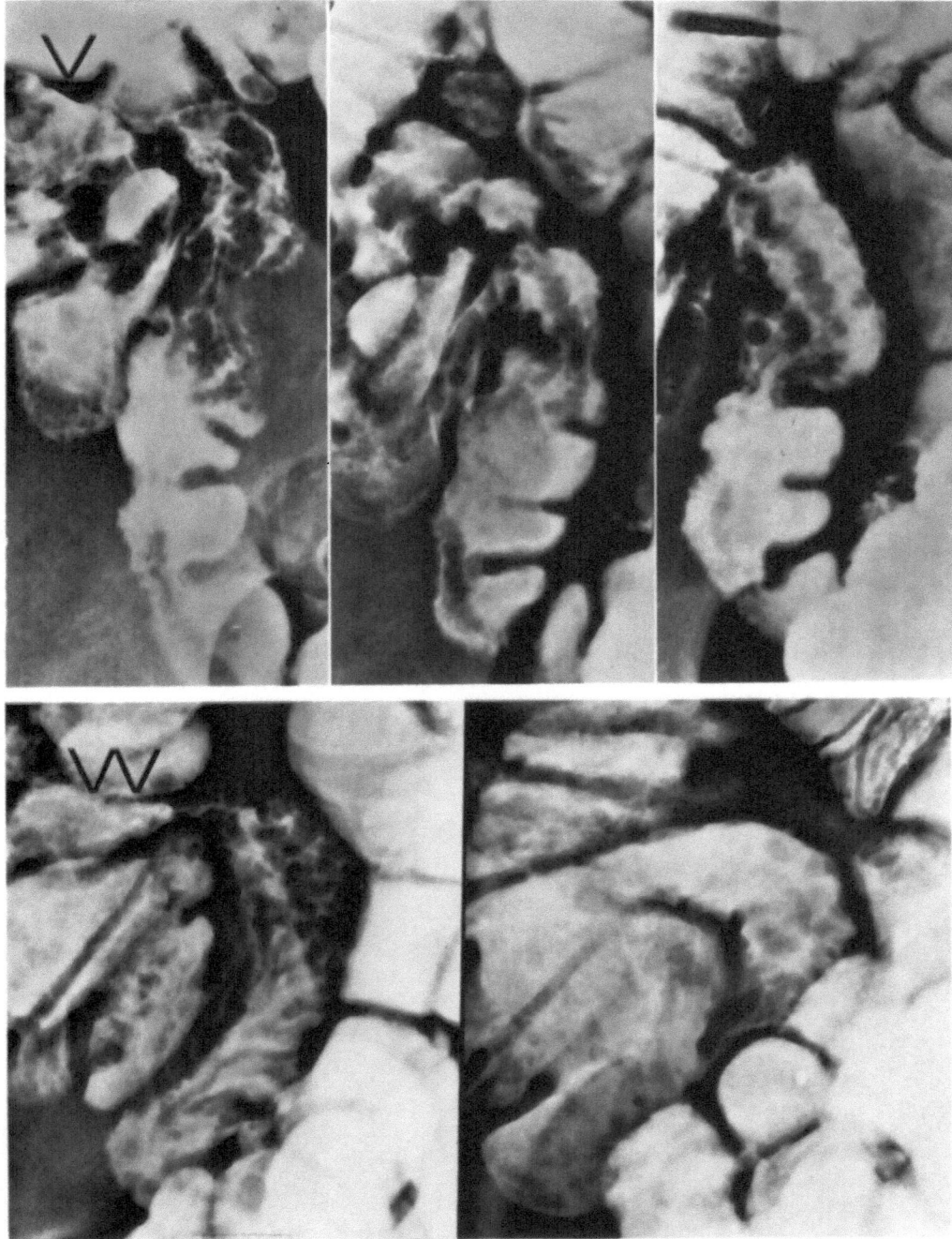

*Fig. 8.2*vw. Thick folds with twisting in the distal ileum, due to *Yersinia EC* infection.

nounced mucosal folds, then these will swell so markedly that they will lie very close together and transverse grooves will form in between. The combination of the longitudinal and transverse grooves, which enclose islands of highly swollen mucosa, produces the so-called railroad track configuration of the cobblestones. It should be obvious that the circulation of blood and lymph will be disturbed mainly in these grooves so that it will be here that ulcerations will develop.

If the edema is mainly superficial, as in the so-called ileitis associated with ulcerative colitis, neither cobblestones nor a railroad track pattern will be visualized. The mucosal folds in such a case never swell so markedly and only superficial erosion-like changes will be observed that ultimately disappear altogether (fig. 8.3A, top right).

Edema is almost always easier to see when the intestine is moderately filled with contrast medium; this cannot be predicted in the case of ulcerations. It

124

Formation of Cobblestones
through edema

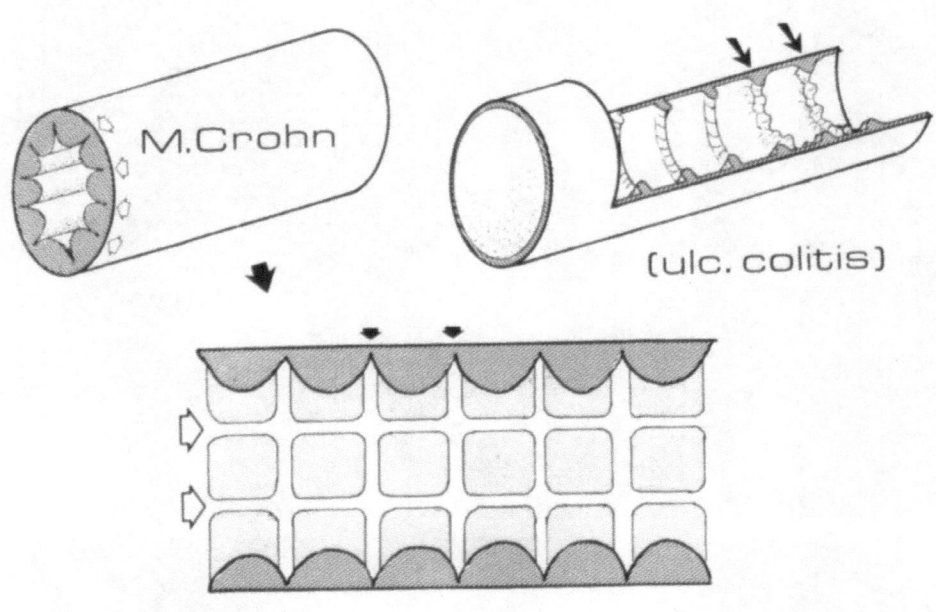

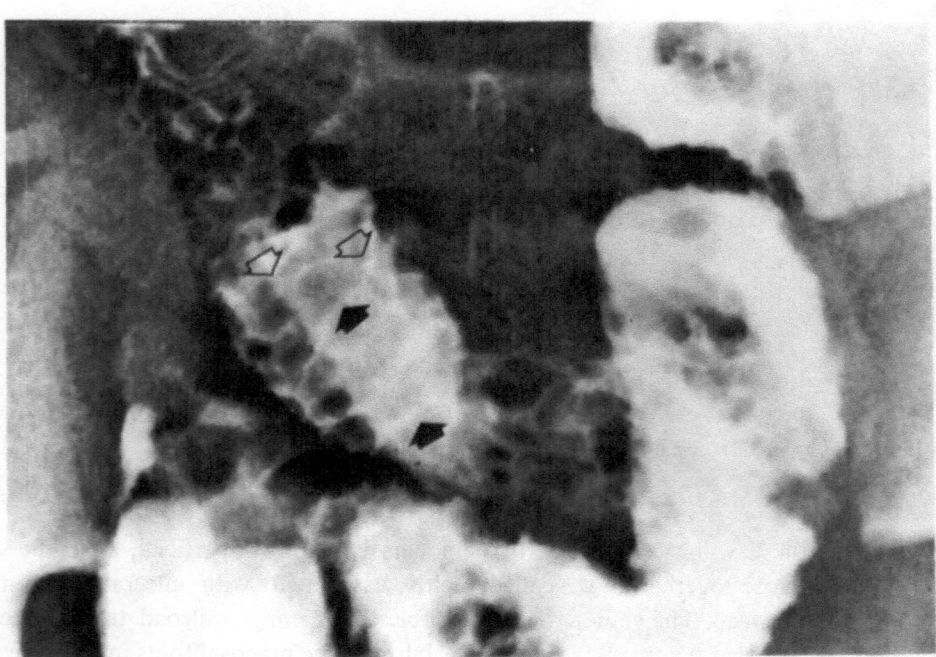

*Fig. 8.3*A. So-called 'trolley track' pattern in Crohn's disease. The longitudinal rails (open arrows) develop because the superficial mucosa is too spacious and must assume smaller dimensions when the mucous membrane swells (see drawing). The ties (solid arrows) are formed by the narrow grooves between the markedly swollen mucosal folds. Between rails and ties is a regular cushion-like pattern (cobblestones).

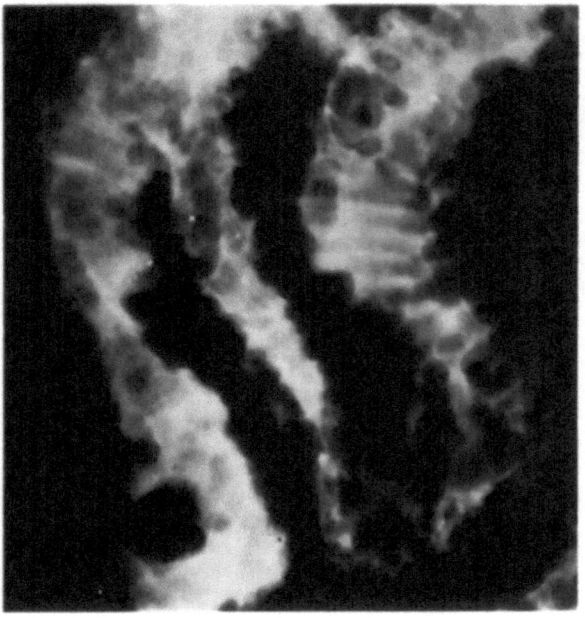

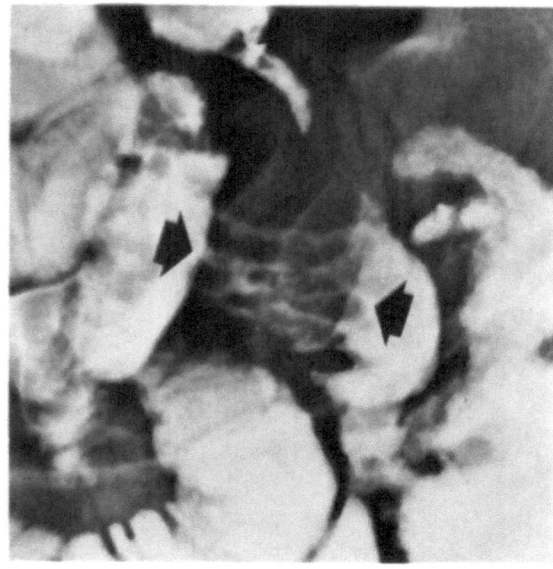

*Fig. 8.3*B. So-called cobblestone relief in Crohn's disease caused by longitudinal and transverse grooves in the edematous swollen mucosal surface.

Fig. 8.4. Cobblestone pattern in the distal ileum as a result of periarteritis nodosa.

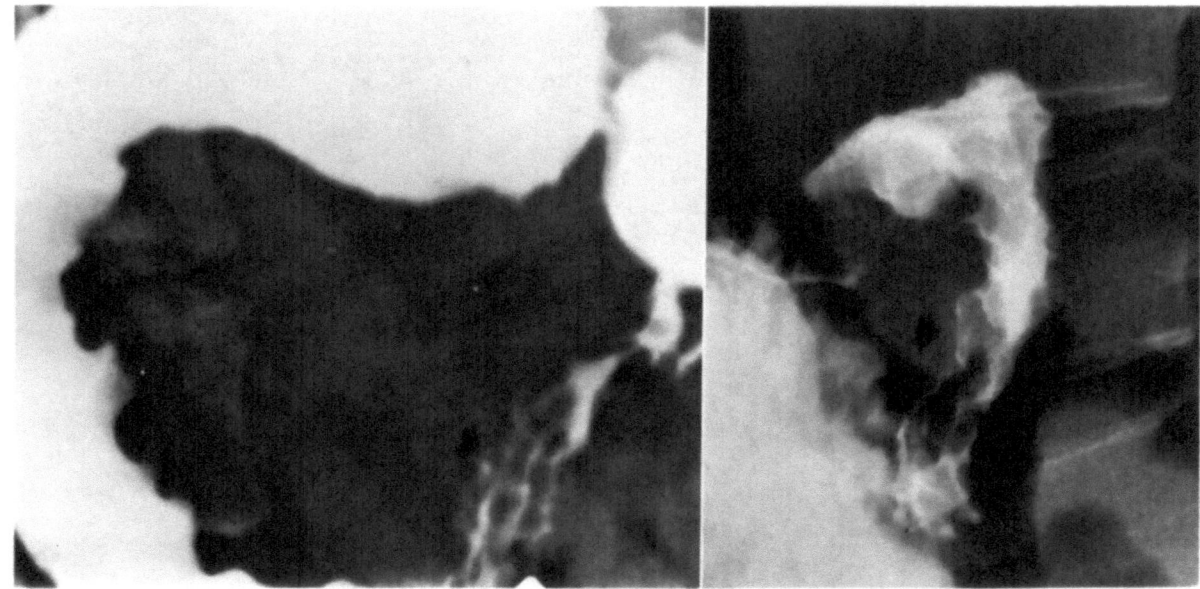

Fig. 8.5. Cobblestone pattern in the duodenum due to a lymphoreticular malignancy.

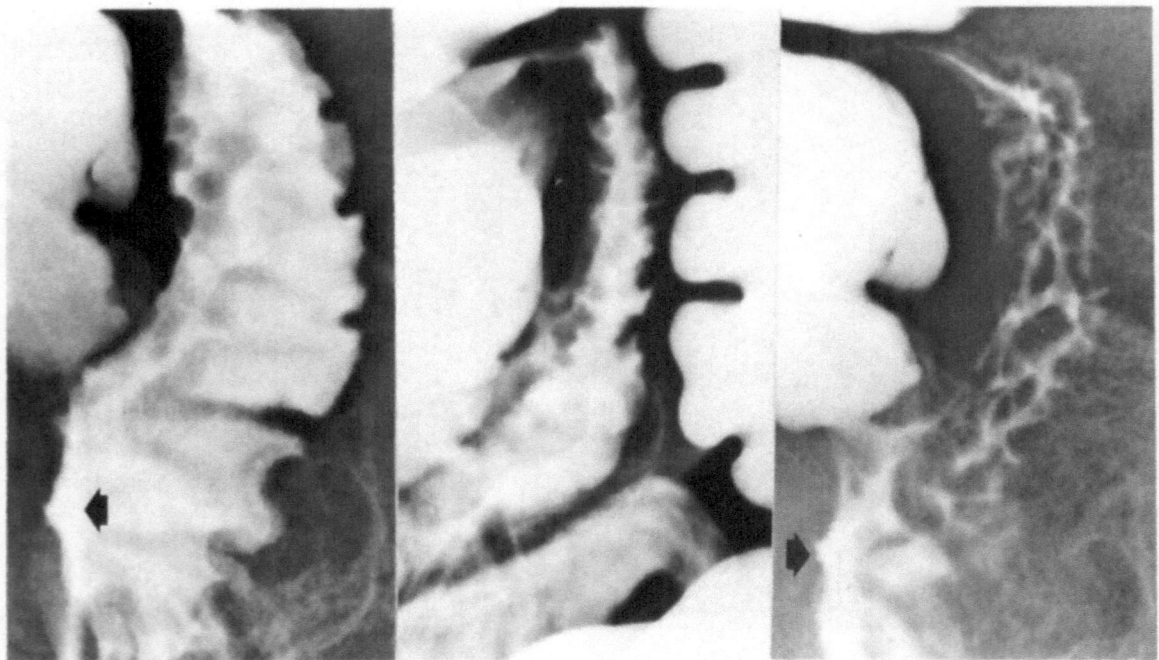

*Fig. 8.6*A. Coarse irregular mucosal relief in the distal ileum with a solitary ulcer (arrow). In this case the abnormalities are clearly visible in the well-filled as well as the empty state and are difficult to evaluate when the intestine is moderately filled. The nature of the abnormality is unknown. X-rays taken two months after removal of a healthy appendix.

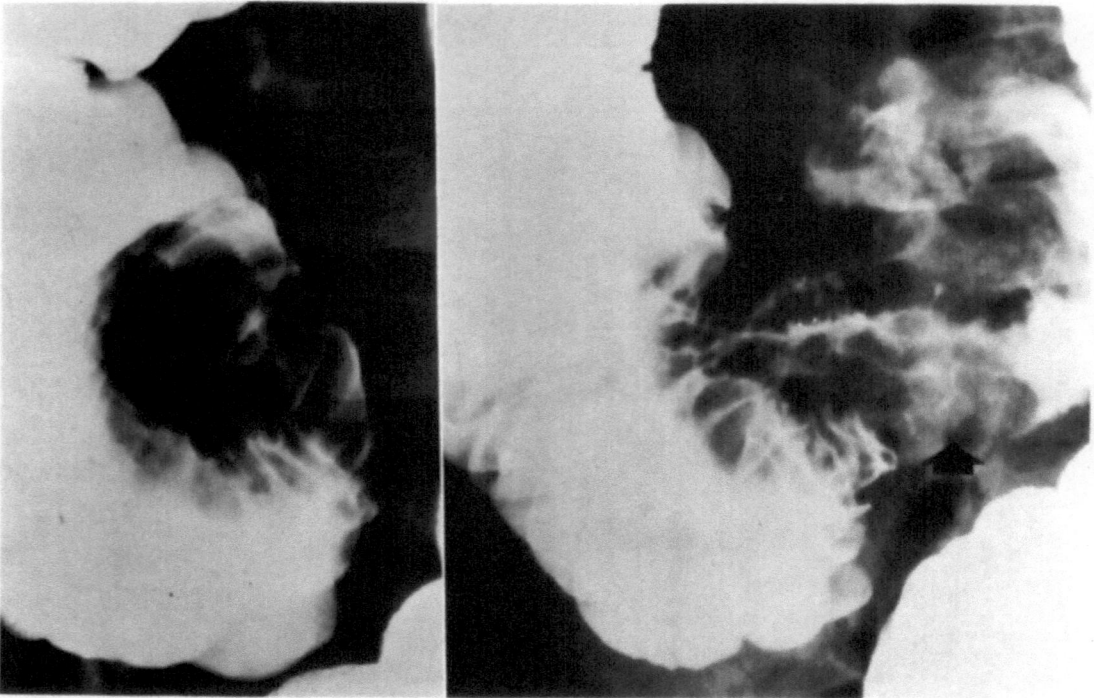

*Fig. 8.6*B. Cobblestone relief in the distal ileum and edematous swollen Bauhin's valve after repositioning of an ileocolic intussusception.

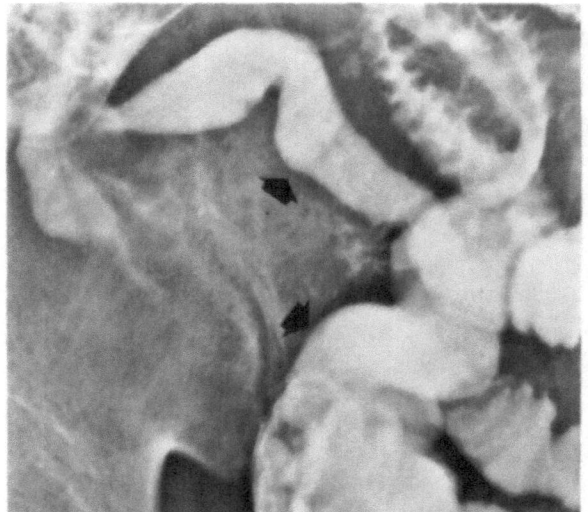
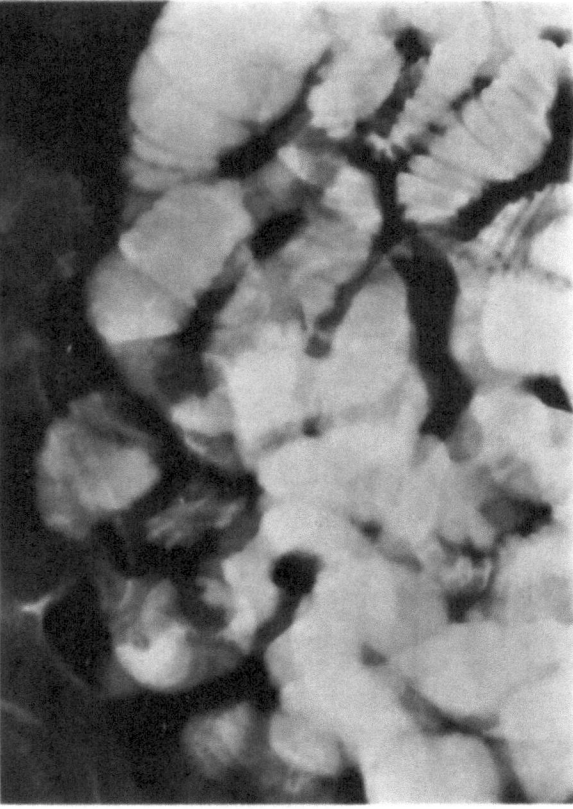

Fig. 8.7. Rigid, somewhat thickened, intestinal wall and clearly outlined smooth mucosal surface in the ileum as a result of a lymphoreticular malignancy (right), and Hodgkin's disease (left).

is therefore essential that in all cases the intestine should be visualized in various degrees of filling (fig. 8.6A).

Because the folds of Kerkring are thinner and farther apart in the ileum than in the jejunum, a slight edematous swelling of this part of the intestine may be indicated by a completely smooth intestinal wall with decreased peristaltic movements (fig. 8.7).

In lymphedema, the lymphatic channels in the mucosa and submucosa are dilated, usually because drainage is impeded somewhere in the mesentery or the paralumbar region. The cause can be congenital – the lymphatic channels in the mesentery and the extremities are then hypoplastic – or it may result from an inflammatory process, tumor growth, or irradiation fibrosis. The space between two adjacent intestinal loops increases slightly as a result of the edematous swelling of the intestinal wall; the lumen is usually somewhat dilated. The mucosal folds become thicker and shorter; the space in between clearly decreases. As a result the mucosal surface in the jejunum can even appear spiculated and may be compared with a coarsely toothed saw (fig. 8.8). When there is lymphedema, the swollen intestine appears somewhat stiff and tube-like; on the x-rays as well as under fluoroscopy it is obvious that the contractions are impeded and less frequent. Lymphedema is accompanied by considerable leakage of serum albumin from the digestive tract. Histologically little or no inflammatory reaction is seen – in contrast, in regional enteritis the lymphatic channels are dilated and there is also an obvious inflammatory reaction.

Rigidity and reduced peristalsis, thickened mucosal folds, and larger spaces between the intestinal loops are also associated with vascular disorders of the intestinal wall. In comparison with lymphedema, however, the following radiological differ-

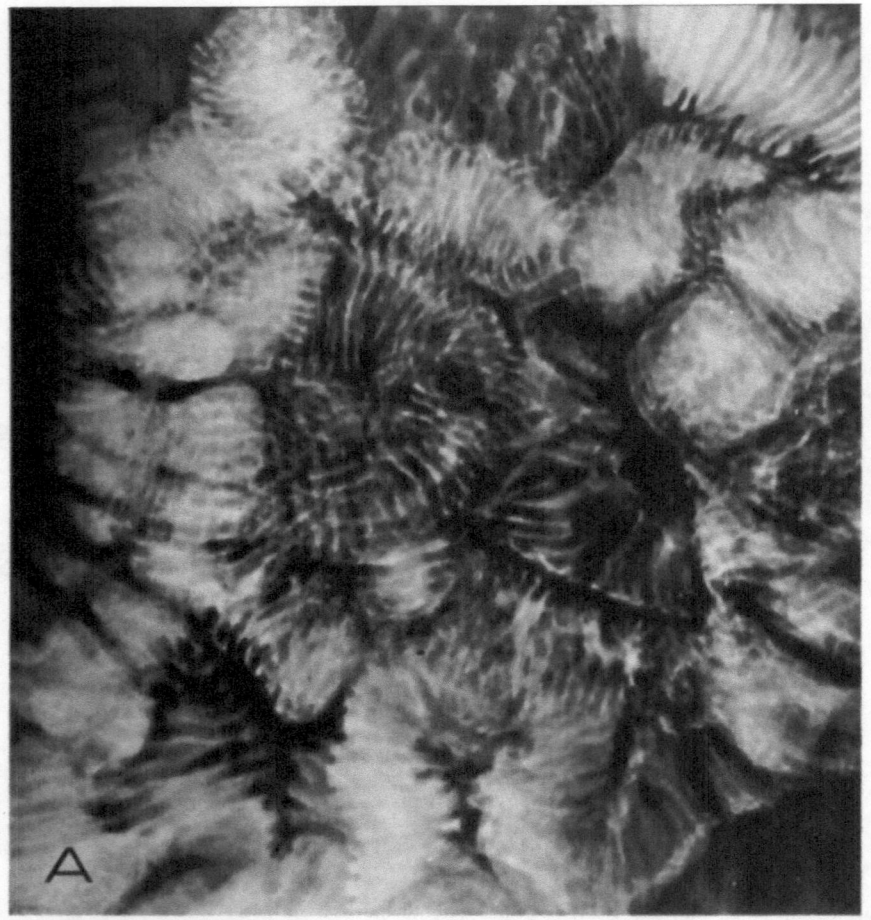

*Fig. 8.8*A. Lymphedema of a congenital origin. It may be difficult to differentiate this pattern from certain forms of celiac disease (fig. 8.62). In celiac disease, however, there is an increased motility, and if there is no hypoalbuminemia or secondary infection, then the mucosal folds are not thickened.

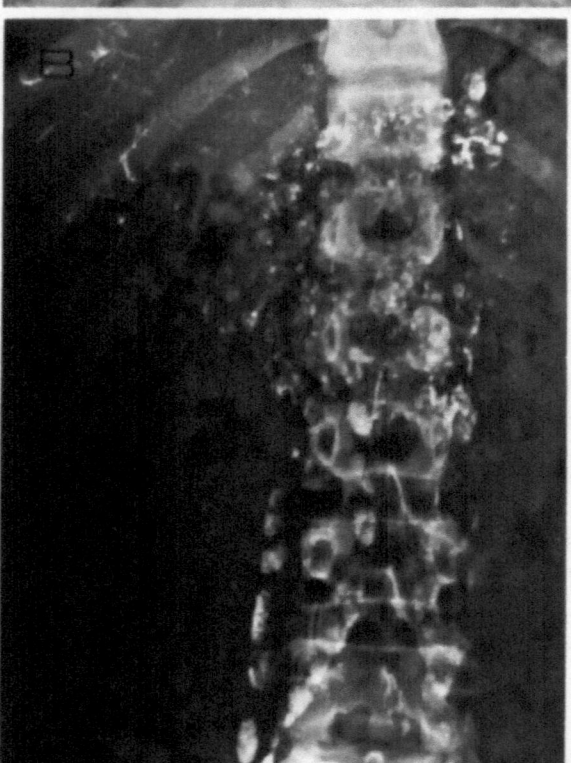

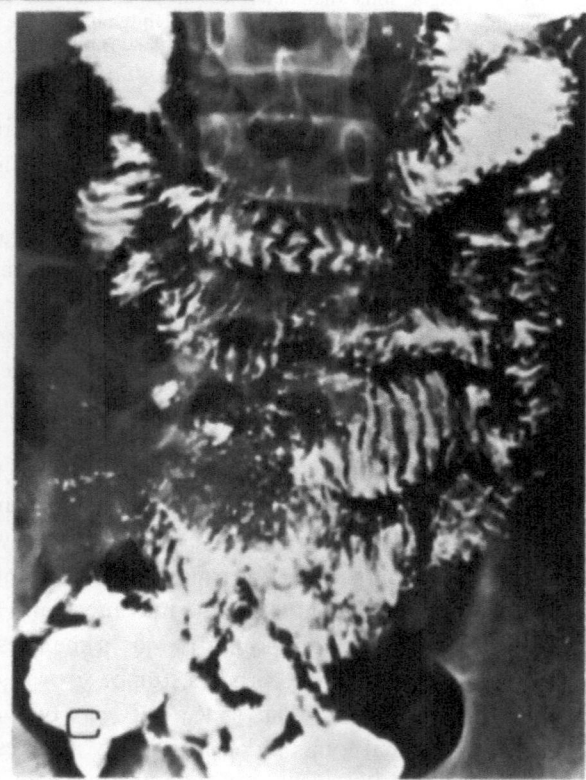

*Fig. 8.8*B. Lymphography, showing numerous collateral lymph vessels in the paralumbar region and toward the liver. There was a hypoplasia of the lymph vessels in the legs.

*Fig. 8.8*C. Conventional examination of the patient in fig. 8.8A.

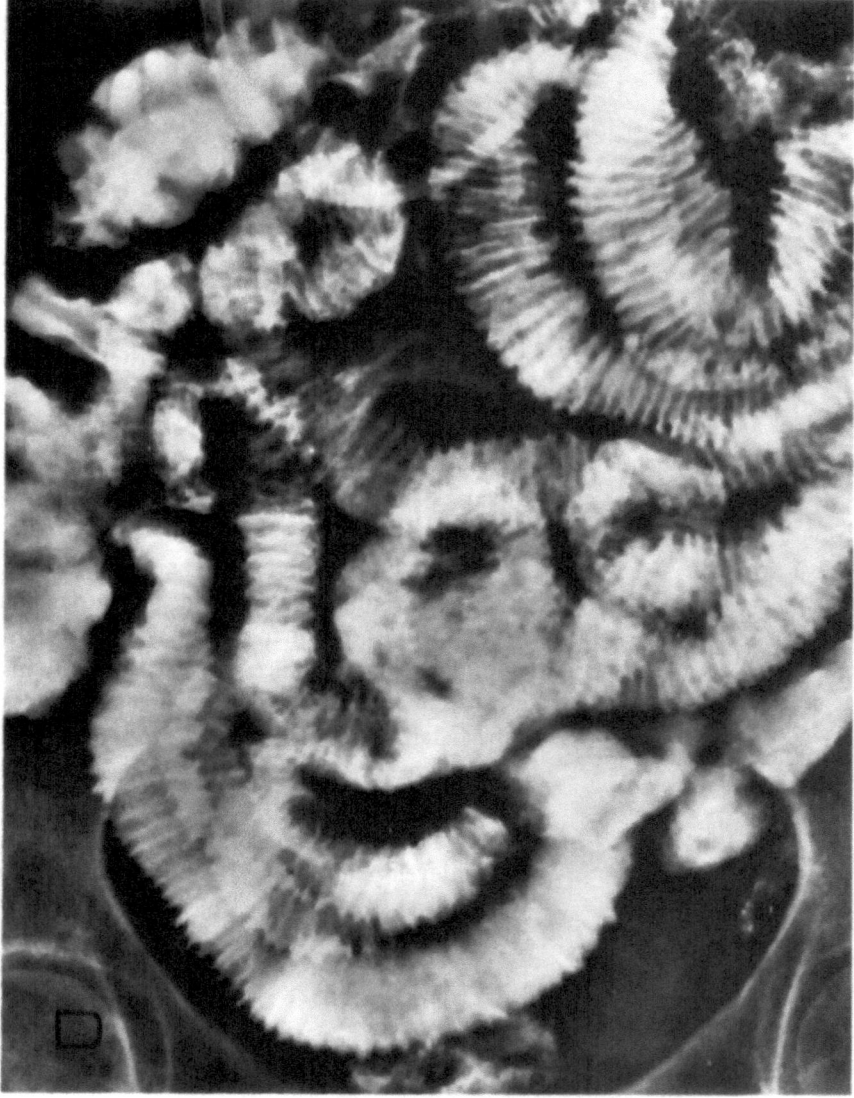

*Fig. 8.8*D. Postirradiation lymphedema. Because this edema has developed in a much shorter time than a congenital lymphedema, the mucosal folds are thicker, the wall of the intestine is more rigid, and therefore there is less peristaltic activity.

ences are found:

1) Thickening of the folds is as a rule much more prominent, the spaces between the folds are smaller and very pointed, and the folds are wider so that the coarse sawtooth effect is even more pronounced than in lymphedema (fig. 8.9D), which develops more gradually.

2) Because multiple hematomas are found in the mucosa, the swollen fold relief often appears highly irregular; in addition, multiple swellings that bulge out into the intestinal lumen may be visible (fig. 8.9E).

3) The intestinal wall may be markedly thicker than in lymphedema so that the spaces between the loops appear on the x-ray to be larger and, as a result of the hematomas, can very greatly in shape and size.

4) The intestinal lumen is often narrower instead of dilated.

5) In contrast to lymphedema, a vascular accident and celiac disease (fig. 8.9F) affect only a restricted segment of the intestine varying in length from 25 to 50 cm.

6) As a result of inflammatory phenomena in necrotic tissue, the mucosa can show superficial ulcerations (fig. 8.10) and the intestinal wall may contain gas (fig. 8.11P). It is obvious that these gas accumulations will often have ragged contours in contrast to the misleading patterns of

130

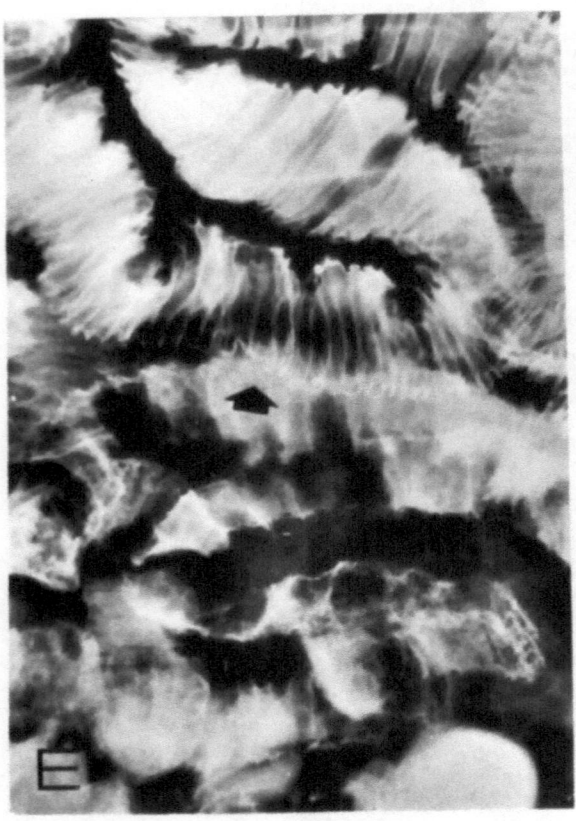

Fig. 8.8ᴇ. Pronounced edema and clearly thickened wall of the intestine in a case of lymphoreticular malignancy.

gas sometimes seen (fig. 8.11ǫ). Moreover, if the gas pattern is misleading, the adjacent mucosal folds appear quite normal.

1.2. Atrophy

Atrophy of the mucosal folds is a common, although somewhat incorrect, term used in all those cases when the fold relief has partly or completely disappeared, leaving a more or less smooth intestinal wall. Most cases, however, do not involve a true atrophy but instead a destruction of the mucosal surface as a result of an inflammatory process or disturbed circulation.

In the ileum where the folds are thinner, shorter, and also less numerous than in the jejunum, such a process will lead sooner, as well as more often, to a smooth mucosal surface than in the jejunum. The most frequent cause of a smooth ileal wall is a very superficial 'reflux ileitis' (fig. 8.12ꜰ) in conjunction with an ulcerative colitis. In those cases of Crohn's disease whereby the inflammatory process is fairly superficial, a completely smooth wall can sometimes develop in the small intestine after several years (pages 9 and 217). These patients often also

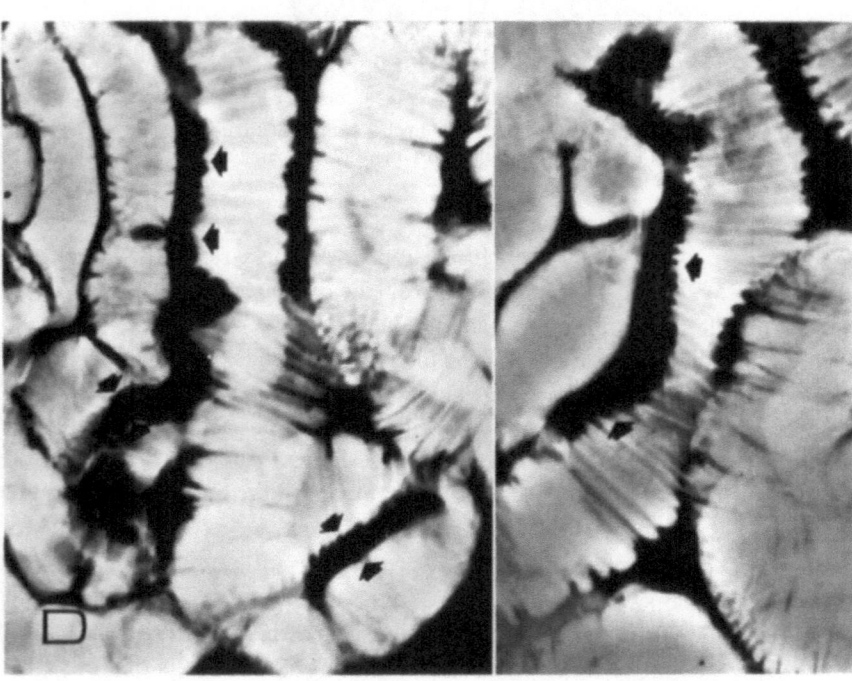

Fig. 8.9ᴅ. Exceedingly swollen mucosal folds in the jejunum as a result of ischemia. Pronounced swelling of the intestinal wall.

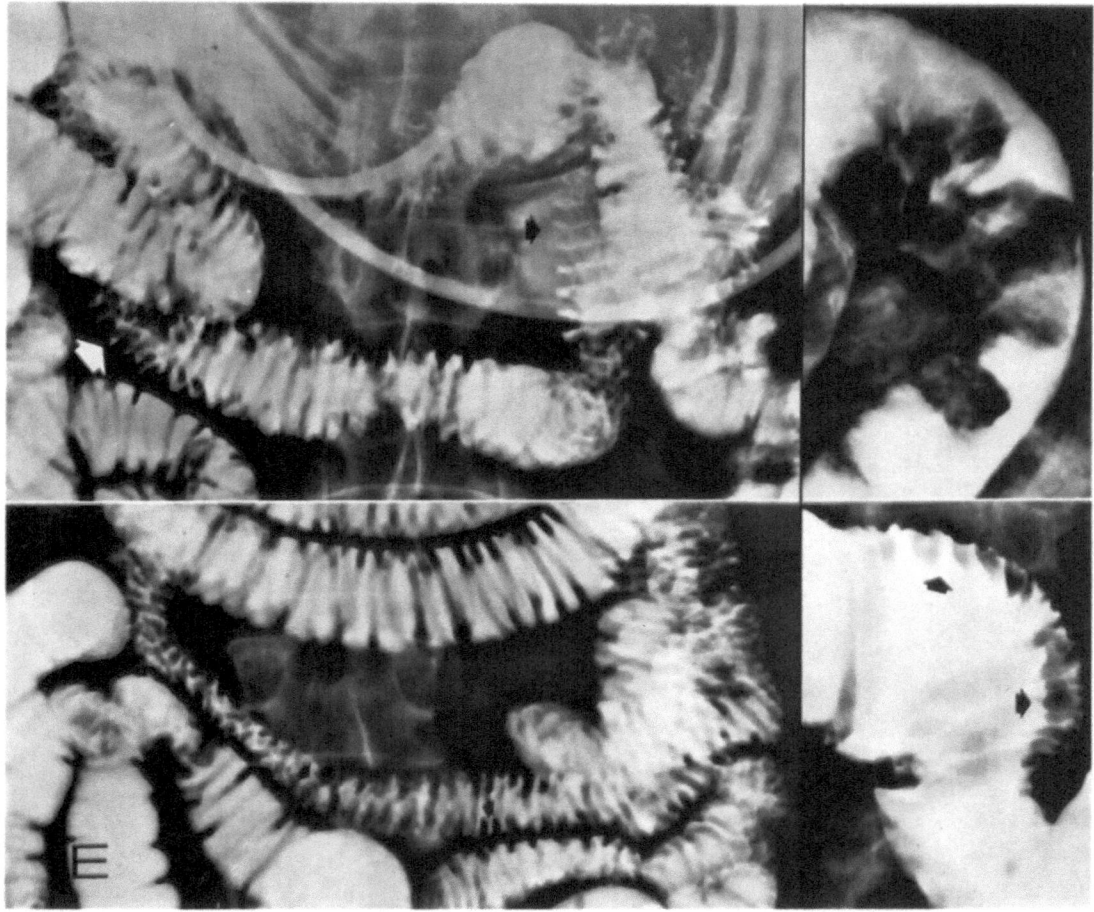

Fig. 8.9E. When anticoagulant therapy is too drastic, mucosal bleeding can cause very thick mucosal folds (left) and multiple swellings that bulge out into the intestinal lumen (right).

show abnormalities due to Crohn's disease in the cecum or throughout the entire colon so that differentiation from a cured ulcerative colitis can cause considerable difficulty. However, in Crohn's disease the segment of atrophied ileum is often significantly longer than in ulcerative colitis (fig. 8.12G). A moderate anoxia of the intestinal wall, for example as a result of a diffuse vasculitis or after irradiation, can also lead to abnormalities of the same nature. In the ileocecal region this is particularly difficult to differentiate from Crohn's disease (fig. 11.1AB, page 322). If the entire colon or mainly the right half of the colon and a large or small segment of the adjacent ileum are atrophied, this can also be caused by prolonged intoxication from certain laxatives (fig. 8.12H). It is strange that the cecum in these patients is dilated rather than

shriveled as in the cases mentioned above. When the abnormalities described here are observed, it is essential that a history be taken with care. Finally the mucosal folds can disappear when the circulation is disturbed due to a functional disturbance or a diffuse process in the intestinal wall, such as for instance in amyloidosis or a superficial lymphoreticular malignancy. In lymphoma, the intestinal wall is obviously thickened; in amyloidosis, this thickness may vary greatly and the colon may also be involved.

It is a worldwide misconception that longitudinal folds in an intestinal segment are indicative of normal mucosal relief. This is true only when these folds develop during the contraction phase. The lumen then decreases and the circular folds disappear as the longitudinal muscles relax. As soon as

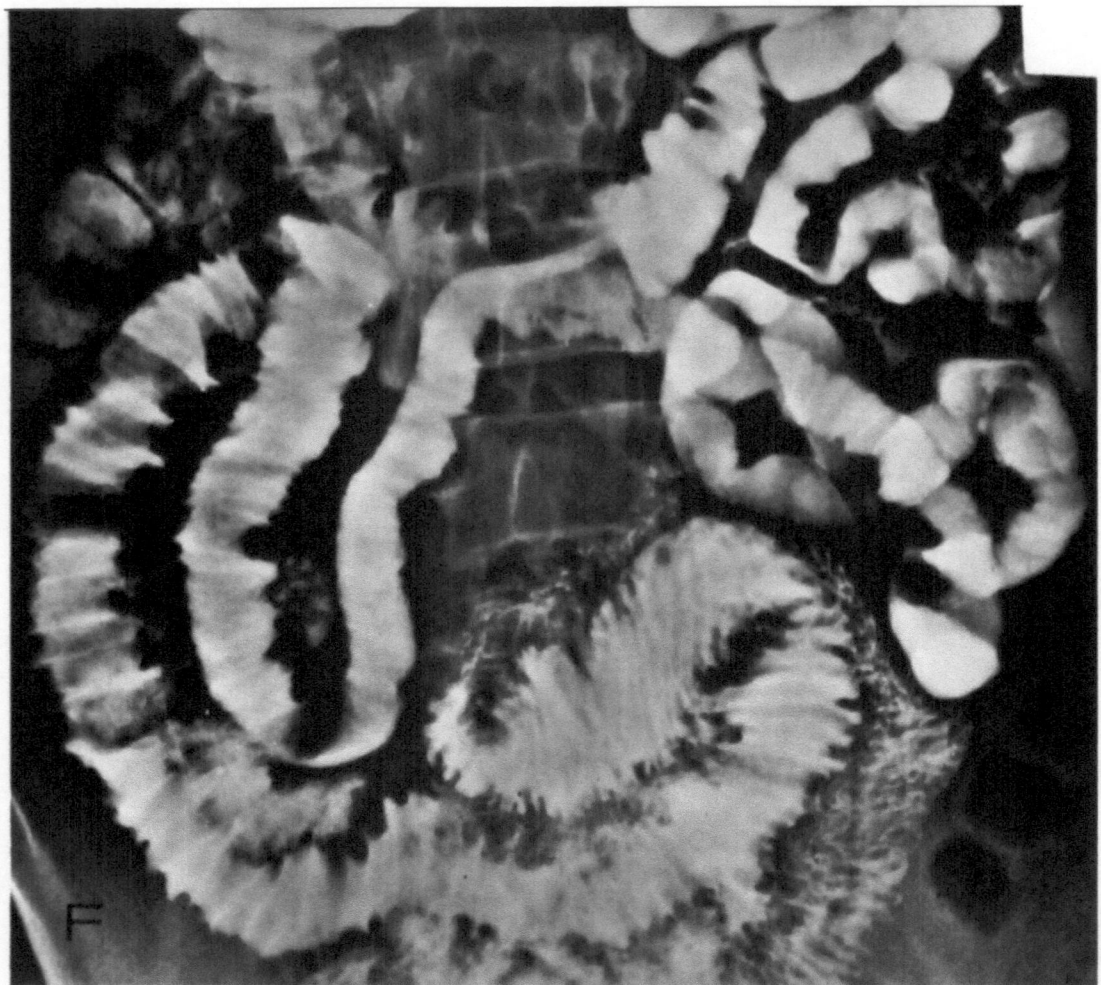

Fig. 8.9F. Broad mucosal folds in celiac disease and thickened intestinal wall due to a concomitant paratyphoid infection.

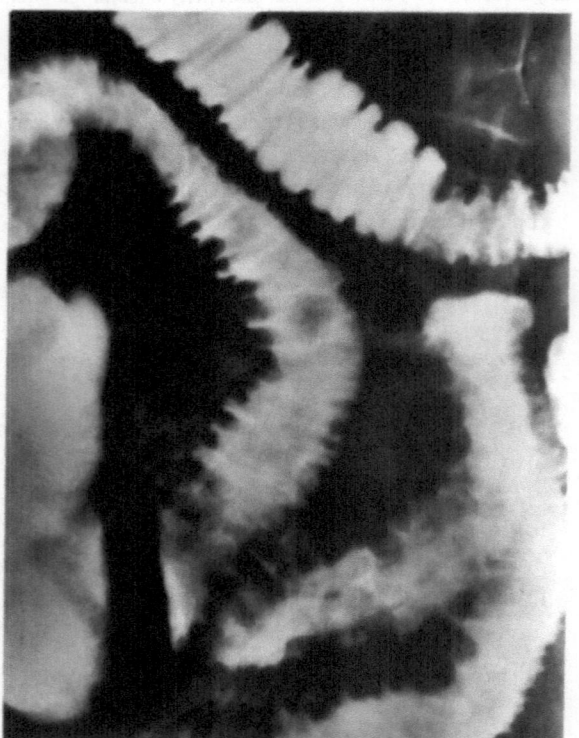

the contraction phase has passed, the circular muscles relax and the longitudinal muscles regain their tone so that the folds of Kerkring are once again clearly visible. When the intestinal lumen is dilated, contraction does not take place and therefore circular folds are never seen; when the segment is well filled, the contrast column will be completely smooth without wrinkles (fig. 2.9B, page 9). In general in these cases there is not only a loss of mucosal relief but also of tone in the longitudinal and possibly also the circular muscles.

In the event of atrophy of the mucosal folds in the jejunum it is noted that they first become shorter and that the transition to the intestinal wall has become more rounded. A rare case of atrophy of the mucosal folds in the duodenum and proximal jejunum is shown in fig. 8.13A. Many years ago this patient underwent irradiation of keloids in the skin

← *Fig. 8.10.* Swollen mucosal folds, thickened intestinal wall, and superficial ulcerations in radiation enteritis.

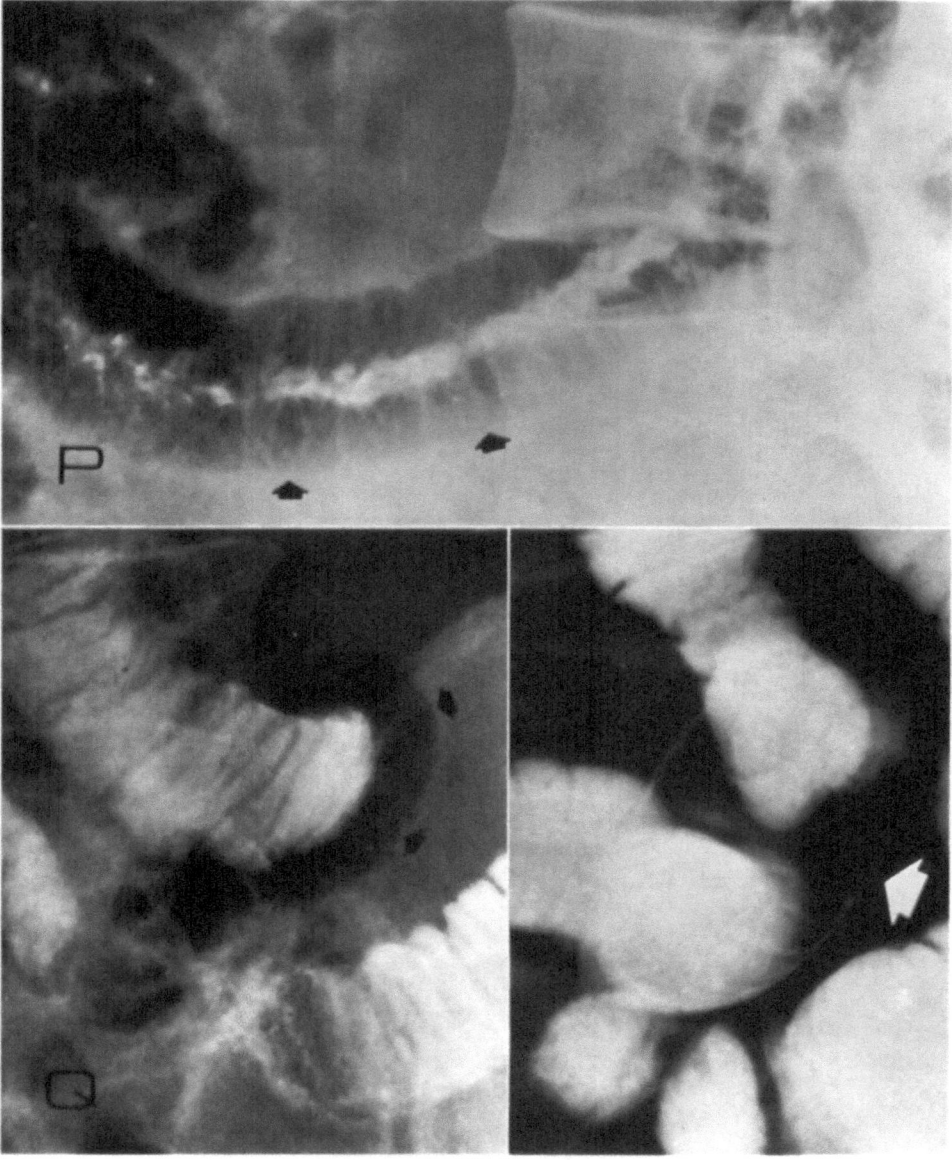

Fig. 8.11. (P) Gas in the intestinal wall due to necrosis in a case of thrombosis of the superior mesenteric vein. The contours of these gas configurations are often ragged. (Q) Misleading pattern of gas in the small intestine with sharply defined margins.

overlying this fixed duodenal loop. The other loops in this region are sufficiently mobile so that they are much less likely to be affected by radiation. Similarly the distal ileal loops in the minor pelvis, which are often also fixed in position, are more susceptible to the hazards of radiation than the more mobile proximal ileal loops. In celiac disease (see chapter 12), there is no dilatation of that part of the jejunum containing the atrophied folds; furthermore, the distance between the folds increases (fig. 8.13B). If there are no complications, then this superficial obliteration of the folds or true atrophy is not accompanied by thickening of the intestinal wall. A

thickened intestinal wall can, however, be seen in amyloidosis whereby the folds in the jejunum become highly irregular due to the numerous deposits. In other cases the mucosal folds are only broadened and flatter and assume a more or less undulating course (fig. 8.14).

1.3. Abnormal course

When otherwise completely healthy mucosal folds enclose a triangular plateau without fold relief, then this can be caused only by a triple junction in the small intestine. This must be the omphalomesenteric duct – even if the large or small sack-like mouth of

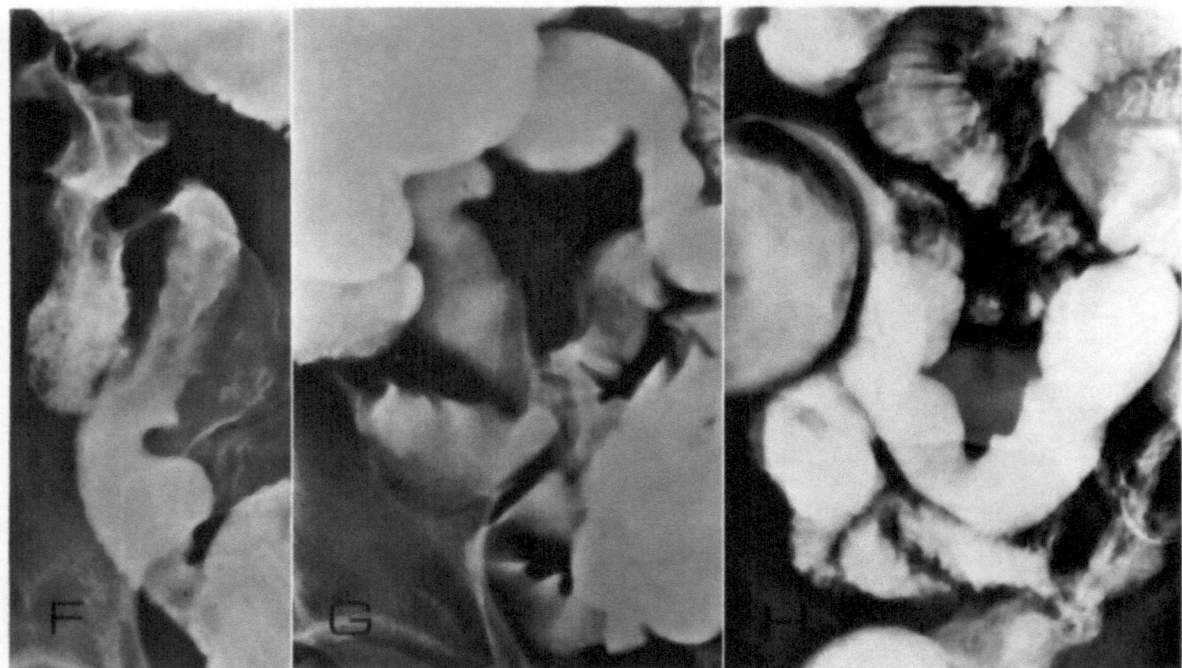

Fig. 8.12. (F) Colitis with reflux ileitis. That segment of the ileum containing the atrophied mucosa is usually only about 15 cm long. (G) Smooth mucosal surface in the ileum and cecum 30 years after Crohn's disease in the ileocecal region was cured. (H) Quite pronounced atrophy of the mucosa in the ileocecal region as a result of the chronic use of drugs. The cecum is highly dilated, which is not the case after an ileocolitis.

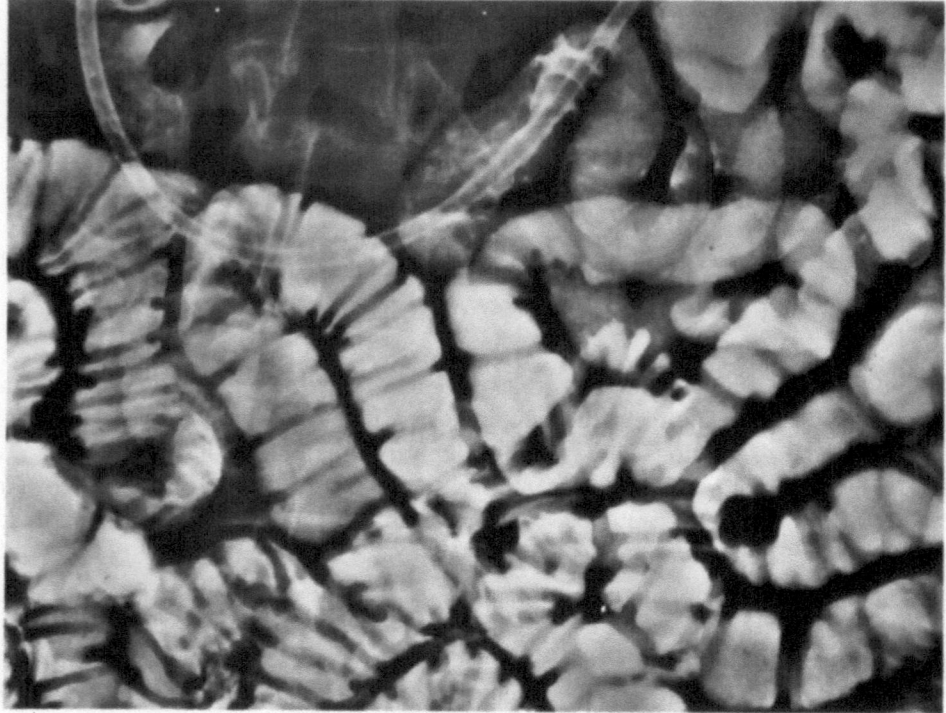

*Fig. 8.13*B. Atrophy of the mucosal folds in the jejunum in celiac disease. The folds are shorter than normal and are farther apart; the transition from fold to intestinal wall is more rounded than normal. Broadening of the folds and thickening of the wall of the intestine are probably due to a hypoalbuminemia.

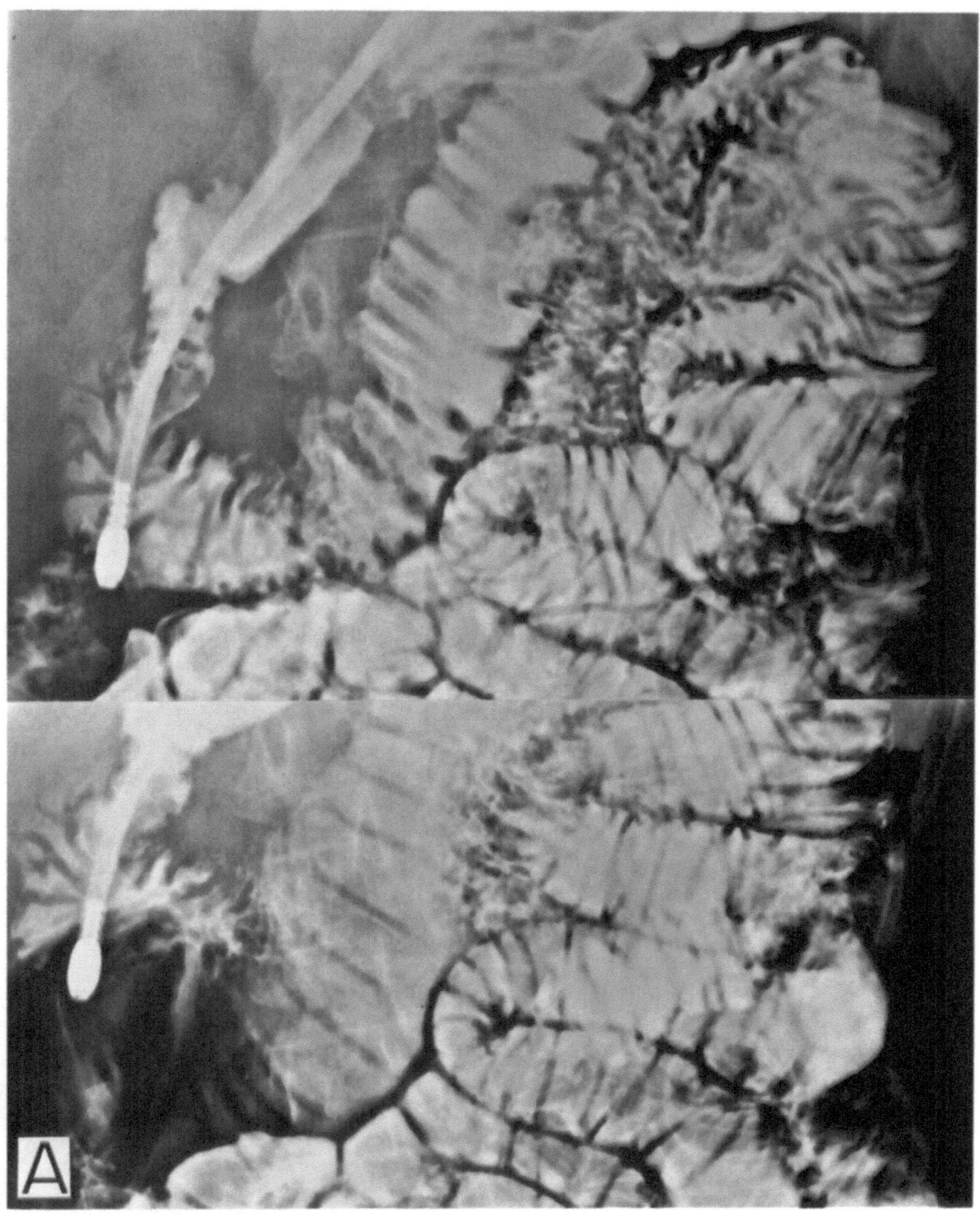

*Fig. 8.13*A. Flattened mucosal relief in the fixed duodenum as the result of irradiation of keloids in the skin above this loop many years ago. The loop is obviously wider than normally seen in patients with celiac disease and no abnormalities were demonstrated in the rest of the small bowel.

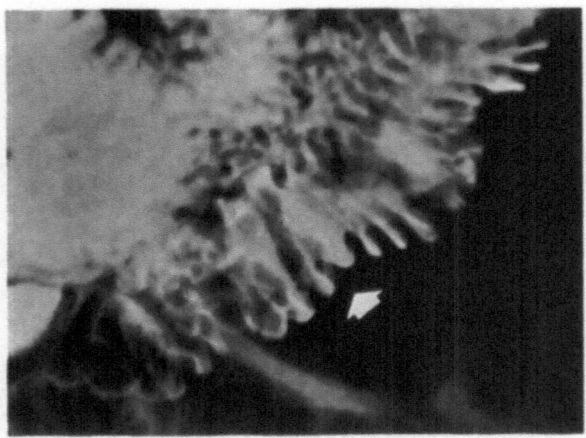

Fig. 8.14. Slightly undulant course or broad and highly irregular folds with a marked thickening of the intestinal wall in amyloidosis.

this Meckel's diverticulum is not visible on the available exposures (fig. 8.15A). Theoretically a duplication could also cause a triple-junction configuration of the fold relief of the intestinal mucosa. It has been shown, however, that as a rule this abnormality develops as a so-called duplication cyst that causes a smoothly defined bulge into the lumen of the intestinal loop or a compression effect on the outside. We have also never seen a triple plateau between the mucosal folds at the mouth of a diverticulum (fig. 8.15B). Mucosal folds that follow an abnormal course but are otherwise intact can also be found at the site of a surgical anastomosis in the intestine. The only way to locate such a suture line – important because it is necessary to determine

whether tumor growth has recurred – is to study the loops in the well-filled state; therefore the rate of flow of the contrast medium must be maintained at about 100–150 ml/min. Since the course of the normal folds is then regular due to stretching, the somewhat confusing usual configuration at the stenosis will be clearly visible (fig. 8.16).

In a mucosal surface with ulcerations, the folds of Kerkring can completely disappear locally. When the inflammatory process is arrested by treatment, the pock-marked surface of these flat ulcers can show a fairly smooth outer zone with such a fine granular surface that it is barely or not visible on the x-rays. The mucosal folds that are still intact terminate abruptly – sometimes more or less gradually – at the plateau of the healed ulcer (fig. 8.17). Later the fibrous tissue that is formed during the healing process shrivels, thus reducing the original surface of the ulcer. The still intact mucosal folds then assume a radial course with the ulcer on one side (fig. 8.18).

One long segment of the small intestine containing irregularly broadened mucosal folds and an intestinal wall that is also irregularly thickened are indicative, if there are no signs of destruction, of deposits such as those seen in primary amyloidosis (fig. 8.14).

Local absence of mucosal folding together with an obvious thickening of the intestinal wall, recognized as a bulge in the lumen or an enlargement of the space between adjacent intestinal loops, suggests tumor growth (fig. 8.19). If the sites are

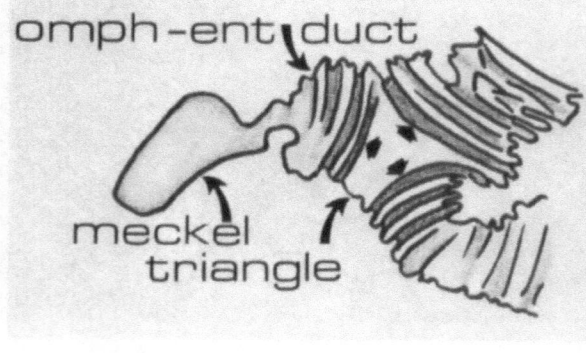

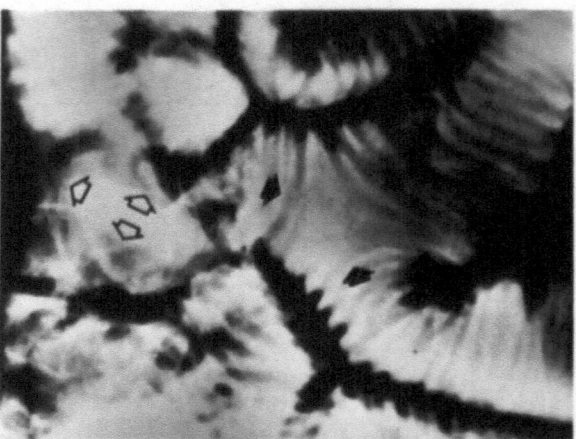

Fig. 8.15A. Triangular configuration in the mucosal pattern at the mouth of the omphalomesenteric duct (Meckel's diverticulum).

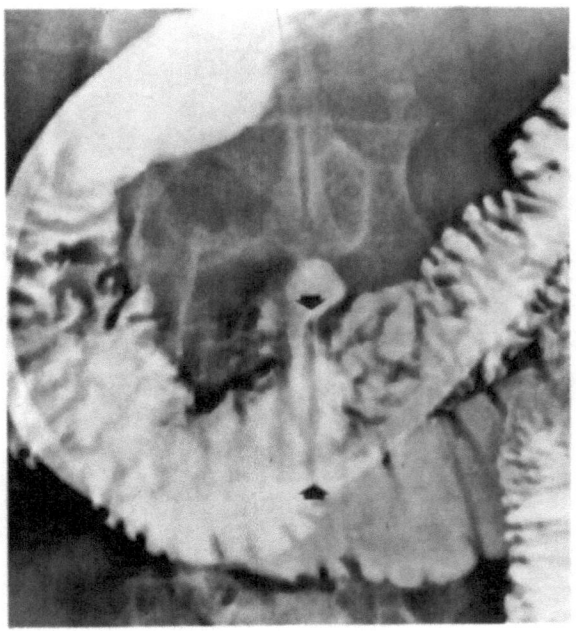

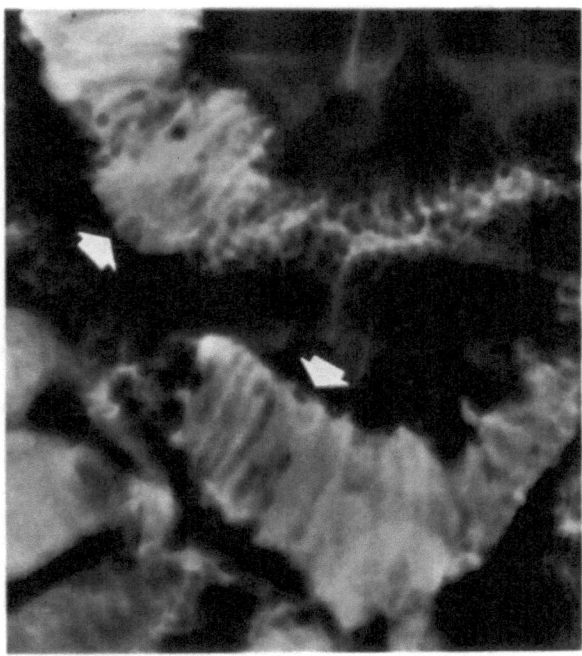

*Fig. 8.15*ʙ. Mucosal pattern at the mouth of a normal diverticulum. The mucosal folds of the intestine extend into the neck of the diverticulum (arrows).

*Fig. 8.17*ᴀ. Mucosal folds terminate abruptly at the plateau of a healed superficial ulceration in Crohn's disease.

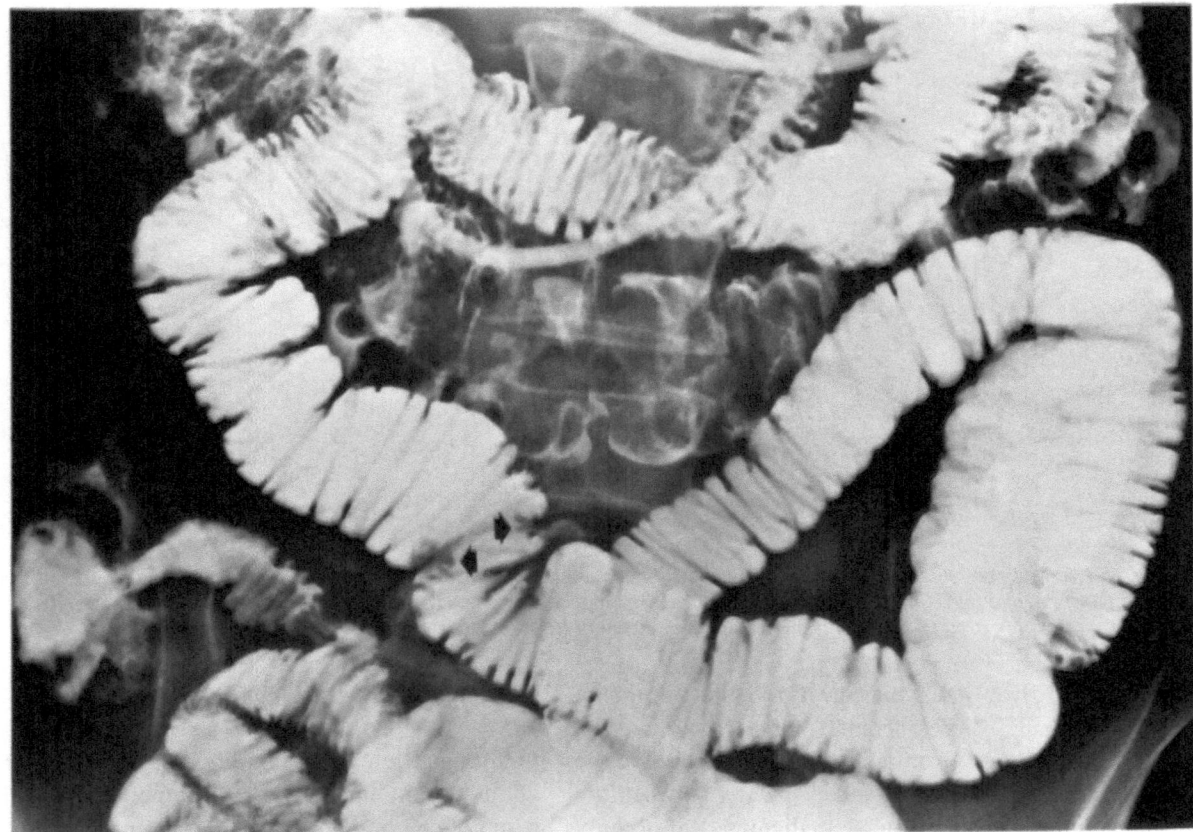

Fig. 8.16. Very local irregular but intact mucosal relief that causes a moderate stenosis at an intestinal suture line after a resection.

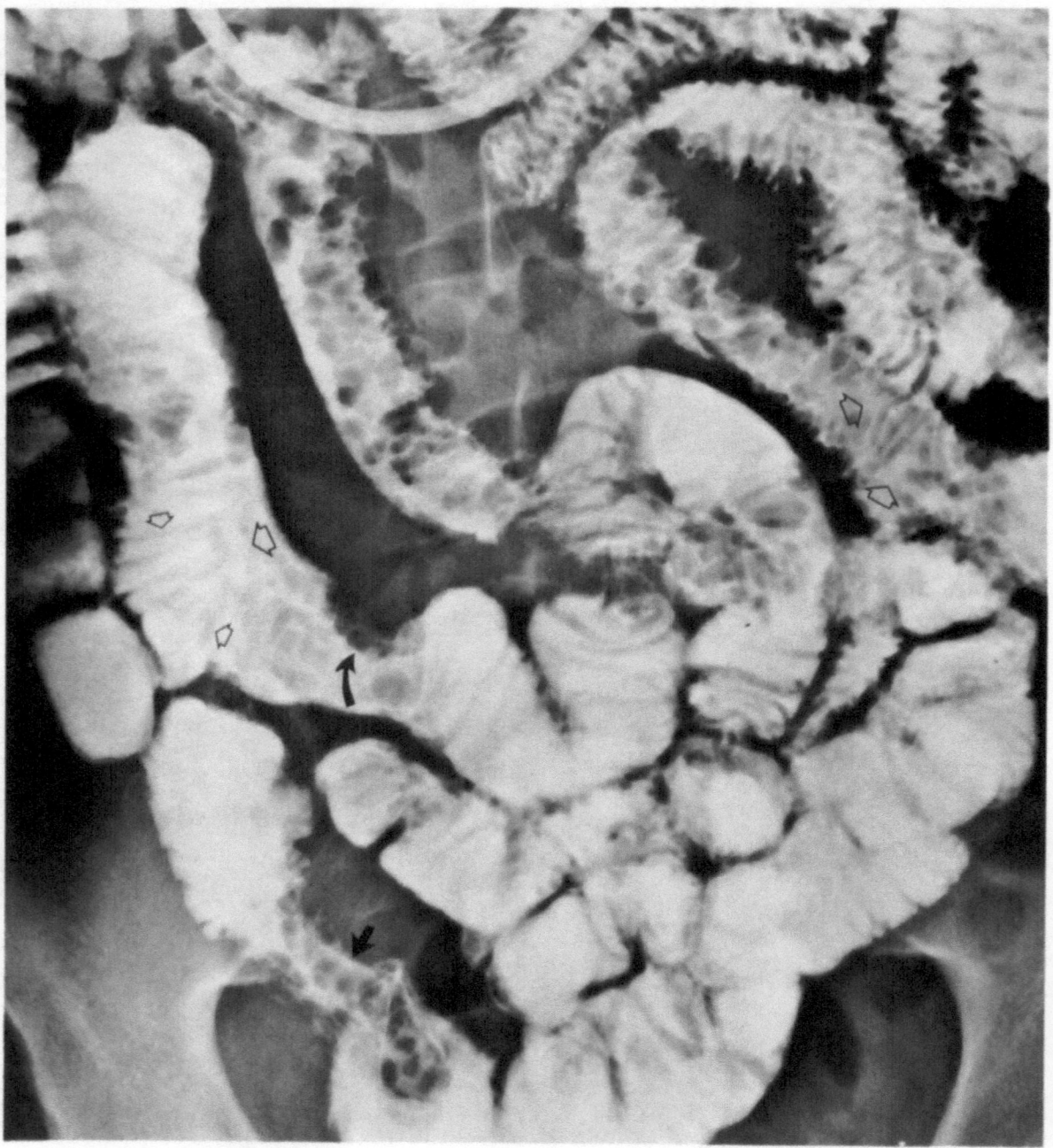

*Fig. 8.17*ʙ. Mucosal relief in Crohn's disease showing obliteration of the mucosa as a result of ulceration that is now healed (large open arrows), and folds that radiate from the old ulcer (small open arrows). A local lesion bulges out into the intestinal lumen (long solid arrow) and an ulcer extends in the longitudinal direction (short solid arrow).

multiple, then leukemia or a reticuloendothelial tumor should be considered. Total destruction of the mucosal pattern, pronounced local stretching of the folds, adhesions and irregular spacing between the intestinal loops indicate a malignant tumor only (fig. 8.20).

2. Lymph follicles – nodules – polyps

Under pathological conditions, lymph follicles about 2 mm in diameter, common in the distal ileum of children and sometimes even young adults, are also found in older adults. These occur in other

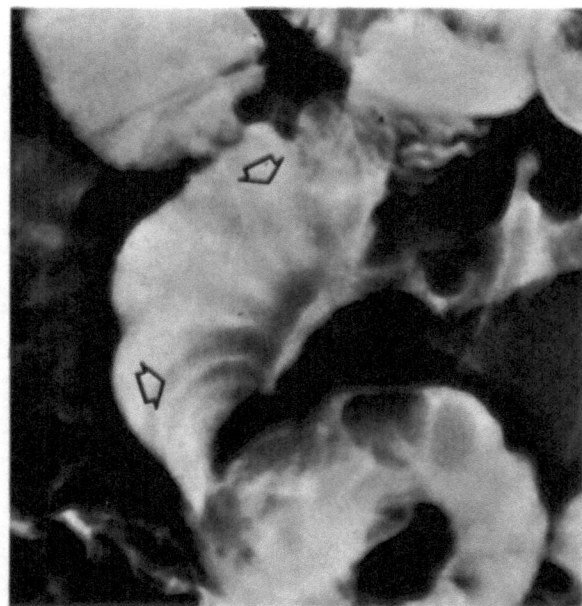

*Fig. 8.18*A. More or less concentric course of the mucosal folds is directed toward the site of the ulceration in the intestinal wall.

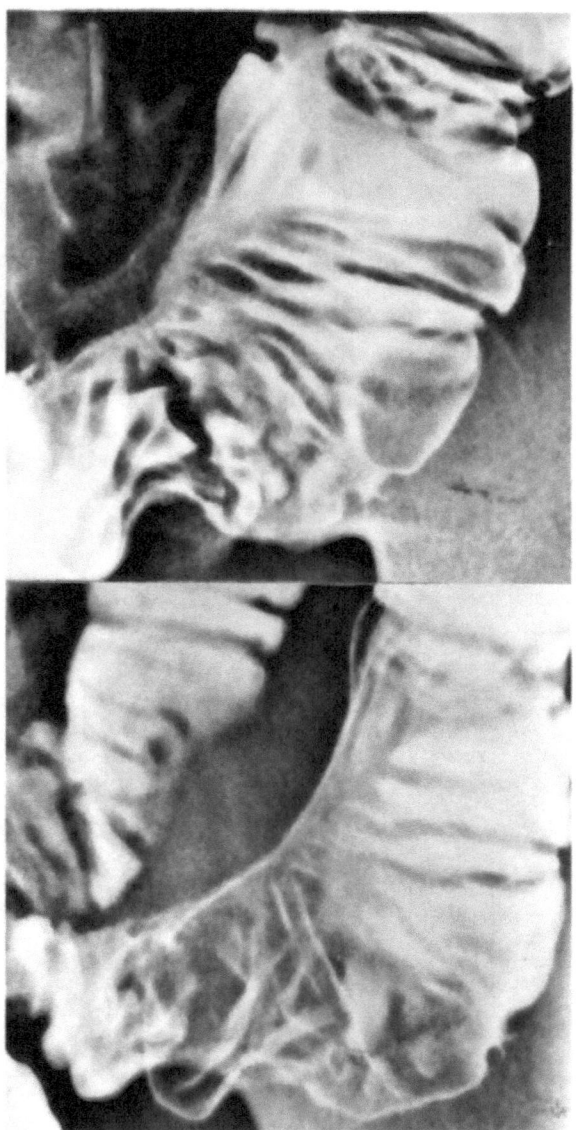

*Fig. 8.18*B. In a patient with Crohn's disease, the remnants of the mucosal folds in a proximal jejunal loop radiate slightly toward the shriveled mesenterial side where a cured ulcer must be located. On the lower exposure, some gas is visible in the intestinal loop. It can be seen clearly that the folds of the upper wall, as in the gastric examination, are visualized only as thin lines. The folds of the lower wall form dark lines 2–3 mm thick with a puddle of contrast fluid inbetween.

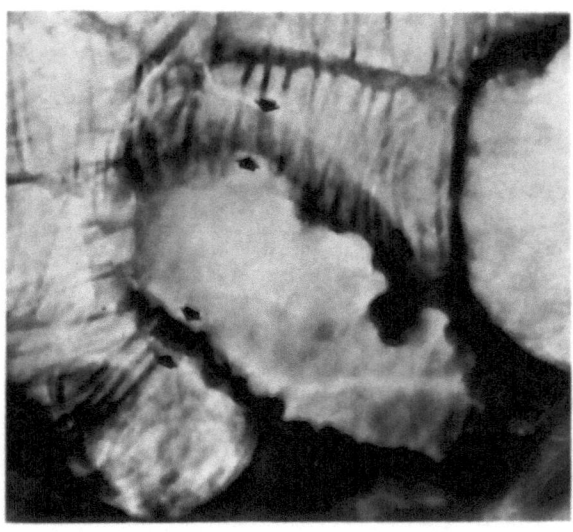

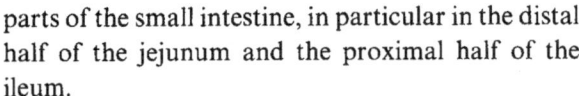

Fig. 8.19. Thickening of the intestinal wall and local absence of mucosal folds due to tumor growth.

parts of the small intestine, in particular in the distal half of the jejunum and the proximal half of the ileum.

In congenital or acquired protein synthesis disorders accompanied by an IgA or IgM deficiency, the mucous membrane in the small intestine can be covered with 1- to 3-mm hyperplastic nodular lymph follicles arising from the lamina propria (fig. 8.21). Sometimes they are also seen in the colon. Although it appears that more than half of these cases of so-called dysgammaglobulinemia are accompanied by lambliasis, the latter probably can-

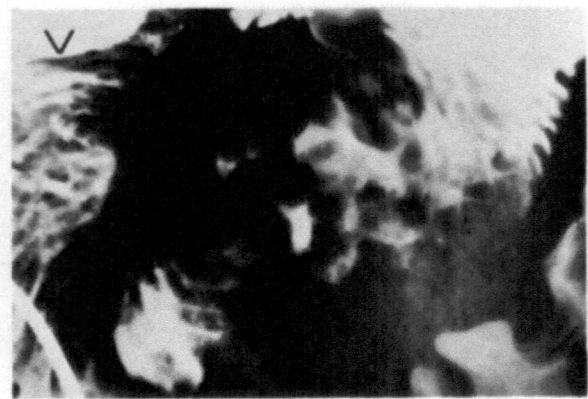

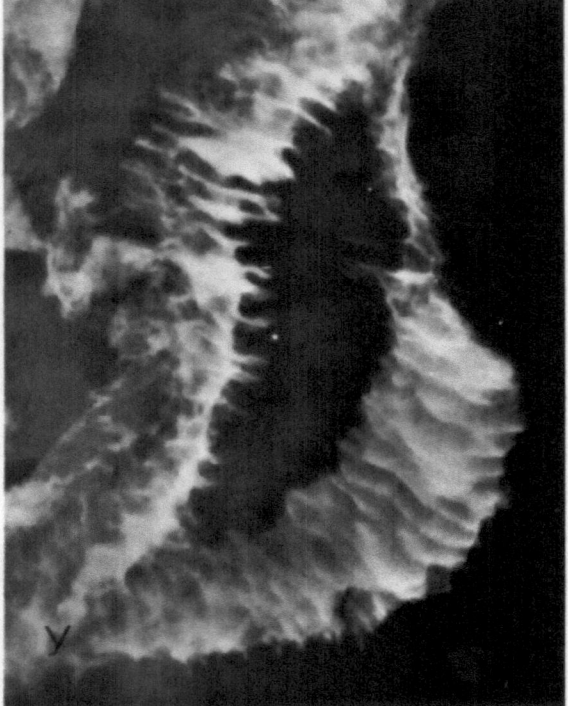

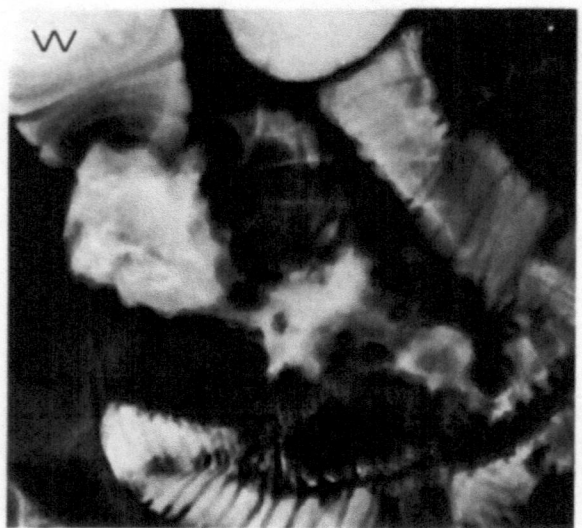

Fig. 8.20. Total destruction or completely irregular course of the mucosal folds in the event of a tumor: (v) adenocarcinoma; (w) lymphosarcoma; (x) malignant lymphoma; (Y) liposarcoma; (z) reticulum cell sarcoma.

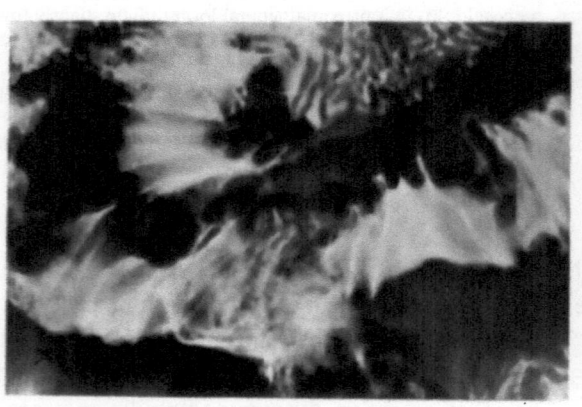

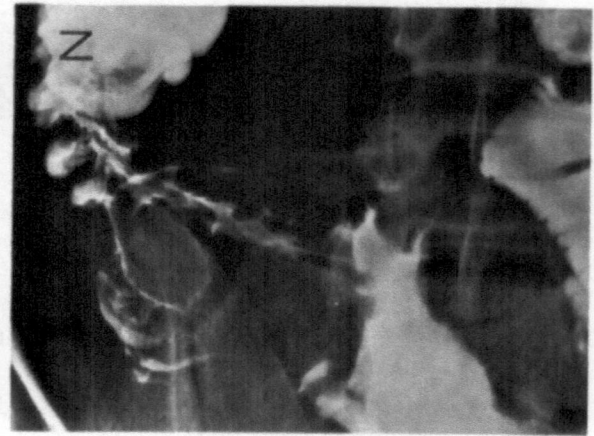

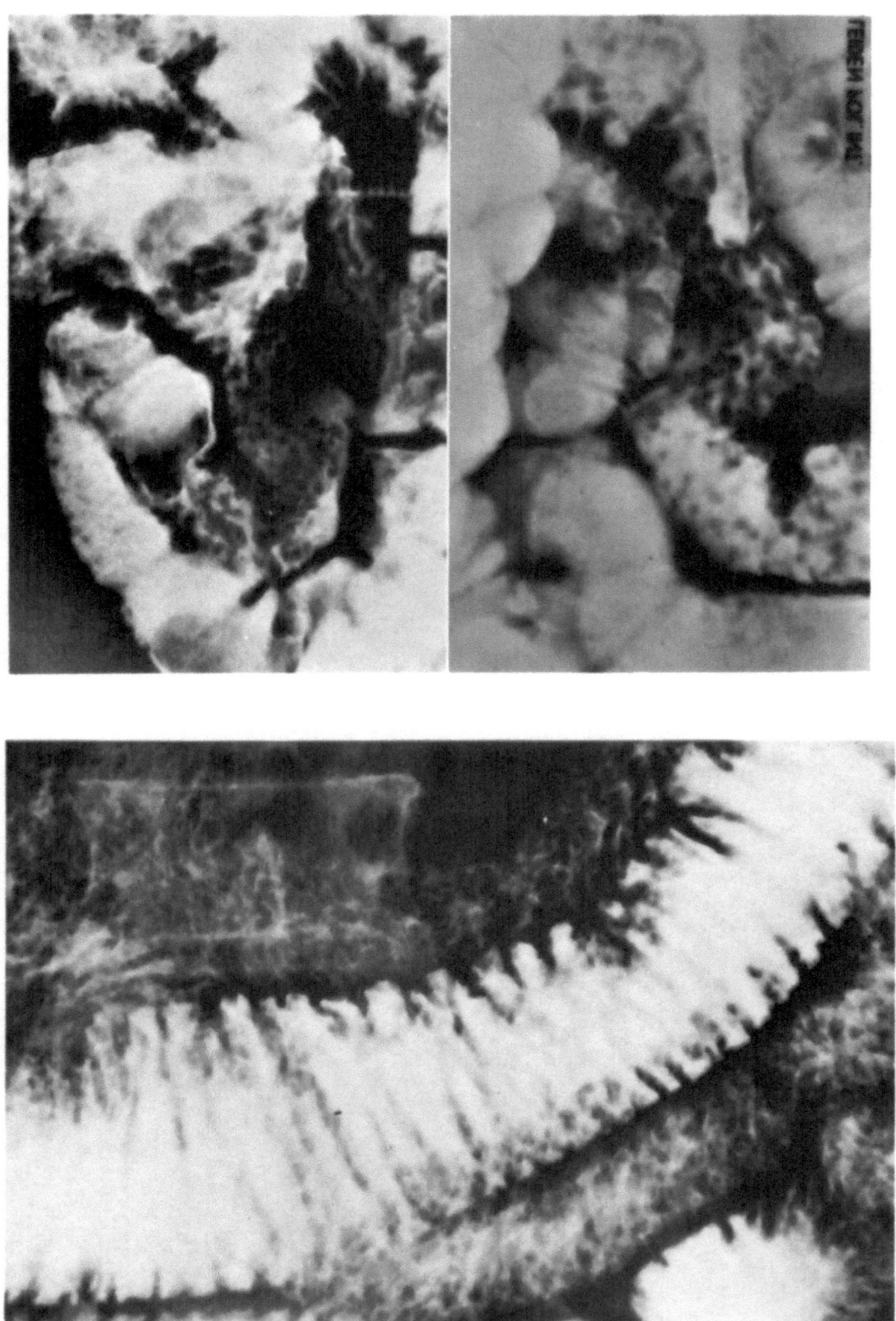

Fig. 8.21. Lymphoid nodular hyperplasia. Multiple filling defects in the contrast fluid, 1–3 mm across.

142

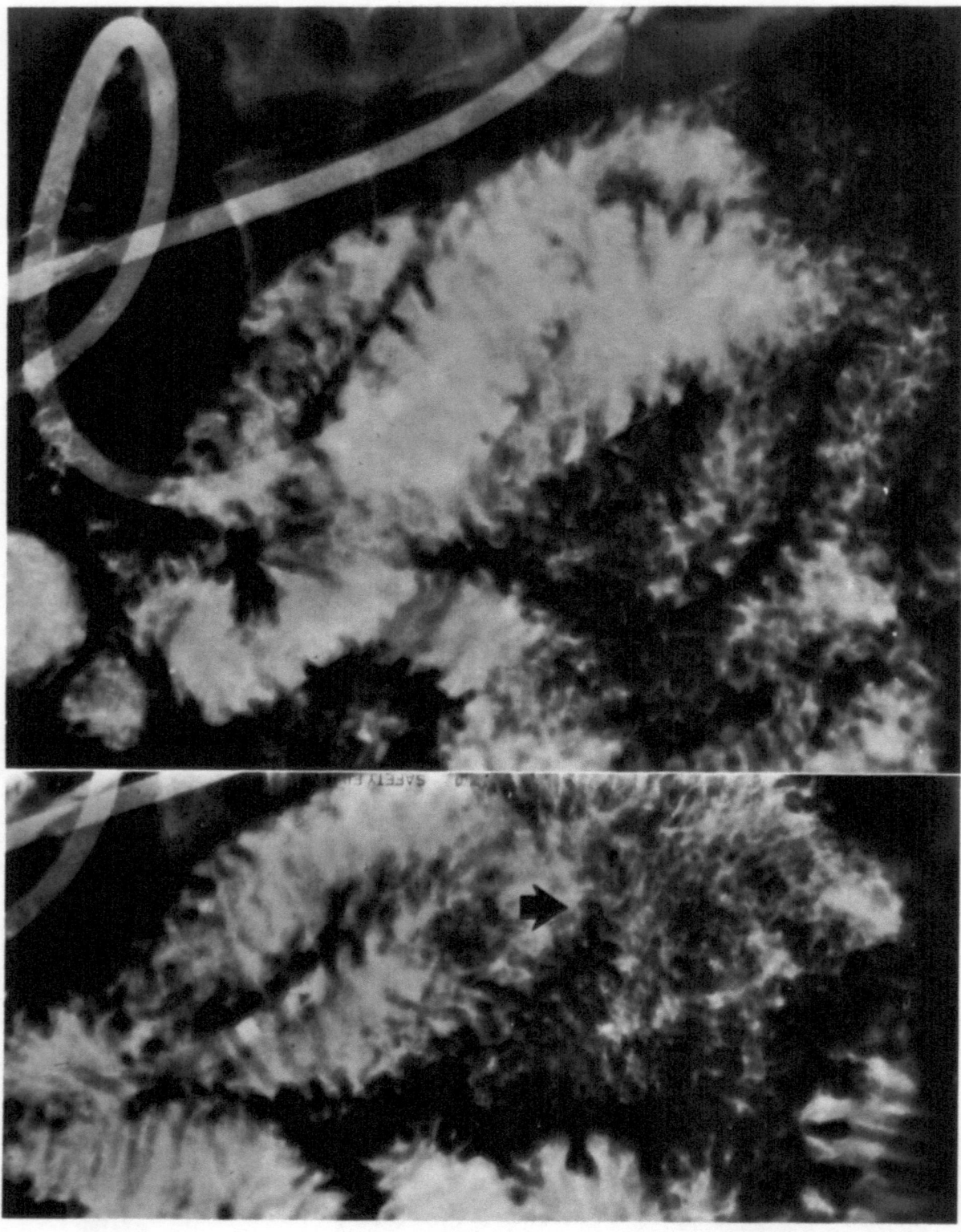

Fig. 8.22. Mucosal pattern in an irritable jejunum of a patient infected with *Giardia lamblia* (top). Rapid disintegration after 1 min (right) although 900 ml contrast fluid was administered through the tube (bottom).

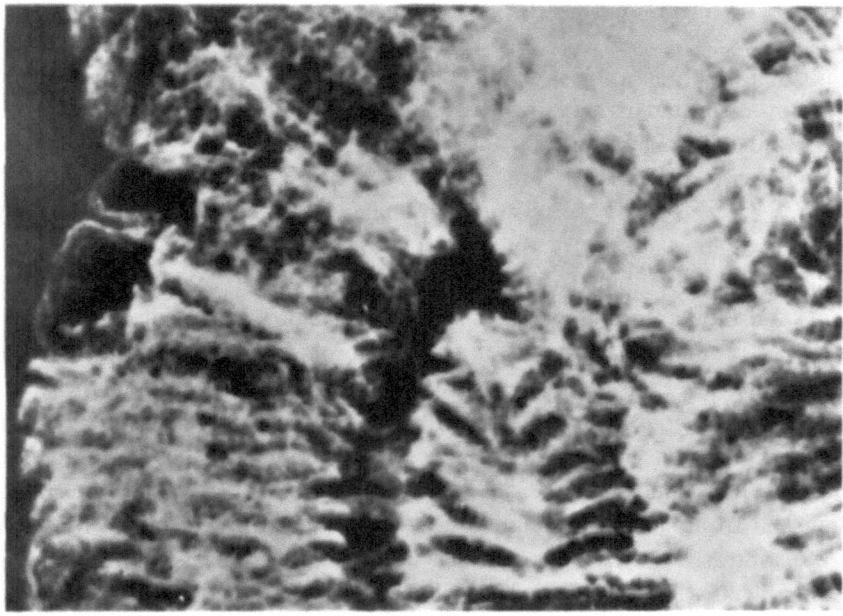

Fig. 8.23. Foamy aspect in the jejunum due to abnormal swelling of the villi in a patient with Whipple's disease.

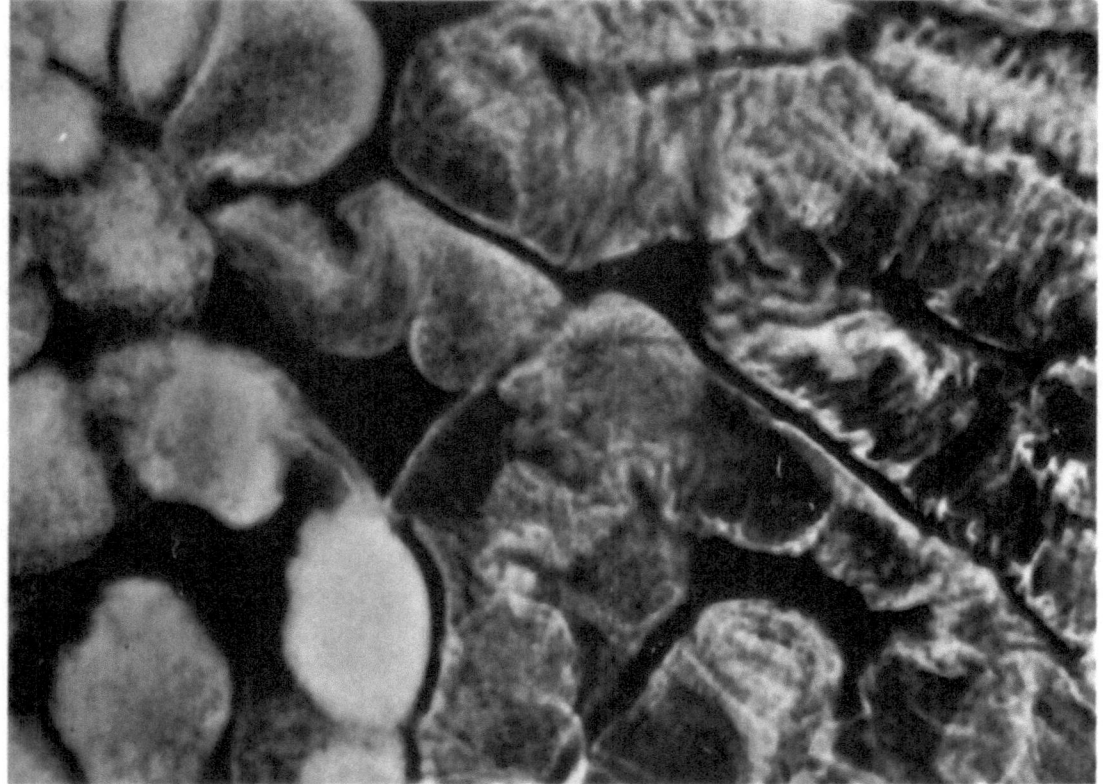

Fig. 8.24. Gas bubbles in the contrast fluid that are the same size as the villi in fig. 8.23 are due to foaming of the barium suspension. The margins of the contrast column are not interrupted by the bubbles as in 8.23.

not be considered as an etiological factor in this so-called lymphoid nodular hyperplasia.

The small intestine is then often highly irritable so that adequate filling with contrast fluid is extremely difficult. The mucosal folds are fairly thin instead of thickened, and lie close together (fig. 8.22).

Very small nodular elevations in the mucosa of the duodenum and proximal jejunum combined with a fairly coarse fold relief and moderate dilatation of the intestinal lumen can occur in Whipple's disease. In such cases the nodular aspect is due to villi that are so swollen that they are visible to the naked eye during endoscopic examination of the mucous membrane (fig. 8.23). On the films these swollen villi must be distinguished from small gas bubbles that develop when the contrast fluid does not contain enough antifoaming agent (fig. 8.24).

Multiple, stalked, or sessile filling defects in the contrast column, many of them much more than 2 or 3 mm long, usually can be attributed to the rare forms of familial polyposis, but in other cases they may be indicative of a lymphoreticular malignancy. In polyposis, they occur more frequently in the stomach and especially in the colon than in the small intestine. Histologically they are found to be adenomas (Gardner's syndrome) or hamartomas (Peutz-Jeghers syndrome) (fig. 8.25).

It is particularly important that the small nodules or polyps described here are not mistaken for multiple gas bubbles of the same size in the contrast fluid. Although not always valid (arrows), it may help to remember that gas bubbles lie very close together and do not interrupt the contour of the intestinal mucosa (fig. 8.26). Follicles or polyps are usually further apart and when they lie along the margin of the contrast column, it can sometimes be seen that they interrupt the contour.

Finally, very small nodules along the margins of a well-filled loop should not be confused with the regular serrated puckers in the mucosa due to contractions of the muscularis (see page 14). Somewhat larger, usually slightly ovoid, nodular elevations in an ulcerative mucosal surface without folds can be seen in Crohn's disease. Sometimes these lumps are widespread and have a broad base at the intestinal wall. Like the larger cobblestones and so-called pseudopolyps in the colon, they often consist of the edematous swollen mucosal residue

from an otherwise totally destroyed mucosal surface (fig. 8.27). Since a mucosal surface destroyed by ulceration can be very smooth during the healing process, correct classification can be difficult.

3. Foreign bodies and filling defects in the contrast fluid

The specific gravity of the foreign body is usually lower than that of the barium suspension; it is therefore visible as a filling defect in the contrast fluid. The most frequently encountered foreign body is without a doubt undigested food residue. Food residue is seen almost exclusively in the distal half of the ileum since transit is most likely to be disturbed in this section because the cecum is so often full. Food residue can also be found when the patient has eaten shortly before the radiological examination, gastric emptying is mechanically impeded, or there is disturbed motility (see page 361). This type of foreign body usually causes a conglomeration of relatively small bright spots in the barium suspension (fig. 8.28KL). However, sometimes for example an undigested bean pod can also produce a sharply defined filling defect and then it will be necessary to examine the feces carefully for several days (fig. 8.28M). The pattern caused by the food residue after rice has been eaten is particularly misleading (fig. 8.28N). These filling defects are small and round and have to be differentiated from those caused by lymph follicles or air bubbles. Now and then, one or more elongated filling defects will be found in the intestinal loops that are caused by tapeworms or roundworms (fig. 8.29A). The intestine then often also exhibits enhanced motility locally. Sometimes there is even a tendency toward flocculation of the contrast medium, probably as a result of enhanced secretion. Misleading patterns of worms can be caused by the sacroiliac joint, threads of mucus, and superposition of mucosal folds in other intestinal loops (fig. 8.29B).

Without a doubt, the filling defect seen in fig. 8.30 is exceedingly rare: diagnosed by many as an invagination, it was in fact caused by a piece of surgical gauze that was 70 cm long. The patient occasionally suffered vague complaints indicative of obstruction. One year ago a sigmoidal resection had been performed as a result of diverticulosis.

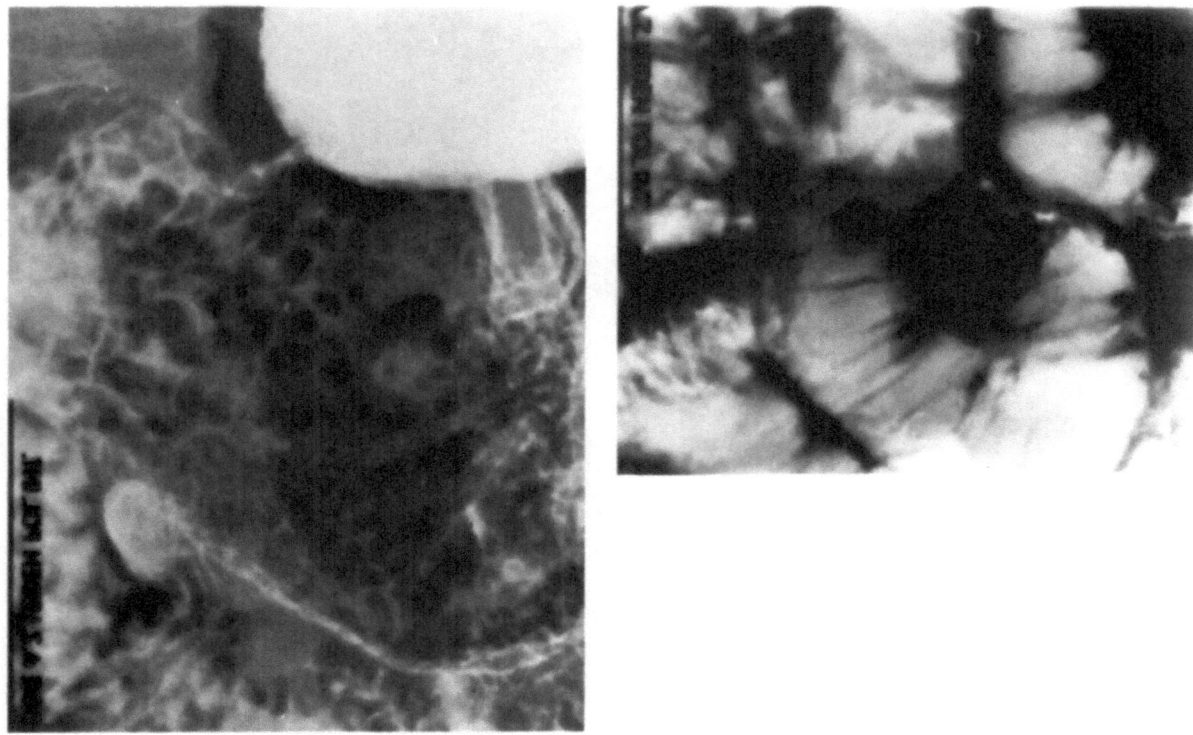

Fig. 8.25. Polypoid or nodular filling defects in the contrast fluid in a patient with familial polyposis. If the filling defects in the small intestine are numerous and much smaller than the one seen here, differentiation from a lymphoid nodular hyperplasia is not really possible on strictly radiological grounds.

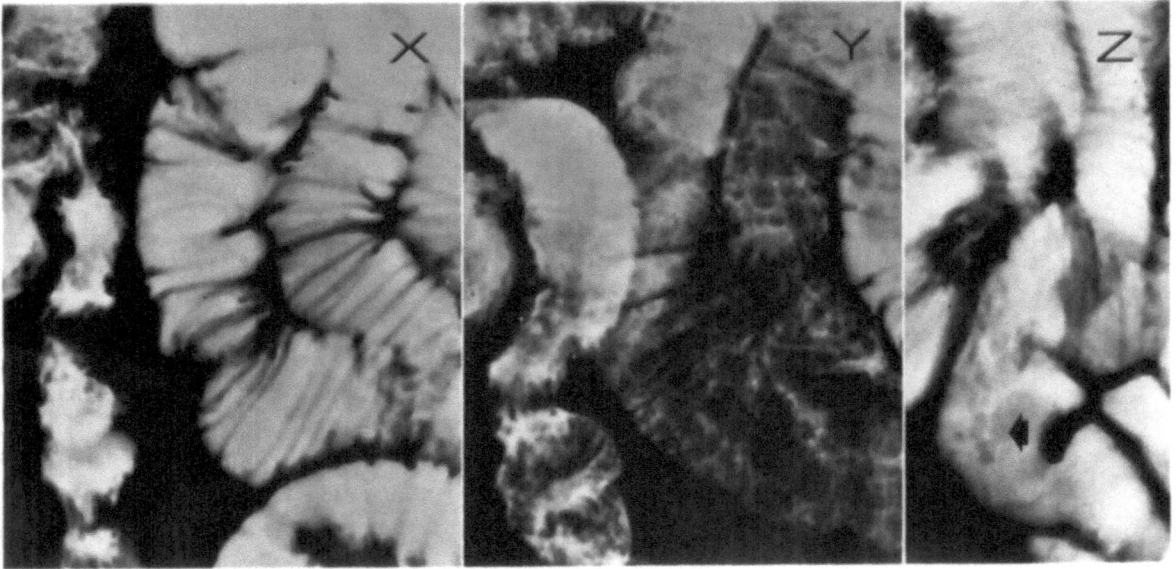

Fig. 8.26. Filling defects 2–3 mm across in the contrast fluid due to gas bubbles (the same loops in x and y). Highly similar to lymph nodules (z).

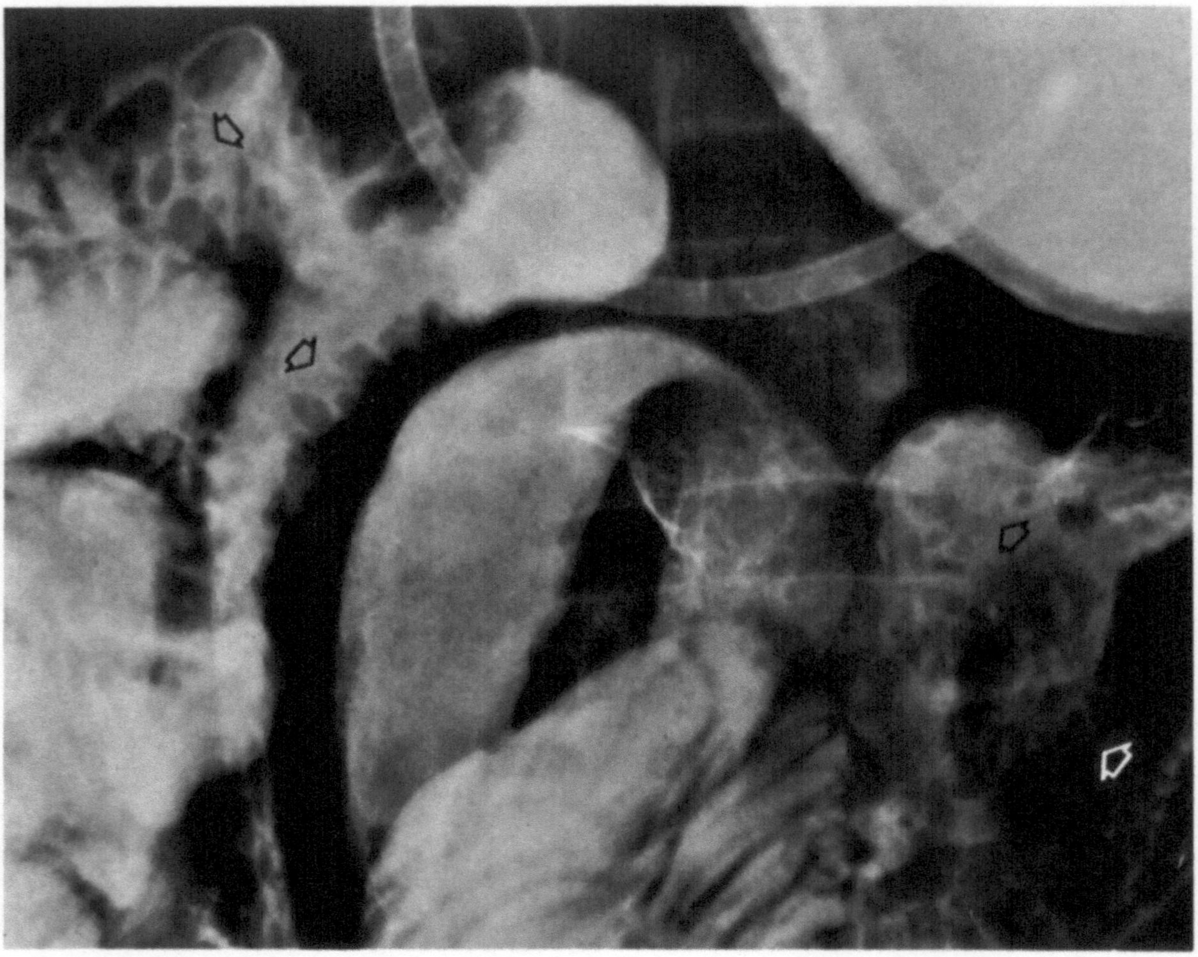

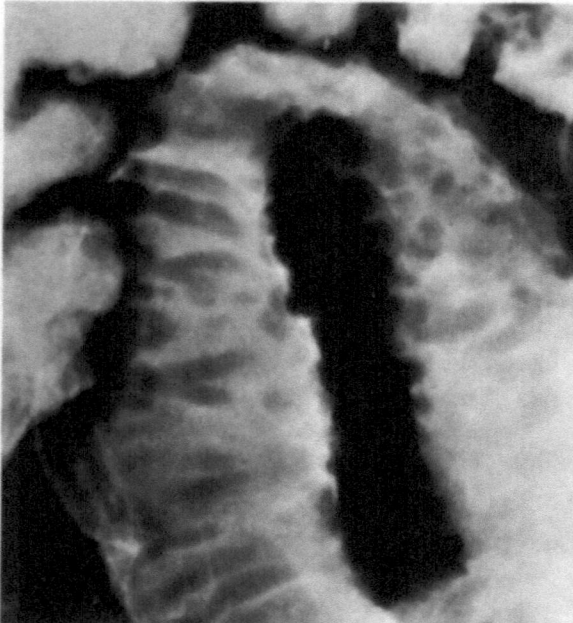

Inflammation and necrosis must have caused the gauze left behind in the abdominal cavity to perforate into the lumen of the small bowel. The discrepancy between the widespread abnormalities and the vague clinical signs made the diagnosis of invagination highly unlikely. Moreover, the barium streamer that should be seen in the event of an invagination could not be found anywhere.

4. Ulcerations

It is very difficult to recognize superficial ulcerations in the small intestine – even more so than in all other parts of the digestive tract. Their presence can be demonstrated only indirectly since the mucosal relief is more or less destroyed and the surface

Fig. 8.27. Round, oval, or elongated clarifications in the contrast fluid caused by residual mucosal folds in an otherwise atrophied mucosal surface in Crohn's disease.

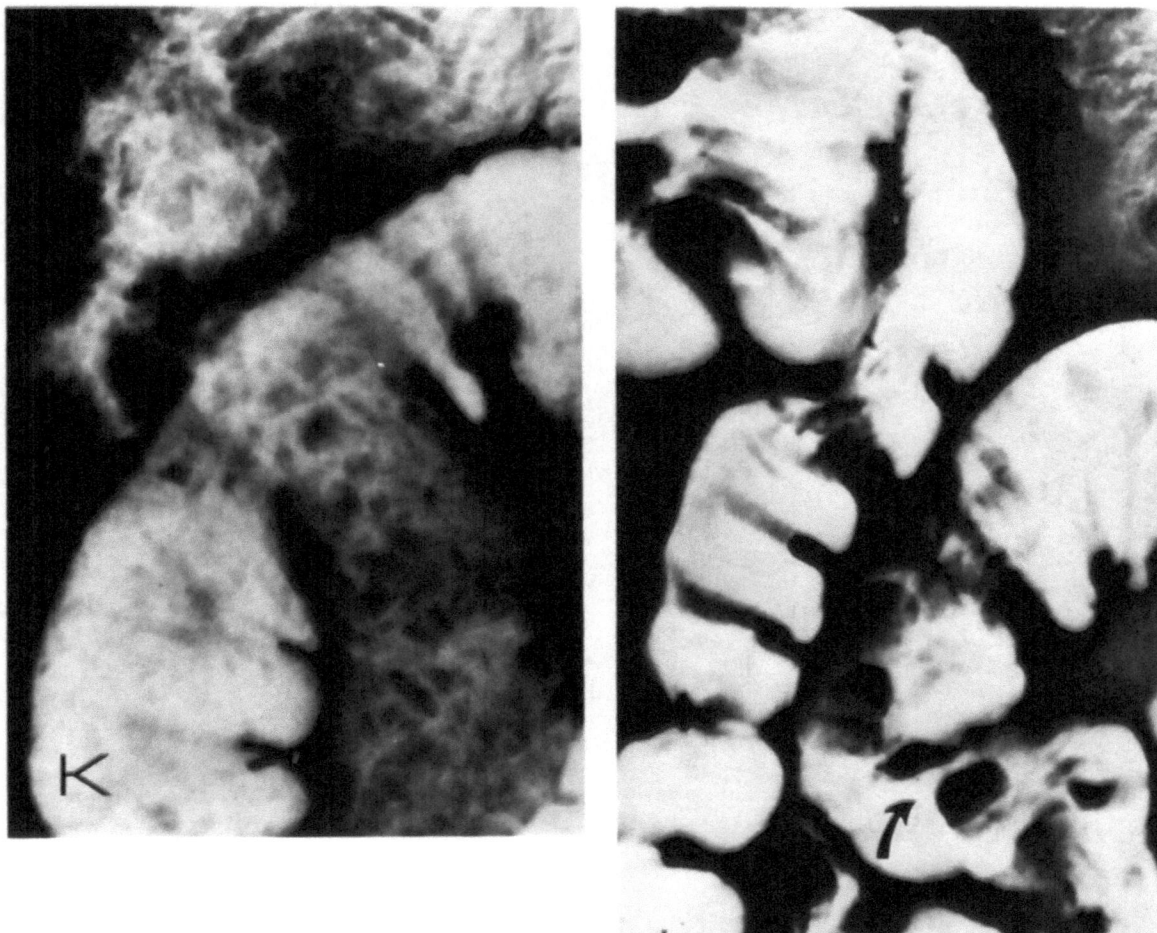

Fig. 8.28. (K) Most common aspect of food residue in the distal ileum. (L) Filling defects resembling fruit pits.

irregularly defined (fig. 8.31). Locally the intestinal wall is somewhat thicker and stiff and is not affected by peristalsis. In this initial stage, ulcer craters can seldom or never be demonstrated, unless they are obviously very deep (arrows). Differentiation between extensive and rather superficial inflammatory processes and a lymphoreticular malignancy is of course difficult and often is possible only several months later on the basis of a follow-up examination. In the case of an inflammatory process, the abnormalities have as a rule obviously changed, and usually improved. In a lymphoreticular malignancy, they have increased or are practically unchanged.

If there are small mucosal infiltrates, then differentiation is based predominantly on the consideration that the relationship between the depth and the surface distribution is different for an infiltrate and a malignancy. An inflammatory process will spread out over the surface whereas the difference between growth in depth and growth in width will be much less pronounced in a tumor. Clinically, too, differentiation may be possible. A tumor can exist for some time without symptoms so that a radiological examination is in fact never carried out in such an early stage of development. On the other hand in spite of the fact that there are only minor radiological abnormalities, inflammatory processes can be preceded by months of vague complaints.

Finally it is statistically much more likely that the abnormalities are due to an inflammatory process rather than a tumor; this factor can also play a role in establishing the probable diagnosis. As soon as

148

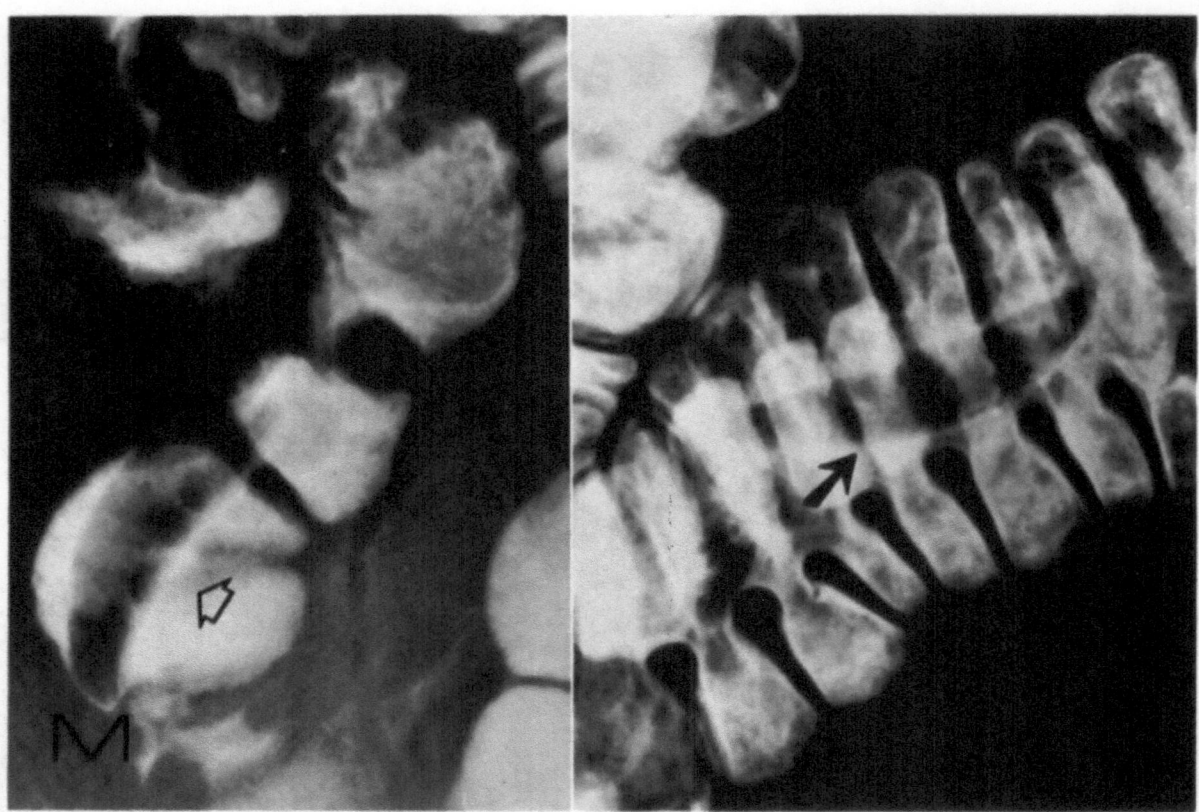

*Fig. 8.28*M. Undigested bean pod.

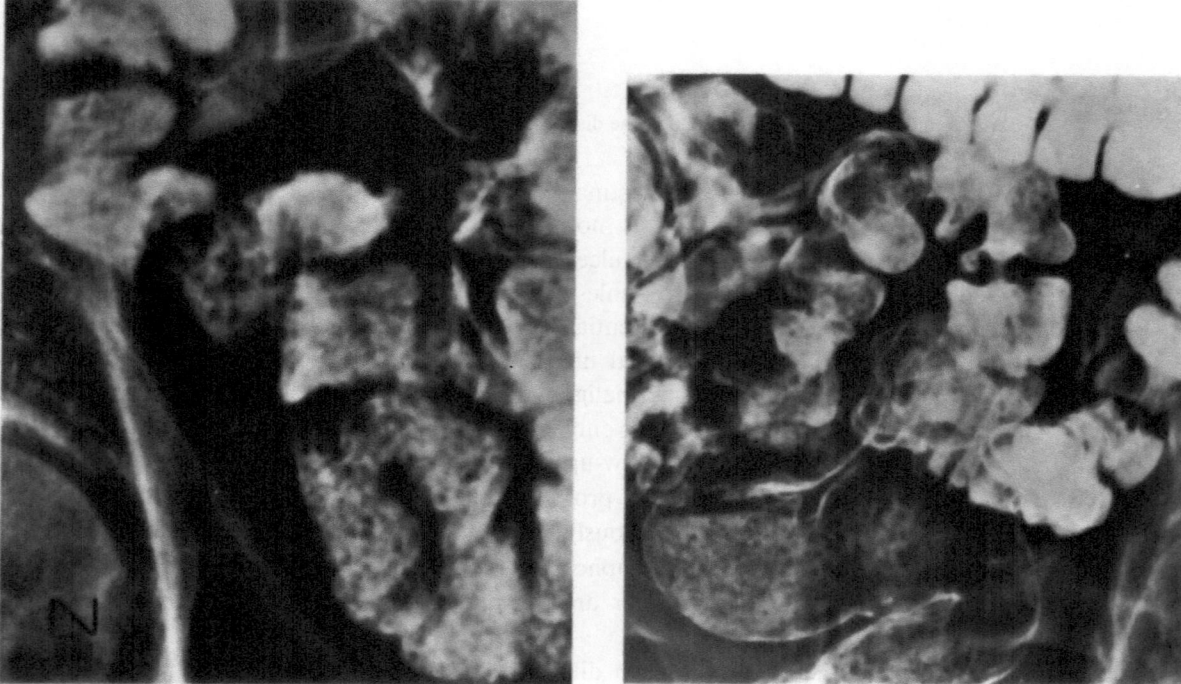

*Fig. 8.28*N. Round filling defects due to undigested rice.

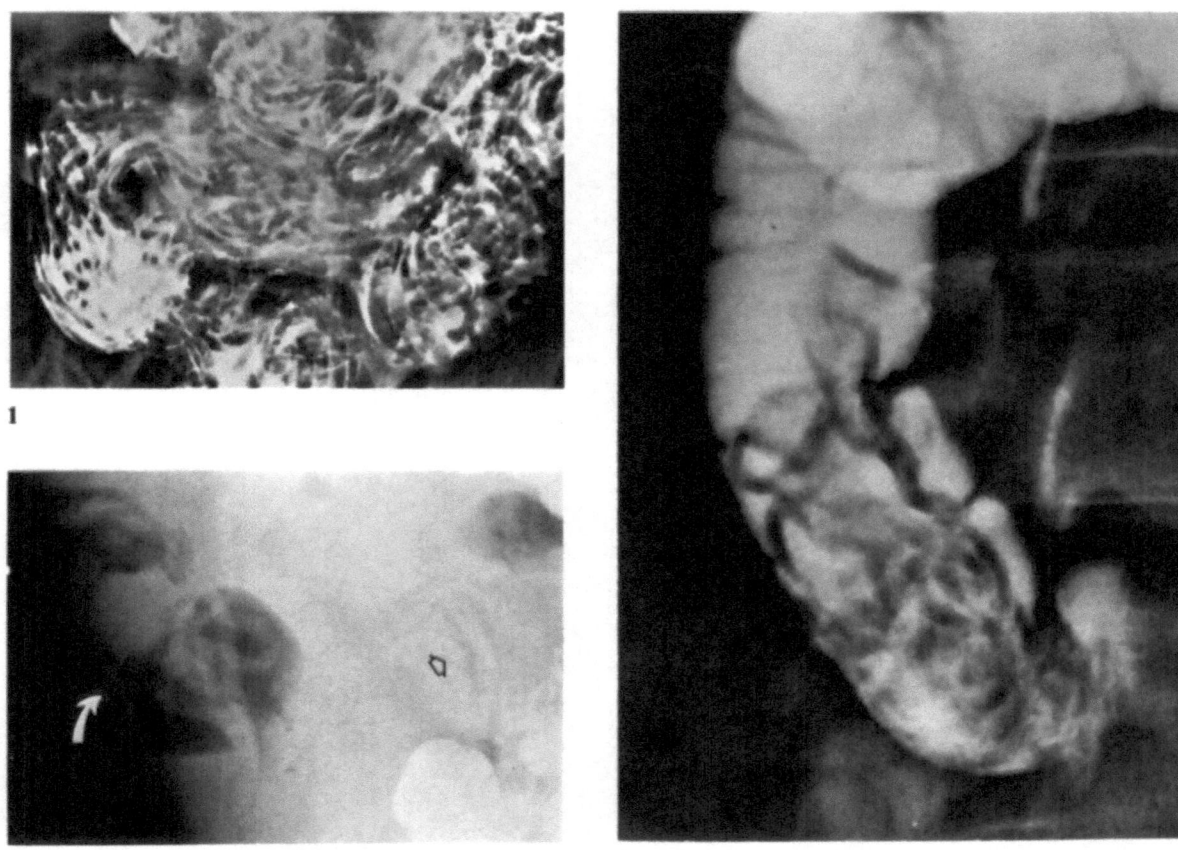

1

*Fig. 8.29*A(1–5). Several examples of filling defects in the contrast fluid caused by Ascaris or tapeworms. The worms are sometimes seen as a tangled mass; in other cases they are even visible on a survey exposure of the abdomen. (See also pages 150 and 151.)

the ulcers become larger or acquire a more or less mushroom-like shape, radiological recognition is not difficult (fig. 8.32). It must be noted that it is easier to discover these ulcers when they are located along the margin of the contrast column. On the other hand, however, they can sometimes be over-exposed so that they are barely visible. In Crohn's disease, if the ulcers are surrounded by a zone of cobblestone-like mucosal swelling and are viewed en face, they may appear identical to metastases of melanoma or other tumors with necrosis in the center (fig. 8.33). Although the differential diagnosis will seldom be a problem in this respect, these small granulomas with ulcer craters can in no way be considered specific in other inflammatory processes. We have for instance observed them in *Yersinia EC* infections. We have occasionally been confronted with a misleading pattern somewhat

similar to that of an aphthous ulcer (fig. 8.34). Comparison of the same intestinal loop during other stages of contraction soon provided the answer. In addition to very local penetrating ulcer craters in granulomatous inflammatory processes, deep elongated ulcers can also develop between the folds of edematous swollen mucosa when the circulation of blood and lymph is disturbed. Moreover, these fissure-shaped ulcers also can not be considered specific, as in the case of the above-mentioned aphthous ulcers. Although in practice on the basis of statistical evidence it will be seen that they usually indicate Crohn's disease.

Split-like ulcers between the folds of the edematous swollen mucosa can also penetrate deep into all layers of the wall of the small intestine. They extend in a longitudinal as well as a transverse direction and cause the characteristic irregular stripe (fig.

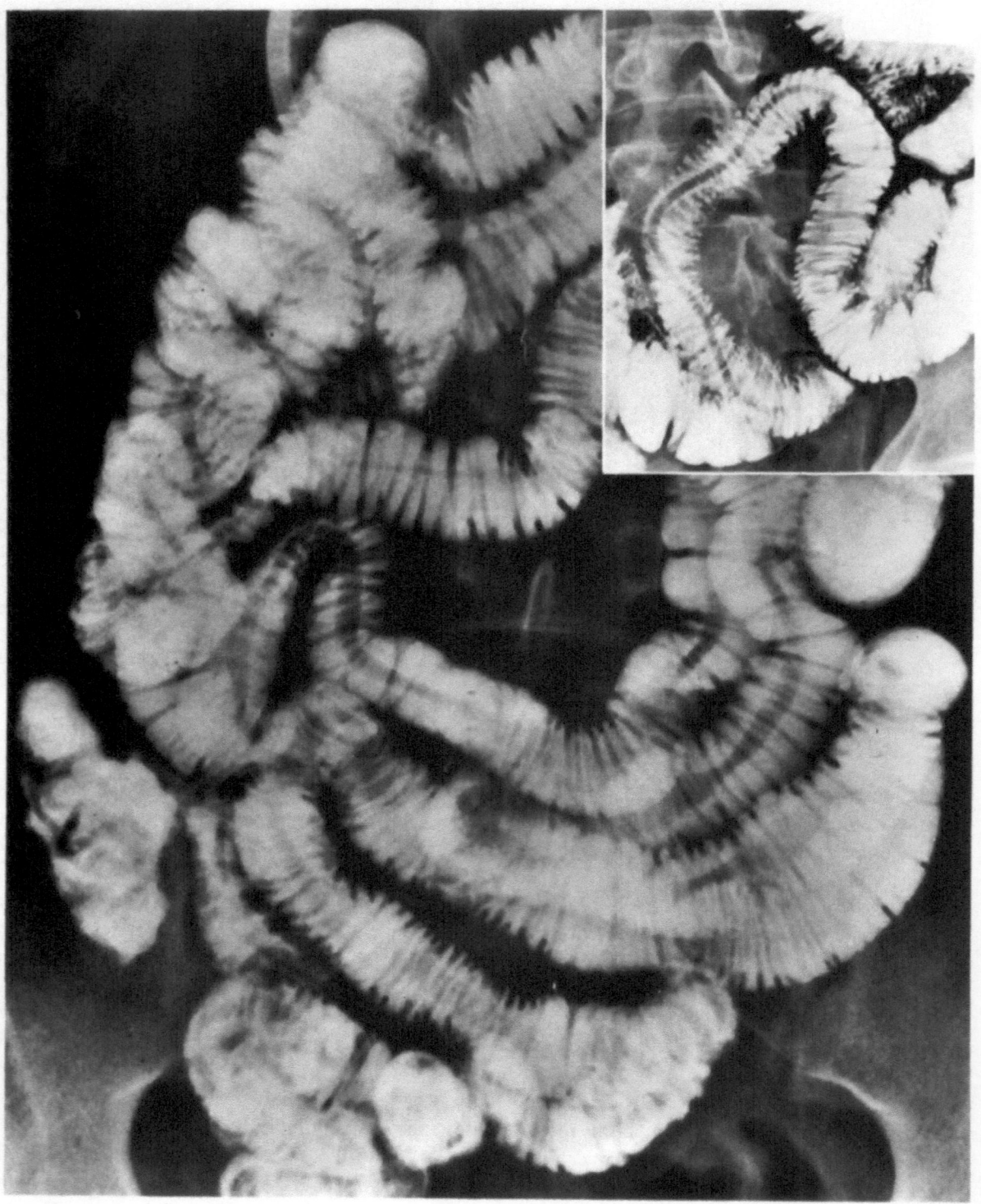

*Fig. 8.29*A (4). See legend on page 149.

151

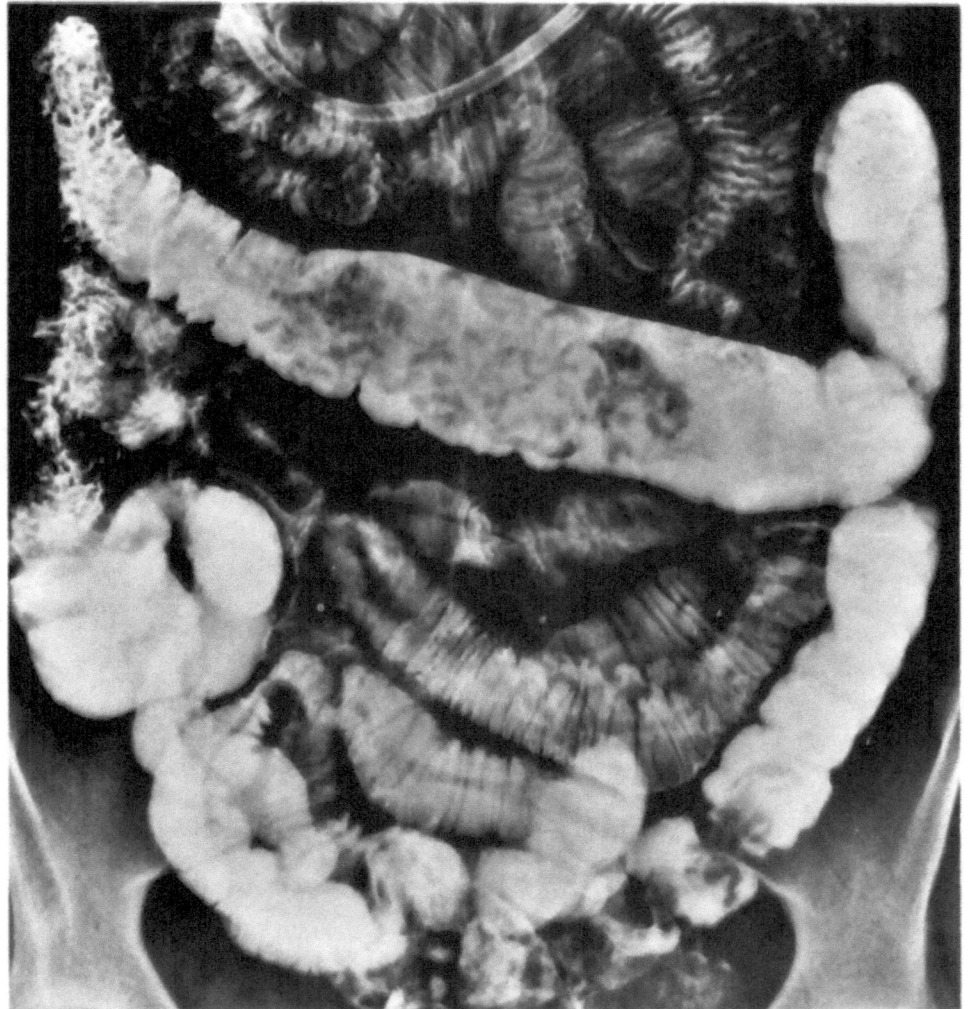

*Fig. 8.29*A (5).
See legend on
page 149.

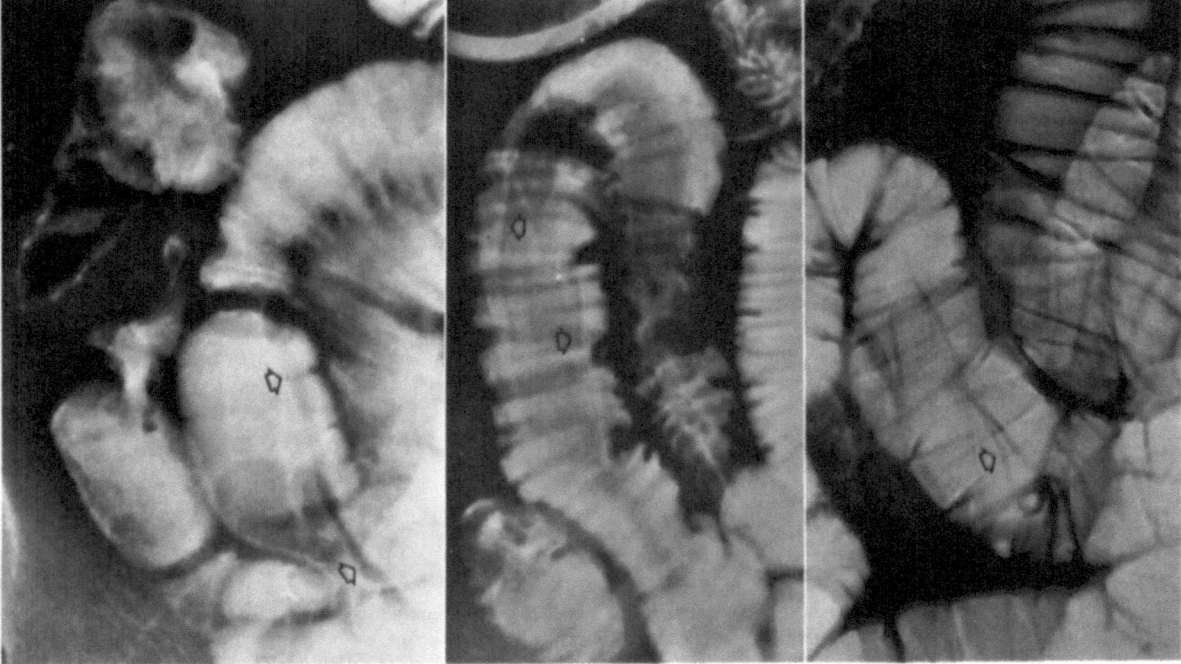

*Fig. 8.29*B. Misleading pattern of worms caused by sacroiliac joint, threads of mucus, and mucosal folds in other intestinal loops.

152

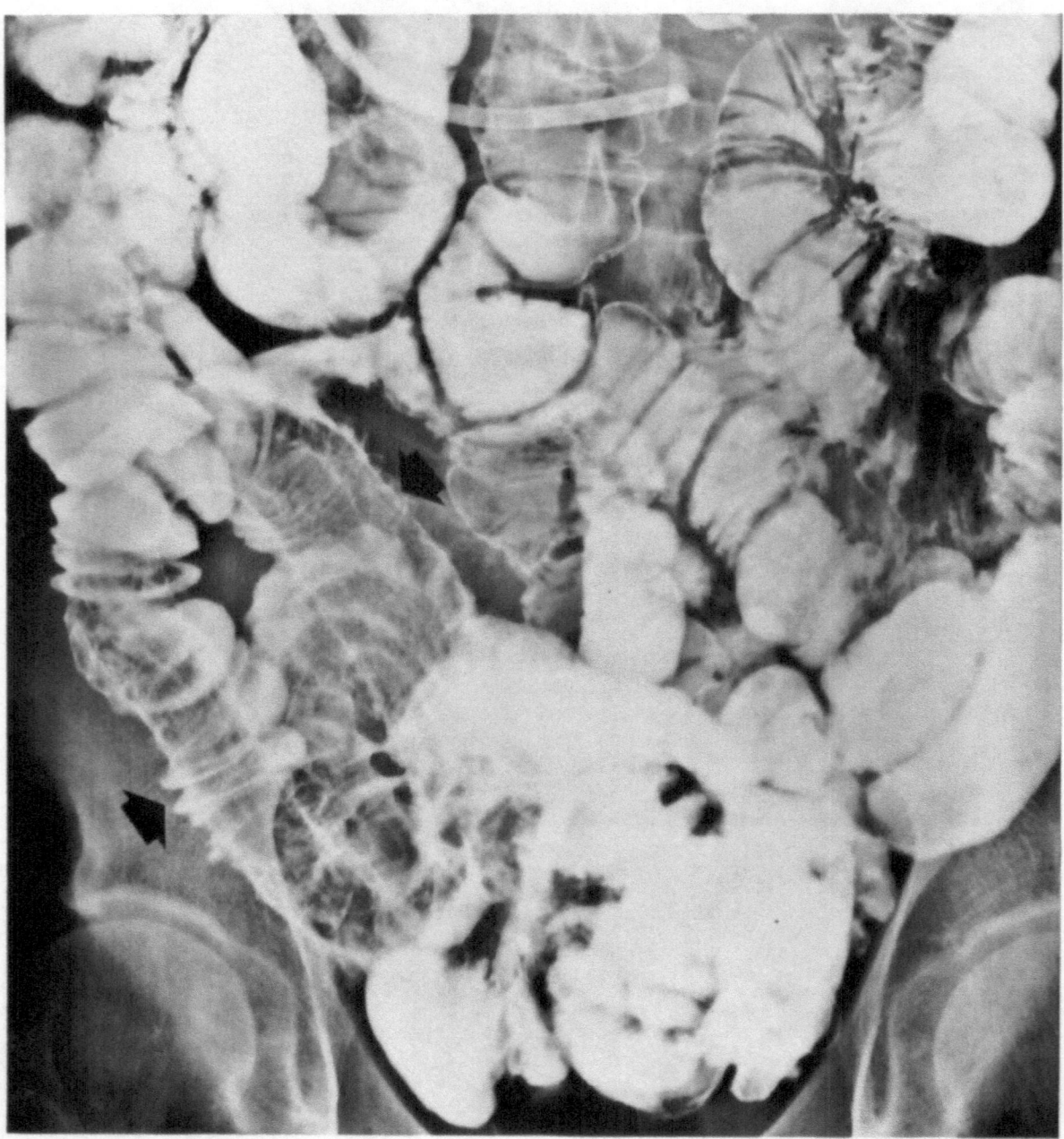

Fig. 8.30. Deceptive pattern of an invagination caused by a surgical gauze 70 cm in length that was left behind in the abdominal cavity and perforated into the intestinal lumen. (Courtesy of Dr. G. Coerkamp – Haarlem.)

Fig. 8.31. Locally stiff and thickened wall of the small intestine due to an inflammatory process. A very long section of the contrast column has ragged margins. Deep ulcerations are observed most easily along the margin of the intestine (arrows). If the film density is too high, they can no longer be seen because of overexposure. Vaguely defined intestinal wall is due to purulent secretion on an ulcerated mucosal surface.

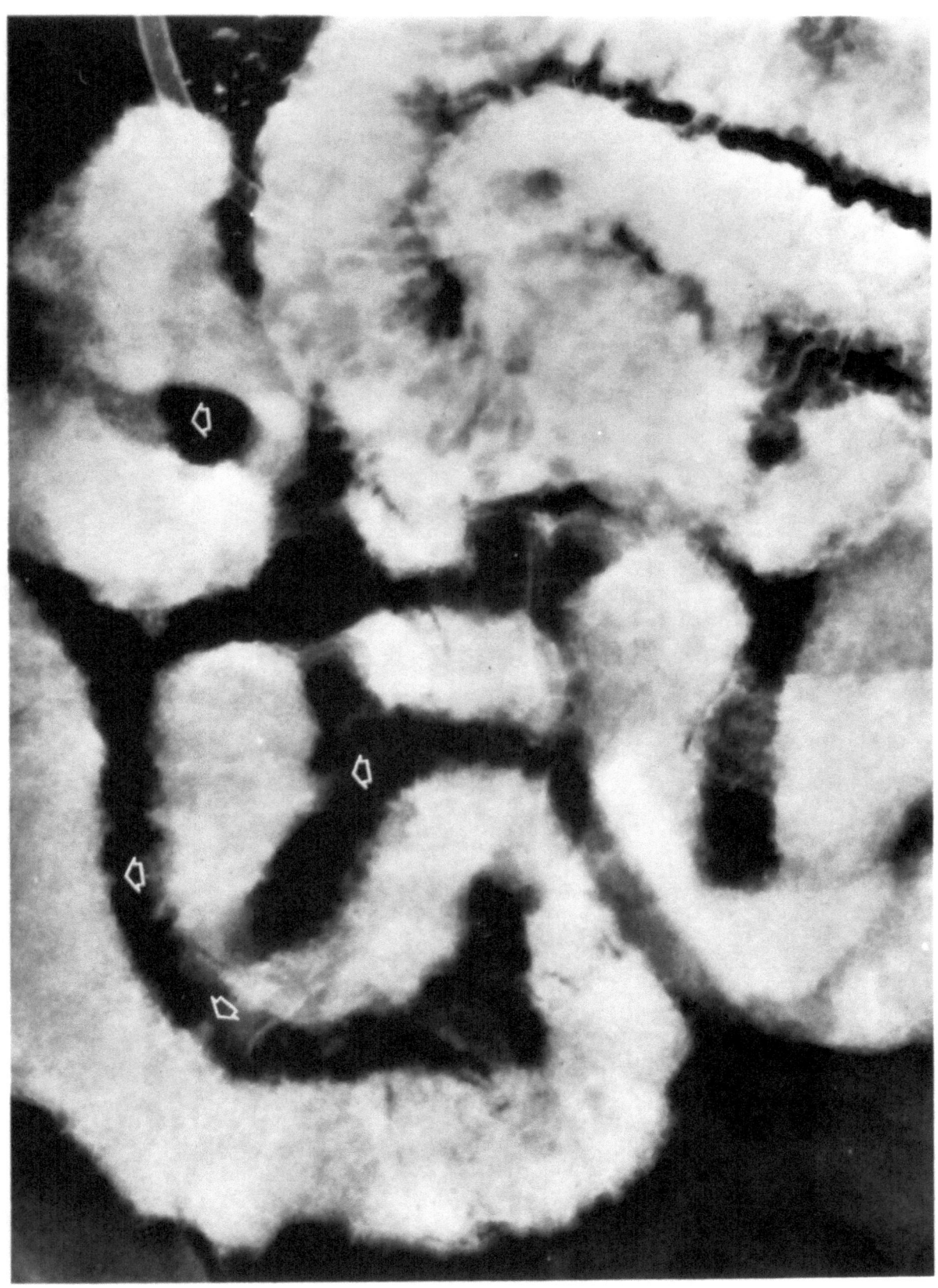

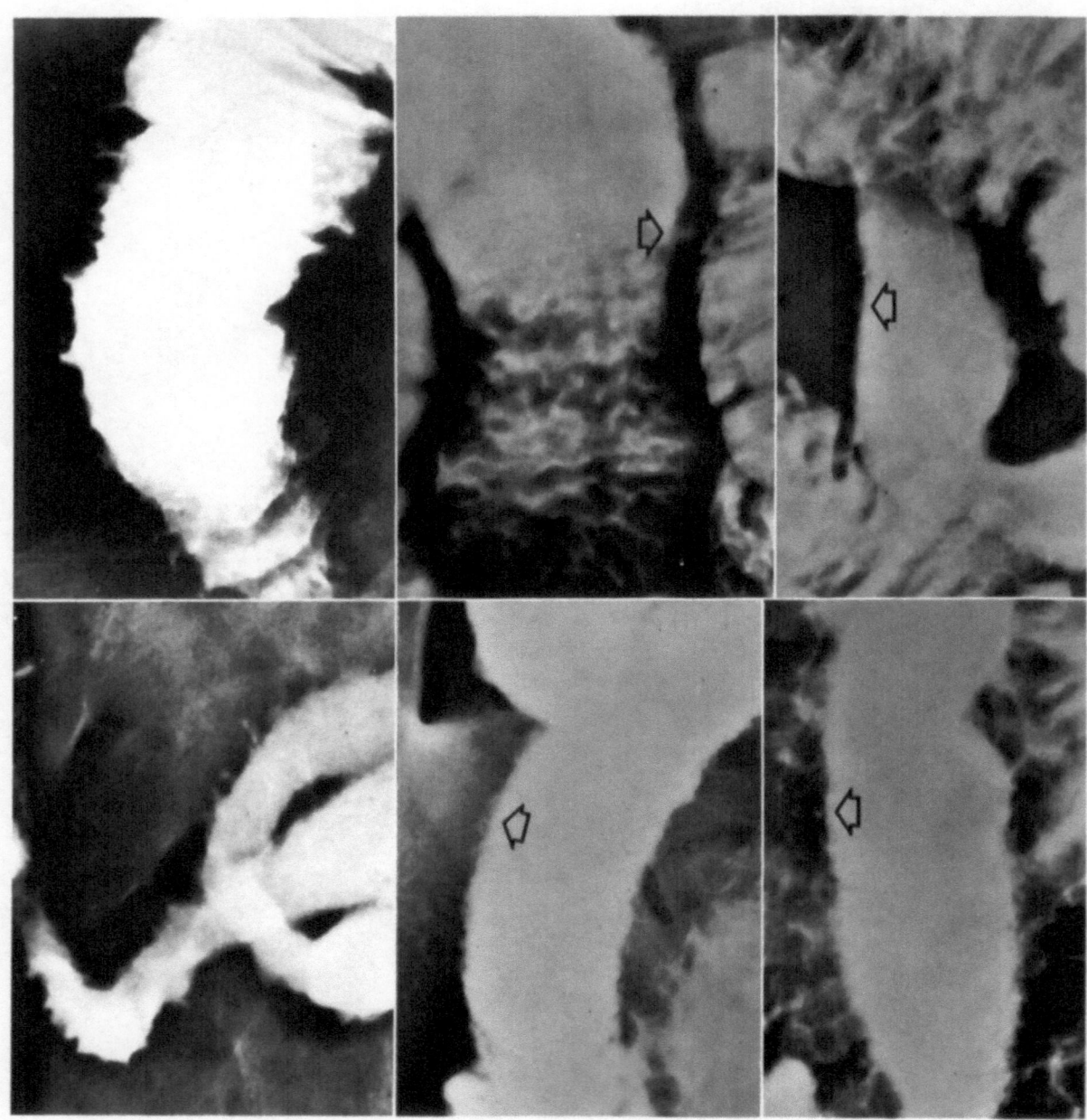

Fig. 8.32. Ulcers in Crohn's disease, some of them mushroom-shaped (arrows).

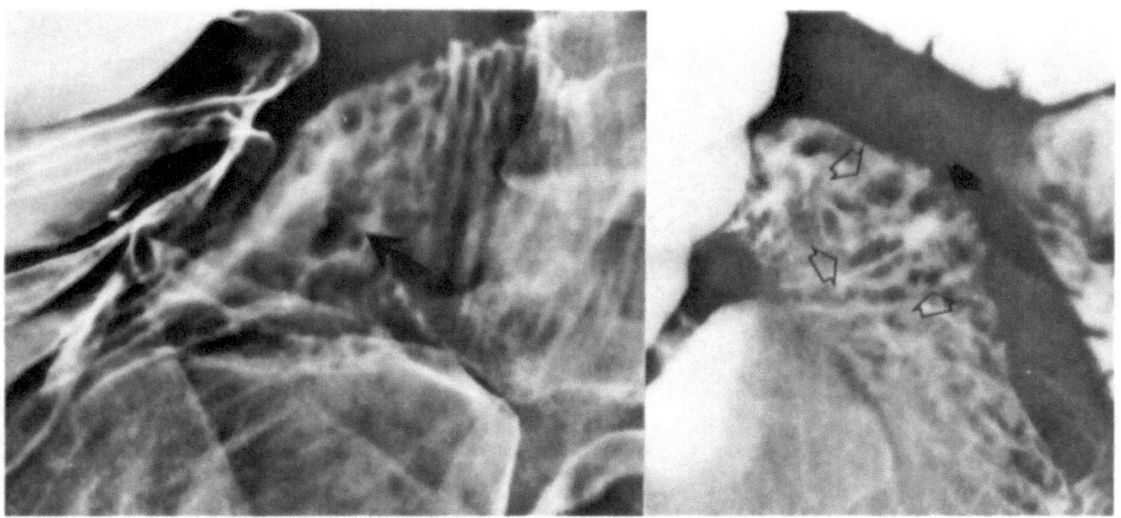

*Fig. 8.33*A. Suspected solitary round ulcer of unknown origin in distal ileum.

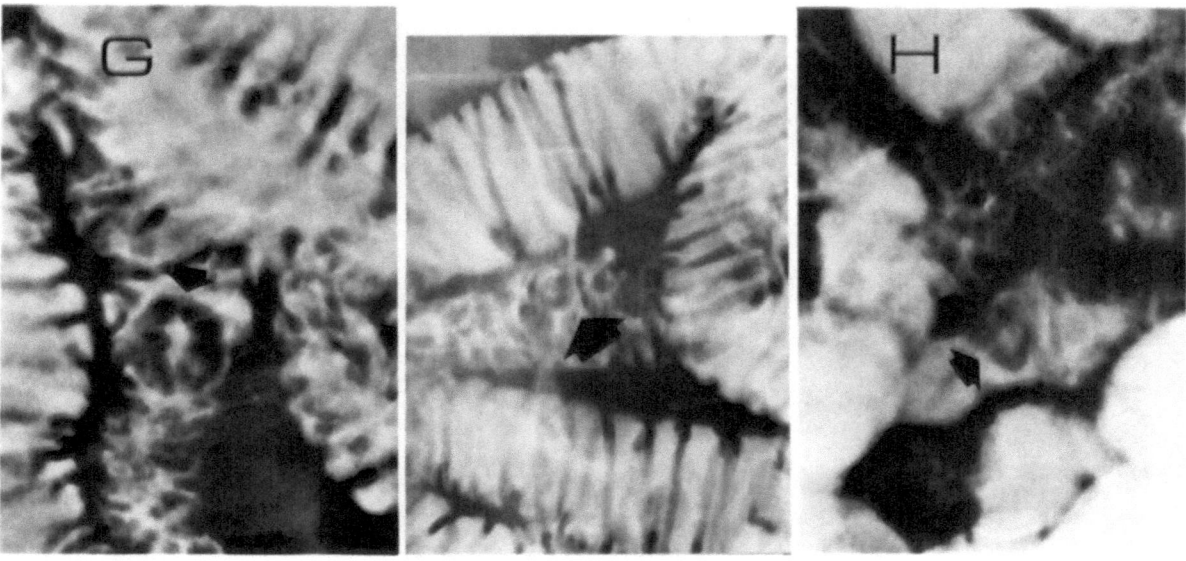

*Fig. 8.33*B. Crater-shaped ulcers in the center of 4-to 8-mm inflammatory granulomas in Crohn's disease (F). Similar granulomas are seen in other inflammatory processes. The x-ray closely resembles those of metastasis of melanoma (G) or reticulum cell sarcoma (H) with central necrosis. (See also page 156.)

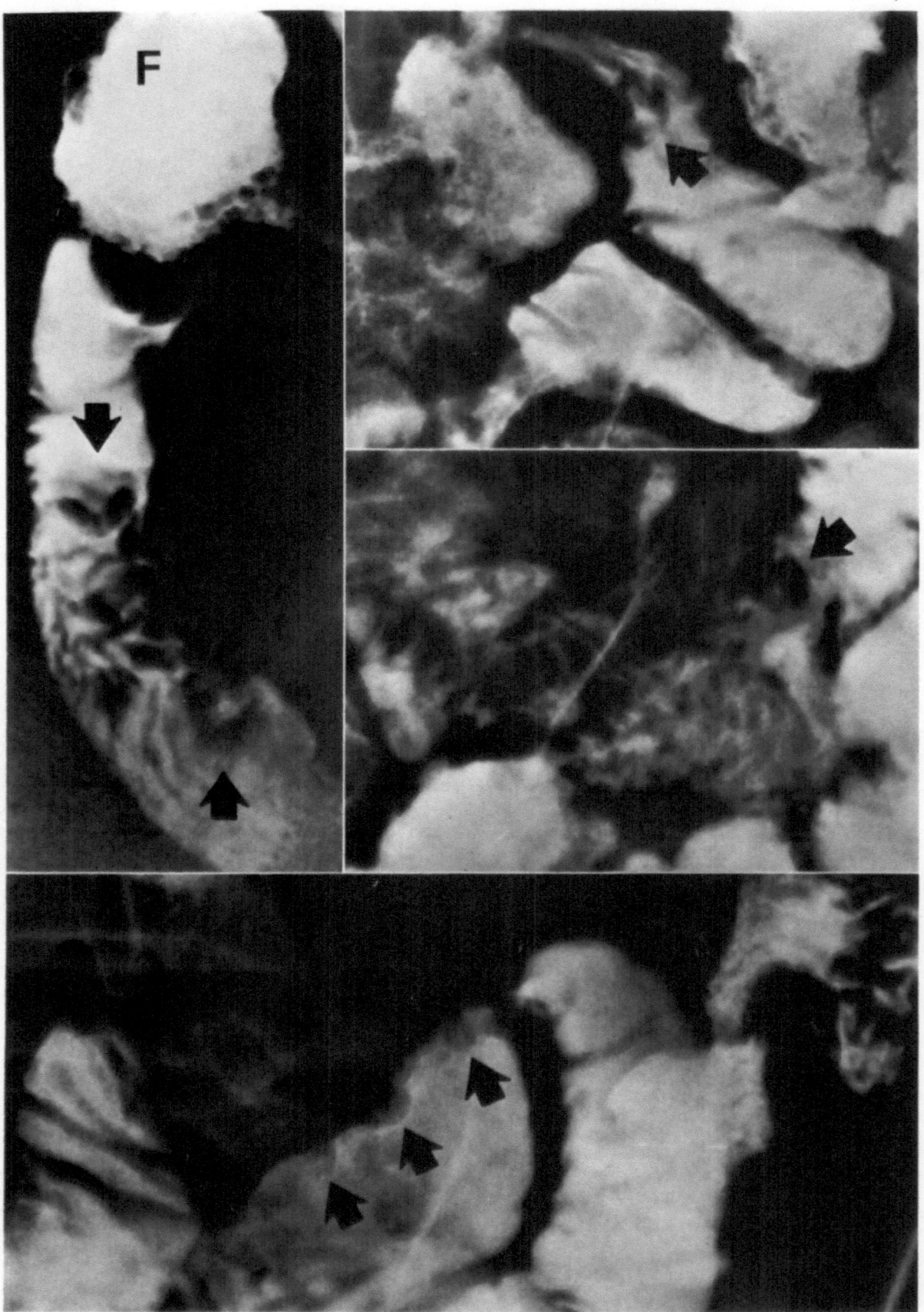

*Fig. 8.33*B. See legend on page 155.

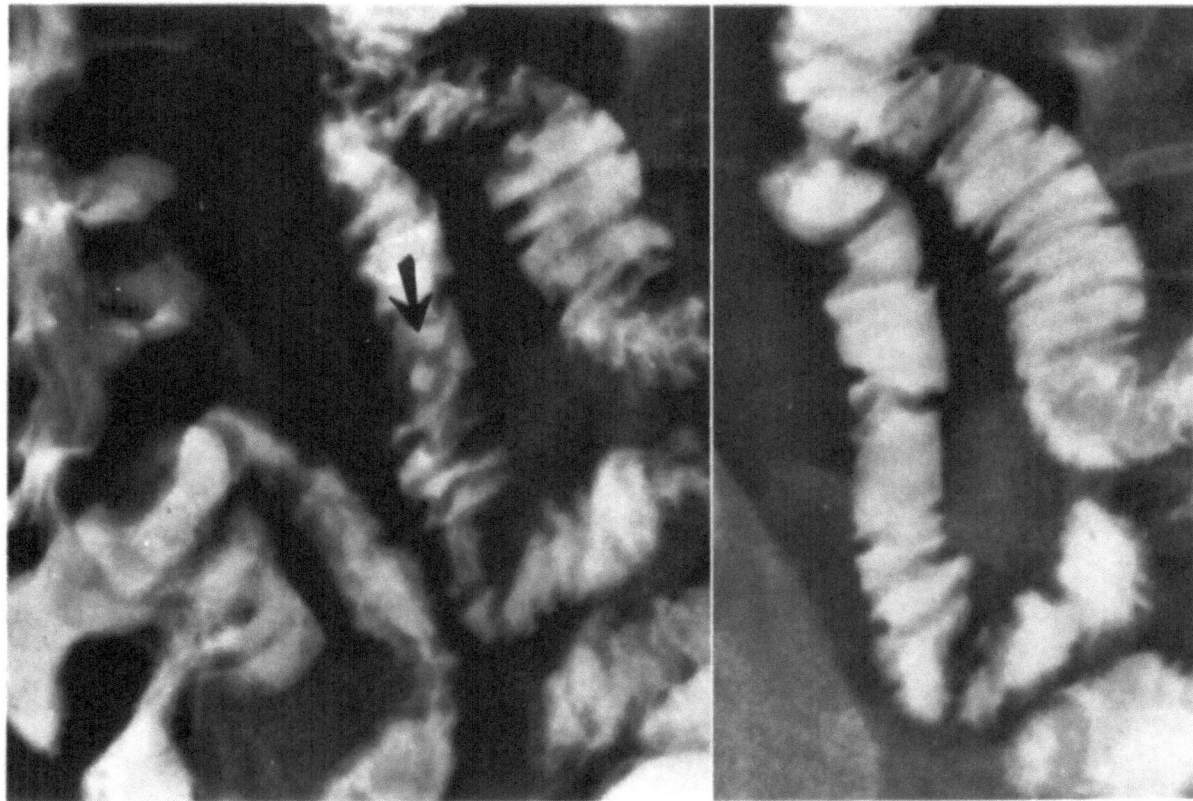

Fig. 8.34. Misleading pattern of an aphthous ulcer (arrow).

8.35R) or cushion-like cobblestone pattern (fig. 8.35s) that is seen in Crohn's disease. Because of the greater number of mucosal folds in the jejunum, the cobblestones in the proximal small intestine (fig. 8.35T) are much more pronounced than in the ileum, where the folds are relatively scarce. It is often difficult to obtain a sharp pattern at the site of an ulcerative surface since the intestinal wall is coated with purulent mucus that is not easily flushed away (fig. 8.31).

If the ulcerations are located predominantly on one side of the intestinal wall, usually the mesenteric side, the opposite wall of the bowel will sometimes show spastic contractions. Not only can the diagnosis of the very small ulcer be difficult but also that of very large ulcers. Often the segment containing the large ulcer will show extensive abnormal infiltrations and erratically defined filling defects. Then it is impossible to identify the normal anatomy as well as the presence of an ulcer crater. An example of this is seen in fig. 8.37: Meckel's diverticulum with a large ulcer, extended infiltration, adhesions, growths, and fistula formation between the adjacent intestinal loops.

In other cases, solitary ulcers, either specific (see fig. 9.9, page 202) or aspecific (fig. 8.36), may cause only irregular mucosal relief in a segment one to several centimeters long without any indication of a crater. Differentiation from local tumor growth is practically impossible.

5. Deformation of the intestine

5.1. Adhesions

It is seldom possible to demonstrate adhesions or fusion of intestinal loops with survey films alone. The finding of two intestinal loops that appear to lie close together in the same manner on all x-rays has turned out to be useless as a sign of adhesions. Many times we have been able to force the two apparently fused loops apart by using compression. If two intestinal loops are truly fused, then this should also be clearly visible on the spot photographs taken during compression. Compression must therefore be considered indispensable. In such

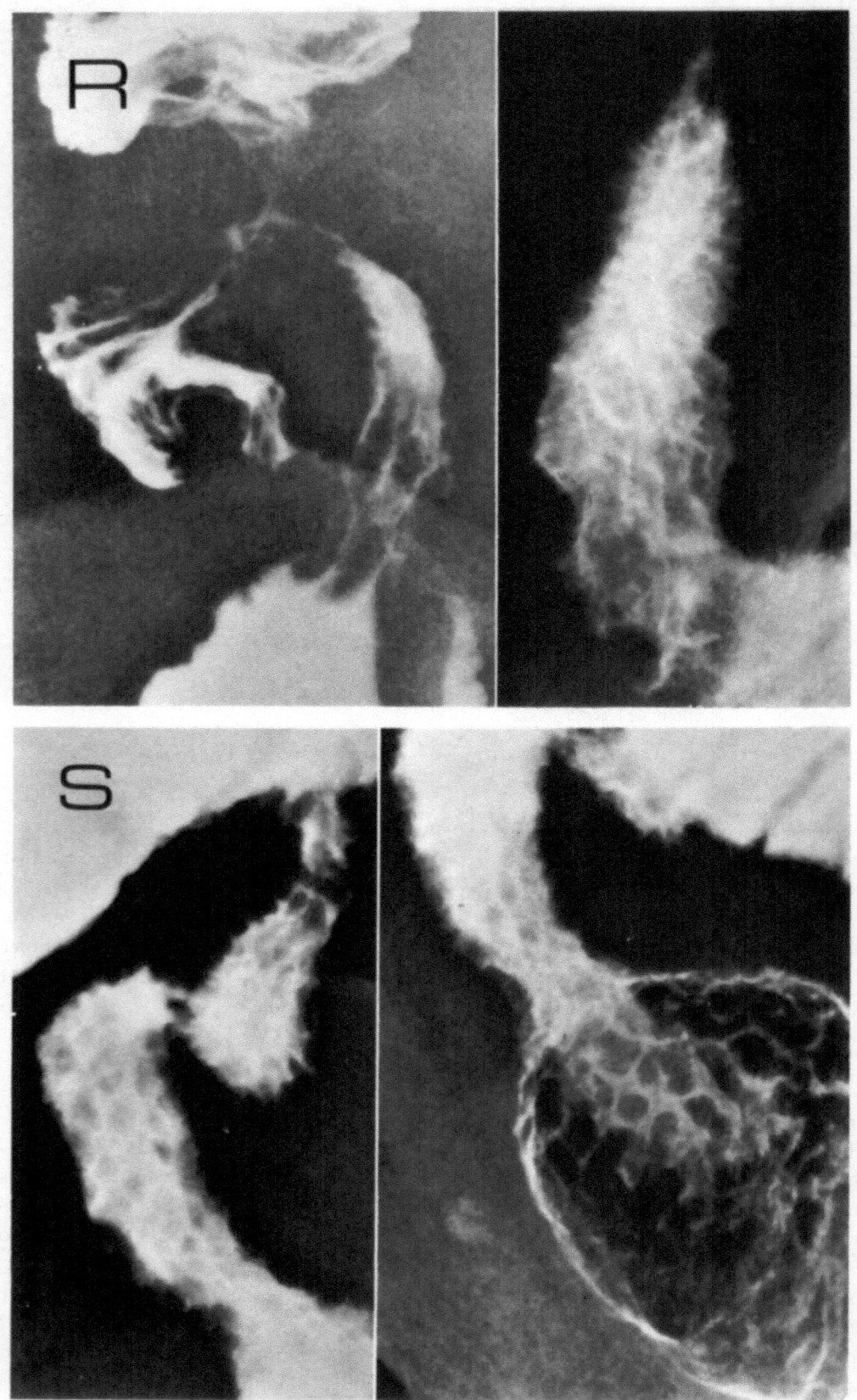

Fig. 8.35. Irregular stripe (R) or cobblestone-like (ST) patterns in Crohn's disease.

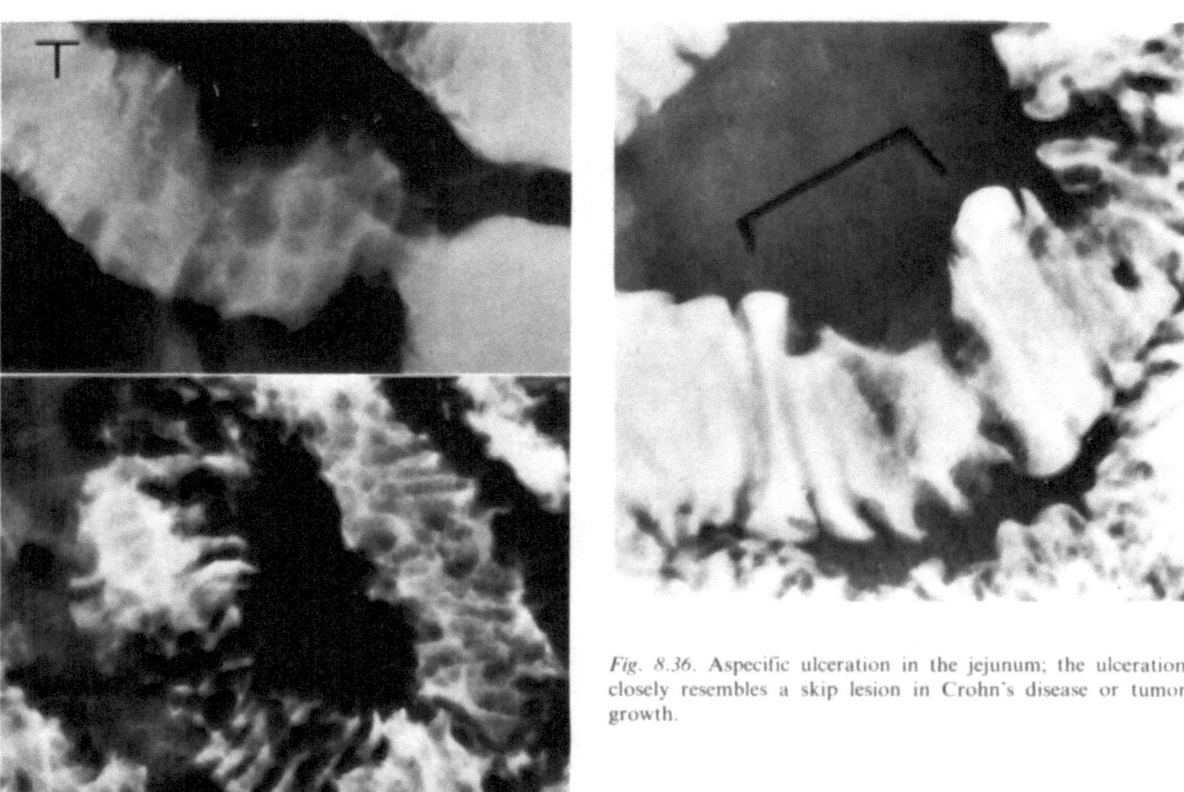

Fig. 8.36. Aspecific ulceration in the jejunum; the ulceration closely resembles a skip lesion in Crohn's disease or tumor growth.

← Fig. 8.35T

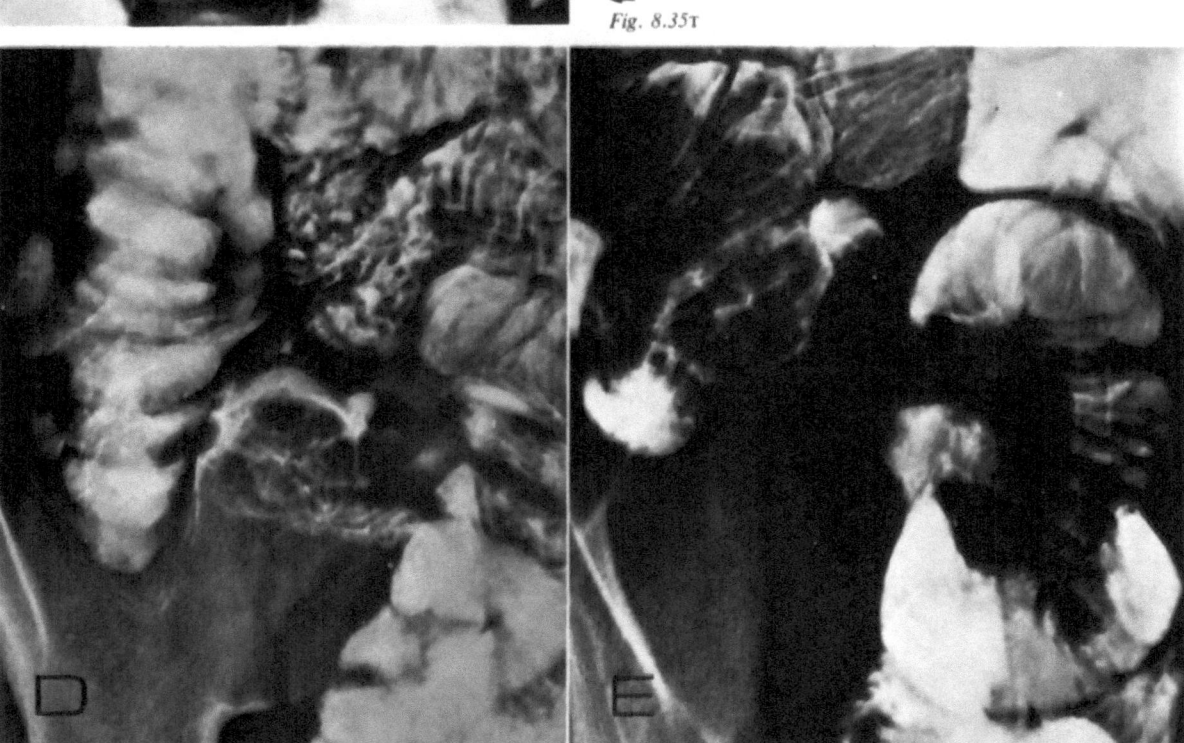

Fig. 8.37. Large ulcer in the ileocecal region that upon surgery turned out to be an ulcerating Meckel's diverticulum. This was not recognized as such on the roentgenogram. X-ray E was taken two months after x-ray D.

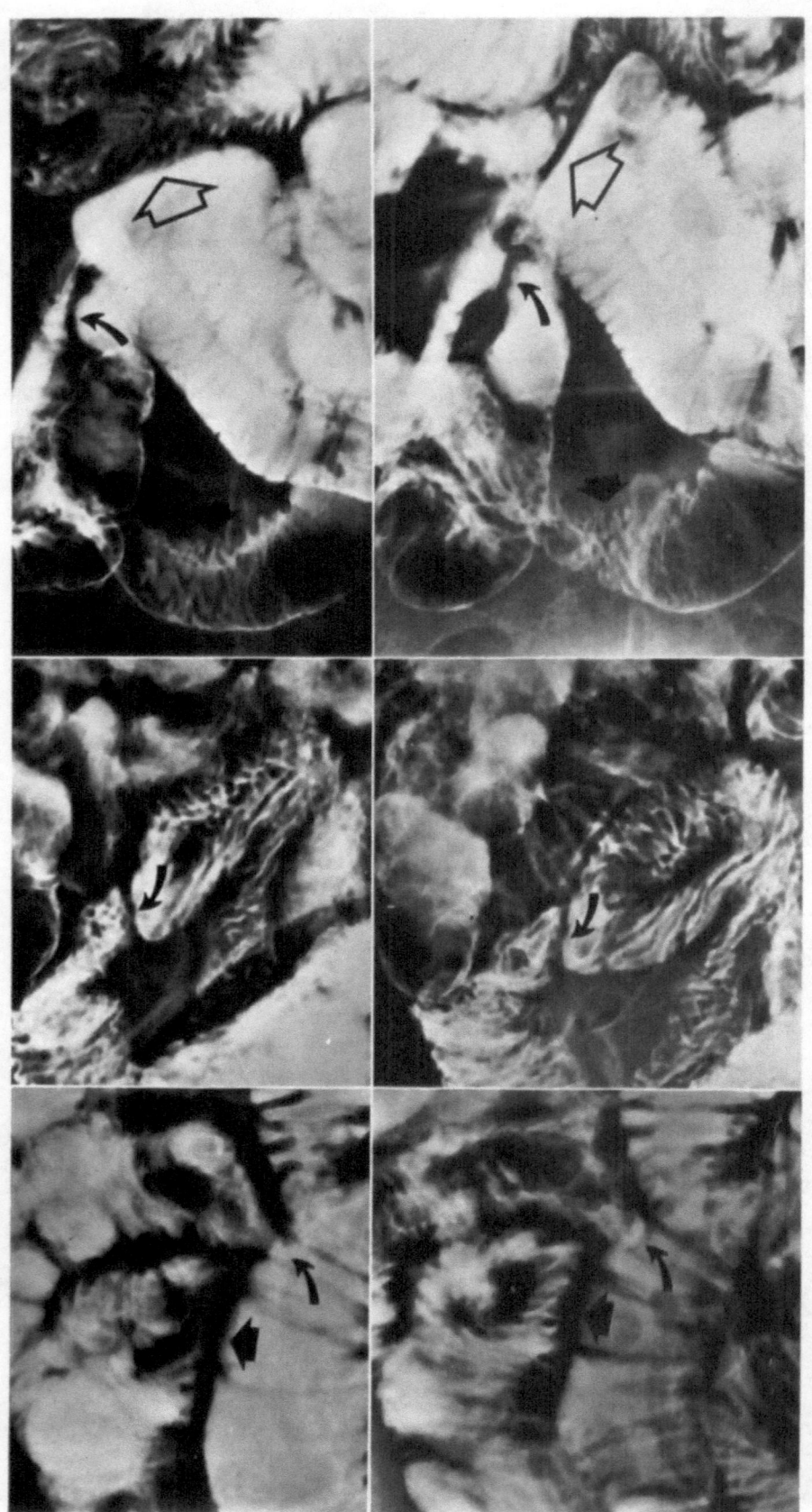

*Fig. 8.38*A. Several examples of adhesion and fusion of adjacent intestinal loops. The tent-shaped bulges in the intestinal loops are seen consistently on all x-rays; in addition certain sections of the intestinal loops cannot be forced apart by compression. Short planes of contact between two intestinal loops or one loop and the surrounding tissue are indicated by arrows.

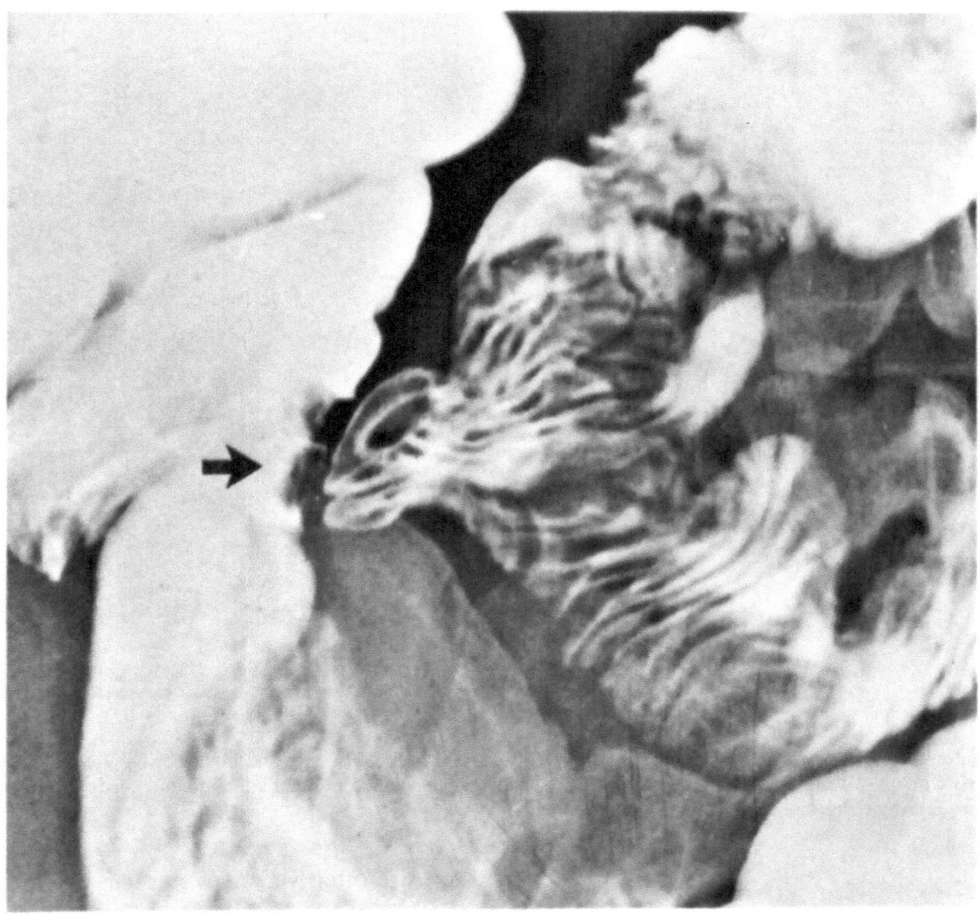

*Fig. 8.38*B. Tent-shaped bulge caused by adhesion but interpreted by some as a Meckel's diverticulum. The circular mucosal folds however continue through the neck of the 'diverticulum' so that it could not possibly be part of the omphalomesenteric duct (compare fig. 13.36, page 408).

cases we see tent-shaped bulges in the intestinal loops (fig 8.38). If the adhesion extends over a somewhat longer distance, the termination of the plane of contact of the two intestinal loops is rather abrupt or sharply angular (thin curved arrows). The mucosal pattern in intestinal loops that have fused with surrounding tissue is always intact, but during dilatation of the loop, induced for example by air insufflation, a very local slightly serrated or wrinkled contour can be seen at the site of the adhesion.

This is because the intestinal wall there cannot stretch with the rest of the wall (thick arrows). Contrary to crossing bands, adhesions rarely cause any restriction of the passage of the contrast fluid. Another aspect of adhesion is that the intestinal loops follow an abrupt and bizarre course because they have fused with their surroundings. It is also striking that, in spite of a minimal degree of filling,

highly stretched folds can still be seen since the relevant loop is passively stretched as a result of this fusion with the adjacent loops (fig. 8.38B). A zigzag course of mucosal folds indicates that these folds are unable to stretch, as a rule because of fusion with surrounding tissue, for example in cases of nearby tumor growth (fig. 10.27M).

5.2. Fistulas

The differentiation between a bulge due to an adhesion and one caused by a fistulous tract is rarely difficult. A fistulous tract is a very long canal that often follows a tortuous course and is irregularly defined. As a rule it does not broaden at the junction with the intestinal loop but passes through as a narrow opening or wide canal. There is often an infiltrate in the neighborhood and the mucosal relief at the site where the fistulous tract originates has changed pathologically. Since fistu-

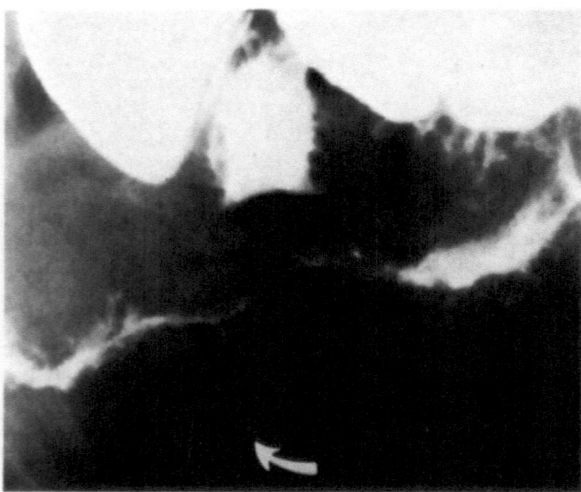

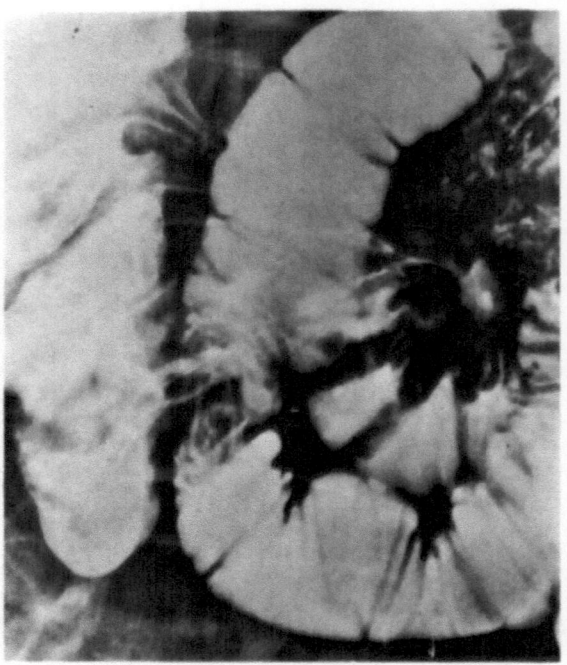

*Fig. 8.39*A. Thin fistulous tracts can best be demonstrated with a contrast fluid of low viscosity and high specific gravity. They are visualized most clearly with a low tube voltage and also a low film density (left). A combination of adhesion and a fistulous tract in a patient suffering from herringworm disease (right).

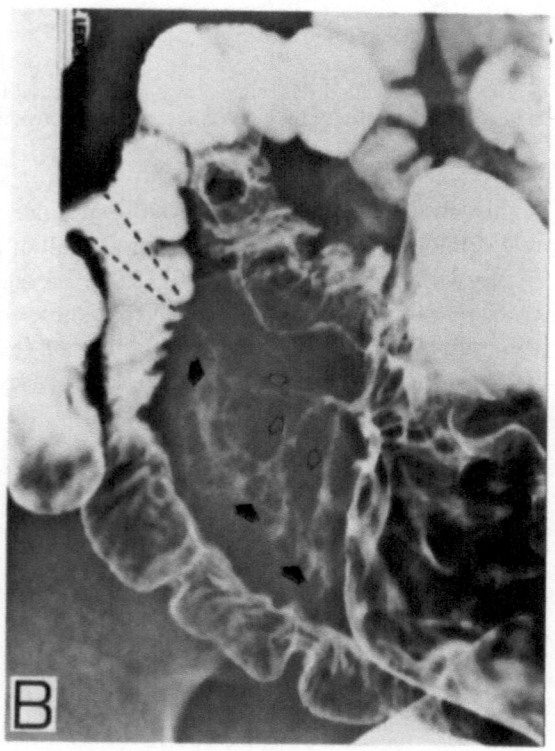

lous tracts are often very narrow, it is possible to visualize them only when the contrast fluid is still thin and there is as yet no increase in the viscosity due to dehydration. Careful projection in order to distinguish them from adjacent intestinal loops and underexposure with a low tube voltage ($\pm$ 80 kV) are also essential in order to be able to demonstrate these final canals (fig. 8.39).

5.3. Fibrosis and shriveling

Fibrotic shriveling of the intestinal wall can cause circular strictures with a completely healthy intestine and normal mucosal relief on either side. If the stricture is about 0.5 cm long, then either a healed ulcer of aspecific origin (fig. 8.40K) or shriveling as a result of carcinoid (fig. 8.40L) must be considered especially. In Crohn's disease when a skip lesion has healed with the formation of fibrosis, or after a cured ischemia with secondary ulceration, the stenosis is as a rule somewhat longer (fig. 8.40M). Multiple short stenoses, like those in fig. 8.40K, due to Crohn's disease are highly unusual (fig. 9.37B). In some cases an adenocarcinoma of

*Fig. 8.39*B. Three fistulous tracts between the ileum (barely visible) and the rectosigmoid, made better visible by rectal air insufflation. Crohn's disease.

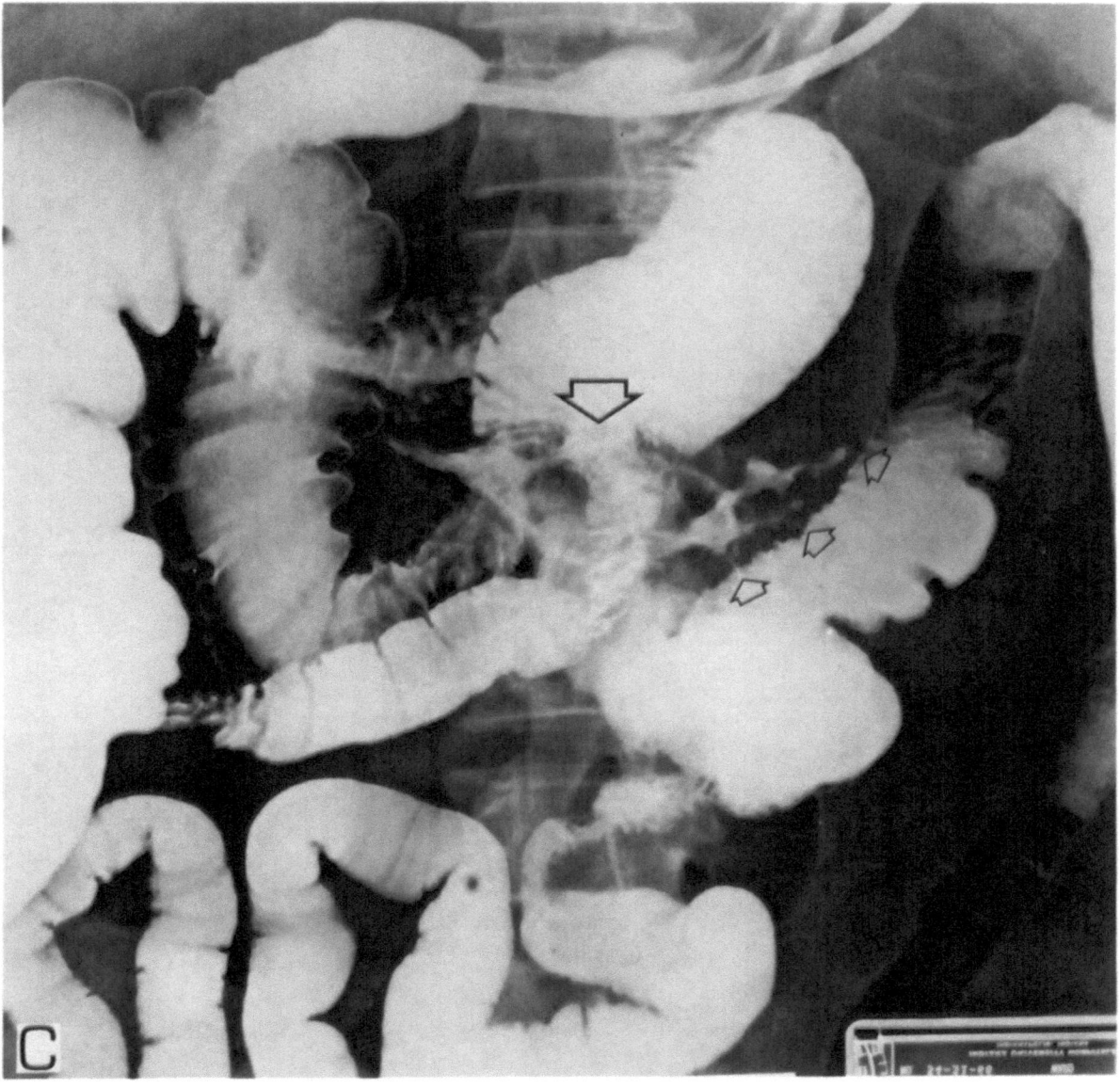

Fig. 8.39c. Enteroclysis examination of a patient weighing 450 pounds who underwent bypass surgery whereby the jejunum and the ileum were connected to combat obesity. Physical examination was impossible. It appeared that at the site of the anastomosis (arrow), fistulization had developed, including three canals to the transverse colon (120 kV in this patient).

the small intestine can also appear as a smooth-walled circular stenosis (fig. 8.40N). However, then the transition between the stenosis and the healthy small intestine is biconvex and not nozzle-shaped as in the case of a healed ulcer. In addition the tumor can cause a small space-occupying process outside the stenosis. In the event of shriveling, this generally does not occur although, here too, the wall can be thickened due to an increase in muscular and especially fibrotic tissue.

Ulcers directed along the length of the intestinal wall and therefore perpendicular to the mucosal folds, as so often seen in Crohn's disease, heal in a completely different manner. At the site of the ulcer, usually on the mesenteric side of the intestine, there is plaque-like fibrosis with secondary shriveling so that the mucosal folds on the other side of the intestinal lumen acquire a more or less concentric

164

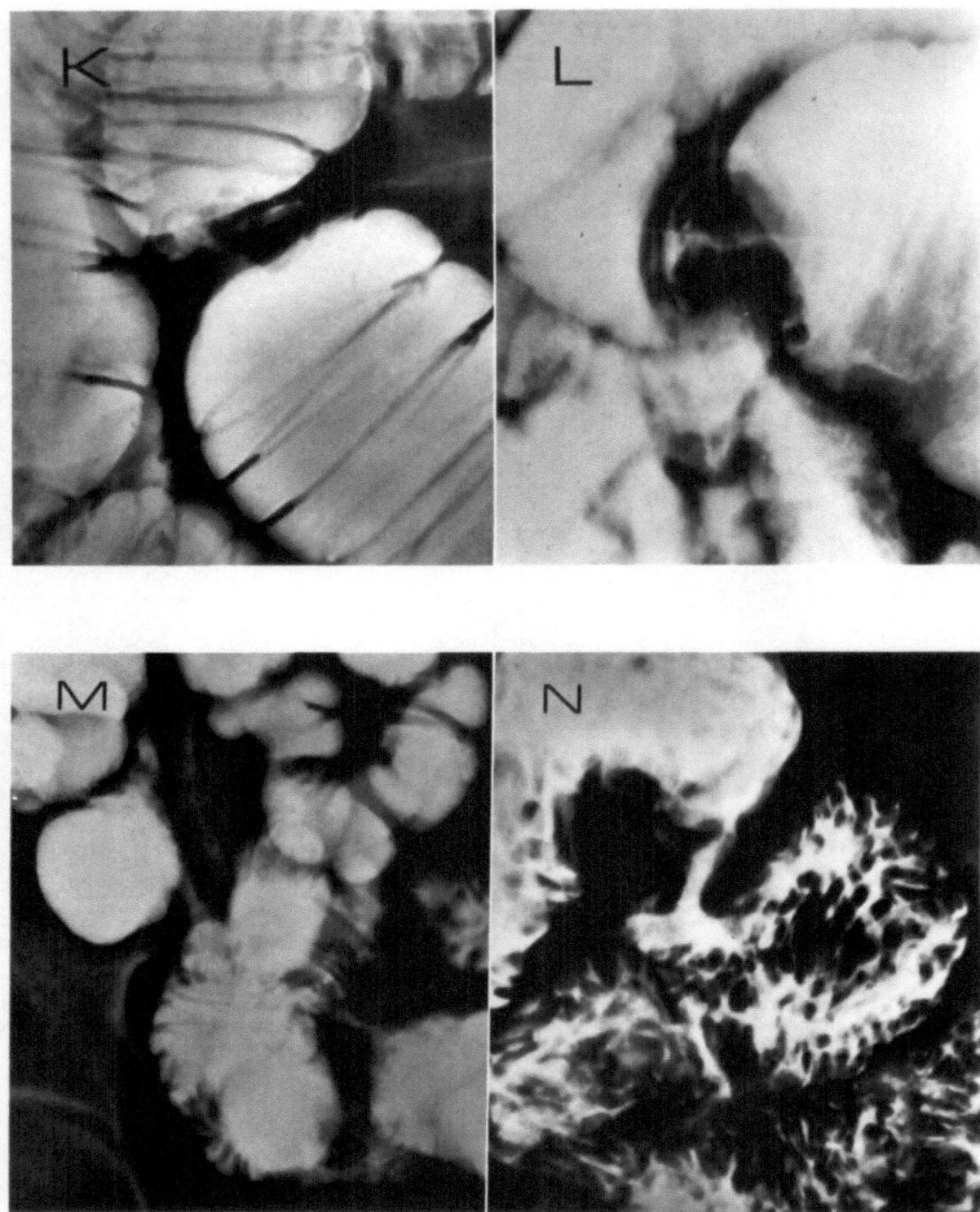

Fig. 8.40. Stenosis in the small intestine, 0.5–1.0 cm long, as a result of an aspecific ulceration (K) and a carcinoid (L). In both cases fibrosis is pronounced. Stenoses in the small bowel more than 1 cm long due to a skip lesion in Crohn's disease (M) and an adenocarcinoma (N).

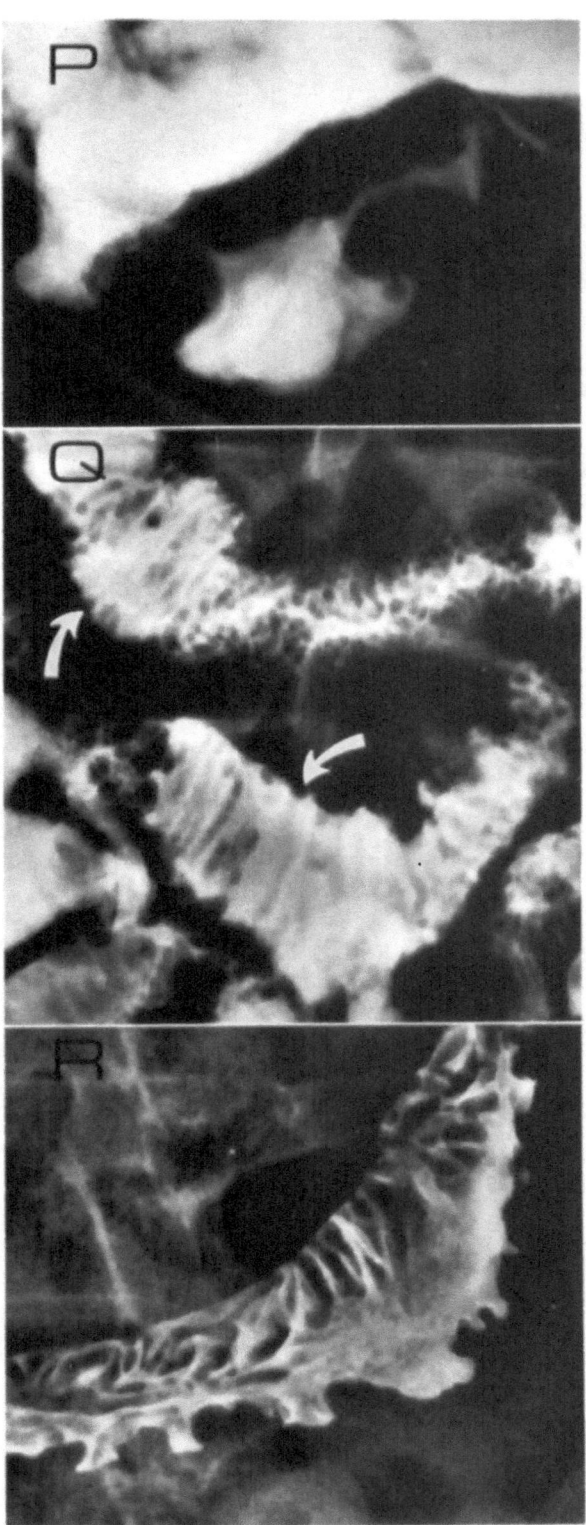

Fig. 8.41. (P) Concentric course of mucosal folds due to asymmetric shriveling as a result of an ulceration on one side of the intestine. (Q) Plaque without mucosal relief in the intestine, not yet shriveled. (R) The same pattern can be seen in the colon.

course directed toward the healed ulcer (fig. 8.41P). Figure 2.10B shows a misleading pattern of an elongated ulcer in the distal ileum; this was caused by the appendix, which is pressed up against the ileum. Note that there are no signs of mucosal abnormalities in the wall opposite the 'ulcer'. In other cases of healed ulcerations, we can find sclerotic plaques in the intestine (fig. 8.41Q). A highly similar pattern can be seen in the rare case of metastasis in the wall of the small intestine from a linitis plastica of the stomach. The shriveling can, however, be much less pronounced or even practically missing. As a result of shriveling on one side, so-called pseudodiverticula can also develop. They sometimes have a broad base at the intestinal wall and may change continuously in size and shape during the various stages of the examination (fig. 8.42). Fibrosis due to carcinoid lesions where the mesentery is attached to the intestine causes marked deformation of the intestinal lumen, sometimes with strictures. In the literature this is called kinking (fig. 8.43). Surgical anastomoses for the purpose of intestinal resection generally do not cause such deformations of the intestine. This obvious alternative diagnosis need not be considered when this phenomenon is observed (fig. 8.44). Kinking or angulation of intestinal loops as well as extensive mutual fusion or adhesions can also be seen in so-called retractile or sclerosing mesenteritis. This is a rare disorder that is accompanied by pronounced fatty degeneration and postinfectious shriveling of the mesentery (fig. 8.45).

As a result of the pronounced shortening and increased thickness of the mesentery, there are then only a few intestinal loops in the center of the abdomen that sometimes follow a more or less taut polycyclic convex course extending outward to the periphery. The decreased lumen of the intestine can vary in size. It is striking that in spite of all of these changes the mucosal relief is still relatively unchanged. The space between the separate intestinal loops is sometimes obviously greater. This phenomenon, although less pronounced, can sometimes also be seen in obese patients. This is possibly due in part to an intraabdominal autocompression of the intestinal loops in the prone position caused by the voluminous greater omentum (fig. 2.26).

In Crohn's disease, as a result of the increase in mesenteric fat, large empty spaces between the

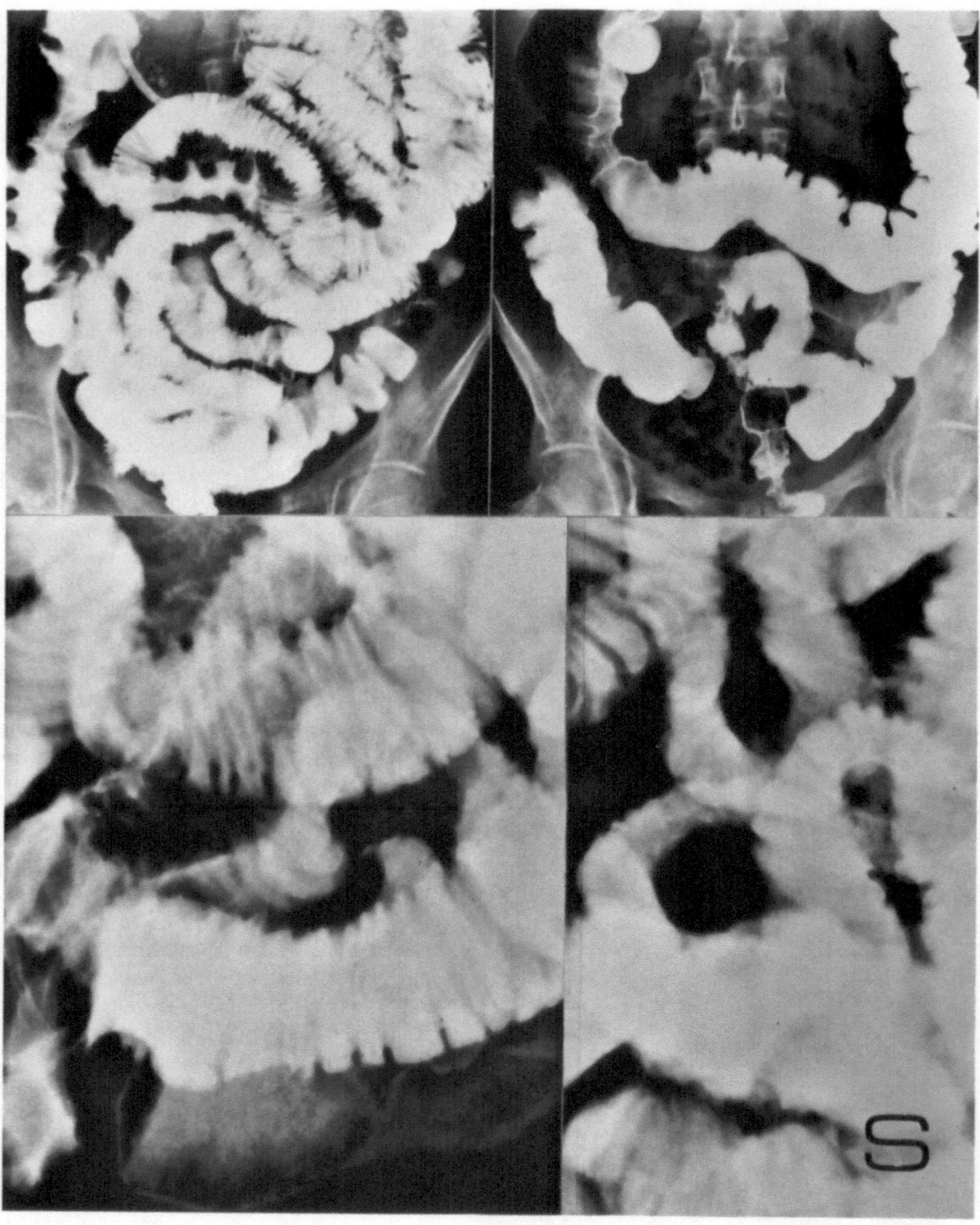

*Fig. 8.41*s. Innumerable plaques with shriveling and loss of mucosal relief throughout the entire digestive tract. These abnormalities could be attributed to metastasis of linitis plastica.

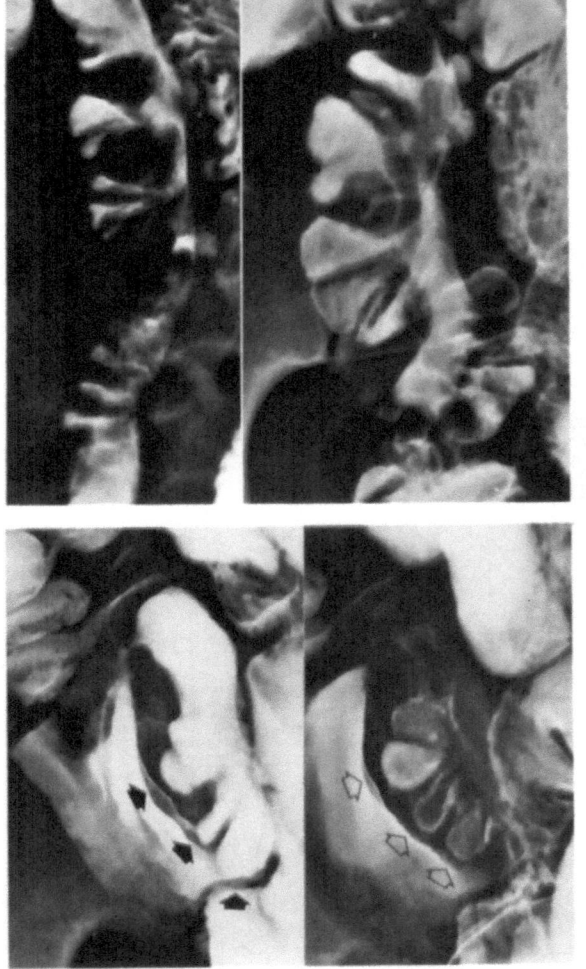

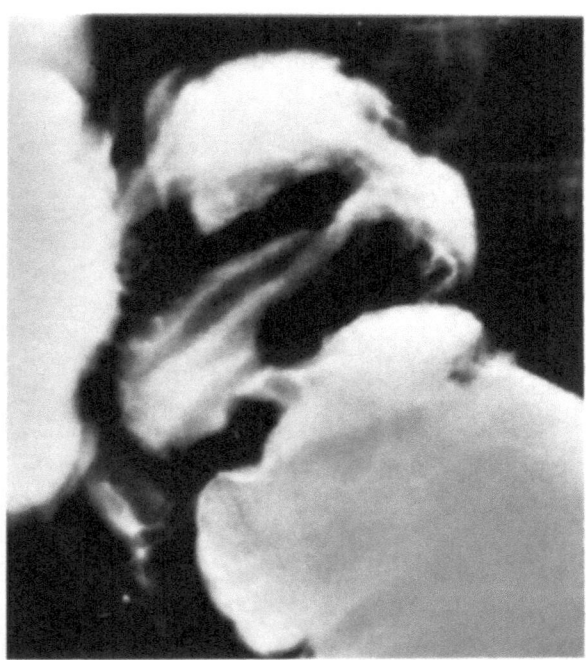

Fig. 8.43. Sudden changes in the caliber of the lumen and direction of the longitudinal axis of the intestine as a result of shriveling at a carcinoid site (so-called kinking).

Fig. 8.42. Opposite stretched, shriveled longitudinal ulcerations, pseudodiverticula in the intestine develop as a result of spastic or partially fibrotic constrictions. They vary in shape and size. Crohn's disease (top) and vasculitis (bottom).

intestinal loops may sometimes also be seen usually in the lower right quadrant (fig. 8.46). If, however, in Crohn's disease the intestinal loops also follow a taut extended course, and there is a varying but marked narrowing of the lumen, then this is definitely accompanied by an obviously abnormal mucosal pattern.

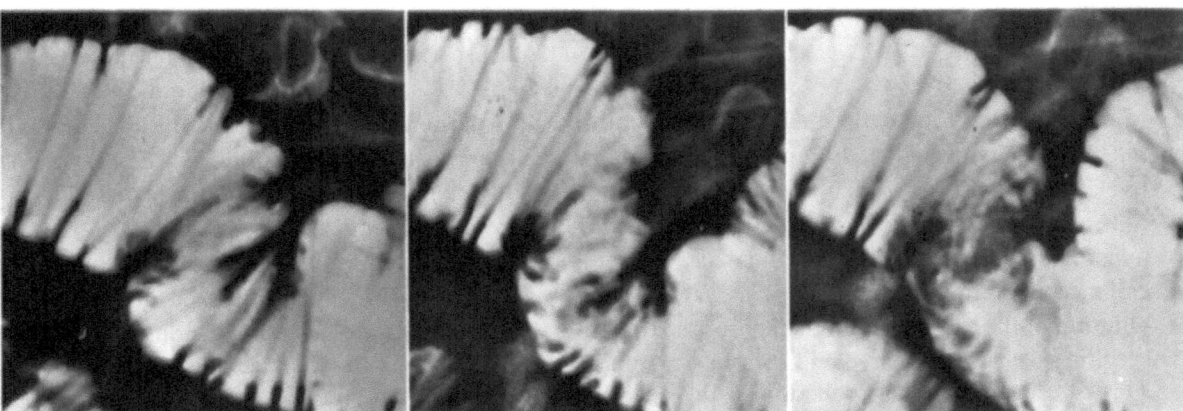

Fig. 8.44. Relatively stenotic area at a surgical anastomosis in the jejunum, made visible by stretching of the intestine. Moderately disordered mucosal pattern.

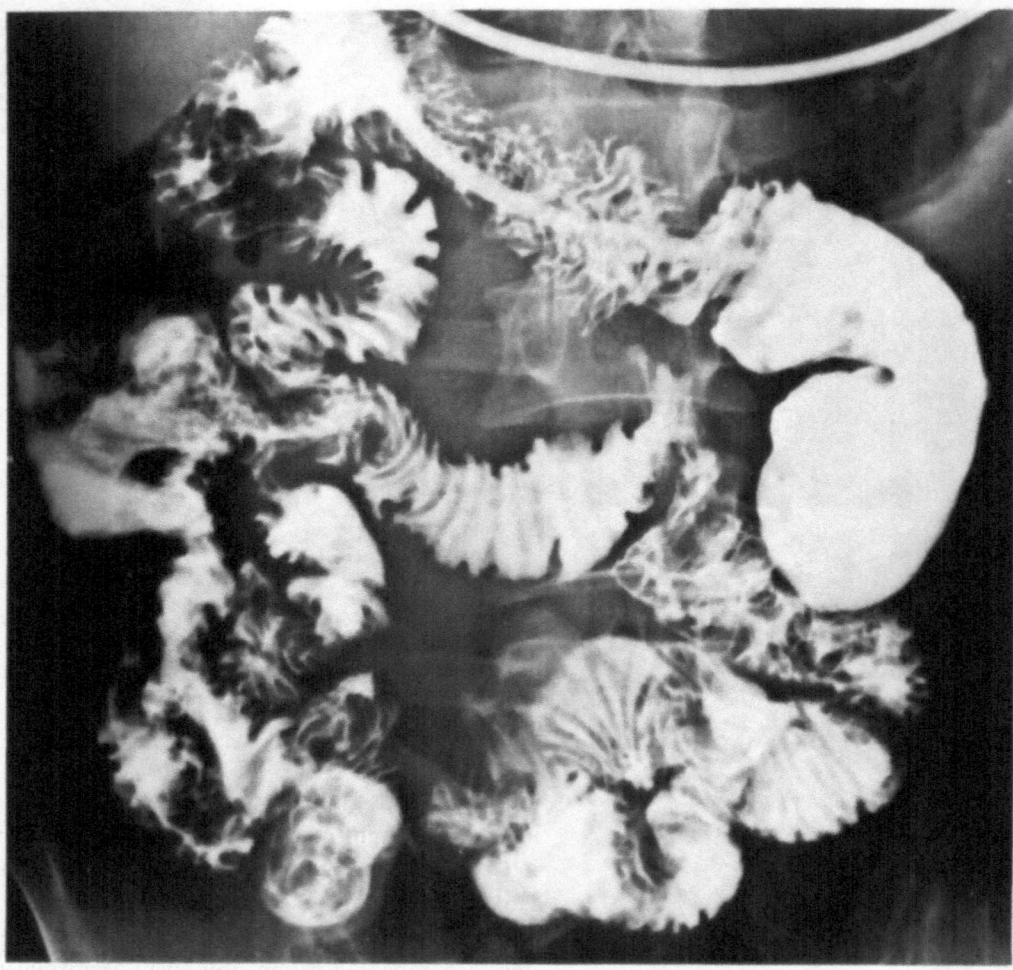

Fig. 8.45. Proven case of mesenteric fibrosis. There are stenotic areas and kinking-like configurations with an empty space in the middle of the abdomen. Short bowel because of a resection a few years previously.

6. Dilution of the contrast fluid – haziness – mucus secretion

Maximum adhesion to the mucosa and therefore the sharpest patterns are obtained when the contrast fluid flows past a 'dry' intestinal wall. Addition of glucose products or other substances with hyperosmotic characteristics or a high caloric value enhances secretion of digestive juices and mucus. Dilution of the contrast fluid then occurs so that the specific gravity is decreased and contrast is reduced. This of course means a reduction in the apparent sharpness of the pattern. This is clearly demonstrated by comparing two examinations of the same patient carried out within a few days of each other.

Figure 8.47D shows a jejunum x-ray when 40 g glucose was added to the 600 ml barium suspension; fig. 8.47E shows the same without any additives in the barium suspension. The differences that are clearly visible here would have been even greater if both examinations had been carried out in the conventional manner.

When the intestinal wall is coated with mucus that is not immediately flushed off by a contrast fluid with a lower viscosity, the outer margins of the contrast column are also less sharp. Within the layer of mucus there is a gradual decrease in the specific gravity of the contrast fluid from 1.25 to 1.0. The vague reproduction of the intestinal mucosa that results from this decrease in specific

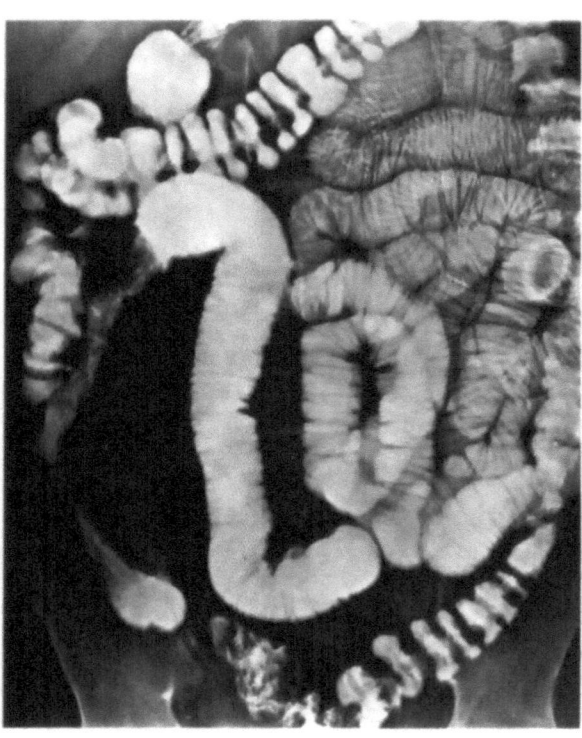

Fig. 8.46. Large empty spaces in the lower right quadrant in a patient with Crohn's disease due to fatty degeneration and shriveling of the mesentery, an extensive layer of fat around the involved intestine, and in some cases also due to infiltration abnormalities. No indications of an infiltrate could be found in this patient.

gravity can be enhanced by dilution of the contrast fluid and by a decrease in sharpness due to hypermotility of the intestinal wall. This is called 'haziness' in the literature (fig. 8.48).

If the viscosity of the mucus coating is very high, which sometimes occurs in inflammatory processes, the mucus is often impossible to flush from the intestinal wall in spite of the administration of large amounts of contrast fluid. The patterns then remain vague (fig. 8.36). Under normal circumstances it can sometimes be seen that the difference in viscosity between the barium suspension and mucus is so great that mixing does not occur. The mucus then remains visible as poorly defined threads that are carried off distally in toto (fig. 8.49).

In other cases, for instance in the event of mechanical obstructions, the intestinal wall is not coated with mucus; instead large quantities of watery fluid are found in the intestinal lumen. There is complete mixing, right up to the intestinal wall, of the barium suspension with the thin fluid in the

intestine. The specific gravity of the former decreases but the sharp delineation of the intestinal wall is retained.

7. Disintegration and misleading patterns

Flocculation of the contrast fluid is a phenomenon that is still seen regularly in a conventional follow-through examination, even when the most stable barium suspension is used, in cases of severe malabsorption. As soon as flocculation occurs, anatomical representation of the intestinal mucosa is impossible and the radiological examination should be terminated (fig. 8.50). In an adequately executed enteroclysis examination, flocculation of the contrast fluid is never encountered within the period required for the actual examination – even in cases of severe malabsorption. If, however, a water infusion is administered after the contrast medium infusion, flocculation may occur at the end of the contrast column where the water column and the barium suspension meet and mix (fig. 7.22). The same phenomenon can occur at the beginning of the contrast column under certain circumstances (fig. 8.51). The first quantity of barium suspension administered has, after all, the most intense contact with the contents of the intestine. Local enhanced secretion of digestive juices, heightened mucus production, fluid absorption, or dehydration due to disturbed resorption of hyperosmotic food particles can sometimes cause disintegration of the first 50 or 100 ml barium suspension. However, the small quantity of disintegrated contrast fluid is quickly forced onward by the rapidly flowing fresh barium suspension. This disintegration of the contrast fluid is observed only when there is sufficient penetration of the contrast fluid by the roentgen rays. It can be masked entirely by underexposure (fig. 4.8). A contrast medium that has flocculated is much more viscous than an intact barium suspension and is no longer able to retain the impression of the folds of the soft intestinal mucosa. Never forget therefore that disintegration of the barium suspension leads to apparent coarsening of the fold relief (fig. 4.9). Failure to recognize this fact will lead to thoroughly incorrect conclusions.

In the proximal part of the jejunum the tendency to reproduce the mucosal folds more coarsely than

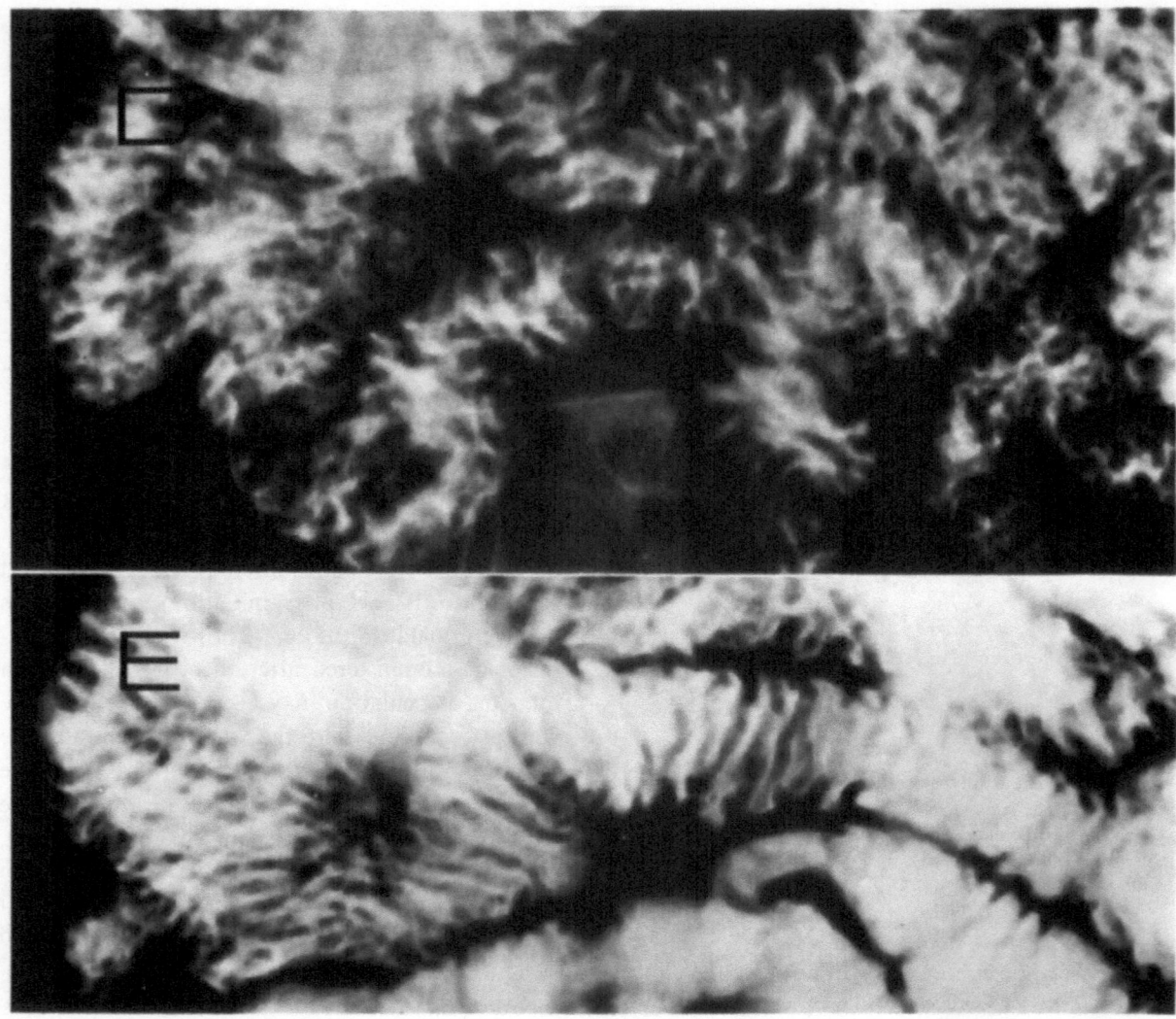

Fig. 8.47. Spot films of the jejunum of same patient as seen in fig. 7.13. (D) Glucose added to the contrast fluid. (E) Repeat examination without glucose.

they truly are is enhanced when there is only moderate filling of the intestinal loops because of hypermotility. The drawing in fig. 8.52 and the in vitro experiment illustrated in fig. 8.53 show that the mucosal folds appear coarser in a moderately filled intestine than in a well-filled intestine. This same phenomenon can be encountered in vivo. Figure 8.54P shows mucosal folds in the jejunum that seem to be very coarse; they appeared quite different in a second examination taken after hypotonia had been induced (fig. 8.54Q). Endoscopic examination and biopsy studies revealed no abnormalities. In our opinion, supported by our experience, the coarse mucosal patterns in Whipple's disease that are mentioned so often in the

literature are also mainly due to an artifact – at least in most cases. In practice an increased tendency toward flocculation and hypermotility often coincide, resulting in an accumulation of unfavorable factors. Evaluation of the shape of the mucosal folds should therefore not be based on the patterns obtained at the beginning nor at the end of the contrast column, and certainly not if it is obvious that the contrast fluid lost its original structure. In exceptional cases, for instance after irradiation of the lower abdomen, we can see quite local and randomly situated spots of disintegrated barium suspension in the middle of the contrast column soon after the infusion is terminated (fig. 8.55A). It should now be apparent that local abnormalities of

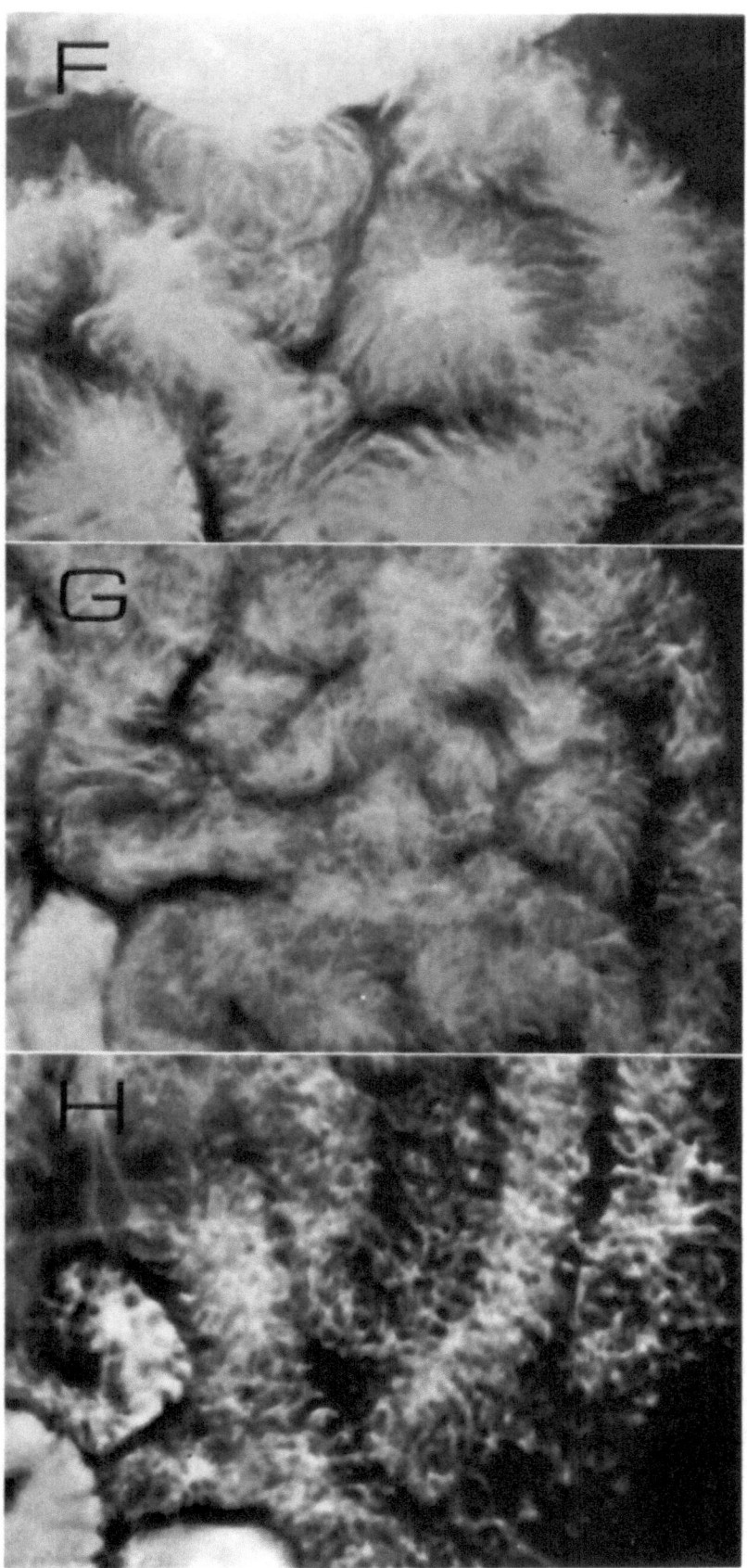

Fig. 8.48. Contrast column with vague margins due to a combination of movement of the intestinal wall, caused by hypermotility, and dilution of the contrast fluid, caused by hypersecretion or disturbed resorption of fluids (F and G). With the infusion technique this vagueness or haziness is less pronounced (H) (same patient).

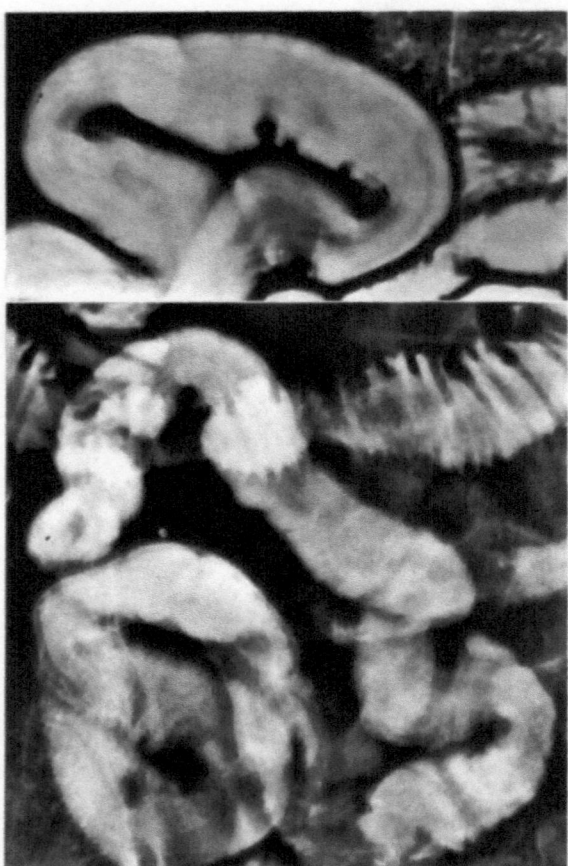

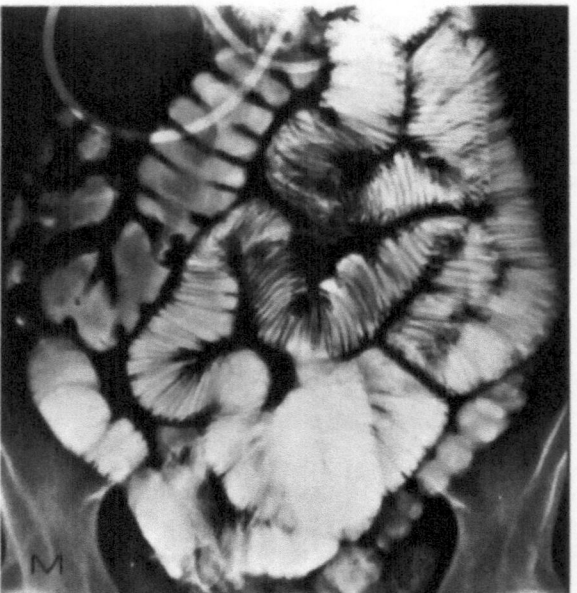

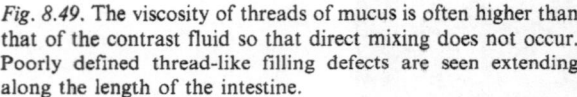

Fig. 8.49. The viscosity of threads of mucus is often higher than that of the contrast fluid so that direct mixing does not occur. Poorly defined thread-like filling defects are seen extending along the length of the intestine.

an inflammatory nature or local enhanced secretion must be involved. For evaluation of the mucosal patterns therefore, it is better to use the films taken during the infusion, and preferably those toward the end of the series.

When an examination has to be prolonged for any reason, changes in the structure of the contrast fluid can also occur in the distal ileum where dehydration leads to thickening of the barium suspension. One then sees a crackle pattern consisting of haphazardly arranged thin bright lines throughout the barium column (fig. 8.55B). These lines can probably be ascribed to residual fold impressions of the more proximal loops where the contrast fluid was less thick only a short time before. As a result of the kneading action in the intestine, these lines become haphazardly arranged.

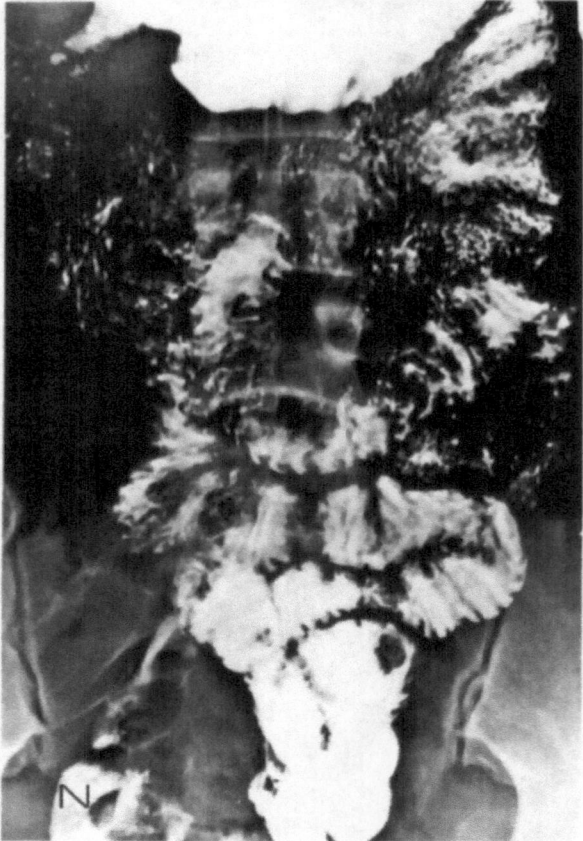

Fig. 8.50. (KM) Enteroclysis films of the small intestine of two patients with a clinical malabsorption syndrome. (LN) The films of the conventional examination carried out one week earlier showed clear disintegration of the contrast medium so that a true reproduction of the intestinal mucous membrane could no longer be obtained.

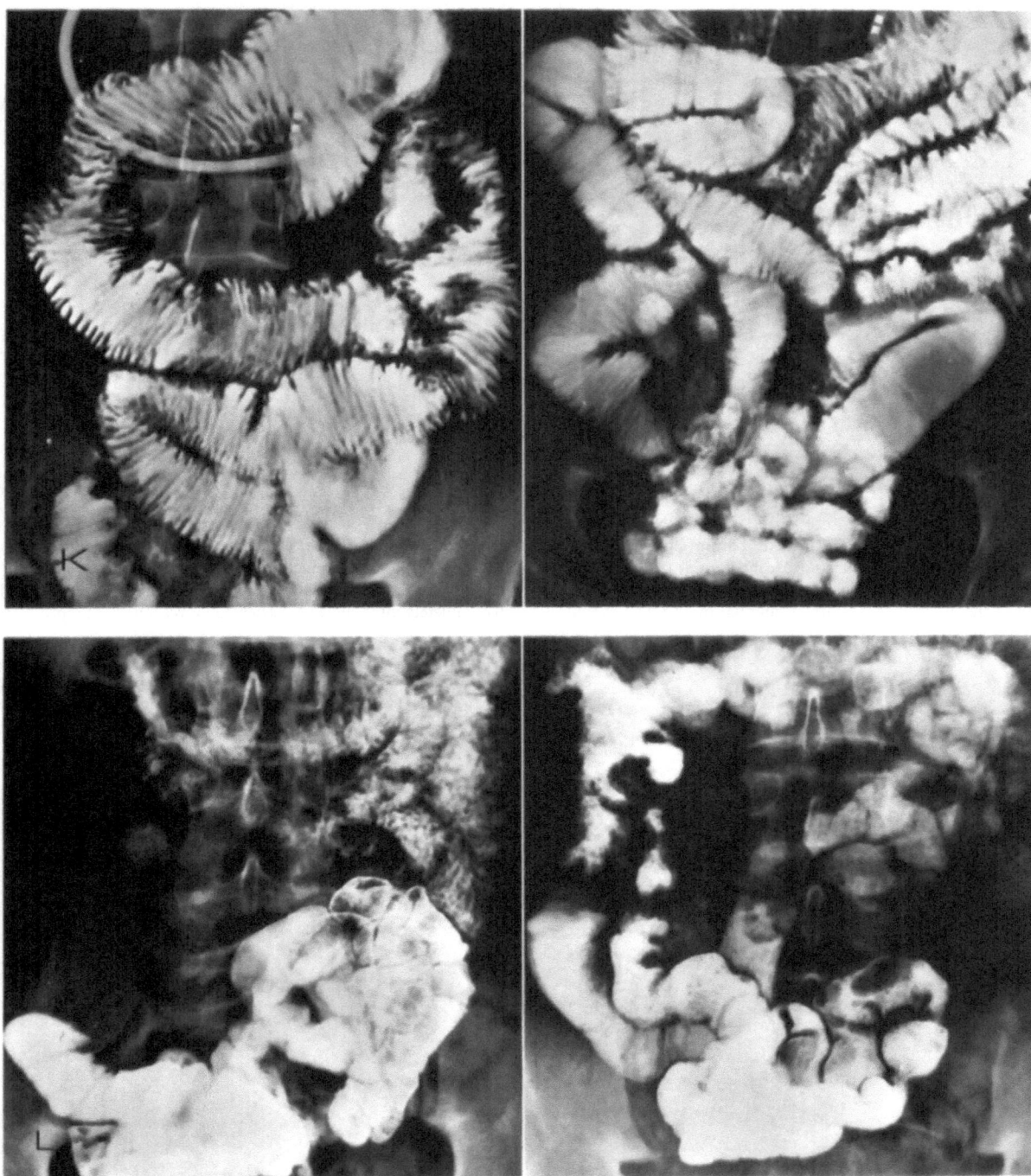

Fig. 8.50. See legend on page 172.

They are thin because they no longer contain folds. An argument in favor of this theory is the fact that often such lines lie perpendicular to the longitudinal impression that is still just visible at the margin.

If during an adequately executed enteroclysis examination the structure in the distal ileum is grainy or inhomogeneous, then each of the following causes should be considered:

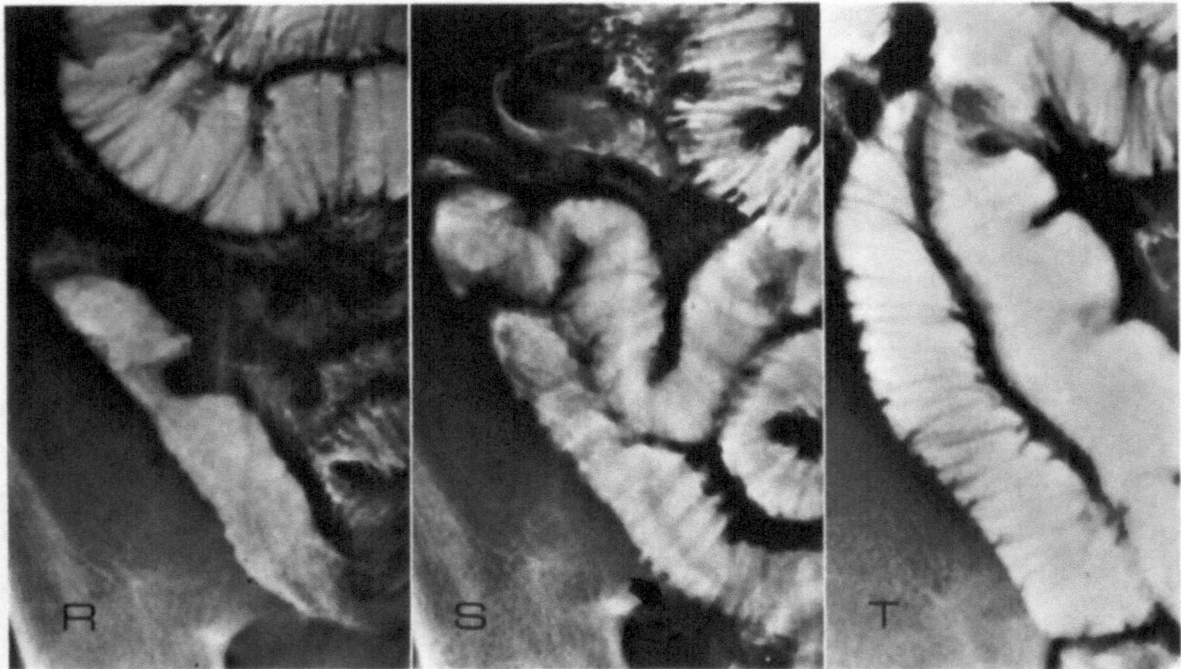

Fig. 8.51. Disintegration of the barium suspension can sometimes occur at the head of the contrast column. Because of the increase in the viscosity of the contrast medium, it is no longer possible to obtain a good reproduction of the mucosal folds (R). At the same location but several minutes later, disintegration is less and vague impressions of the mucosal folds can already be seen (s). Still later the disintegrated contrast fluid has moved distally and the fresh completely intact barium suspension gives a normal reproduction of the fold relief (T).

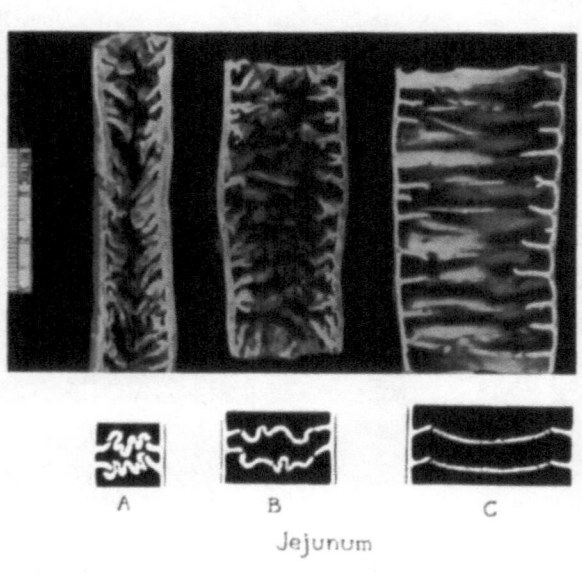

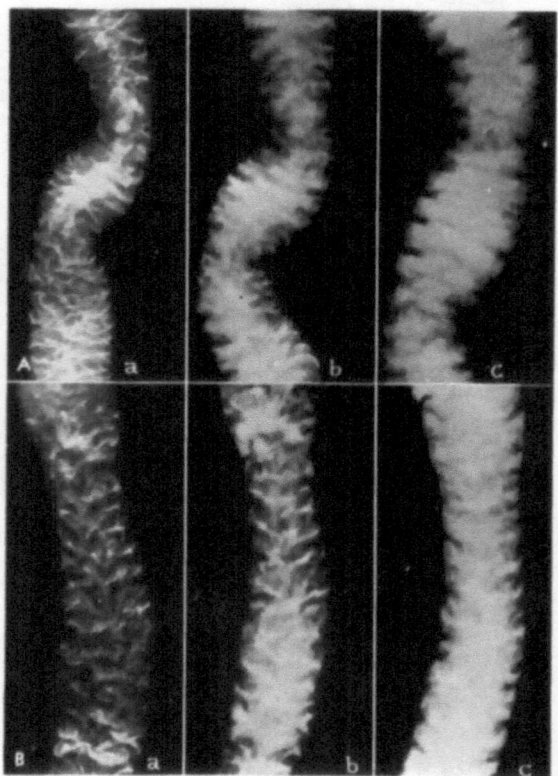

Fig. 8.52. Schematic representation of a stretched and a contracted intestinal loop. Stretched mucosal folds probably cause thinner clarification lines on the x-ray than those which are more or less folded together [220].

Fig. 8.53. Sloan's experiments in vitro showing that mucosal folds appear coarser when the intestinal loops are moderately filled with contrast fluid than when the loops are well filled.

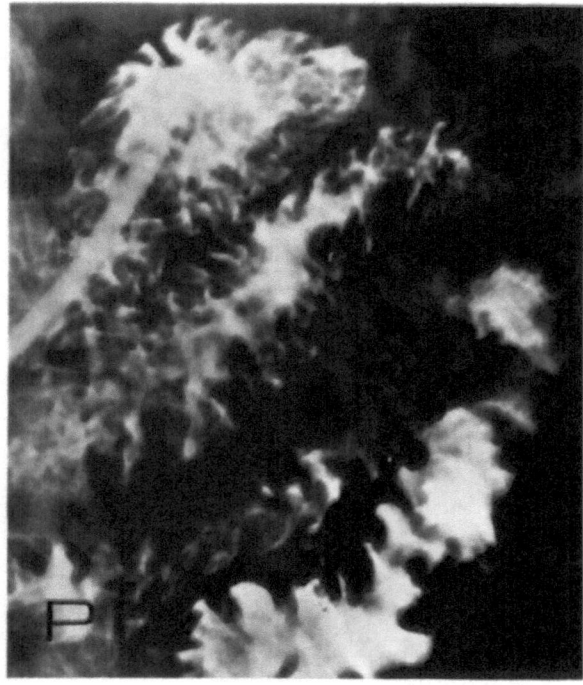 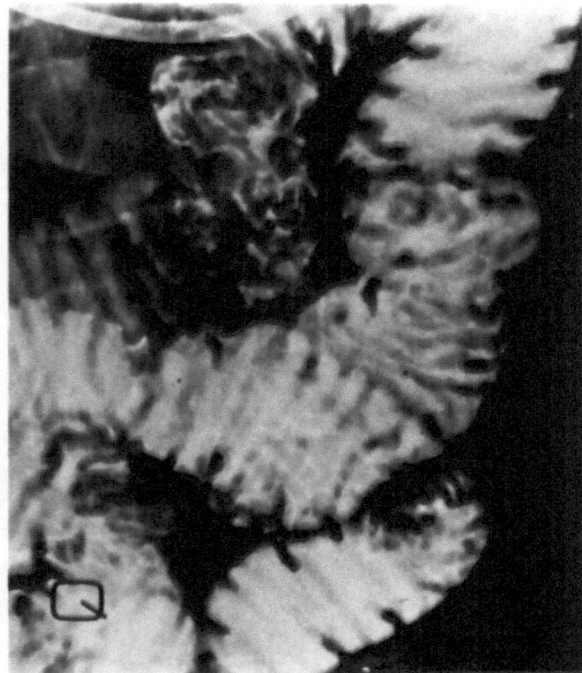

Fig. 8.54. These mucosal folds in the jejunum were judged definitely too coarse (P). Before the repeat examination, a hypotonic agent was administered. The folds are now seen to be completely normal (Q).

1) beginning of the contrast column (fig. 8.51);
2) food residue as a result of atony of the small intestine due to chronic use of tranquilizers, sedatives, or antispasmodics (fig. 8.28);
3) the stomach was not empty;
4) reflux of the contents of the cecum due to an inadequate Bauhin's valve in ulcerative colitis (fig. 7.23).

8. Malabsorption

A great deal has been written in the past about malabsorption, and today it is still the subject of an occasional article. For older radiologists it is a diagnosis frequently encountered in the course of their career, since until recently the contrast medium very often flocculated. In fact, malabsorption does accompany 50–100 disorders of the small intestine so that this diagnosis was seldom incorrect. One wonders therefore why radiodiagnosis of the small intestine is regarded with such disfavor. If desired, malabsorption can be subdivided into three categories that with a little effort could include practically all existing disorders of the small intestine:

1) Disturbed digestion of food, irrespective of whether this is caused by a bacterial infection or a deficiency of digestive juices or enzymes.
2) Disturbed food transport either because transit is too rapid or too slow or because the intestine is too short after repeated resections.
3) Truly disturbed resorption of the partially digested food particles as a result of various disorders that more or less damage the intestinal mucosa or, as in edema, impede its function.

Radiology can only offer an extremely modest contribution to the differentiation between the many diseases with the malabsorption syndrome. In a number of cases, radiological differential diagnosis is in principle not possible. This is because there are many histological and biochemical abnormalities of the small intestinal mucous membrane without macroscopic abnormalities. There remain, however, many diseases with malabsorption for which a morphological examination can be highly valuable. This applies for:

1) Diseases with gross anatomical abnormalities: anastomoses, fistulas, blind loops, short bowel, strictures, adhesions; diverticula.

176

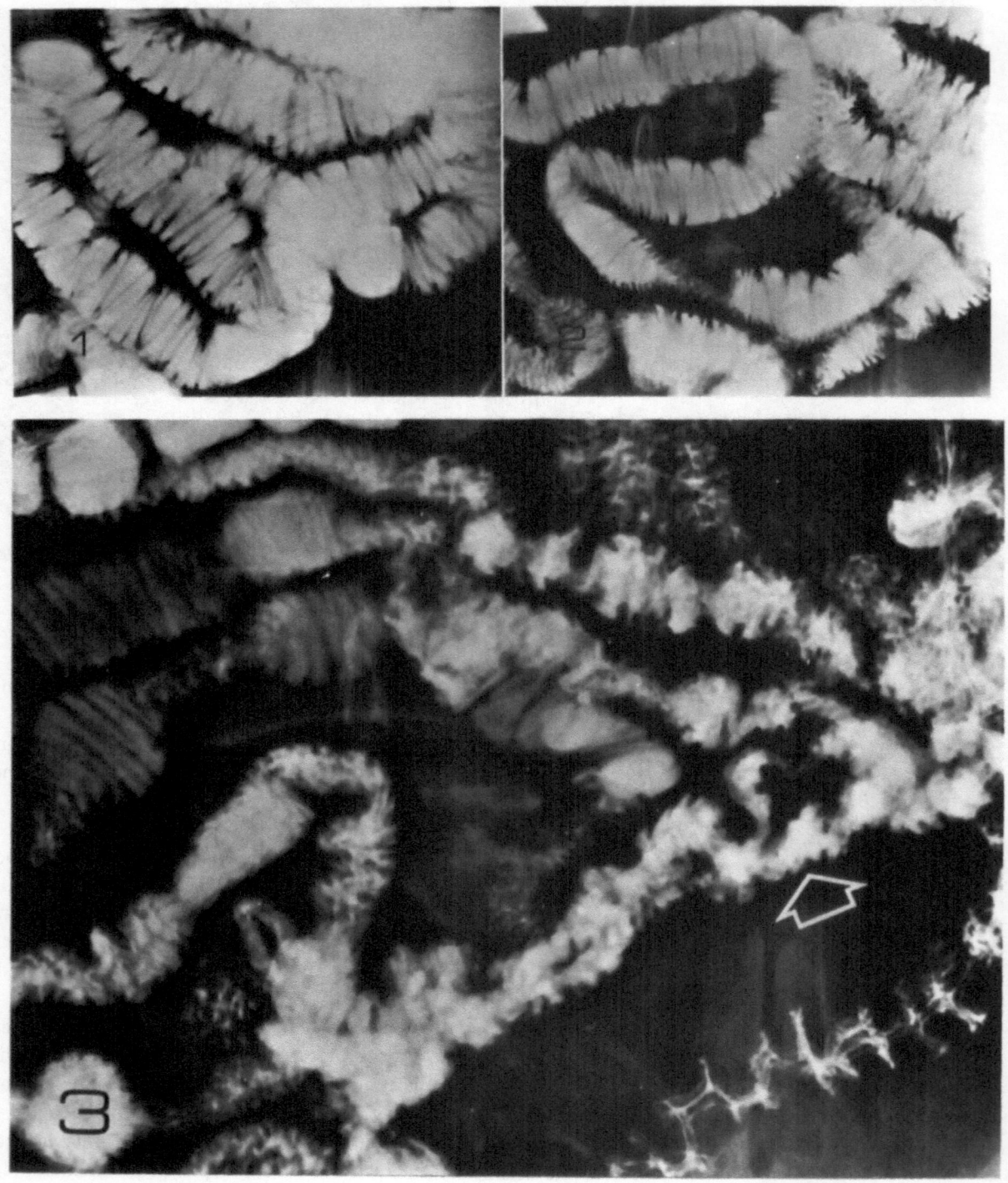

*Fig. 8.55*A. Local spasticity of the intestine and disintegration of the barium suspension in the middle of the contrast column, soon after the infusion was terminated. Three x-rays taken at 2-min intervals. The cause of these abnormalities in this patient remained unknown.

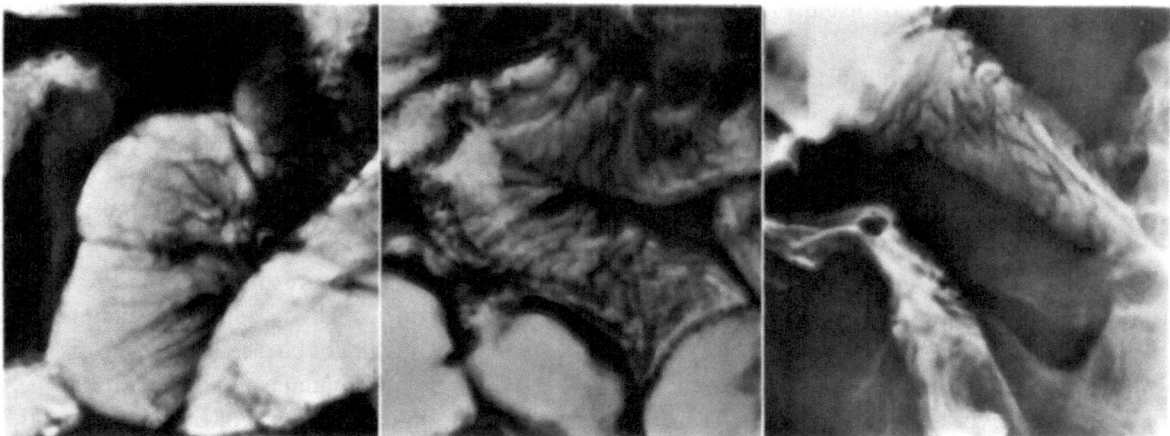

*Fig. 8.55*B. Crackle-like configuration of bright lines in the contrast fluid in the distal ileum. We have seen these lines as yet only in the ileum; presumably they are caused by residual fold impressions in a thickened barium suspension.

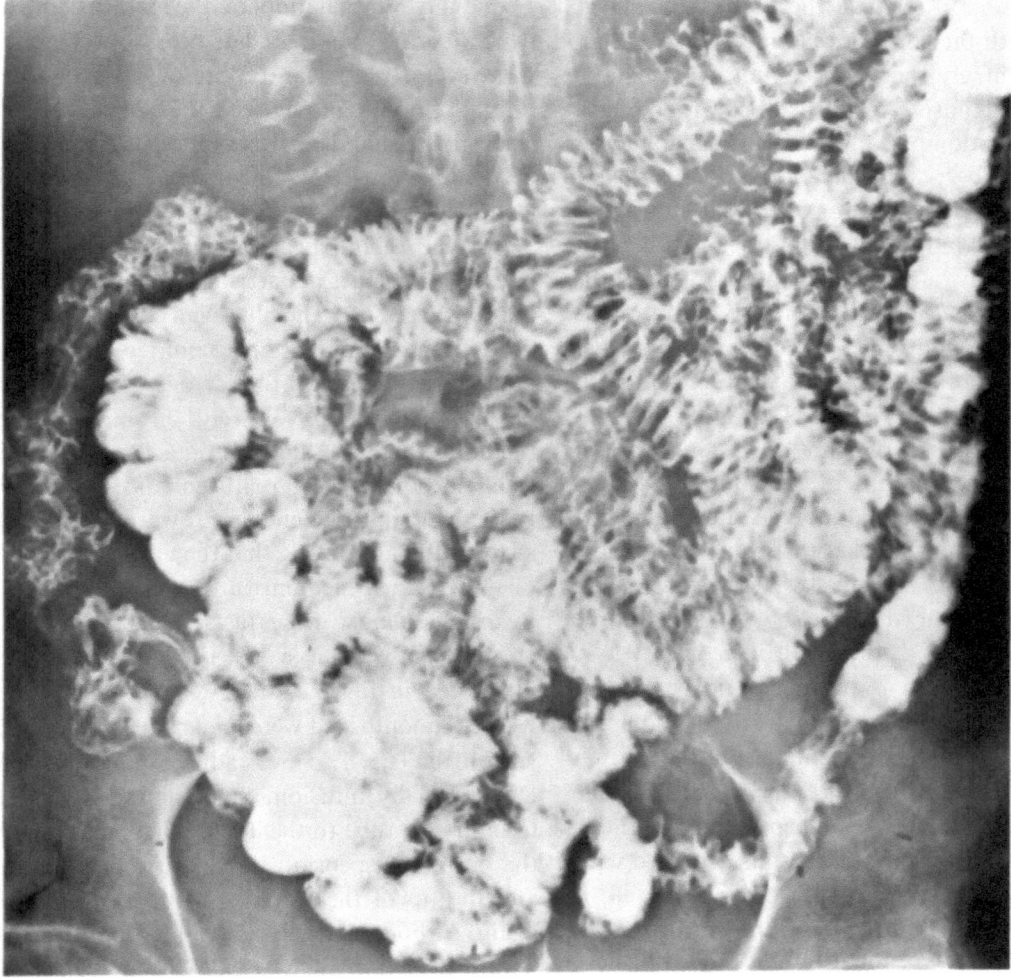

Fig. 8.56. Highly thickened mucosal folds in the jejunum and hypermotility of the small intestine in a patient with mixed collagen disease. A marked malabsorption was apparent clinically. The hypermotility and the edema could be due to anoxia as a result of vasculitis.

2) Diseases with local, usually rather gross, mucosal abnormalities:
   leukemia, Hodgkin's disease, lymphosarcoma; intramural bleeding; local edema due to venous congestion (e.g. thrombosis) or lymphatic obstruction (irradiation).
3) Diseases with more general mucosal abnormalities:
   edema due to lymphangiectasis, allergic reactions, protein-losing enteropathy; amyloidosis, Whipple's disease, scleroderma.
4) All those diseases accompanied by such a pronounced hypermotility that there is insufficient time for resorption of the nutriments, as for example in collagen diseases (fig. 8.56).

For some of these diseases, the radiologist is the only one who can provide the correct diagnosis. However, with the conventional methods of examination still in use, he often cannot even make a differential diagnosis. He must suffice with a report that malabsorption probably exists. This opinion is based on the observation of flocculation as well as the eventual disintegration of the barium into segment clumps in the small intestine. This conclusion incidentally is seldom important since the referring specialist is usually already aware of the malabsorption syndrome on the basis of other evidence. As soon as flocculation occurs, morphological evaluation of the small intestine becomes impossible because there is no longer any relationship between the margins of the contrast column and those of the intestinal mucous membrane.

The flocculation is usually irreversible and the flocculi continue to grow in size until segments are formed. In addition, when the rate of transit of the contrast fluid through the small intestine is slow, this clump formation is promoted further in the distal ileum by the absorption of fluids from the intestine. In the colon, segmentation of the barium column is the natural end of every normal passage through the small intestine. When various methods of examination as well as the results obtained with diverse brands of contrast media are analyzed, it becomes apparent that the development of flocculation is highly dependent upon both of these factors. As a result, one radiologist will observe flocculation frequently and another only when

there is a serious malabsorption. The highly illogical situation then arises that a radiologist can only interpret to a limited degree the small intestine examination of a colleague. Even if there are signs of a pronounced and relatively early flocculation on the x-ray film of a patient with a known malabsorption, the radiologist will not be able to express his opinion about the severity of the malabsorption. Therefore an observed flocculation and segmentation must be reported such that faulty conclusions will not be drawn. This means that each radiologist accumulates experience exclusively for himself, based on the use of one specific method of examination. This experience cannot be transferred to someone else. Should he change one or both of these factors, then he has lost his experience in this respect and he must start again.

Actually, flocculation of the contrast medium, which for the most part has been overcome in the past several years, can be caused by many factors that have nothing to do with the clinical concept of resorption. Clinical malabsorption therefore cannot be demonstrated on x-rays, but must instead be identified by means of fecal examination.

For the radiological examination of the small intestine, in babies in particular – which fortunately is a rare necessity – the physician should realize that an optimum examination technique is essential to obtain useful results. Babies only several months old are fed almost entirely on milk products; therefore there is a high lactic acid content in the small intestine, which greatly enhances flocculation. In these infants, the tendency toward flocculation is so exceptionally strong that the natural rate of flow of the contrast medium through the stomach and pylorus is almost never fast enough to prevent it, even when a very large dose is administered. This is illustrated in fig. 6.2; these x-rays of babies who were 3–8 months old were made after 400 ml barium suspension (s.g. 1.15) was administered at a rate of 80 ml/min by infusion. Since it was not possible to insert the tube to the Treitz's ligament, reflux of the barium suspension into the stomach occurred and the tip of the tube ended up in the stomach again. Although another 200 ml barium suspension as well as several ml metoclopramide were given before the tube was removed, the natural rate of gastric emptying was too slow to prevent floccu-

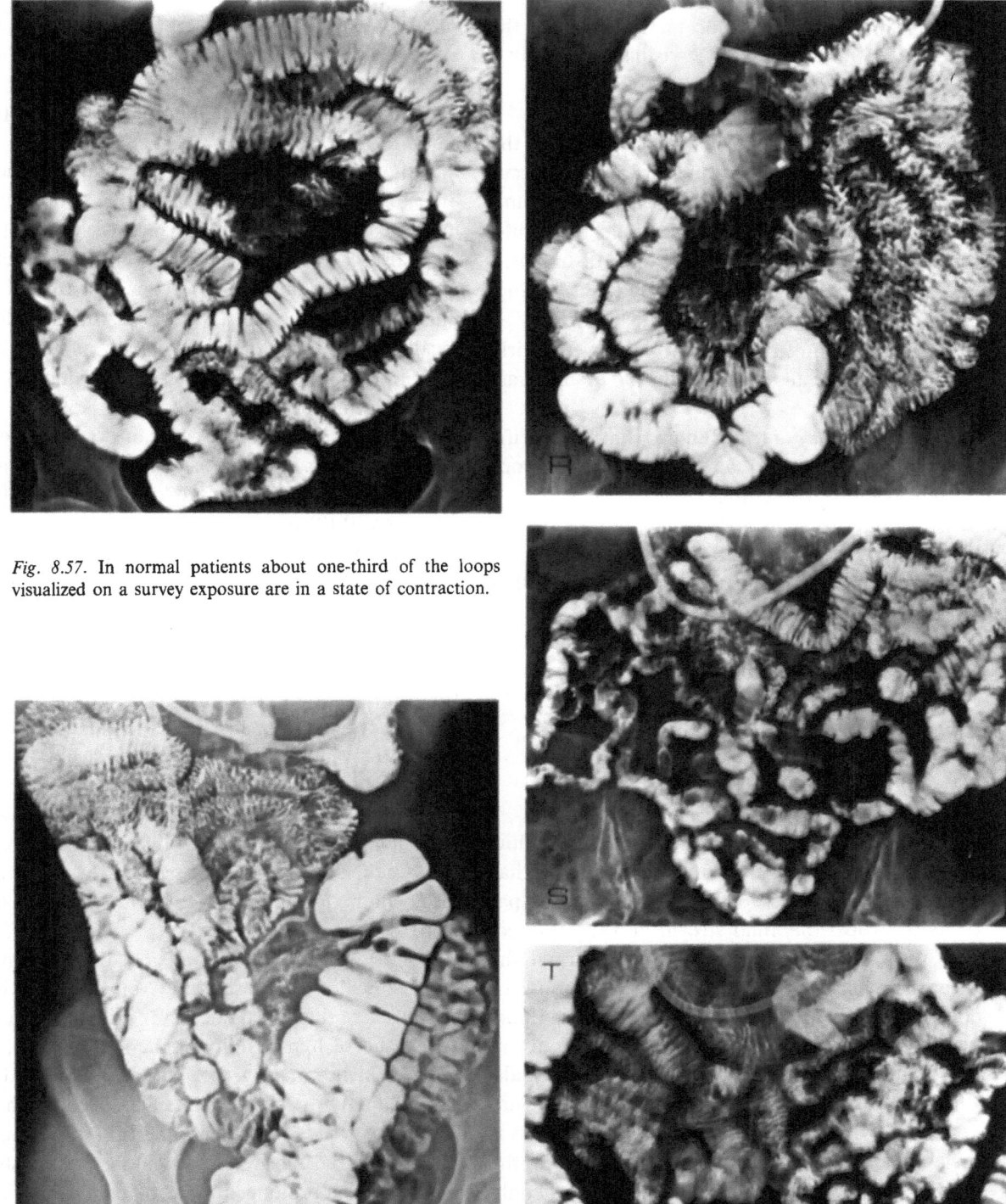

Fig. 8.57. In normal patients about one-third of the loops visualized on a survey exposure are in a state of contraction.

Fig. 8.58. In the event of hypermotility of the intestine, about two-thirds of the loops (R) and sometimes even more (ST) are in a state of contraction and the diameter of the intestine is usually somewhat smaller than normal. In patient U, the hypermotility was only transient and may have been caused by a diminished vascular supply due to the rotation anomaly.

lation. The next x-rays (fig. 6.2ʙ), taken several minutes later, show total flocculation, whereas the mucosal pattern was clearly visible on the first x-rays.

Hypersecretion of mucus or digestive juices in the small intestine, a phenomenon that leads to flocculation and segmentation in a conventional examination, is accorded too much diagnostic significance by many. Hypersecretion can be distinguished in an enteroclysis examination by the following:

1) Disintegration of the contrast fluid over a fairly large segment at the beginning of the contrast column.
2) Dilution of the contrast fluid so that the specific gravity is decreased and the intestinal loops appear more transparent.
3) There may be signs of 'haziness'.
4) Rapid disintegration of the barium suspension at the end of the contrast column after termination of the flow of contrast medium. This can be determined easily by taking several films after the actual examination is completed, for instance 15 or 30 min later.

9. Motility

The enteroclysis technique, whereby the rate of flow of the contrast fluid is the same for all patients, has enabled us to compare the ability of various patients to propel this fluid stream in a distal direction. We have found that if peristalsis is normal, the cecum is reached in 6–10 min and the amount of contrast fluid required is 600–900 ml. During fluoroscopy it is noted that peristalsis is most active in the jejunum, particularly in the proximal half. Furthermore when these peristaltic movements are abnormal, whether overactive or diminished, this is easiest to see in the jejunum. A change in the motility of the intestine is easily established not only under fluoroscopy but also on the roentgenograms. On the survey films taken during the enteroclysis examination, it appears that in normal patients about one-third of the jejunal loops are in a state of contraction (fig. 8.57). In cases of so-called 'intestinal hurry' the cecum is reached in much less than 6 min and frequently less than 600 ml of

contrast fluid is required. Moreover, on the x-rays it can be seen that the intestinal loops are on the average several millimeters narrower than normal and that two-thirds, and sometimes even more, of the jejunal loops are in a state of contraction (fig. 8.58).

Although by far less common than a general 'intestinal hurry' that involves the entire small intestine, and often also the colon, a local hyperperistalsis can sometimes be seen on the roentgenograms as well as during fluoroscopy. The tone of the musculature of the intestinal wall is then also high locally; the intestinal lumen is narrow and the folds of Kerkring lie close together, producing an exceedingly fine feathered pattern (fig. 8.59ᴀ).

This type of local spasticity can be encountered for example in cases of parasitosis, allergic reactions to food substances, adjacent carcinoids (see figs. 8.55ᴀ and 10.19), and inflammatory processes. A local hyperperistalsis also occurs in those diseases that are accompanied by a slight anoxia such as minute or moderate vascular occlusions, intermittent herniation, and after local radiotherapy. Adhesions and bands, however, are without doubt the most frequent cause of local hyperperistalsis. An impaired oxygenation, caused by a disturbance in the arterial or venous blood flow, is most likely to be the reason for this phenomenon (fig. 8.59ʙ).

Often local stimulation of the intestine is also accompanied by an enhanced mucus production in the same region. This can be seen on the x-rays as a local clump formation in the contrast fluid (fig. 8.55).

A local spasticity of a completely different nature is the so-called 'string sign' in Crohn's disease (fig. 8.60ᴘ). Here the intestinal wall is greatly thickened as a result of hypertrophy of the musculature; the mucous membrane has been totally destroyed by the inflammatory process and has become an ulcerating surface. There is no question of peristalsis in this case; the involved intestinal segment exists as a whole in a prolonged state of contraction and relaxes only slightly every once in a while. This then is not a true stenosis, as believed previously. Moreover, the prestenotic dilatation is also missing. It should be obvious that the chance of visualizing the string sign is considerably greater in the contraction phase than during a dilatation. The fluoroscopic findings can therefore be very important in establishing

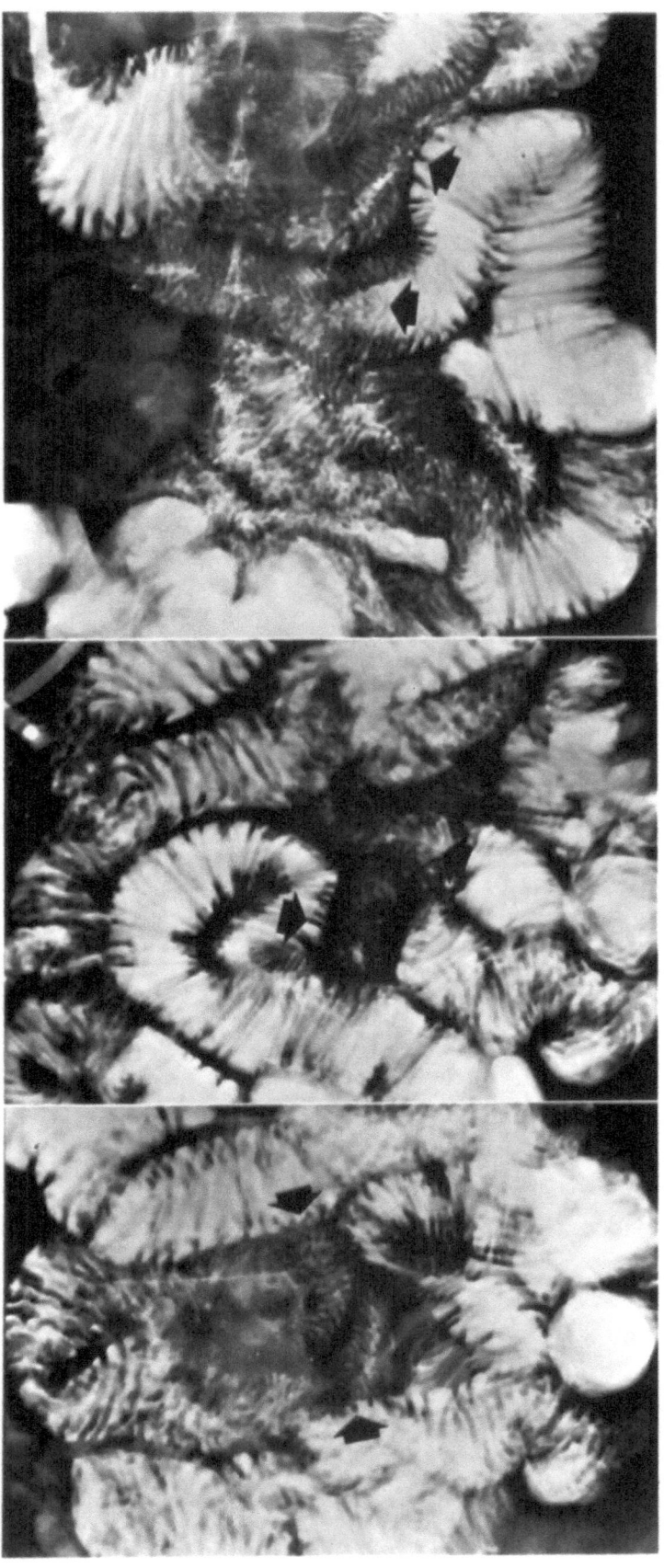

*Fig. 8.59*A. Three examples of local spasticity of the intestine with feathery mucosal folds.

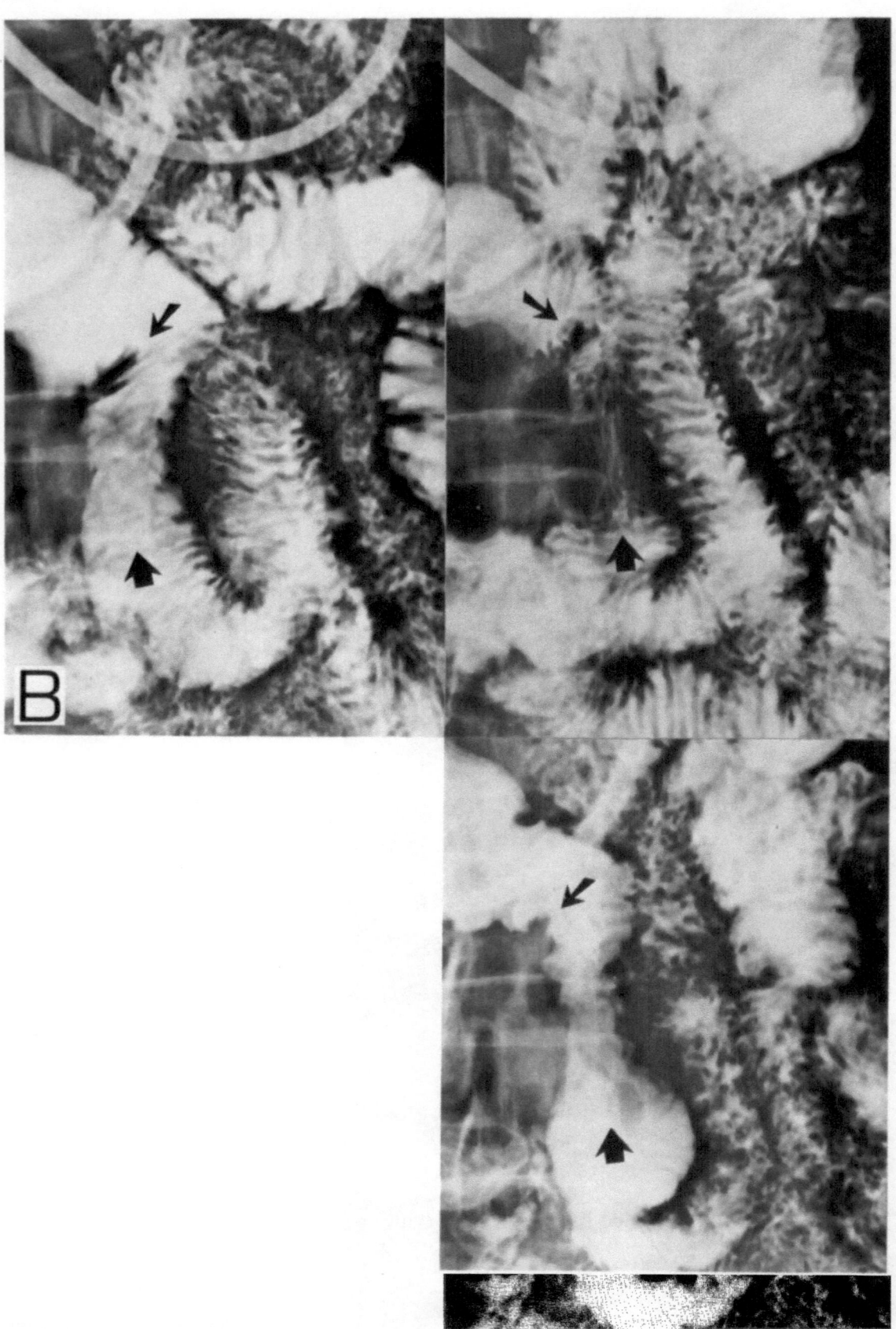

B

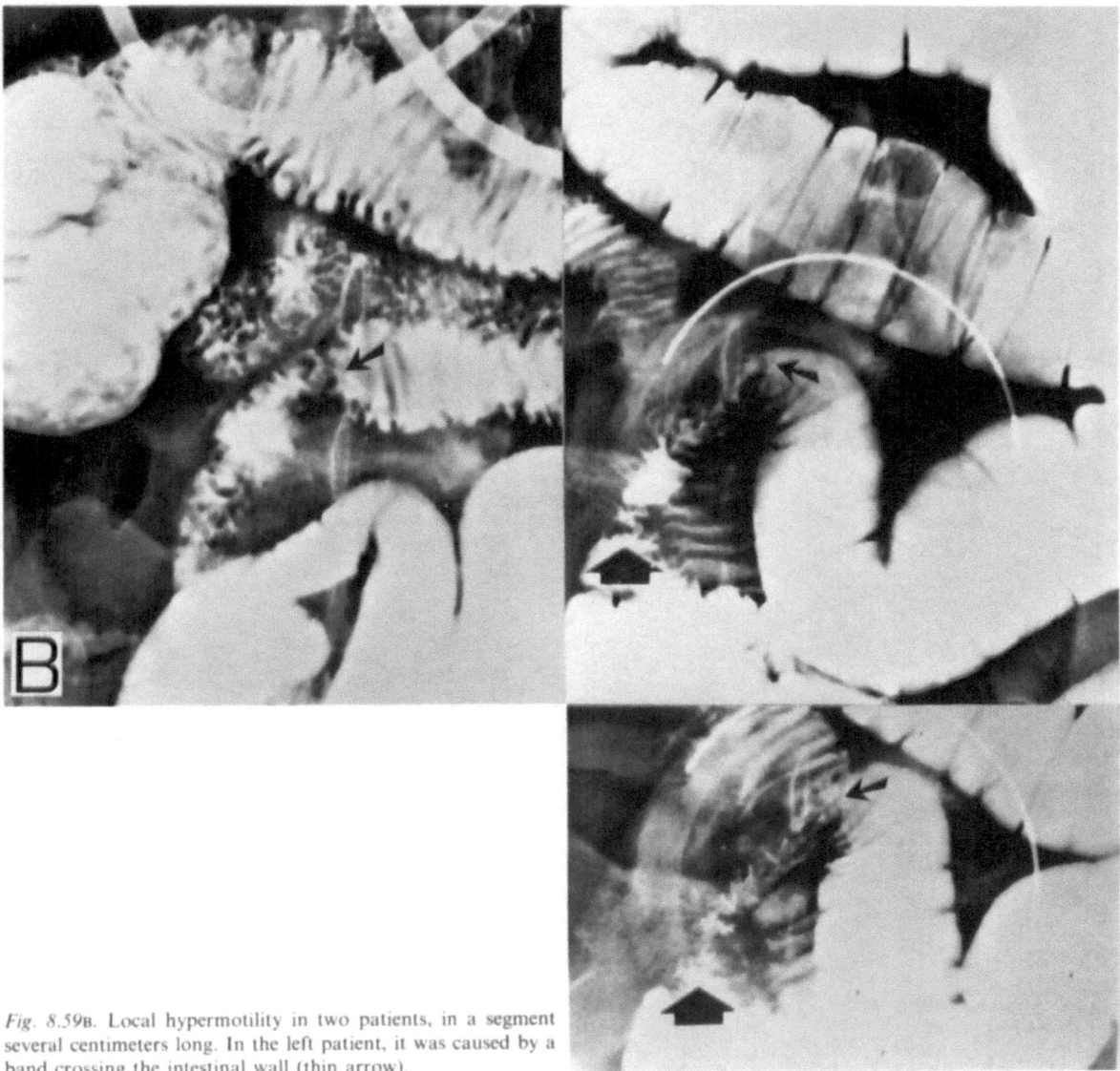

Fig. 8.59ʙ. Local hypermotility in two patients, in a segment several centimeters long. In the left patient, it was caused by a band crossing the intestinal wall (thin arrow).

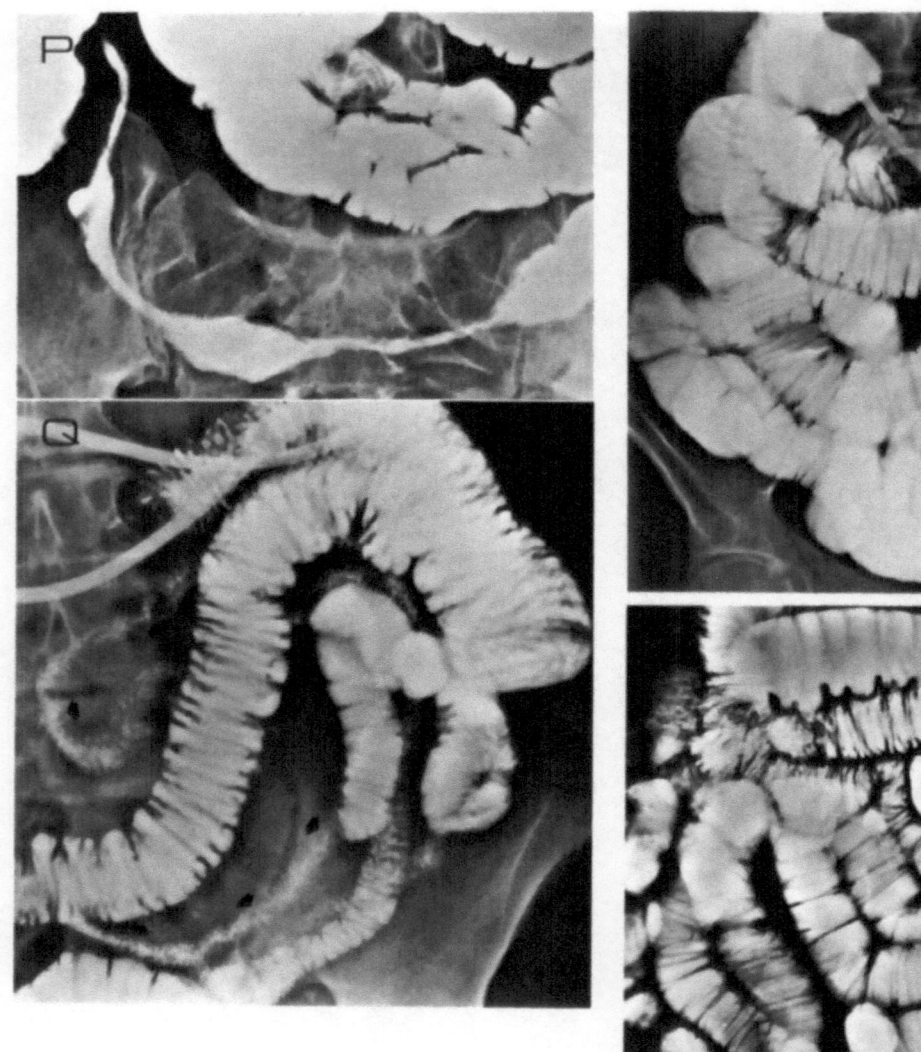

Fig. 8.60. (P) Local spasticity or 'string sign' in Crohn's disease. (Q) Spasms of an entire intestinal segment are rare in the jejunum. No abnormalities of the mucosa or intestinal wall could be seen in this patient. Etiology unknown.

Fig. 8.61. In hypomotility of the intestine, very few loops are in a state of contraction and in addition the lumen of the intestine is clearly dilated. Both patients had used vagotonics for years.

the true nature of the apparent stenosis. Prolonged contractions of an entire intestinal segment are rare in the jejunum, especially when no other abnormalities can be demonstrated in the intestinal wall or the mucosa (fig. 8.60Q). The reverse, decreased motility and a somewhat larger average diameter of the intestinal lumen, is seen more often than intestinal hurry (see also chapter 12). It then takes

much longer for the contrast medium to reach the cecum and the amount required is also considerably greater. On the x-ray it is obvious that only a few loops are in a state of contraction (fig. 8.61). If the decrease in, or even absence of, peristaltic movements and the dilatation are only local, or if the dilatation shows sacculations, the possibility of scleroderma must also be considered. This is true

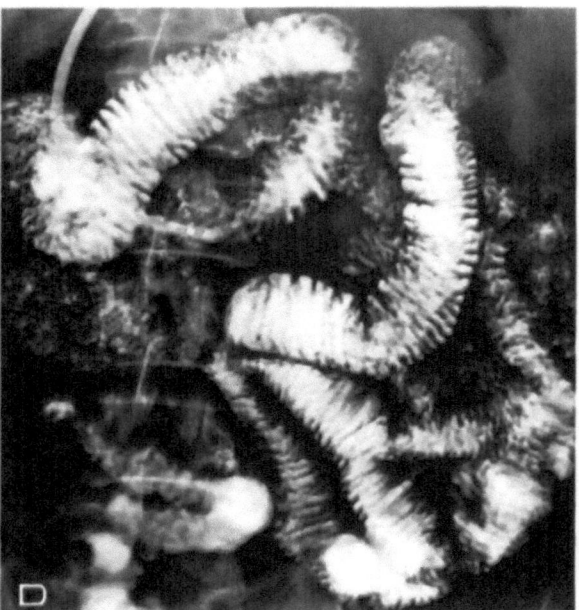

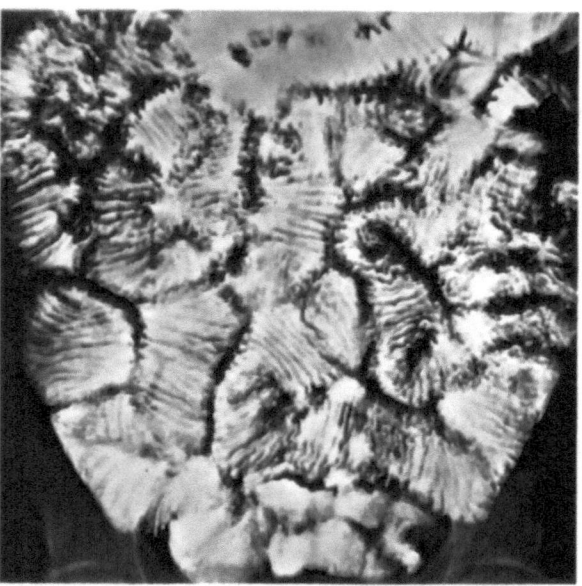

Fig. 8.63. Pattern characteristic of certain cases of celiac disease. Increased motility and obviously dilated loops.

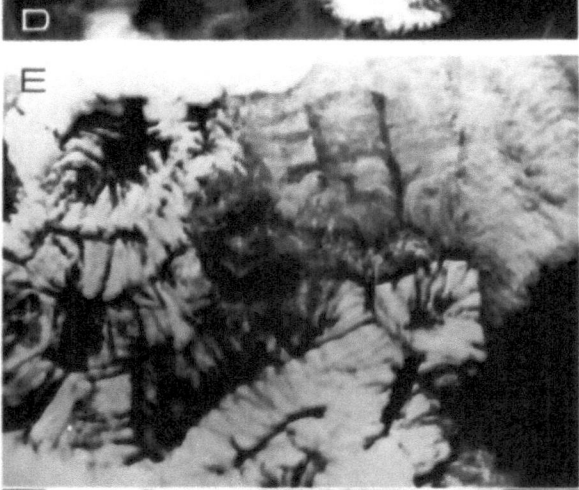

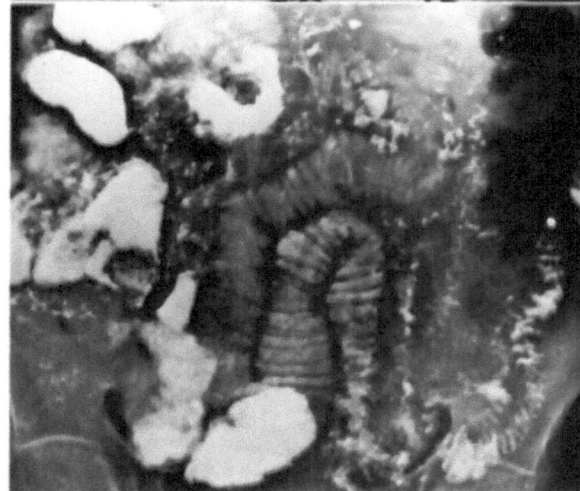

Fig. 8.62. Hypermotility of the intestine accompanied by a dilated lumen in pancreatogenic steatorrhea (D). The conventional examination of the same patients showed only dilution and marked flocculation of the contrast fluid (E).

even if none of the abnormalities characteristic of this disease are found in the esophagus and even if no ectodermal abnormalities can be discerned.

It should be clear that decreased peristalsis and dilated intestinal loops, as well as a highly contractile intestine and a narrow caliber, will as a rule occur together. This is, however, not true in Whipple's disease, pancreatogenic steatorrhea (fig. 8.62) and in particular in certain cases of celiac disease (see page 376) when there is a highly active peristalsis and obviously dilated intestinal loops. In celiac disease, this causes a very characteristic x-ray pattern (fig. 8.63) that is observed almost exclusively with enteroclysis since total flocculation usually occurs when the contrast medium is administered orally. We have found that intestinal hurry is accompanied by only a small caliber when the hyperperistalsis is either neurogenic or humoral in origin.

If, on the other hand, a true malabsorption exists, i.e. a diminished resorption of food substances, then the hyperperistalsis is found together with a dilated lumen. This hyperperistalsis is probably due to an increase in the intestinal contents that in turn is a result of the absorption of fluid from the intestinal wall and the enhanced secretion of intestinal juices.

BIBLIOGRAPHY: CHAPTERS 1–8

1. Abbott O, Pendergrass EP (1936) Intubation studies of the human small intestine. Am J Roentgenol 35: 289–299.
2. Adam A (1932) Kontrastmittel und Innenwanddarstellung des Verdauungstraktes. Fortschr R 45: 385–396.
3. Adlersberg D, Marshak RH, Colcher H, Drachman SR, Friedman AI, Wang CI (1954) The roentgenologic appearance of the small intestine in sprue. Gastroenterology 26: 548–581.
4. Adolph W, Taplin GV (1950) Use of micropulverized barium sulfate in x-ray diagnosis. A preliminary report. Radiology 54: 878–883.
5. Alexander GH, Alexander RE (1950) The use of gastric mucin as a barium suspension medium. Radiology 54: 875–877.
6. Alister WH Mc, Anderson S, Bloomberg GR, Margulis AR (1963) Lethal effects of tannic acid in the barium enema. Report of three fatalities and experimental studies. Radiology 80: 765–773.
7. Ament ME, Rubin CE (1972) Relation of giardiasis to abnormal intestinal structure and function in gastrointestinal immunodeficiency syndromes. Gastroenterology 62: 216–226.
8. Anderson ChM, Astley R, French JM, Gerrard JW (1952) The small intestine pattern in coeliac disease. Br J Radiol 25: 526–530.
9. Ardran GM, French JM, Mucklow EH (1950) Relationship of the nature of the opaque medium to small intestine radiographic pattern. Br J Radiol 23: 697–702.
10. Arens RA, Mesirow SD (1937) Gastric mucosal relief. A modified sedimentation method, using a colloidally suspended barium sulphate. Radiology 29: 1–11.
11. Astley R, French JM (1950) The small intestine pattern in normal children and in coeliac disease. Its relationship to the nature of the opaque medium. Br J Radiol 24: 321–330.
12. Balthazar EJ, Gade MF (1976) Gastrointestinal edema in cirrhotics. Gastrointest Radiol 1: 215–223.
13. Barclay AE (1938) The practical importance of mechanics in digestion. Am J Roentgenol 40: 325–334.
14. Barden RP, Thompson WD, Ravdin IS, Frank JL (1938) The influence of the serum protein on the motility of the small intestine. Surg Gynecol Obstet 66: 819–821.
15. Beerstecher HJP (1973) De ileo-rectale anastomose bij de chirurgische behandeling van colitis ulcerosa. Thesis, Leiden University.
16. Bendick AJ (1954) Diagnostic advances in gastrointestinal roentgenology. New York.
17. Berger G (1968) Erfahrungen über die Verwendung von Visotrast in der Kinderklinik. (In der Magen-Darm-Diagnostik bei Kindern.) Dtsch Gesundheitswes 23: 356–360.
18. Berkovits L, Javor T (1965) Über die Untersuchung des Dünndarms mit Enteramin. Fortschr R 103: 60–62.
19. Berman CZ, Avnet NL (1960) The use of water soluble urographic contrast media in paediatric G.I. studies. Br J Radiol 33: 92–97.
20. Bilbao MK, Frische LH, Dotter ChT, Rösch J (1967) Hypotonic duodenography. Radiology 89: 438–443.
21. Bourdon R, Hummel J (1956) Base de la radiologie du grêle. J Radiol Electr 37: 210–215.
22. Bouslog JS (1937) The gastro-intestinal tract in children. Radiology 28: 683–692.
23. Bouslog JS (1942) The normal stomach and small intestine in the infant. Radiology 39: 253–260.
24. Braeckman P (1947) Over suspensies met bariumsulfaat. Pharm Weekbl 49/50: 709–719.
25. Brown FO (1959) On routine barium examination of the small bowel. Lancet 2: 530–533.
26. Brown GR (1963) High-density barium-sulfate suspensions; an improved diagnostic medium. Radiology 81: 839–846.
27. Buffard P (1952) Le diagnostic des tumeurs de l'intestin grêle est-il possible dans la pratique radiologique quotidienne? J Radiol Electr 33: 64–66.
28. Buffard P, Crozet L (1952) Zur Dünndarmallergie. Fortschr R 76: 497–507.
29. Bugyi B (1955) Praktische Beiträge zur röntgenologischen Untersuchung der Verdauungsorgane. Roentgenblaetter 8(4): 107–111.
30. Bulatao E, Carlson AJ (1924) Contributions to the physiology of the stomach. Influence of experimental changes in blood sugar level on gastric hunger contractions. Am J Physiol 69: 107–115.
31. Burhenne JH, Vogelaar P, Arkoff RS (1966) Liver function studies in patients receiving enemas containing tannic acid. Am J Roentgenol 96: 510–518.
32. Busscher G de (1950) Étude radiologique du grêle au cours de diverses affections. Acta Gastroenterol Belg 13: 295–350.
33. Caldwell WL, Floch MH (1963) Evaluation of the small bowel barium motor meal with emphasis on the effect of volume of barium suspensions ingested. Radiology 80: 383–391.
34. Caldwell WL, Swanson VL, Bayless ThM (1965) The importance and reliability of the roentgenographic examination of the small bowel in patients with tropical sprue. Radiology 84: 227–240.
35. Cameron AL (1938 II) Primary malignancy of the jejunum and ileum. Ann Surg 108: 203–220.
36. Chamberlin GW (1939 II) The roentgen anatomy of the small intestine. JAMA 113: 1537–1541.
37. Clure CW Mc, Reynolds L, Schwartz CO (1920) On the behavior of the pyloric sphincter in normal man. Arch

188

Intern Med 26: 410–423.

38. Cole et al. (1932) Findings observed in the gastro-intestinal tract. Radiology 18: 886–941.

39. Crohn BB, Ginzburg L, Oppenheimer GD (1932) Regional ileitis. A pathologic and clinical entity. JAMA 99: 1323–1329.

40. Crowley RT, Johnston ChG (1946) Physiological principles in intestinal obstruction. Surg Clin North Am 1427–1439.

41. Cummack DH (1969) Gastro-intestinal X-ray diagnosis. Edinburgh: Livingstone.

42. Cummins AJ, Almy TP (1953) Studies on the relationship between motility and absorption in the human small intestine. Gastroenterology 23: 179–190.

43. Deucher WG (1949) Über die Variabilität der Dünndarmschleimhaut. Radiol Clin (Basel) 18: 265–272.

44. Diner WC (1968) Small intestinal edema in cirrhosis; its disappearance with diuresis. Radiology 91: 792–794.

45. Donato H, Mayo HW Jr, Barr LH (1954) The effect of peroral barium in partial obstruction of the small bowel. Surgery 35: 719–723.

46. Ekberg O (1977) Double contrast examination of the small bowel. Gastrointest Radiol 1: 349–353.

47. Embring G, Mattsson O (1966) An improved physiologic contrast medium for the alimentary tract. Acta Radiol [Suppl] (Stockh) 4: 105–109.

48. Embring G, Mattsson O (1968) Barium contrast agents. Acta Radiol [Diagn 3] (Stockh) 7: 245–256.

49. Epstein BS (1957) The use of a water soluble contrast medium (Hypaque) for gastrointestinal roentgenography. JAMA 165: 44–46.

50. Ettinger AJH (1949) Small intestinal pattern in sprue and similar deficiency diseases. Am J Roentgenol 61: 658–670.

51. Fabian M, Lakos A, Feher I (1966) Passagebeschleunigende Methoden zur röntgenologischen Untersuchung des Darmtraktes. Roentgenblaetter 19: 58–64.

52. Figiel SJ, Figiel LS (1964) Tumors of the terminal ileum. Diagnosis by retrograde filling during barium enema study. Am J Roentgenol 91: 816–818.

53. Fischer AW (1925) Über die Röntgenuntersuchung des Dickdarms mit Hilfe einer Kombination von Lufteinblasung und Kontrasteinlauf. ('Kombinierte Methode'.) Arch Klin Chir 134: 209–269.

54. Fisher ChH, Oh KS, Bayless ThM, Siegelman SS (1975) Current perspective on giardiasis. Am J Roentgenol 125: 207–217.

55. Flach A (1949) Vergleichende Untersuchungen über die Viskosität, Oberflächenspannung und Grenzflächenspannung verschiedener Kontrastmittel. Roentgenblaetter 2: 303–310.

56. Floch MH, Caldwell WL, Sheehy TW (1962) A histopathologic basis for the interpretation of small bowel roentgenography in tropical sprue. Am J Roentgenol 87: 709–716.

57. Forssell G (1923) Studies of the mechanism of movement of the mucous membrane of the digestive tract. Am J Roentgenol 2: 87–104.

58. Forssell G (1939) Role of autonomous movements of the gastrointestinal mucous membrane in digestion. Am J Roentgenol 41: 145–165.

59. Foubert F, Robert F (1951) Intérêt d'un nouveau support de produit de contraste dans le radiodiagnostic digestif: la Carboxy-Méthyl-Cellulose. J Radiol Electr 32: 925.

60. Frazer AC, French JM, Thompson MD (1949) Radio-graphic studies showing the induction of a segmentation pattern in the small intestine in normal human subjects. Br J Radiol 22: 123–136.

61. French JM (1950) Further studies in the radiology of the small intestine. Gastroenterologia (Basel) 76: 343–345.

62. Friedenberg MJ, Alister WH Mc, Margulis AR (1962) Roentgen study of the small bowel in adults and children with neostigmine. Am J Roentgenol 88: 693–701.

63. Friedman J (1954) Roentgen studies of the effects on the small intestine from emotional disturbances. Am J Roentgenol 72: 367–379.

64. Friedman J, Rigler LG (1950) A method of double-contrast roentgen examination of the small intestine. Radiology 54: 365–379.

65. Frik K, Blühbaum Th (1928) Eine neue Anwendungsart der Kolloide in der Röntgendiagnostik. Fortschr R 38: 1111–1120.

66. Friman-Dahl J (1954) The administration of barium orally in acute obstruction; advantages and risks. Acta Radiol 42: 285–295.

67. Furnemont E (1966) l'Utilisation du Sorbitol dans l'exploration radiologique du tractus intestinal. Acta Gastroenterol Belg 24: 779–790.

68. Gershon-Cohen J, Shay H (1947) Experimental studies on gastric physiology in man. A study of pyloric control. The rôle of milk and cream in the normal and in subjects with quiescent duodenal ulcer. Am J Roentgenol 38: 427–446.

69. Gershon-Cohen J, Shay H (1939) Barium enteroclysis. A method for the direct immediate examination of the small intestine by single and double contrast techniques. Am J Roentgenol 42: 456–458.

70. Gershon-Cohen J, Shay H, Fels SS (1938) Experimental studies on gastric physiology in man. The influence of osmotic pressure changes of salt and sugar solutions on pyloric action and gastric emptying in the normal and operated stomach. Am J Roentgenol 40: 335–343.

71. Gershon-Cohen J, Shay H, Fels SS (1940) The relation of meal temperature to gastric motility and secretion. Am J Roentgenol 43: 237–242.

72. Gianturco C (1950) Fast radiological visceral survey. Radiology 54: 59–64.

73. Girand M, Bret P, Pinet F, Roche P (1951) L'examen radiologique du grêle par transit accéléré. J Radiol Electr 32: 583–595.

74. Glaser FH, Kölling HL (1967) Beitrag zur peroralen Magen-Darm-Diagnostik mit Bariumsulfat-Amidotrizoat-Gemischen. Radiol Diagn (Berl) 8: 13–22.

75. Goin LS (1952) Some obscure factors in the production of unusual small bowel patterns. Radiology 59: 177–184.

76. Golden R (1941) Abnormalities of the small intestine in nutritional disturbances. Radiology 36: 262–286.

77. Golden R (1950) Some clinical problems in small intestinal physiology. Br J Radiol 23: 390–409.

78. Golden R. (1951) Advances in gastro-enterological radiology 1937–1950. Br J Radiol 24: 237–245.

79. Golden R (1959) Technical factors in the roentgen examination of the small intestine. Am J Roentgenol 82: 965–972.

80. Golden R (1959) Radiologic examination of the small intestine. Philadelphia: Lippincott, 2nd edn.

81. Good A (1963) Tumors of the small intestine. Am J Roentgenol 89: 685–705.

82. Greenspon EA, Lentino W (1960) Retrograde enterography. A new method for the roentgenologic study of the small bowel. Am J Roentgenol 83: 909–919.

83. Grier T, Miller, Karr WG (1936) Intubation studies of the human small intestine. The influence of variations in the reaction and the motility of the stomach contents on the reaction and the motility of the intestinal contents. Am J Roentgenol 35: 300–305.

84. Gryboski JD, Self TW, Clement A, et al. (1968) Selective immunoglobulin. A deficiency and intestinal nodular lymphoid hyperplasia: correction of diarrhea with antibiotics and plasma. Pediatrics 42: 833–837.

85. Hafter E (1973) Praktische Gastroenterologie. Stuttgart: Thieme.

86. Hanafee W, Weiner M (1967) External guided passage of an intestinal intubation tube. Radiology 89: 1100–1102.

87. Harris PD, Neuhauser EBD, Gerth R (1964) The osmotic effect of water soluble contrast media on circulating plasma volume. Am J Roentgenol 91: 694–698.

88. Hecht G (1934) Heubners Handbuch der experimentellen Pharmakologie, vol. 8. Berlin: Springer, p. 97.

89. Heitzman RE, Berne AS (1961) Roentgen examination of the cecum and proximal ascending colon with ingested barium. Radiology 76: 415–421.

90. Henderson NP (1944) The value of the opaque enema and its modifications. Br J Radiol 17: 140–149.

91. Henderson SG (1942) The gastrointestinal tract in the healthy newborn infant. Am J Roentgenol 48: 302–335.

92. Highman JH (1964) Urinary excretion as a sign of intestinal perforation. Br J Radiol 37: 697–700.

93. Hirsch J, Ahrens E, Blankenhorn DH (1956) Measurement of the human intestinal length in vivo and some causes of variation. Gastroenterology 31: 274–285.

94. Hodges FJ, Rundless RW, Hanelin J (1947)
I. Roentgenologic study of the small intestine. Neoplastic and inflammatory diseases. Radiology 49: 587–602.
II. Roentgenologic study of the small intestine. Dysfunction associated with neurologic diseases. Radiology 49: 659–673.

95. Hodgson JR, Hoffman HN II, Huizinga KA (1967) Roentgenologic features of lymphoid hyperplasia of the small intestine associated with dysgamma-globulinemia. Radiology 88: 883–888.

96. Holt JF, Lyons RH, Neligh RB, Noe GK, Hodges FJ (1947) X-ray signs of altered alimentary function following autonomic blockade with tetraethylammonium. Radiology 49: 603–610.

97. Holzknecht G (1931) Handbuch der theoretischen und klinischen Röntgenkunde. Wien.

98. Howarth FH, Cockel R, Roper BW, Hawkins CF (1969) The effect of metoclopramide upon gastric motility and its value in barium progress meals. Clin Radiol 20: 294–300.

99. Hudak A (1951) Le transit accéléré du grêle. Radiol Clin (Basel) 20: 148–154.

100. Hüpcher N (1961) Het gebruik van bariumsulfaatsuspensies, in het bijzonder tylosebarium in de tractus digestivus. J Belg Radiol 44: 161–169.

101. James WB, Hume R (1968) Action of metoclopramide on gastric emptying and small bowel transit time. Gut 9: 203–205.

102. Janower ML, Robbins LL, Tomchik FS, Weylman WT (1965) Tannic acid and the barium enema. Radiology 85: 887–894.

103. Jeffries GH, Weser E, Sleisinger MH (1964) Progress in gastroenterology. Malabsorption. Gastroenterology 46: 434–466.

104. Johnston CG, Ravdin IS (1935 I) Action of glucose on emptying of stomach. Effect of varying concentrations in both normal stomachs and after various gastric operations. Am Surg 101: 500–505.

105. Jollasse (1907) Zur Motilitätsprüfung des Magens durch Röntgenstrahlen. Fortschr R 11: 47–53.

106. Jones GE, Chalecke WE, Dec J, Schilling JA, Ramsey GH, Robertson HD, Strain WH (1947) Iodinated organic compounds as contrast media for radiographic diagnosis. Studies on tetraiodophthalimidoethanol as a medium for gastrointestinal visualization. Radiology 49: 143–151.

107. Kaestle (1907) Bolus alba und Bismutum subnitricum, eine für die röntgenologische Untersuchung des Magen-Darmkanals brauchbare Mischung. Fortschr R 11: 266–271.

108. Kantor JL (1939) The roentgen diagnosis of idiopathic steatorrhea and allied conditions. Practical value of the 'Moulage sign'. Am J Roentgenol 41: 758–778.

109. Kaufmann HJ (1969) Progress in pediatric radiology, vol. 2: Gastro-intestinal tract. Basel: S. Karger.

110. Khilnani MT, Keller RJ, Cuttner J (1969) Macroglobulinemia and steatorrhea: roentgen and pathologic findings in the intestinal tract. Radiol Clin North Am 7: 43–55.

111. King CE, Arnold L (1922) The activities of the intestinal mucosal motor mechanism. Am J Physiol 59: 97–121.

112. Kirsh IE (1956) Motility of the small intestine with non-flocculating medium; a review of 173 roentgen examinations. Gastroenterology 31: 251–260.

113. Kirsh IE, Spellberg MA (1953) Examination of small intestine with carboxymethylcellulose. Radiology 60: 701–707.

114. Knoefel PK, Davis LA, Pilla LA (1956) Agglomeration of barium sulfate and roentgen visualisation of the gastric mucosa. Radiology 67: 87–91.

115. Knox R (1919) Radiography and radio-therapeutics. London: E and C Black.

116. Korpassy B, Horvai R, Koltay M (1951) On the absorption of tannic acid from the gastrointestinal tract. Arch Int Pharmacodyn Ther 88: 368–377.

117. Kunz B, Lemm M, Haubach D (1965) Die Verwendung von 'Visotrast 370' in der Magen-Darm Diagnostik. Dtsch Gesundheitswes 20: 593–595.

118. Lafontaine A (1965) Danger de l'acide tannique utilisé en lavement. J Belg Radiol 48: 551–555.

119. Laren JW Mc (1960) Modern trends in diagnostic radiology. Series 3: Scott-Harden WG (ed) Examination of the small bowel. London: Butterworths, pp 84–87.

120. Läser S (1966) Verbesserungen der Eigenschaften von Bariumsulfatsuspensionen für die Magen-Darm-Passage durch Zusatz von Polysaccharidlösungen. Schweiz Med Wochenschr 96: 633–638.

121. Laws JW, Neale G (1966) Radiological diagnosis of disaccharidase deficiency. Lancet 2: 139–143.

122. Laws JW, Pitman RG (1960) The radiological investigation of malabsorption syndromes. Br J Radiol 33: 211–228.

123. Laws JW, Shawdon H, Booth CC, Stewart JS (1963) Correlation of radiological and histological findings in idiopathic steatorrhea. Br Med J 1311–1314.

124. Leb A (1951) Eine Röntgen-Digestionsprüfung, Die Röntgenuntersuchung des resezierten Magens mit Eiweiss- und Fett-Bariumkernen. Fortschr R 75: 106–116.

125. Ledoux-Lebard G (1968) Histoire de la radiologie du tube digestif. Gaz Med Fr 75: 209–216.

126. Lehner HH, Märki W, Zimmer EA (1948–49) Ueber ein neues Barium-Kontrastmittel, zugleich ein Beitrag zur

190

Prüfung solcher Substanzen. Gastroenterologia (Basel) 74: 193-208.

127. Lenz H (1962) Weitere Untersuchungen zur Funktions-analyse der Dünndarmperistaltik. Fortschr R 97: 147-159.

128. Lenz H (1962) Die Segmentationsbewegungen des Ileums im Röntgenkinobild. Fortschr R 97: 159-168.

129. Lenz H, Kreppel E (1965) Röntgenkinematographische Untersuchungen über das Verhalten der Dünndarmmoto-rik bei der Katze unter Prostigmin, Pilocarpin und Are-colin. Fortschr R 102: 268-277.

130. Lessman FP, Lilienfeld RM (1959) Gastrografin as water soluble medium in roentgen examination of the G.I. tract. Acta Radiol 51: 170-178.

131. Letters K, Gaul M (1951) Neue Untersuchungen zur Charakterisierung von Röntgenkontrastmittel für Magen und Darm. Fortschr R 74: 229-234.

132. Liere EJ v., Northuys DW, Clifford SJ (1946) The effect of glucose on the motility of the stomach and small intestine. Gastroenterology 7: 218-223.

133. Liu HY, Whitehouse WM, Giday Z (1975) Proximal small bowel transit pattern in patients with malabsorption in-duced by bovine milk protein ingestion. Radiology 115: 415-420.

134. Lönnerblad L (1951) Transit time through the small intestine. A roentgenologic study on normal variability. Acta Radiol [Suppl] 88.

135. Lumsden K, Truelove SC (1965) Radiology of the digestive system. Oxford: Blackwell.

136. Lura A (1951) Radiology of the small intestine. Enema of the small intestine with special emphasis on the diagnosis of tumours. Br J Radiol 24: 264-271.

137. Magnusson W (1931) On meteorism in pyelography and on the passage of gas through the small intestine. Acta Radiol 12: 552-561.

138. Manecke H, Schmidt FW (1962) Die Magen-Darm-Pas-sage mit Karion. Fortschr R 97: 142-146.

139. Maretic Z, Homadovski K, Razbojnikov S, Brecevic V (1957) Barium poisoning. Ein Beitrag zur Kenntnis von Vergiftung mit Barium. Med Klin 52: 1950-1953.

140. Margulis AR (1967) Some new approaches to the exam-ination of the gastro-intestinal tract. Am J Roentgenol 101: 265-286.

141. Margulis AR, Burhenne HJ (1967) Alimentary tract roentgenology. St. Louis: CV Mosby.

142. Margulis AR: Mandelstam P (1961) The use of parenteral neostigmine in the roentgen study of the small bowel. Radiology 76: 223-229.

143. Marshak RH (1961) Roentgen findings in lesions of the small bowel. Am J Dig Dis 6: 1084-1114.

144. Marshak RH, Lindner AE (1966) Malabsorption syn-drome. Semin Roentgenol 1: 138-177.

145. Marshak RH, Lindner AE (1970) Radiology of the small intestine. Philadelphia: Saunders.

146. Marshak RH, Friedman AJ, Wolf BS, Crohn BB (1951) Roentgen findings in ileo-jejunitis. Gastroenterology 19: 383-408.

147. Marshak RH, Wolf BS, Adlersberg D (1954) Roentgen studies of the small intestine in sprue. Am J Roentgenol 72: 380-400.

148. Marshak RH, Wolf BS, Cohen N, Janowitz HD (1961) Protein losing disorders of the gastrointestinal tract: roent-gen features. Radiology 77: 893-905.

149. Marshak RH, Khilnani M, Eliasoph J, Wolf BS (1967) Intestinal edema. Am J Roentgenol 101: 379-387.

150. Marshak RH, Ruoff M, Lindner AE (1968) Roentgen manifestations of giardiasis. Am J Roentgenol 104: 557-560.

151. Marshak RH, Hazzi Ch, Lindner AE, Maklansky D (1975) The small bowel in immunoglobulin deficiency syndromes. Am J Roentgenol 122: 227-240.

152. Martel W, Hodges FJ (1959) The small intestine in Whipple's disease. Am J Roentgenol 81: 623-636.

153. Mattson O, Perman G, Lagerlöf H (1960) The small intestine transit time with a physiologic contrast medium. Acta Radiol 54: 334-344.

154. Mellink JH (1961) Radiophysical aspects of the use of contrast substances in radiodiagnosis. J Belg Radiol 44: 107-126.

155. Menville LJ, Ané JN (1932) An x-ray study of the passage of different foodstuffs through the small intestine of man. Radiology 18: 783-786.

156. Meyers MA (1974) Radiological features of the spread and localization of extraperitoneal gas and their relationship to its source. Radiology 111: 17-26.

157. Meyers MA (1976) Clinical involvement of mesenteric and antimesenteric borders of small bowel loops. Gastrointest Radiol 1: 41-47.

158. Meyers MA, Ghahremani GR, Clements JL, Goodman K (1977) Pneumatosis intestinalis. Gastrointest Radiol 2: 91-105.

159. Miller RE (1965) Barium sulfate suspensions. Radiology 84: 241-251.

160. Miller RE (1965) Complete reflux small bowel examin-ation. Radiology 84: 457-463.

161. Miller RE, Brahme F (1969) Large amounts of orally administered barium for obstruction of the small intestine. Surg Gynecol Obstet 129: 1185-1188.

162. Miller RE, Miller WJ (1966) Inflammatory lesions of the small bowel. Complete reflux small bowel examination. Am J Gastroenterol 45: 40-49.

163. Moreton RD, Yates ChW (1950) The double-contrast study of the colon. A comparative study of barium sulfate preparations. Radiology 54: 541-547.

164. Mori PA, Barrett HA (1962) A sign of intestinal per-foration. Radiology 79: 401-407.

165. Morrison BO, Haley TJ, Payzant AR, Gentner GA, Pagon-Carlo J (1959) Use of Hypaque as contrast medium in G.I. examination. Am J Gastroenterol 31: 398-407.

166. Morrison WJ, Christopher NL, Bayless ThM, Dana EA (1974) Low lactase levels: evaluation of the radiologic diagnosis. Radiology 111: 513-518.

167. Morton JL (1961) Notes on a small bowel examination. Am J Roentgenol 86: 76-85.

168. Müller JHA (1968) Die Röntgendiagnostik des Dünn-darms mit Neostigmine. Dtsch Gesundheitswes 23: 391-397.

169. Munteau E (1951) Experimentelle Grundlagen einer rönt-genologischen Eiweiss Digestionsprüfung. Radiol Aus-triaca 4: 187-199.

170. Murray JP (1966) Buscopan in diagnostic radiology of the alimentary tract. Br J Radiol 39: 102-111.

171. Naumann W (1948) Funktionelle Dünndarmdiagnostik im Röntgenbild. Stuttgart: Thieme.

172. Nelson SW (1972) Extraluminal gas collections due to diseases of the gastrointestinal tract. Am J Roentgenol 115: 225-248.

173. Nelson SW, Christoforidis AJ, Roenigk WJ (1965) Dan-gers and fallibilities of iodinated radiopaque media in

obstruction of the small bowel. Am J Surg 109: 546–559.

174. Nelson SW, Christoforidis AJ (1967) The use of barium sulfate suspensions in the study of suspected mechanical obstruction of the small intestine. Am J Roentgenol 101: 367–378.

175. Nice ChM (1963) Roentgenographic pattern and motility in small bowel studies. Radiology 80: 39–45.

176. Osborn AG, Friedland GW (1973) A radiological approach to the diagnosis of small bowel disease. Clin Radiol 24: 281–301.

177. Pajewski M, Itzchak Y, Profis A (1970) The double contrast examination of the small intestine. Preliminary communication of a new technique. Clin Radiol 21: 83–86.

178. Pansdorf H (1937) Die fraktionierte Dünndarmfüllung und ihre klinische Bedeutung. Fortschr R 56: 627–634.

179. Patterson DE, Rad M, David R, Baker SJ (1965) Radiodiagnostic problems in malabsorption. Br J Radiol 38: 181–191.

180. Paulson M (1969) Gastroenterologic medicine. Philadelphia: Lea and Febiger.

181. Pendergrass EP (1936) The small intestine. JAMA 107: 1859–1861.

182. Pendergrass E, Ravdin IS, Johnston CG, Hodes PJ (1936) The effect of foods and various pathologic states on the gastric emptying and the small intestinal pattern. Radiology 26: 651–662.

183. Perez CA, Friedenberg MJ (1967) Comparison of carboxymethyl-cellulose, tannic-acid and no additive in barium examinations of the colon. Am J Roentgenol 99: 98–105.

184. Pesquera GS (1929) A method for the direct visualization of lesions in the small intestines. Am J Roentgenol 22: 254–257.

185. Pirk F, Vulterinová M (1964) The x-ray picture of the small intestine and impaired absorption. Radiol Clin (Basel) 33: 249–267.

186. Pirk F, Stáhlavska A, Cerná M (1967) Vergleich der Eigenschaften einiger Bariumkontrastmittel verschiedener Herkunft. Radiol Diagn (Berl) 8: 773–780.

187. Pock-Steen OC, Lorenzen J (1968) Gluten-intolerance and food allergy. Clinical signs and radiological changes of the small intestine. Radiol Clin (Basel) 37: 65–78.

188. Porcher P, Caroli J (1957) Un accélérateur inattendu du transit intestinal (grêle et colon). Arch Mal Appar Dig Mal Nutr 46: 663–665.

189. Portis SA (1941) The clinical significance of the roentgenological findings of the small intestine. Radiology 37: 289–293.

190. Preger L, Amberg JR (1967) Sweet diarrhea. Roentgen diagnosis of disaccharidase deficiency. Am J Roentgenol 101: 287–295.

191. Prévôt R (1940) Ergebnisse röntgenologischer Dünndarmstudien unter besonderer Berücksichtigung der Morphologie. Fortschr R 62: 341–388.

192. Pygott F (1958) Modern trends in gastroenterology. London: Butterworths.

193. Pygott F, Street DF, Shellshear MF, Rhodes CJ (1960) Radiological investigation of the small intestine by small bowel enema technique. Gut 1: 366–370.

194. Raiford ThS (1931) Tumors of the small intestine. Their diagnosis, with special reference to the x-ray appearance. Radiology 16: 253–270.

195. Reidell H (1937) Vergleichende Untersuchungen an Magen-Darmkontrastmitteln. Fortsch R 56: 653–662.

196. Reinhardt K (1960) Untersuchungen über den Wert einer Sorbitolbeimischung zum Bariumbrei für die Röntgendarstellung des Darmtraktes. Fortschr R 92: 78–84.

197. Reinhardt JF, Barry WF (1962) Scleroderma of the small bowel. Am J Roentgenol 88: 687–692.

198. Reynolds L, Macy IG, Hunscher H, Olson MB (1940) The gastro-intestinal response of average, healthy children to test meals of barium in milk, cream, meat and carbohydrate media. Am J Roentgenol 43: 517–532.

199. Rice RP, Roufail WM, Reeves RJ (1967) The roentgen diagnosis of Whipple's disease (intestinal lipodystrophy). Radiology 88: 295–301.

200. Rieder H (1904–5) Beiträge zur Topographie des Magen-Darmkanals beim lebenden Menschen, nebst Untersuchungen über den zeitlichen Ablauf der Verdauung. Fortschr R 8: 141–172.

201. Robbins LL (1969) Golden's diagnostic radiology. Section 5: Digestive tract. Baltimore: Williams and Wilkins.

202. Robinson D, Levene JM (1958) Oral Renografin: a new contrast medium for gastrointestinal tract. Am J Roentgenol 80: 79–81.

203. Rosen RS, Jacobson G (1965) Visible urinary tract excretion following oral administration of water-soluble contrast media. Radiology 84: 1031–1032.

204. Rubin RJ, Ostrum BJ, Dex WJ (1960) Water-soluble contrast media. Their use in the diagnosis of obstructive gastrointestinal disease. Arch Surg 80: 495–500.

205. Sack GM (1963) Die orale Schnellpassage des Darms. Fortschr R 99: 337–342.

206. Schatzki R (1943) Small intestinal enema. Am J Roentgenol 50: 743–751.

207. Schönbauer E (1955) Mitteilung über die Verwendung von Baridol in der Magen-Darmdiagnostik. Roentgenblaetter 8: 8–15.

208. Scott-Harden WG, Hamilton AR, McCall Smith S (1961) Radiological investigation of the small intestine. Gut 2: 316–322.

209. Sears AD, Hawkins J, Kilgore BB, Miller JE (1964) Plain roentgenographic findings in drug induced intramural hematoma of the small bowel. Am J Roentgenol 91: 808–813.

210. Seijss R (1961) High kV technique for gastro-intestinal diagnosis. Roentgenblaetter 14: 54–56.

211. Shay H, Gershon-Cohen J (1934–36) Experimental studies in gastric physiology in man. A study of pyloric control. The rôles of acid and alkali. Surg Gynecol Obstet 58: 935–955.

212. Shehadi WH (1960) Orally administered water-soluble iodinated contrast media. Am J Roentgenol 83: 933–941.

213. Shehadi WH (1963) Studies of the colon and small intestines with water-soluble iodinated contrast media. Am J Roengenol 89: 740–751.

214. Shimkin PM, Waldman TA, Krugman RL (1970) Intestinal lymphangiectasia. Am J Roentgenol 110: 827–841.

215. Shufflebarger HE, Knoefel PK, Telford J, Davis LA, Pirkey EL (1953–55) Some factors influencing the roentgen visualization of the mucosal pattern of the gastrointestinal tract. Radiology 61: 801–805.

216. Sidaway ME (1964) Use of water-soluble contrast medium in paediatric radiology. Clin Radiol 15: 132–138.

217. Sielaff HJ (1970) Die radiologische Diagnostik der Dünndarmerkrankungen. Therapiewoche 20: 3207–3215.

218. Sinclair DJ, Buist TAS (1966) Instrumental and technical notes. Water contrast barium enema using methyl cellulose. Br J Radiol 39: 228–232.

192

219. Sleisenger MH, Fordtran JS (1973) Gastrointestinal disease. Philadelphia: Saunders.
220. Sloan RD (1957) The mucosal pattern of the mesenteric small intestine; an anatomic study. Am J Roentgenol 77: 651–669.
221. Sloan RD, Brock JW, Fant WM (1961) Non-strangulating distal ileal obstruction, the rôle of hydration. An experimental study correlating pathologic and radiologic findings. Radiology 76: 407–414.
222. Snell AM, Camp JD (1934) Chronic idiopathic steatorrhea. Roentgenologic observations. Arch Intern Med 53: 615–629.
223. Sövényi E, Varró V (1959) Über eine neue Methode zur Röntgenuntersuchung des Dünndarms. Fortschr R 91: 269–270.
224. Spencer RP (1961) Microvilli and intestinal surface area: an evaluation. Gastroenterology 41: 313–314.
225. Stacy GS, Loop JW (1964) Unusual small bowel diseases. Methods and observations. Am J Roentgenol 92: 1072–1079.
226. Stecken A, Richter K, Weiss U (1961) Zur Kontrastmitteldarstellung des Magen-Darm-Traktes. Ergebnisse von 117 Untersuchungen mit Gastrografin und Gastrografin-Bariumsulfat Gemischen. Fortschr R 95: 172–188.
227. Steinbach HL, Burhenne J (1962) Performing the barium enema: equipment, preparation and contrast medium. Am J Roentgenol 87: 644–654.
228. Sussman ML, Wachtel E (1943) Factors concerned in the abnormal distribution of barium in the small bowel. Radiology 40: 128–138.
229. Swischuk LE, Welsh JD (1968) Roentgenographic mucosal patterns in the 'malabsorption syndrome'. A scheme for diagnosis. Am J Dig Dis 13: 59–78.
230. Tachev T, Hadjidekov G, Nedkova-Bratanova N, Ijanev S (1967) Radiologic stigmata of allergic enteropathies. Acta Gastroenterol Belg 30: 209–224.
231. Thorner RS (1955) The effect of exclusion of the bile upon gastrointestinal motility. Am J Roentgenol 74: 1096–1122.
232. Tosch R (1961) Untersuchungen über die Resorption von I 131 markiertem Gastrografin aus dem Magen-Darm Kanal. Fortschr R 95: 189–192.
233. Truelove SC, Reynell PC (1972) Diseases of the digestive system. Oxford: Blackwell.
234. Tulley TE, Feinberg SB (1974) A röntgenographic classification of diffuse diseases of the small intestine presenting with malabsorption. Am J Roentgenol 121: 283–290.
235. Underhill BML (1955) Intestinal length in man. Br Med J 49/50: 1243–1246.

236. Vest B, Margulis AR (1962) Roentgen diagnosis of postoperative ileus-obstruction. Surg Gynecol Obstet 115: 421–427.
237. Weel JGA v., Wouters JO (1963) Het meten van röntgencontraststoffen 'in vitro' door middel van röntgen-stralen. J Belg Radiol 46: 481–489.
238. Weigen JF, Pendergrass EP, Ravdin IS, Machella TE (1952) A roentgen study of the effect of total pancreatectomy on the stomach and small intestine of the dog. Radiology 59: 92–102.
239. Weintraub S, Williams RG (1949) A rapid method of roentgenologic examination of the small intestine. Am J Roentgenol 61: 45–55.
240. Weltz GA (1937) Der kranke Dünndram im Röntgenbild. Fortschr R 55: 20–40.
241. Wilson JP (1967) Surface area of the small intestine in man. Gut 8: 618–621.
242. Wooldman EE (1938) Barium sulphate suspension in colloidal aluminium hydroxide. An improved contrast medium for the roentgenographic diagnosis of gastrointestinal lesions. Am J Roentgenol 40: 705–707.
243. Wolf BS (1959) Functional aspects of gastro-intestinal radiology. Surg Clin North Am 39: 1431–1449.
244. Wolf BS, Faegenburg DH (1963) Progress in gastroenterology. Gastroenterology 44: 886–899.
245. Youmans WB (1944) The intestino-intestinal inhibitory reflex. Gastroenterology 3: 114–118.
246. Zaslon J, Portner JH, Cohen EA, Kremens V, Berger SM (1961) Complete small intestinal obstruction in the absence of positive roentgen findings. Am J Gastroenterol 35: 122–126.
247. Zboralske F, Bessolo RJ (1967) Metastatic carcinoma of the mesentery and gut. Radiology 88: 302–310.
248. Zboralske F, Harris PA, Riegelman S, Rambo ON, Margulis AR (1966) Toxicity studies on tannic acid administered by enema. Studies on the retention of enemas in humans. Review and conclusions. Am J Roentgenol 96: 505–509.
249. Zimmer EA (1948–49) Barium 'Wander'. A new contrast medium with special advantages in examination of the gastro-intestinal tract. Gastroenterologia (Basel) 74: 208–224.
250. Zimmer EA (1951) Radiology of the small intestine. Studies on contrast media for the x-ray examination of the gastro-intestinal tract. Br J Radiol 24: 245–251.
251. Zimmer EA (1954) Die Röntgenologie des Dünndarms. Gastroenterologia (Basel) 70: 113–171.
252. Zollner S (1937) Physiologische Schwankungen in der Motorik des Dünndarms. Fortschr R 56: 644–649.

9. INFLAMMATION AND INFLAMMATORY-LIKE DISEASES

1. General

Inflammatory processes in the wall of the small intestine can be due to, or enhanced by, various highly divergent factors. Several of these are:

1) Direct action on the intestinal mucosal membrane by chemicals or toxins produced by bacteria.
2) Impaired arterial or venous circulation in the involved intestinal segment; intramural bleeding as a result of abdominal blunt trauma; a greatly prolonged coagulation time. Both embolic processes and thrombosis, or intramural hematomas, can lead to necrosis of the intestinal wall.
3) Ulcerations can also develop in mucosa swollen as a result of lymphedema. Lymph drainage can be disturbed by a number of causes such as tumorous growth, inflammatory processes, or fibrotic shriveling. Although rare, congenital lymphedema can also occur.
4) Stimulation of the mucosa by parasites not normally found in the intestine.
5) Lowered resistance of the intestinal mucosal membrane as a result of marked atrophy of the folds of Kerkring can also lead to increased susceptibility to harmful agents.

If the wall of the small intestine is inflamed, it will appear upon examination to be red and swollen. Roentgenologically, one or more of the following phenomena may be observed during the transit examination:

1) The intestine is highly irritable and numerous contractions in rapid succession will be observed. Locally the transit time is greatly accelerated so that antispasmodics must be used in order to obtain an x-ray of the involved loops in a sufficiently well-filled state. Prolonged spasms in intestinal segments with an otherwise normal mucosal pattern, such as can be observed during the colon examination, seldom occur in the small intestine (fig. 8.60Q). In Crohn's disease, however, we can see spastic contractions extending over a length of 5–15 cm. On the roentgenogram, the barium in the involved intestinal segment then sometimes appears to be as thin as a thread. In the loops where this so-called 'string sign' is observed, the mucosal surface has already become highly ulcerous. Pathological-anatomical examination has revealed that under the ulcerous mucosa there is an obviously thickened muscular layer that undoubtedly causes these spasms. If the flow of contrast fluid is sufficiently abundant, then under prolonged fluoroscopy the short periods of relaxation can also be observed. That we are concerned with a temporary spasm and not a manifest stenosis is obvious because there is no sign of a prestenotic dilatation in these cases.

2) As a result of the edematous swelling of the mucosa, the diameter of the lumen of an inflamed intestinal loop can be somewhat smaller than normal during the rest phase. The affected intestinal loops then also show a certain degree of rigidity. They more or less stretch across the abdomen and the number of loops in the affected area are clearly decreased.

3) As a result of multiple ulcerations the normal mucosal pattern can be completely or partially disturbed over a large or small area; sometimes the pattern is completely destroyed.

4) A deep necrosis involving all layers of the intestinal wall can lead easily to the formation of fistulas or adhesion to adjacent intestinal loops. Gas can be found in the intestinal wall and even in the portal vein. This gas is caused by gas-producing bacteria or enters from the lumen of the intestine.

194

These accumulations of gas in the intestinal wall are first visible on the roentgenogram as 1- to 3-mm thin straight or ring-shaped shadows with a somewhat ragged margin along both sides. As a result of the cleavage of the intestinal wall into its layers, these strips of gas often have a sort of fibrillar structure similar to that of muscle bundles. If the gas accumulation is larger, then of course the radiolucent areas are wider, but the ragged margins remain as well as thin offshoots along the edges of the gas shadows.

5) The mucosal surface can appear coarsely nodular or cushion-like. Sometimes these polypoid formations are more or less spread out over the mucosal surface. In such cases they are the sites of inflammatory infiltration or nodules of lymphatic tissue. In other cases, for instance Crohn's disease, the cushion-like mucosal swellings lie adjacent to one another and are separated by deep longitudinal and transverse grooves so that a more or less regular pattern resembling cobblestones is seen. Ulcerations often develop in the depths of the grooves as a result of, or enhanced by, local circulatory disorders.

6) On the roentgenograms, the spaces between the intestinal loops may be increased in the inflamed region. These wider spaces may be due to thickening or fatty degeneration of the intestinal wall, shriveling of the mesentery, or an inflammatory infiltrate.

7) On the mesenteric side of the intestine there may be impressions in the intestinal lumen that are caused by thickening of the mesentery and enlargement of the glands within the mesentery.

A superficial inflammatory process in the mucosa of the small intestine can heal without radiologically visible scarring. If, however, the inflammatory process is not limited to the surface but is transmural in character, which is the case in Crohn's disease, then the mucosa can be completely destroyed. There is no longer any chance of recovery of the fold relief. In such an intestine we will find areas, corresponding more or less to these sites, in which the fold relief has completely disappeared. Such foldless plaques can also be due to metastases from a linitis plastica of the stomach. In spite of the great similarity radiologically between these two very different diseases, differentiation will in prac-

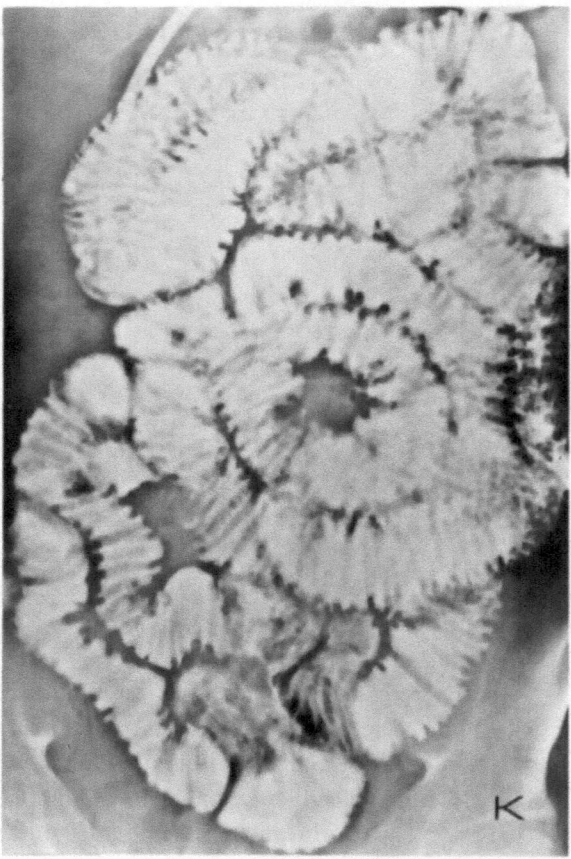

*Fig. 9.1*κ. Generalized edema of the mucosa in the jejunum and ileum due, according to the biopsy, to Crohn's disease. As a rule this stage precedes the superficial ulcerative changes seen in fig. 9.1м.

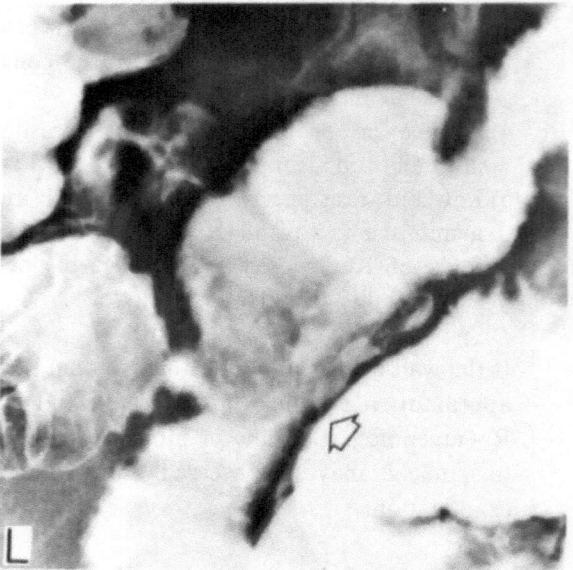

*Fig. 9.1*ʟ. As a result of highly superficial ulcerations in the distal ileum of a patient with Crohn's disease, the margins of the barium column are vague and ragged. Where compression was applied, the deeper ulcers are visible as white dots (arrow).

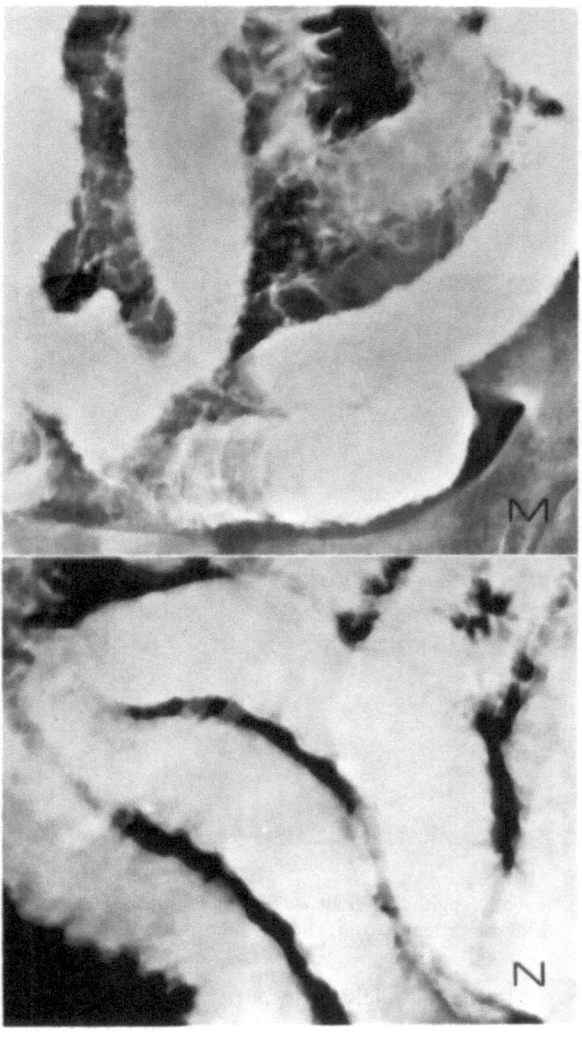

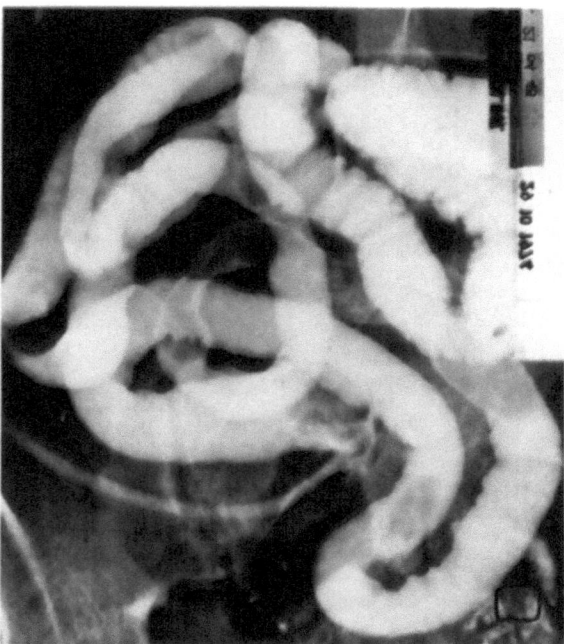

Fig. 9.1. (M) Superficial, more or less merging ulcerations in Crohn's disease slightly similar to the mucosal abnormalities in the colon in a case of ulcerative colitis. There are only a few cobblestones, no skip lesions, and no healthy segments. (N) One year later the ulcerations have disappeared and the intestinal wall is more or less smooth with no visible mucosal relief. (O) Another year later.

tice not be difficult if the patient is examined further and a history is carefully taken. If a previous examination has revealed a widespread inflammatory process, then on a later roentgenogram there will be an extensive area with no circular mucosal folds at all.

Due to the transmural character of the inflammation, the deep-seated muscular layers will be replaced by connective tissue so that the intestine becomes dilated and shows no peristalsis at all. As a result of the passive collapse of these completely atonic loops, only coarse longitudinal folds will be seen. These are formed by the entire intestinal wall and not only by the mucosa, as in an intact intestine. During the fluoroscopic examination, it is

seen that the contrast fluid flowing in the distal direction is passively propelled through these loops. This phenomenon, which is so characteristic of complete atony of the mucosal membrane and the muscular layers, has acquired in our clinic the name 'bike tire phenomenon'. This is because of the similarity to the tire's inner tube (fig. 9.2A). A highly similar pattern of atony, but with a normal circular mucosal relief, is seen when buscopan or glucagon is administered during the examination (fig. 9.2B). In fact, however, the administration of an atony-inducing drug will presumably never be indicated during an enteroclysis examination.

Ulcers in the intestinal wall will heal with the formation of fibrous tissue. As a result of shrivel-

196

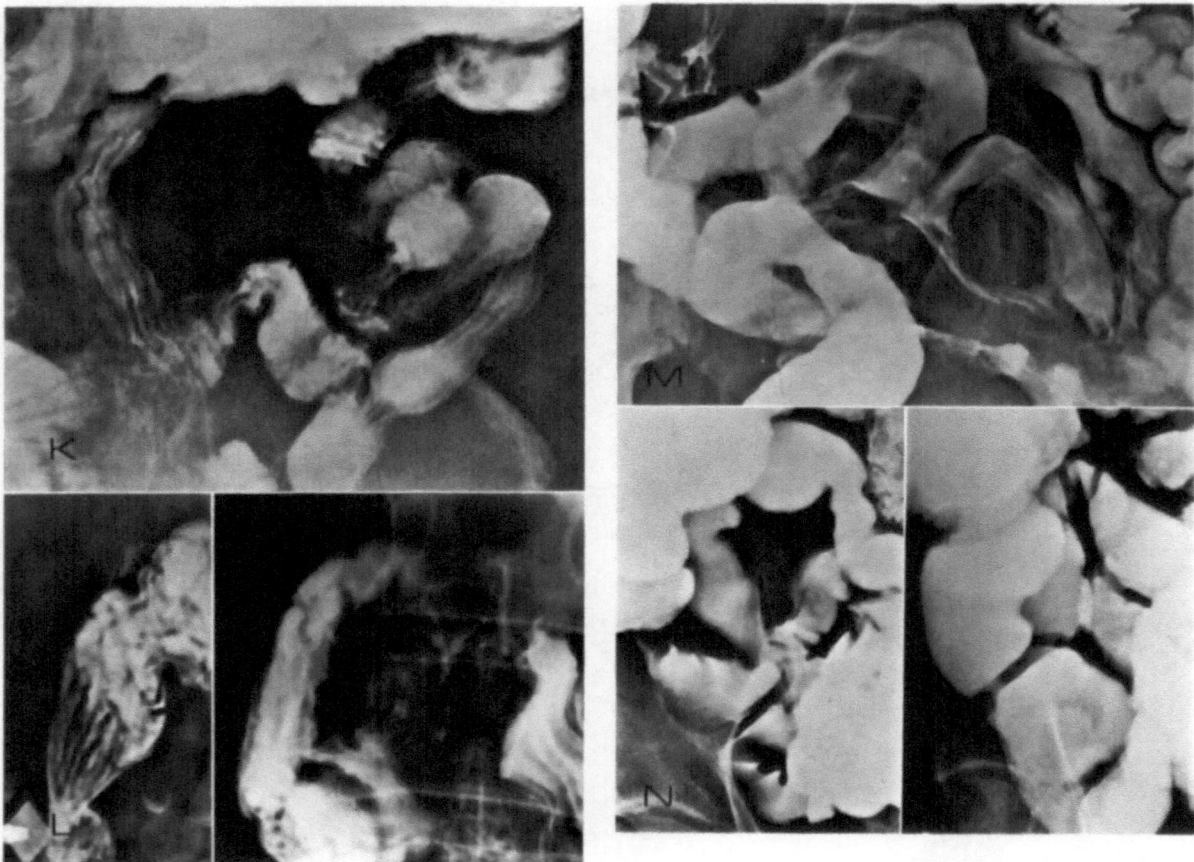

Fig. 9.2A. Four examples of atrophied mucosa after Crohn's disease with longitudinal folds when the intestine is inadequately filled: the so-called bike tire phenomenon; (K) proximal jejunum, (L) distal duodenum, (M) proximal ileum, (N) distal ileum.

ing of this connective tissue, circular strictures may ultimately develop that cause more or less pronounced stenoses.

2. Crohn's disease

In 1932, when most of the inflammatory processes in the small intestine were ascribed to tuberculosis, the internist Crohn and his associates identified a disease that they called regional ileitis. This was because they thought at that time that it would develop only in the terminal ileum. We now know that this disease can involve the entire digestive tract from the mouth to the anus. Moreover, at least radiologically, it canot be distinguished from tuberculosis. Today almost every internist and radiologist believes that Crohn's disease has spread considerably in the past few years. It is difficult to determine with any certainty whether this should be

attributed solely or in part to the greatly improved clinical and radiological diagnostic methods in use today. In any event, regional enteritis or ileitis is definitely now one of the most common diseases of the small intestine. A precise estimate of the frequency is difficult, but it is known that one out of every 10,000 Dutchmen is being treated in a University Hospital for this disease. It can easily be assumed that an equal number is being treated elsewhere.

The question that logically follows is: were some of the cases diagnosed in the past as tuberculosis in fact Crohn's disease? In the numerous publications of the 19th and early 20th centuries, the clinical and in particular the pathological and histological descriptions were so detailed that it has become apparent that the answer is probably yes! In a number of cases it has now even been established definitely. The earliest of this series of publications is that of Morgagni in 1769. In 1920, Tietze col-

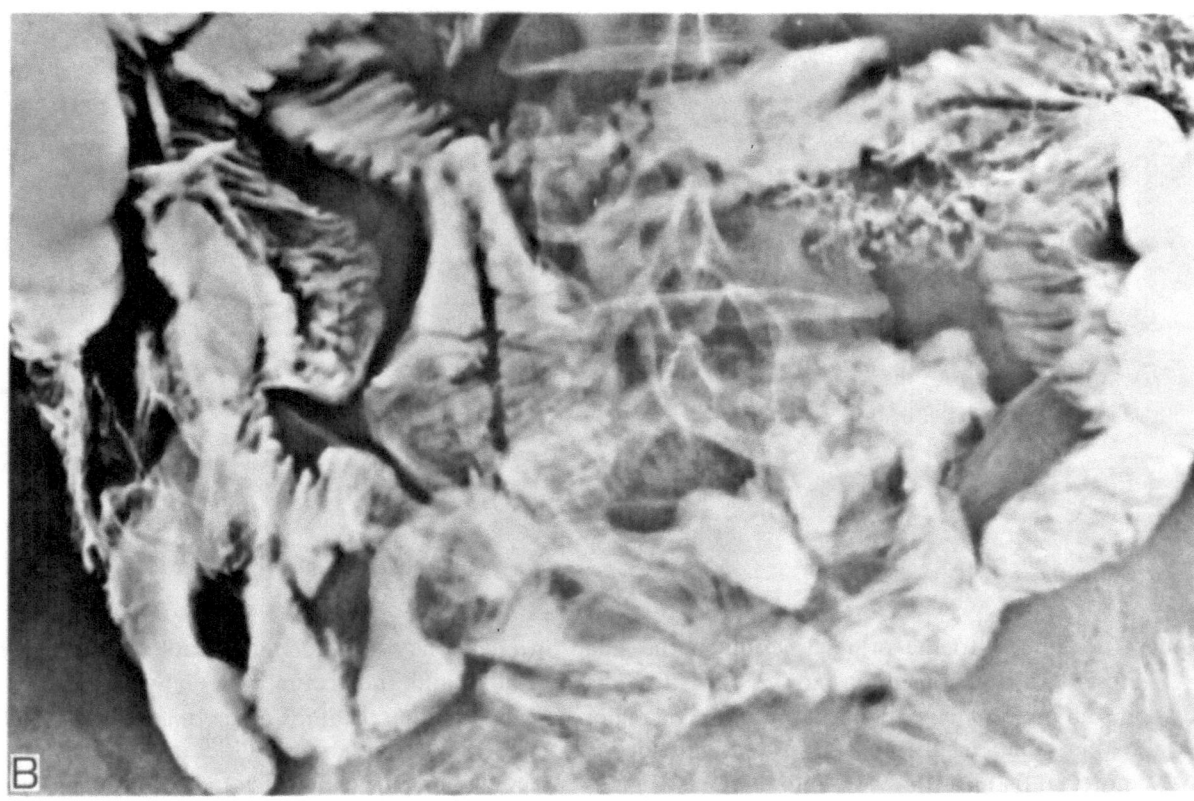

Fig. 9.2b. Atonic intestinal loops with numerous angular margins and sharp bends in the lumen, caused by the administration of glucagon. The mucosal folds have not disappeared. Superficially this is reminiscent of M in fig. 9.2A.

lected some 281 literature references to cases of tb that probably were not tuberculosis. On the basis of the publications that have appeared so far, Crohn's disease appears to occur mainly in western and northwestern European countries and in the northeastern part of North America. There is a possible predisposition for the Jewish race. There is no clear predilection for sex. Occasionally a hereditary relationship can be established. The disease is seen predominantly in young adults between 15 and 40 years of age, is less common in older adults, and only rarely occurs in children under ten years of age. It is not surprising that for a long time the disease was called terminal ileitis because it is this part of the intestine that is involved in four out of five patients. In about 1/5th of these cases the wall of the cecum is also thickened and inflamed so that one could speak of an ileocecal infection.

In general about one out of every ten patients has Crohn-like abnormalities in the colon when the small intestine does not appear to be involved. On the average these patients are somewhat older than the patients with a localization in the small intestine. It has never been established with any certainty how often the abnormalities characteristic of ulcerative colitis occur in the small intestine. It is known that the radiological abnormalities of some of the patients being treated for a probable Crohn's disease are very similar to those of an ulcerative colitis. In the latter case the disease usually starts with a generalized edema (fig. 9.1K). In this early phase of the disease, a radiological examination is seldom carried out. In a later stage, ulcerations develop. They are collar-button shaped and fairly superficial. Sometimes there are no indications of cobblestones, deep longitudinal ulcerations, fistulization, skip lesions, or strictures (fig. 9.1.LM). Upon remission of Crohn's disease, there remains a smooth flaccid thin intestinal wall that shows no peristalsis (fig. 9.1NO). If the intestinal loop is only moderately filled, then the 'bike tire' phenomenon (see page 195) will be observed (fig. 9.2A).

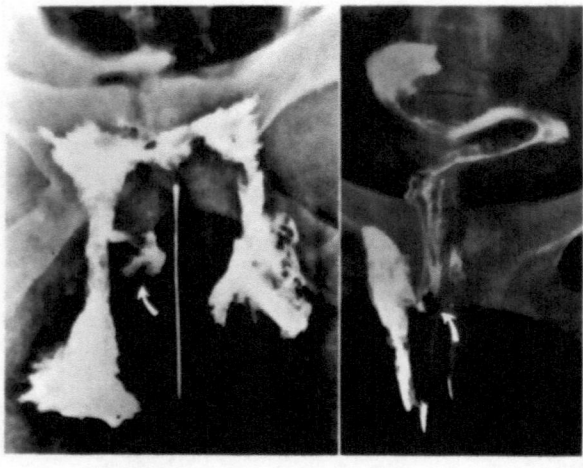

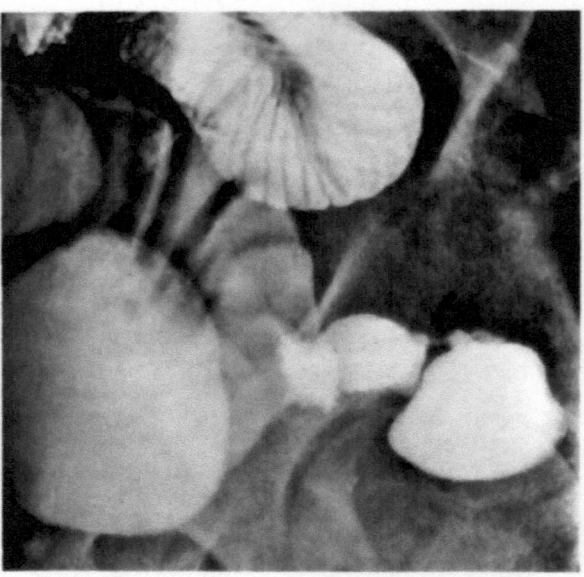

Fig. 9.3. Right-sided ischiorectal fistula in Crohn's disease. At the time the abnormalities in the small intestine were minimal (see fig. 9.9w); now (four years later) they have become extensive.

Fig. 9.4. Abscess in Douglas' pouch in Crohn's disease that communicates via a fistulous tract with the greatly dilated ileum.

In addition to the primary lesion in the small intestine, a mucosal abnormality is also found in one out of every ten patients in the anorectal region. In this same region, anal fissures, right-sided ischiorectal fistulas (fig. 9.3), and abscesses (fig. 9.4) can precede the appearance of the intestinal lesions by many months, sometimes even years. If these fistulas are filled carefully, then it is often possible to demonstrate a communication between these canals and the rectum – usually just inside the sphincter muscle of the anus. In another 10% of the patients, Crohn abnormalities are not encountered in the distal ileum but more proximal in the digestive tract. In one-half of these cases they involve the remaining part of the ileum (fig. 9.5). The other half are localized in the jejunum (fig. 9.6),

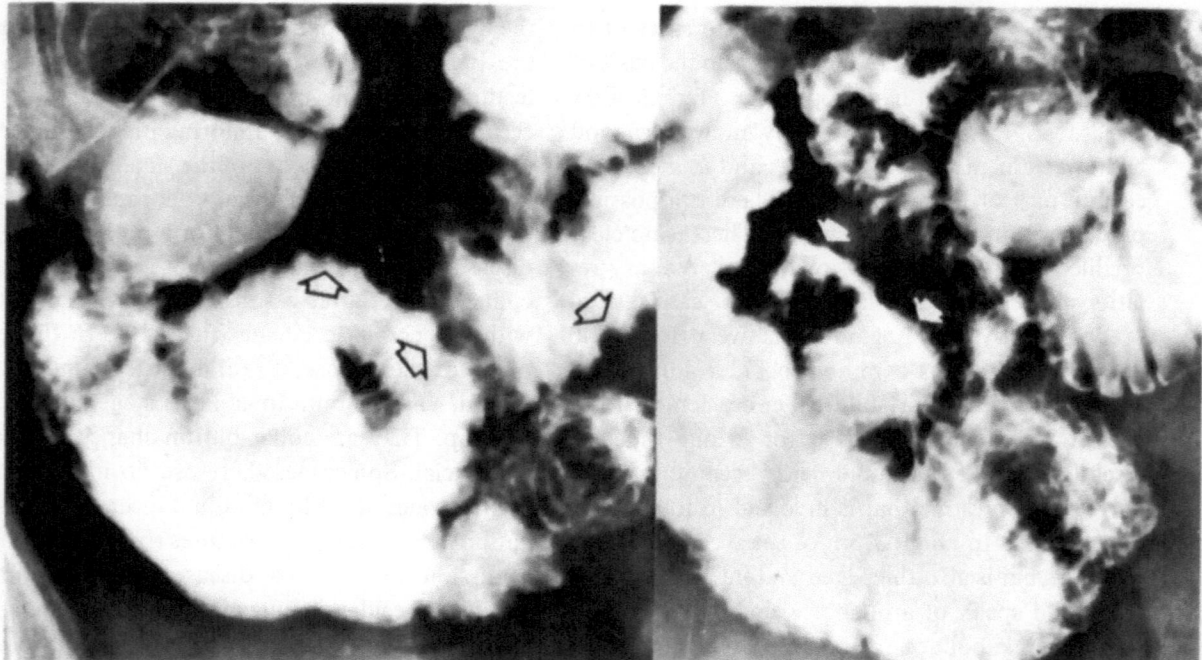

Fig. 9.5. Slight abnormalities in the more proximal part of the ileum in a patient with aphthous stomatitis due to Crohn's disease.

199

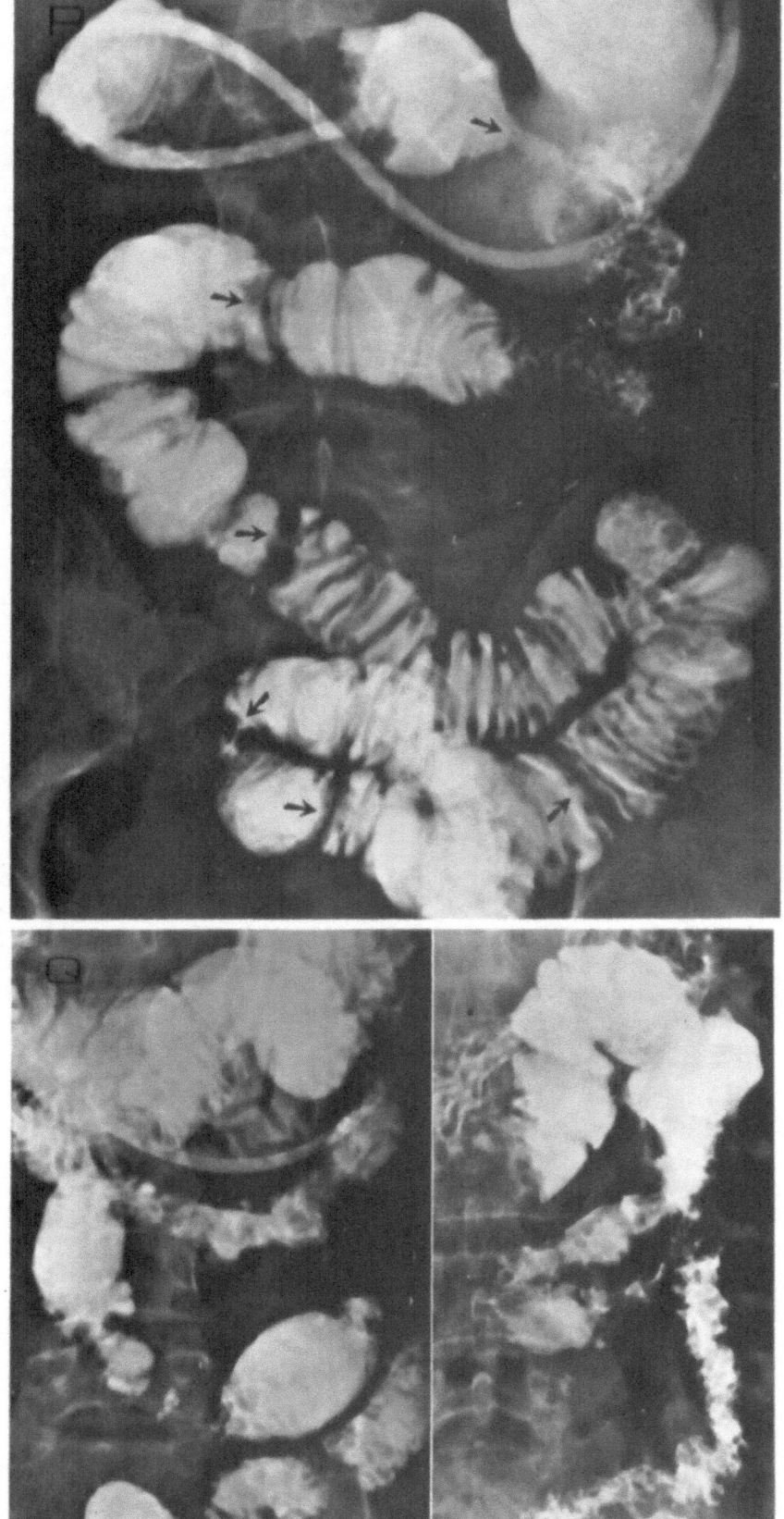

Fig. 9.6. Three patients with Crohn's disease of the jejunum. Longitudinal ulcer (arrows) and multiple more or less constricting skip lesions. The skip lesion at the ligament of Treitz in patient ʀ is visible on only one of the two exposures. Loss of mucosal relief in the proximal duodenum of this patient and edematous thickened folds farther distalward are also visible.

200

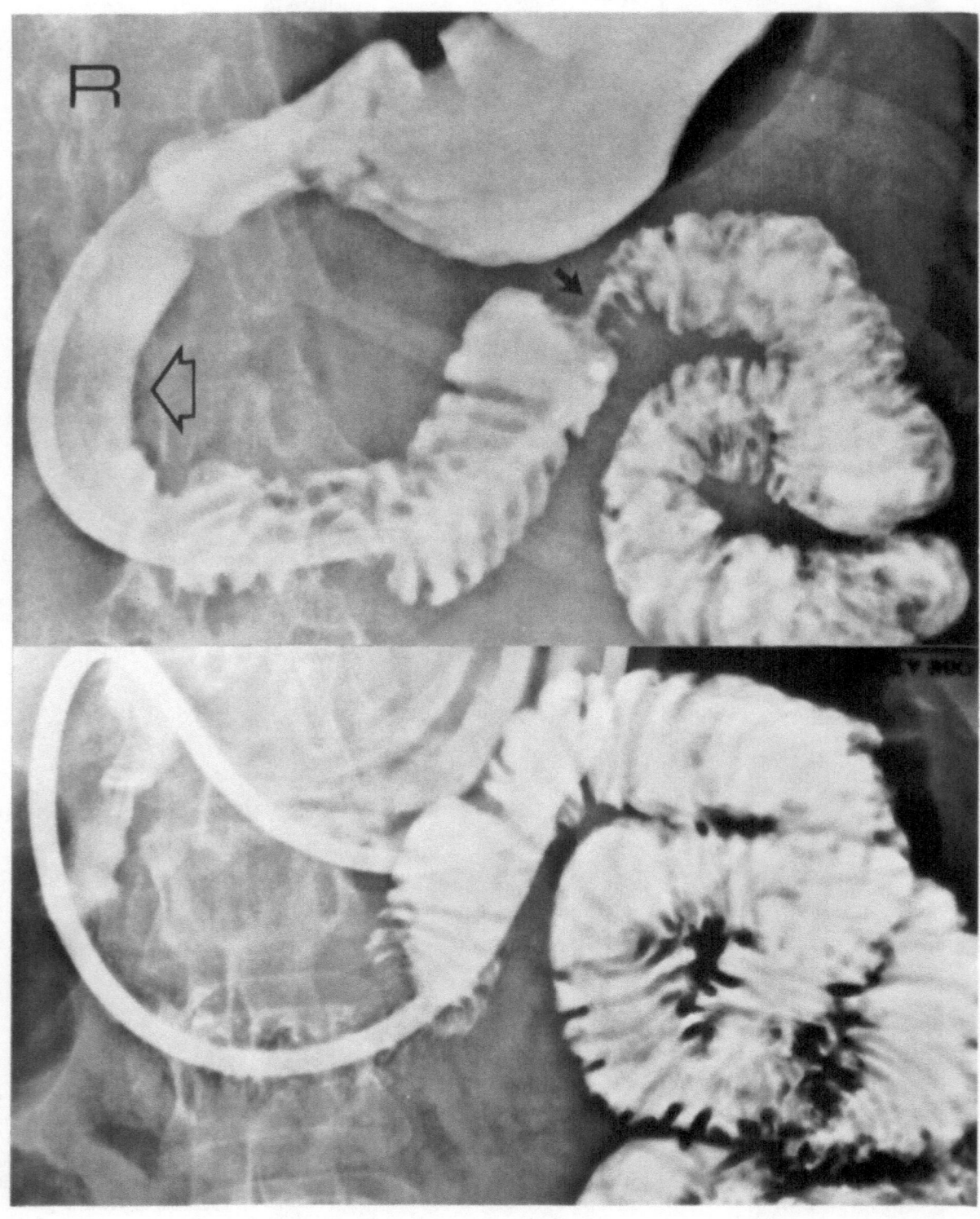

Fig. 9.7. See legend on page 201.

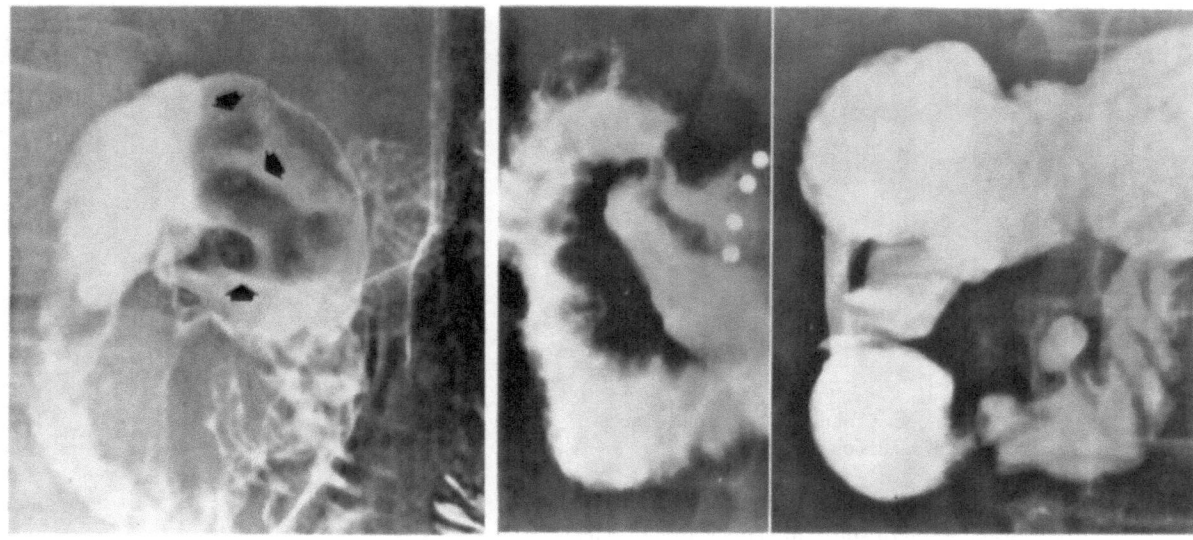

Fig. 9.7. Three patients with Crohn's disease of the duodenum. Aphthoid ulcers (arrows) in the patient on the left. (See also page 200.)

duodenum (fig. 9.7), or stomach (fig. 9.8) with a relative frequency of about 6:3:1, respectively. Prodromic indications of Crohn's disease occur not only in the mucosal membrane of the anus but also in the mouth. Careful inquiry reveals that one out of every ten patients has a history of aphthae. Also of every ten patients with a Crohn's lesion in the small intestine, there is approximately one with one or more 'skip' lesions proximal to the primary lesion. Skip lesions are clearly circumscribed sites in the middle of a fairly normal mucosa (fig. 9.9vw). An intestinal loop affected by Crohn's disease, usually in the last few decimeters of the ileum, appears red and swollen during the acute phase of the infection. Although the diameter of the lumen has decreased slightly, the outer diameter of the

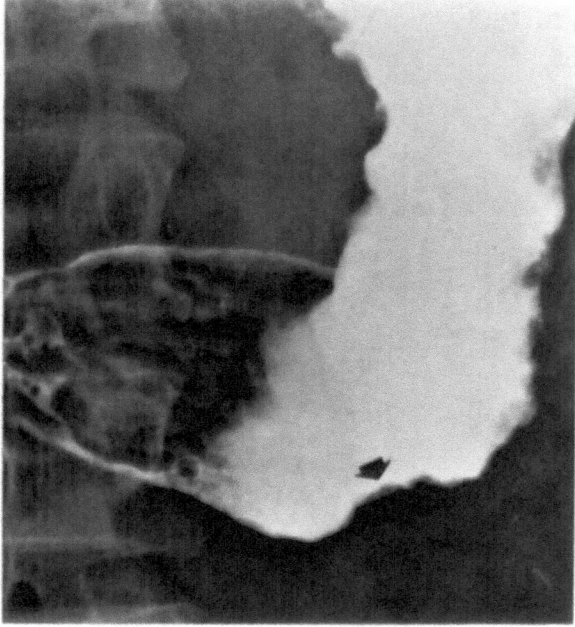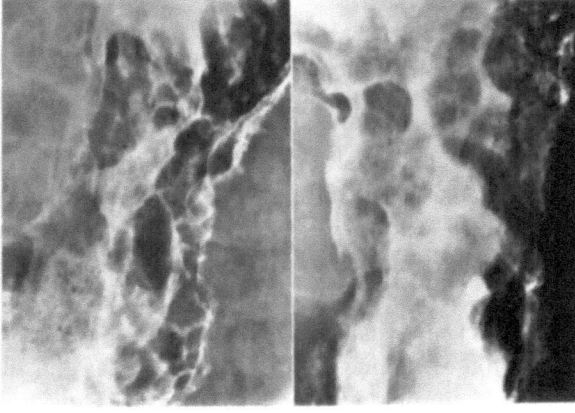

Fig. 9.8. Crohn's disease of the stomach. The mucosal pattern in the stomach somewhat resembles that of a lymphoreticular malignancy, a hypertrophic gastritis, or Zollinger-Ellison disease, except that the thick folds are often interrupted in the transverse direction so that a highly irregular network is observed.

202

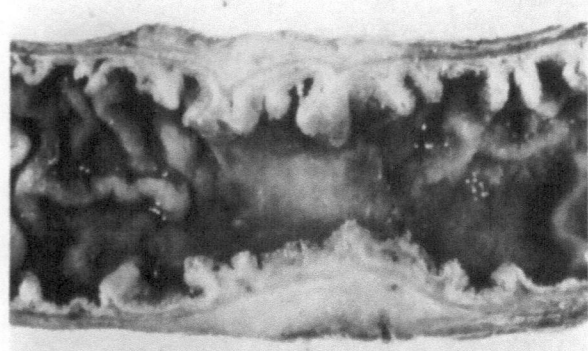

*Fig. 9.9*v. Skip lesions in Crohn's disease; fairly normal mucosa on either side of the lesion.

diseased part of the intestine is still larger due to the pronounced thickening of the wall. This is due in part to the fact that Crohn's disease is often accompanied by a pronounced hypertrophy of the muscular layers in the wall of the intestine. This hypertrophy causes prolonged spasms in the involved intestinal segment so that the contrast fluid appears thread-like on the x-ray. This is the so-called string sign (fig. 9.10). An intraluminal increase in pressure in these loops may lead to herniation of the intact mucosal tissue right through the intestinal wall. Fluoroscopic examination shows that each of these so-called 'false diverticula' alternates in size (fig. 9.11). False diverticula are lined with mucosal tissue only and consequently they are extremely thin-walled. They are situated on the mesenteric side of the intestine, and have to be differentiated from still another type of diverticula, the so-called pseudo-diverticula (fig. 9.12). Pseudodiverticula are usually situated on the antimesenteric side of the intestine, and the wall of these diverticula, indeed, contains all layers of the intestinal wall. They are formed by contractions or fibrotic rings originating in the intact intestinal wall opposite the site of an ulceration at the mesentery attachment that has healed with fibrous degeneration and shriveling. In contrast to the former type of diverticula that are spherical with a narrow and sometimes long neck, the second type usually appear to be much larger, vary in shape, and join the wall of the intestine with a more or less broad base. Figure 9.13 illustrates that this type of shriveling cannot be differentiated from that seen in the colon. Sometimes it is quite obvious that there is little or no fibrosis; the sacculations then change so completely that it

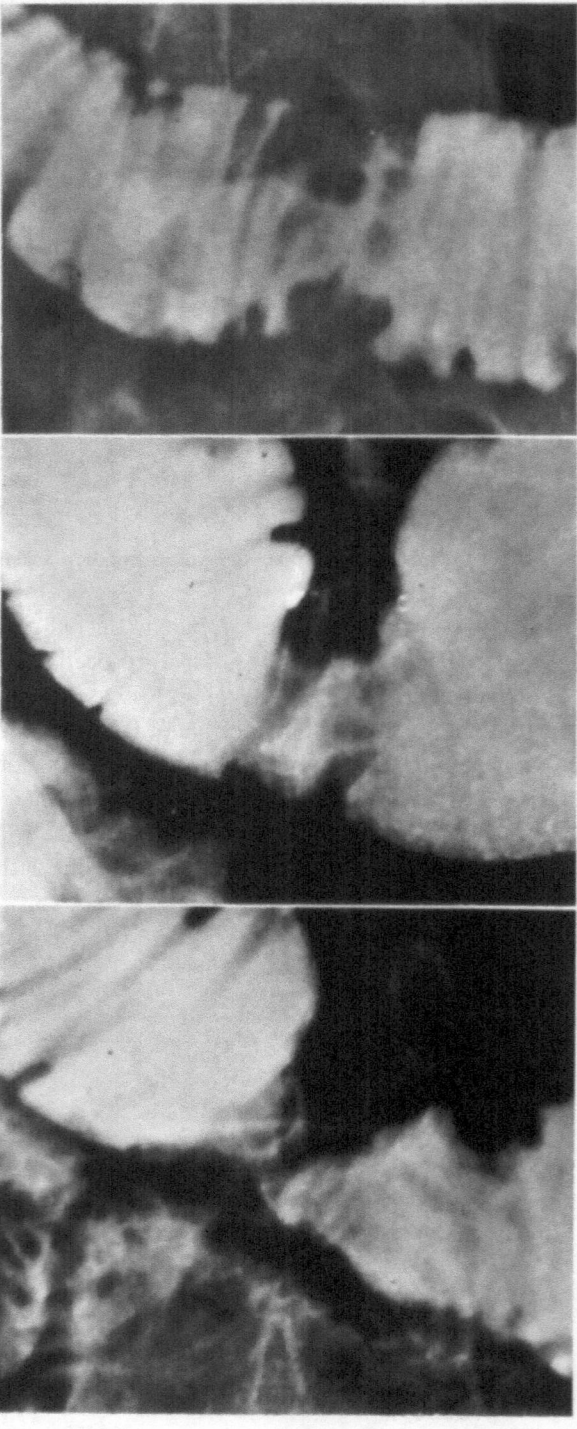

*Fig. 9.9*w. Skip lesions in Crohn's disease: fairly normal mucosa on either side of the lesion.

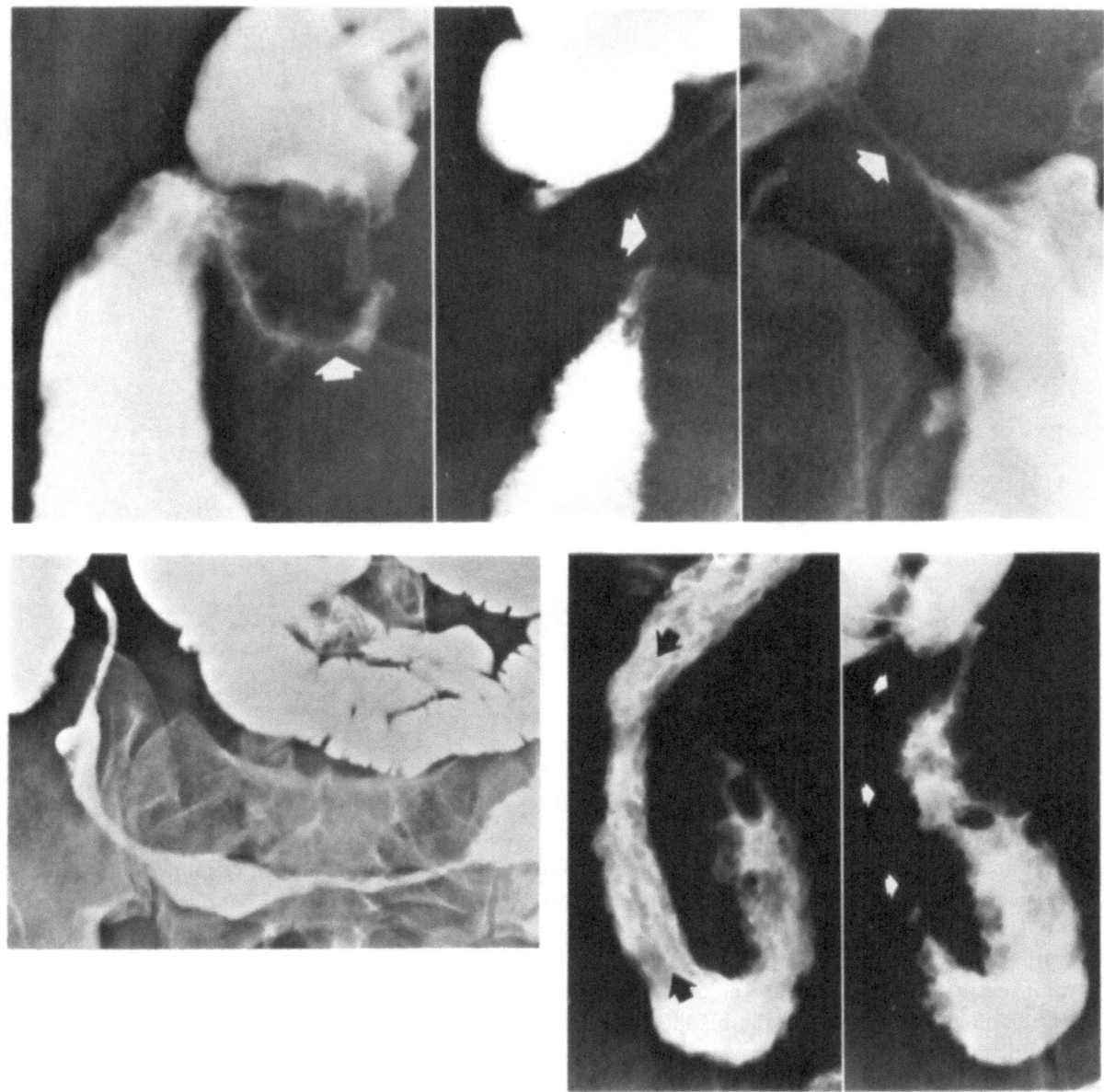

Fig. 9.10. Several examples of the so-called string sign in Crohn's disease caused by spasms due to a marked hypertrophy of the muscular layers. There is no indication of either a stenosis or a prestenotic dilatation.

would be better to call them pseudo-pseudodiverticula (fig. 9.14).

Another factor that can cause thickening of the intestinal wall in Crohn's disease is a thickened mesentery as a result of edema and an increase in the fat tissue that encircles the intestine somewhat like claws (fig. 9.15). The lymph nodes in the mesentery and the retroperitoneal area are often obviously enlarged, but sometimes they show no change at all.

The latter abnormalities are actually never visualized on the films and in any case cannot be recognized as such.

In Crohn's disease the intestinal mucosa is usually swollen and cushion-like, mainly as a result of a lymphedema, an inflammatory infiltrate, and lym-

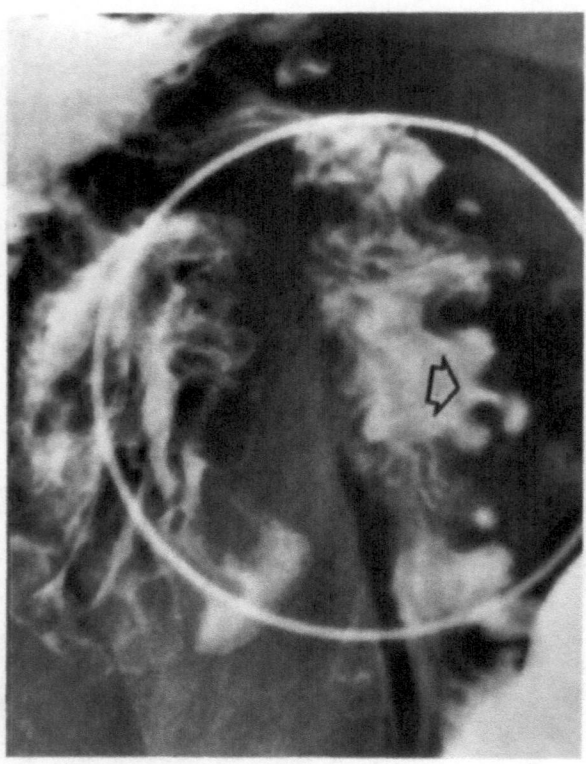

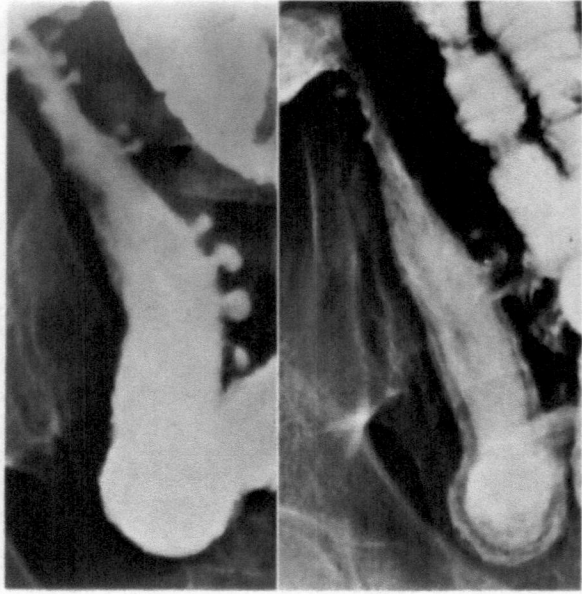

Fig. 9.11. So-called false diverticula in Crohn's disease caused by herniation of the mucosa out through the other layers of the wall. Compare true diverticula that originate in a normal mucosa (arrow).

phoid hyperplasia of the submucosa (fig. 9.16). Between these cushions or 'cobblestones' (fig. 9.17) that are seen as islands of relatively intact mucosal tissue are fissures or ulcers that penetrate deep into all layers of the intestinal wall. Abscesses form within the depths of these fissures and perforate quite easily, forming fistulas to adjacent ileal loops, the sigmoid, or the apex of the bladder (fig. 9.18). Fistulization is not only enhanced by the fusion of adjacent inflamed ileal loops but probably also by minute intestinal infarctions resulting from the frequently concomitant endarteritis.

The ulcerations in the mucosa are found mainly on the mesenteric side of the intestine. They extend along the length of the intestine as well as perpendicular to it, thus sometimes causing a railroad track pattern. Near the ulcers there is often pus as well as an enhanced secretion due to hyperplasia of the mucus-secreting glands so that it can be difficult to obtain a sufficiently sharp film of these ulcerations (fig. 9.19). Due to the richer mucosal folding, the formation of cobblestones and deep linear ulcers is greater in the proximal small intestine than

in the distal segments – independent of the direction of the spread of the disease.

It is assumed that a pure mucosal swelling as a result of a submucosal lymphedema and aphthoid ulcerations are the earliest demonstrable symptoms of an incipient Crohn's disease (fig. 9.20). The formation of cobblestones and fissures does not develop until later. Ulcerations in the fissures then occur because the circulation is highly disturbed as a result of the edema. This hypothesis is based on the observation that with a recurrence after an ileocecal resection, edema of the mucosa is observed first (fig. 9.20B–D). There is a greater chance of finding the earliest symptom of Crohn abnormalities in these patients than in patients who are being examined the first time for unexplained abdominal complaints. After all, surgical patients come back regularly for a checkup even if they have no complaints. The findings of the pathologist and early roentgenological examination of patients with a positive family history have shown, however, that this concept is not always correct.

Furthermore, we have also noted that the ulcer-

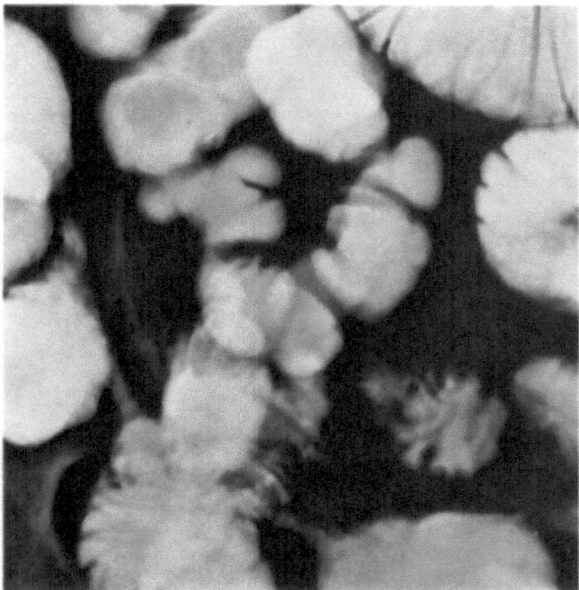

Fig. 9.12

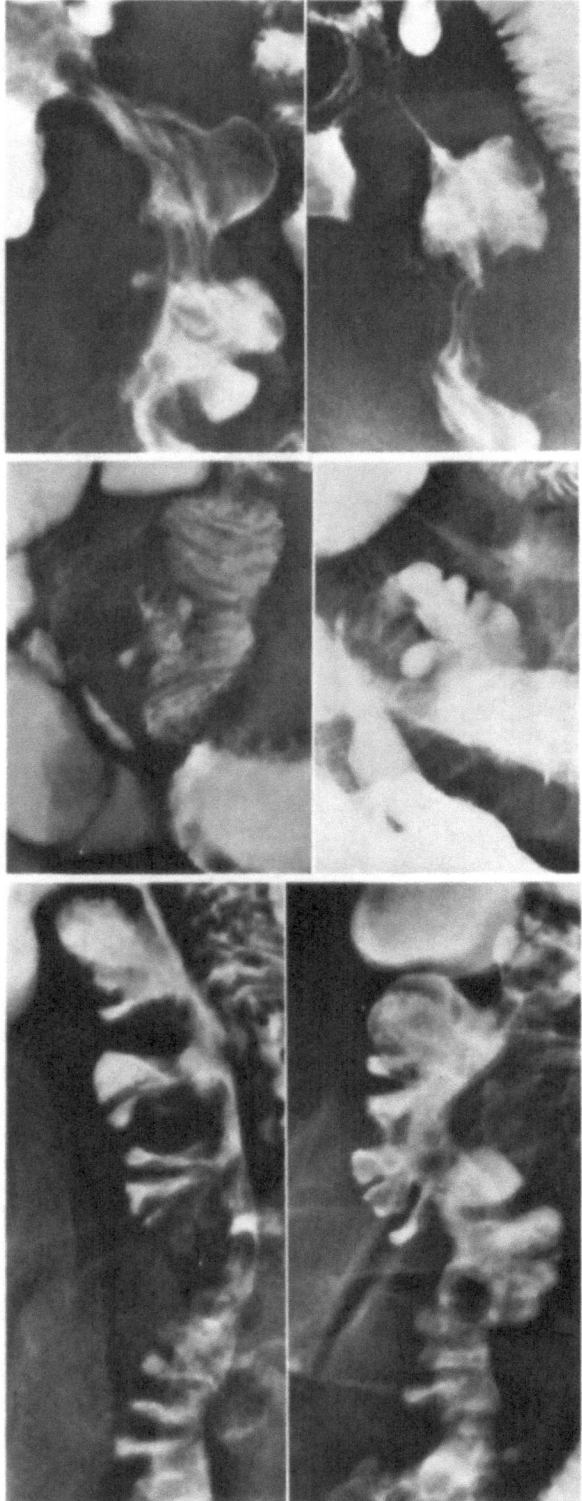

ations can be limited in size, be most superficial (fig. 9.21), and sometimes occur in the center of granulomas in a mucous membrane that shows no signs of submucosal edema (fig. 9.22). In particular this appears to be true in the distal ileum, possibly because the disease occurs there more frequently. This is also true because diagnosis of such subtle abnormalities is somewhat easier in this segment than in the jejunum, where the folds are so much more numerous. Such a loop sometimes feels completely normal when examined during surgery or at autopsy, so that negative findings of this type should not be accorded too much significance. If granulomas or cobblestones are large, they may occasionally be visible in an air-filled loop on a survey exposure of the abdomen (fig. 9.23).

Histologically this type of Crohn's disease is characterized by a chronic inflammatory infiltrate in all layers of the intestinal wall. However, the most pronounced abnormalities in Crohn's disease are found in the submucosa where lymphedema and hyperplasia of the lymphoid tissue are seen. Another characteristic is sarcoid formation manifested as granulomas with Langhan's giant cells that are also found to a lesser extent in Boeck's disease but are more common in tuberculosis. In spite of extensive examination, the pathologist is not always

Fig. 9.12. So-called pseudodiverticula in Crohn's disease are caused by fibrous constrictions and contractions on the healthy side of the intestinal wall opposite a longitudinal ulcer. (See also page 206.)

206

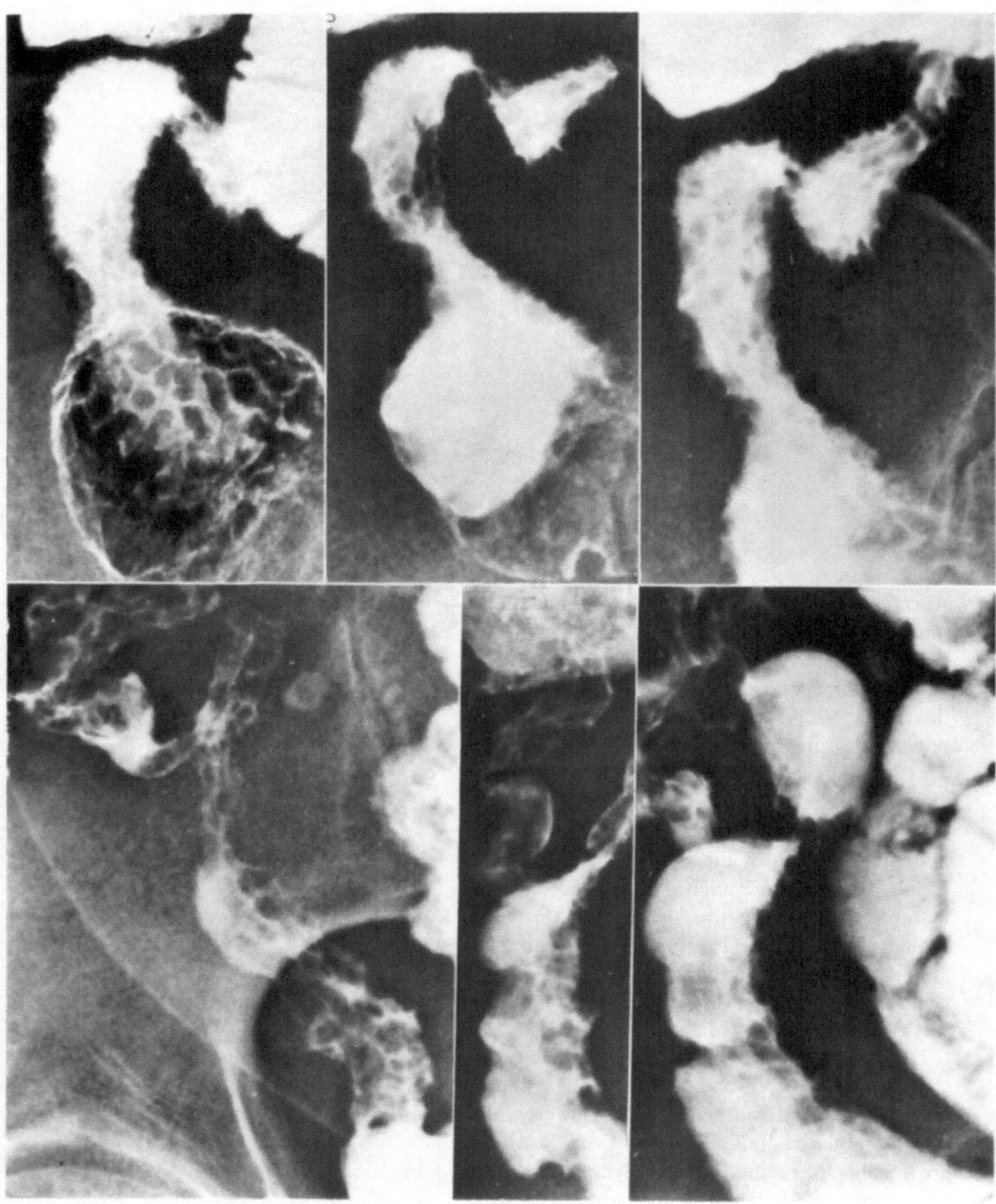

Fig. 9.12. See legend on page 205.

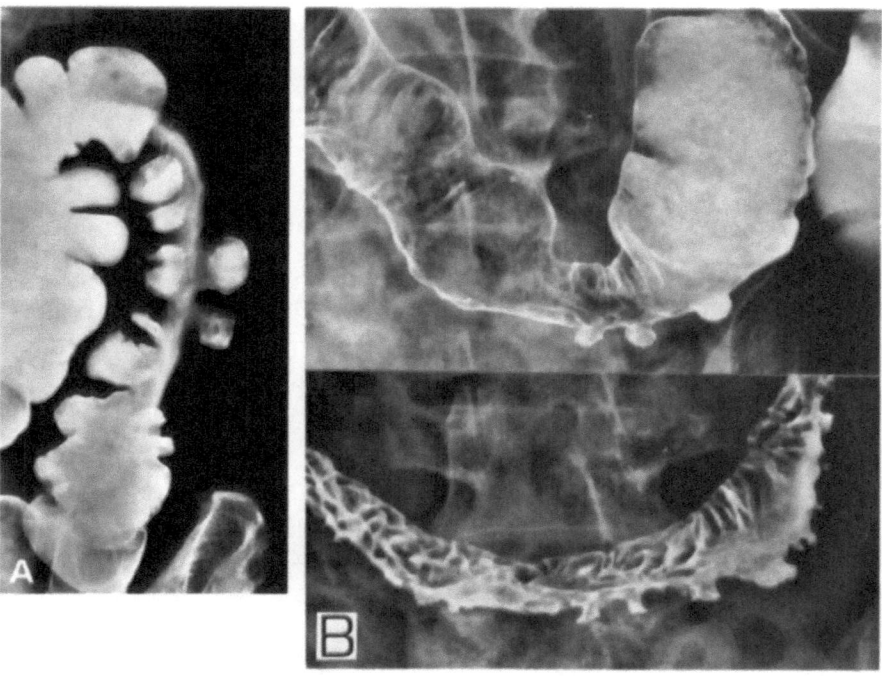

Fig. 9.13. Pseudodiverticula in the colon in Crohn's disease (A) and ischemia (B) cause the same pattern as those in the small intestine.

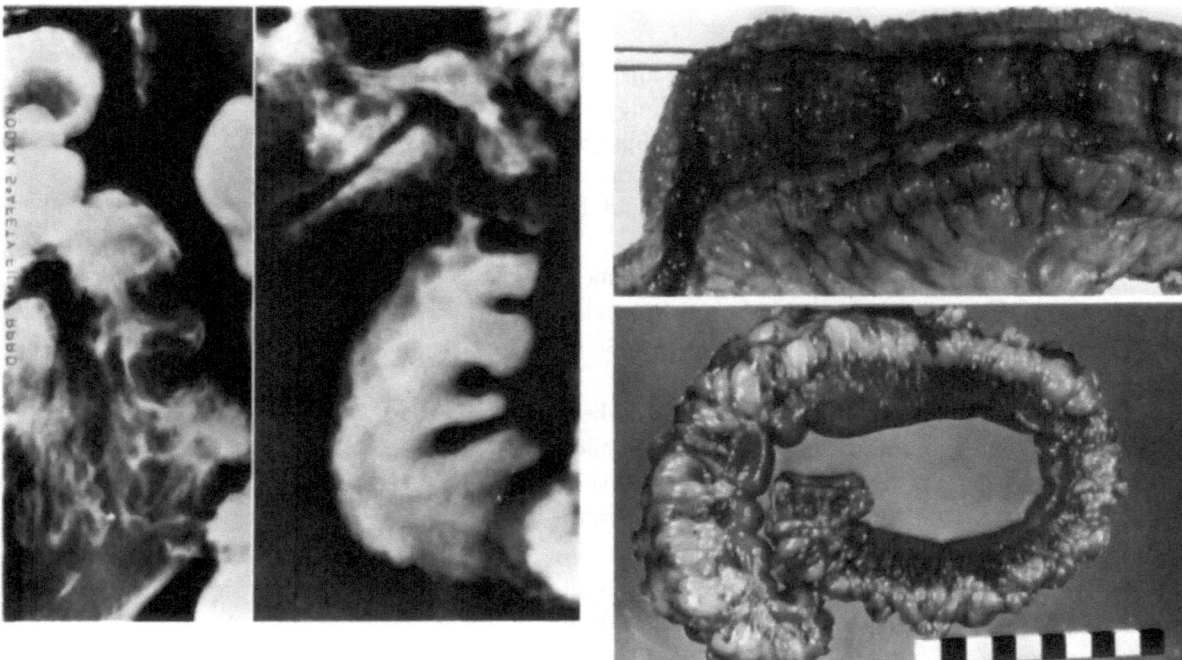

Fig. 9.14. Pseudo-pseudodiverticula in Crohn's disease. The sacculations alternate not only in shape but also in location. Such a pattern is a result of spasms only and not fibrosis.

Fig. 9.15. In Crohn's disease the intestinal wall is thicker due to edema of the mucosa and hypertrophy of the muscular layers, and especially because it is enclosed in a claw-like thick coat of fat originating from the mesenteric attachment.

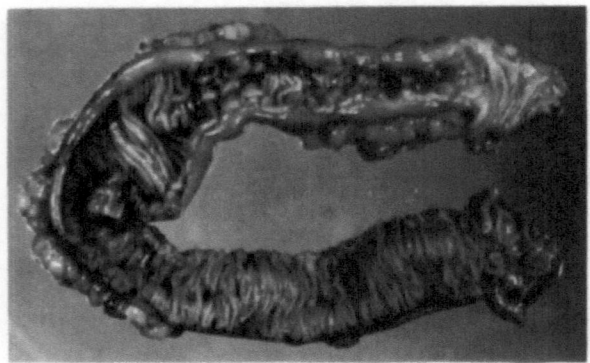

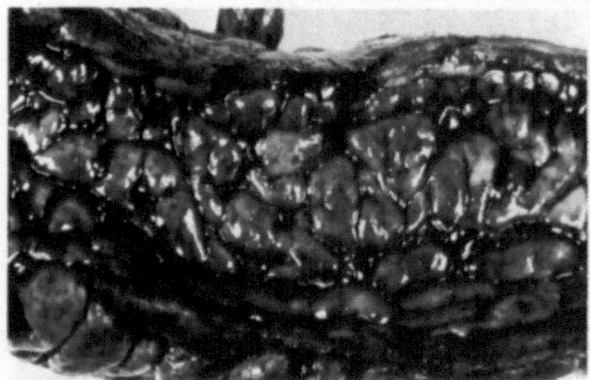

Fig. 9.16. Macroscopic examples of swollen mucosal folds and the cobblestone pattern in Crohn's disease.

able to locate these granulomas with giant cells so that the transmural character of the infection sometimes can be the decisive factor in establishing the diagnosis. In tuberculosis, the acid-fast rods can be demonstrated and the submucosa should be thinner and not thickened by edema.

The resemblance between the pathoanatomical pattern of Crohn's disease and those of Boeck's disease and tuberculosis has not solved the mystery surrounding the etiology of the former.

Moreover, Crohn's disease resembles tuberculosis in that the radiological abnormalities cannot be differentiated from one another, and the skin reaction to purified tuberculin is positive in both cases. Crohn's disease resembles Boeck's disease in that an erythema nodosum, iritis, or uveitis as well as vague complaints in the joints may appear in both.

Partly because of the identical clinical course of Crohn's disease and rheumatoid arthritis, as well as the therapeutic reaction to corticosteroids and immunosuppressive drugs, it is generally assumed that

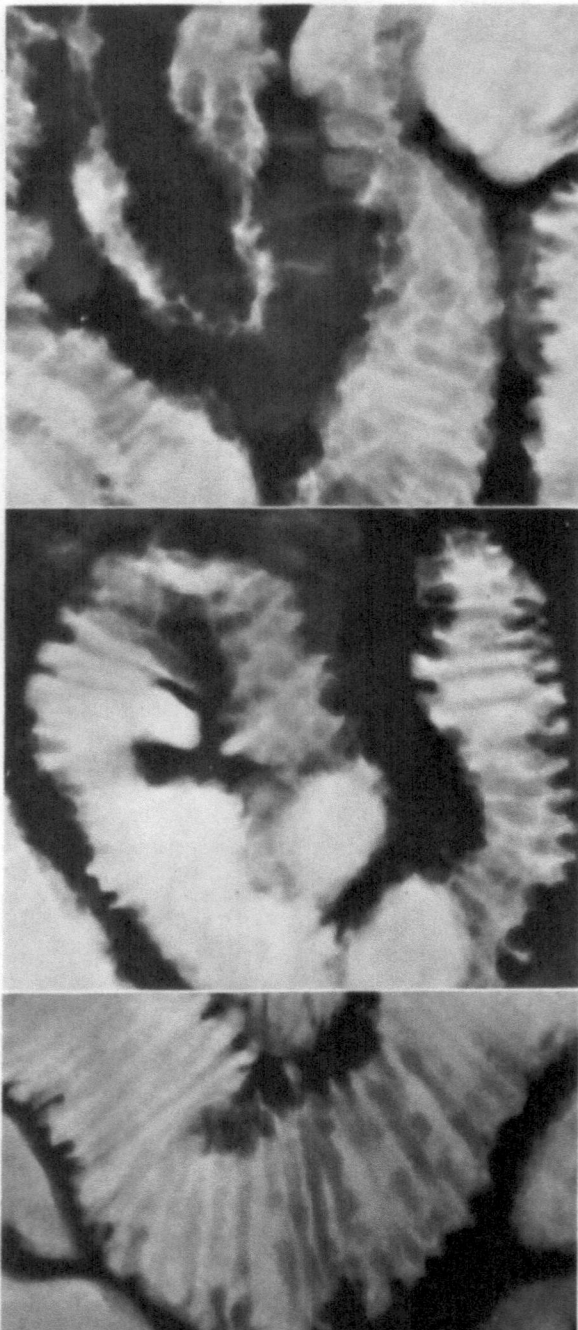

Fig. 9.17. Several examples of the so-called cobblestone pattern in Crohn's disease. The mucosa between the fissure-like ulcerations that penetrate deep into the intestinal wall is swollen like a cushion. Because the mucosal folds are more numerous in the jejunum, the cobblestone relief is more pronounced there than in the ileum.

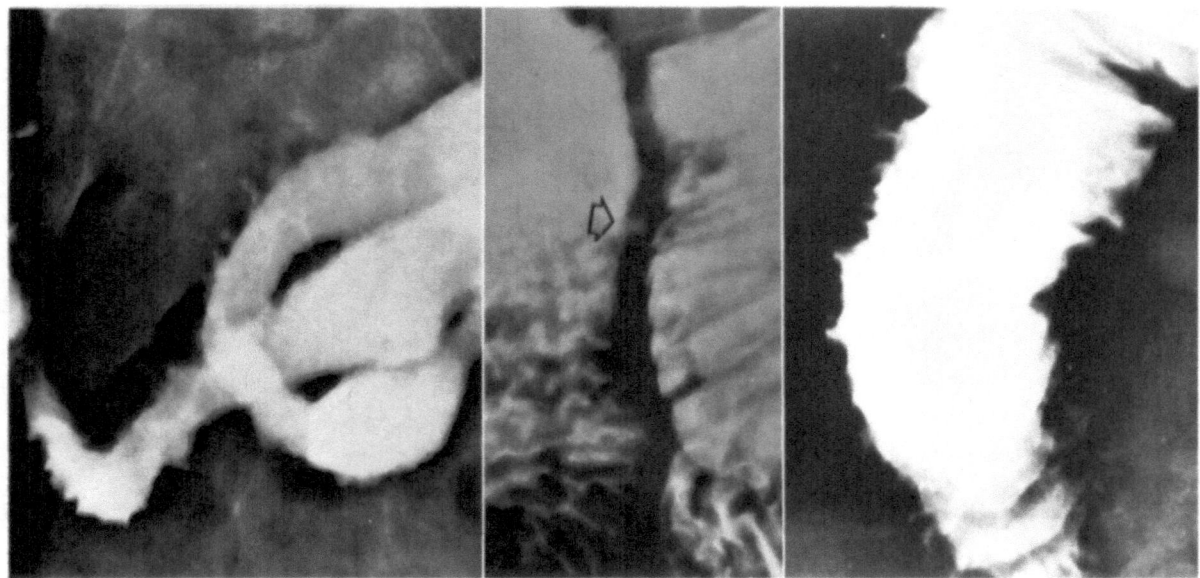

*Fig. 9.18*x. Deep ulcerations in the intestinal wall in Crohn's disease, some clearly mushroom-shaped.

the origin of Crohn's disease is immunobiological.

A history of recurrent skin and joint complaints, in addition to aphthae in the oral cavity and anal fistulas, fissures, or abscesses can be important indications of Crohn's disease. The establishment of this diagnosis at an early stage is often difficult.

The most prominent complaints (abdominal pain, diarrhea, loss of weight, and recurrent high temperatures) are so nonspecific that it can be six months to a year before the diagnosis is definitely established by means of a rectal biopsy or roentgenological examination. In the more advanced stages of Crohn's disease, palpation will reveal a resistance in the abdomen – usually in the lower right quadrant – and fistulas may also be found. Most of the internal fistulas develop between the ileum and another ileal loop, or the sigmoid or the bladder and vagina. In addition to this fistulization, rectovaginal fistulas and, after surgery, fistulas toward the abdominal wall or the surgical scar in particular also occur. In young females frequent painful micturition with pneumaturia can even be the first complaint!

Clinical differentiation from an ulcerative colitis can also be a problem, especially when the radiological abnormalities closely resemble those of the latter. In ulcerative colitis, diarrhea is usually more frequent and is often accompanied by loss of

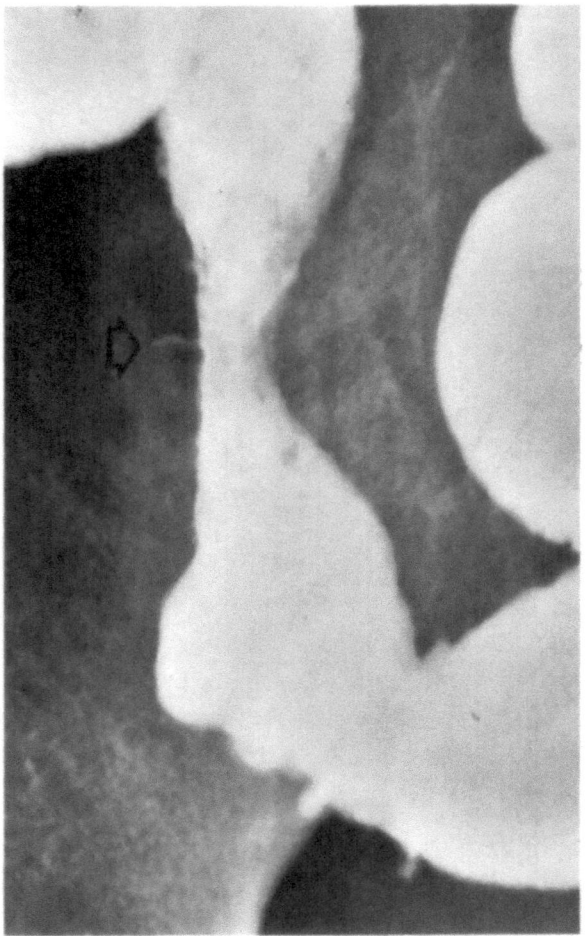

*Fig. 9.18*Y. Probably the beginning of a fistulous tract.

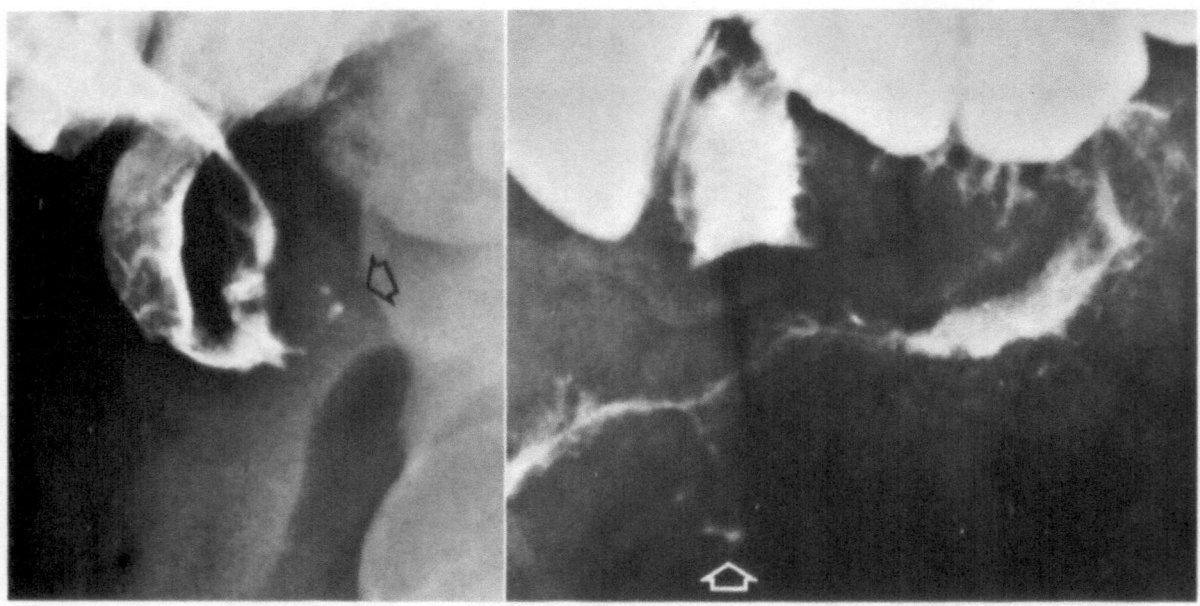

*Fig. 9.18*z. Fistulization toward the bladder.

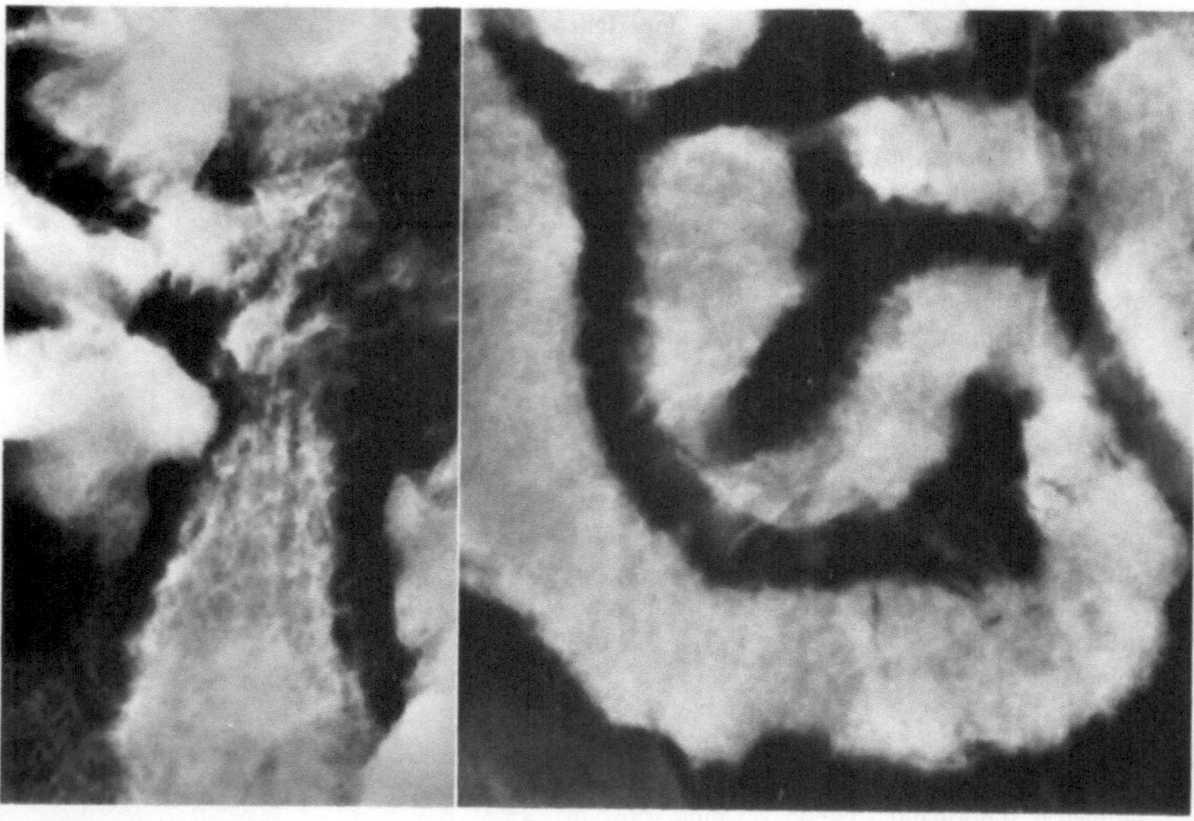

Fig. 9.19. Vague representation of the intestinal wall as a result of the purulent secretion covering the mucosa.

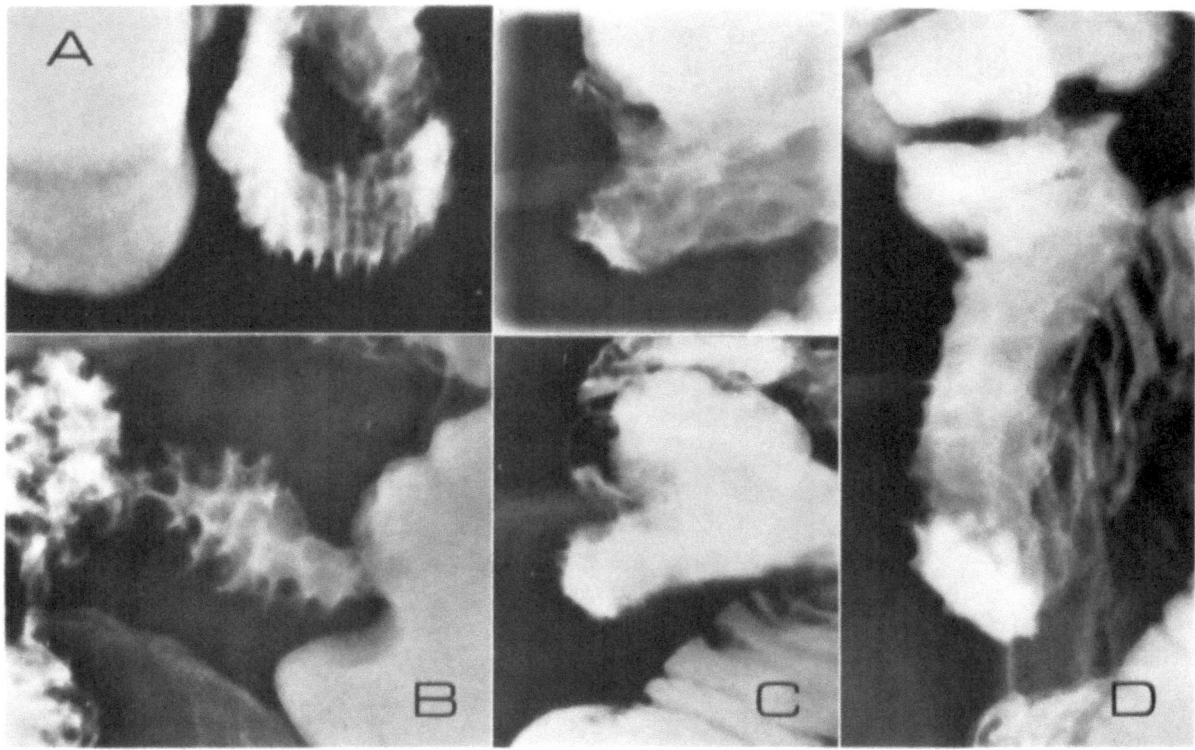

*Fig. 9.20*A–D. Local lymphedema of the intestinal wall, in most cases the earliest demonstrable sign of a beginning Crohn's disease.

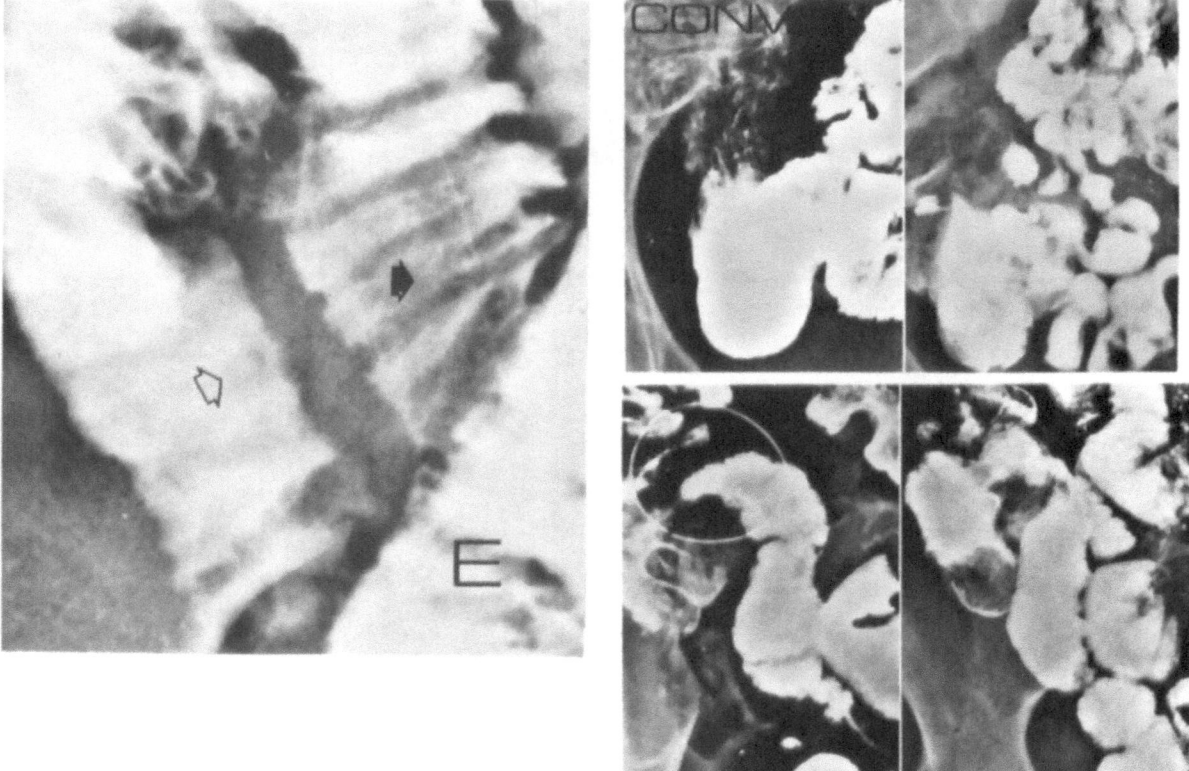

*Fig. 9.20*E. Edematous folds and multiple aphthoid ulcerations in the distal ileum.

*Fig. 9.21*W. See legend on page 212.

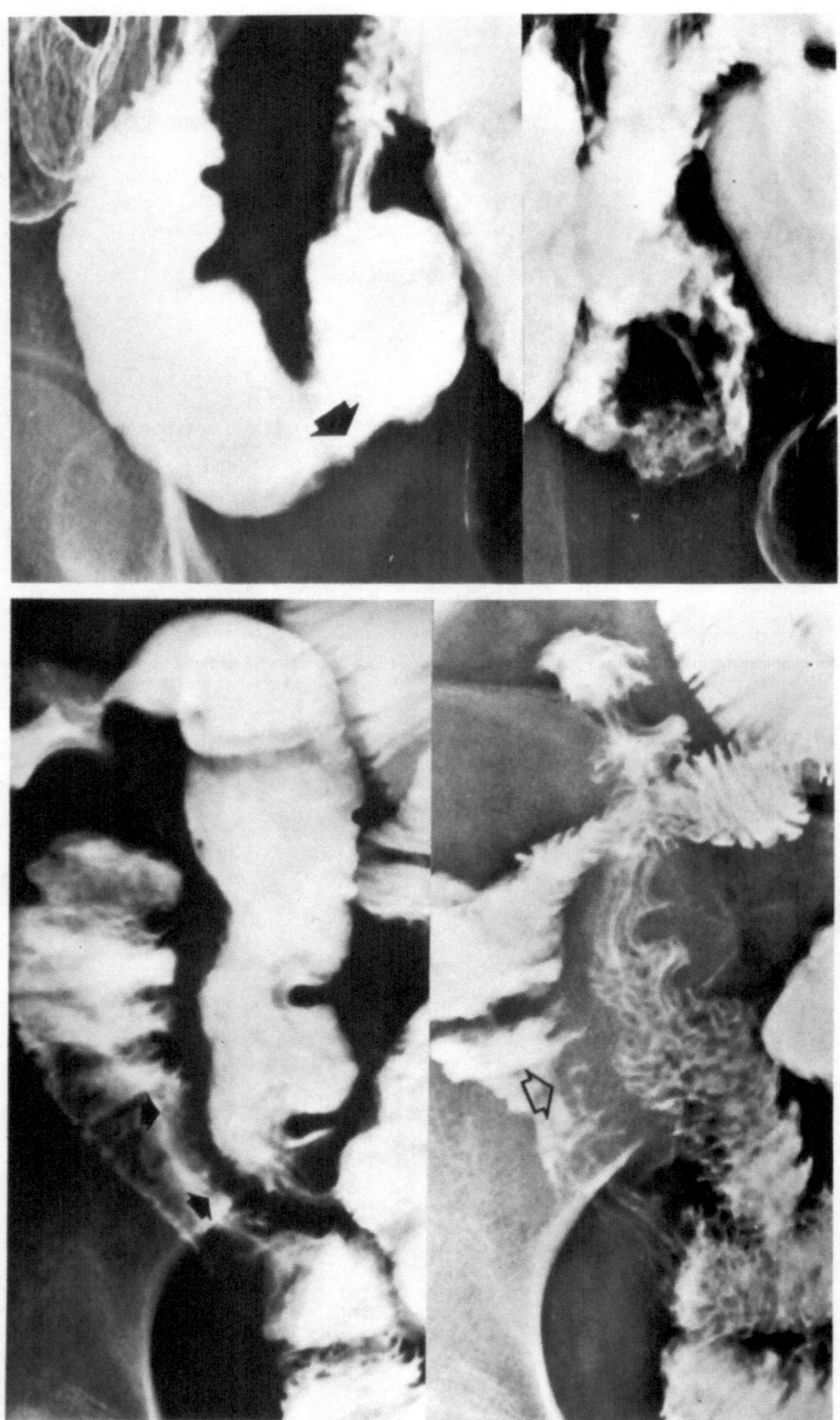

Fig. 9.21. (v) Slight abnormalities of the mucosa without signs of edema in two patients. (w) Several years later an extensive Crohn's disease was demonstrated. In both cases, the conventional examination showed no abnormalities. (see also page 211.)

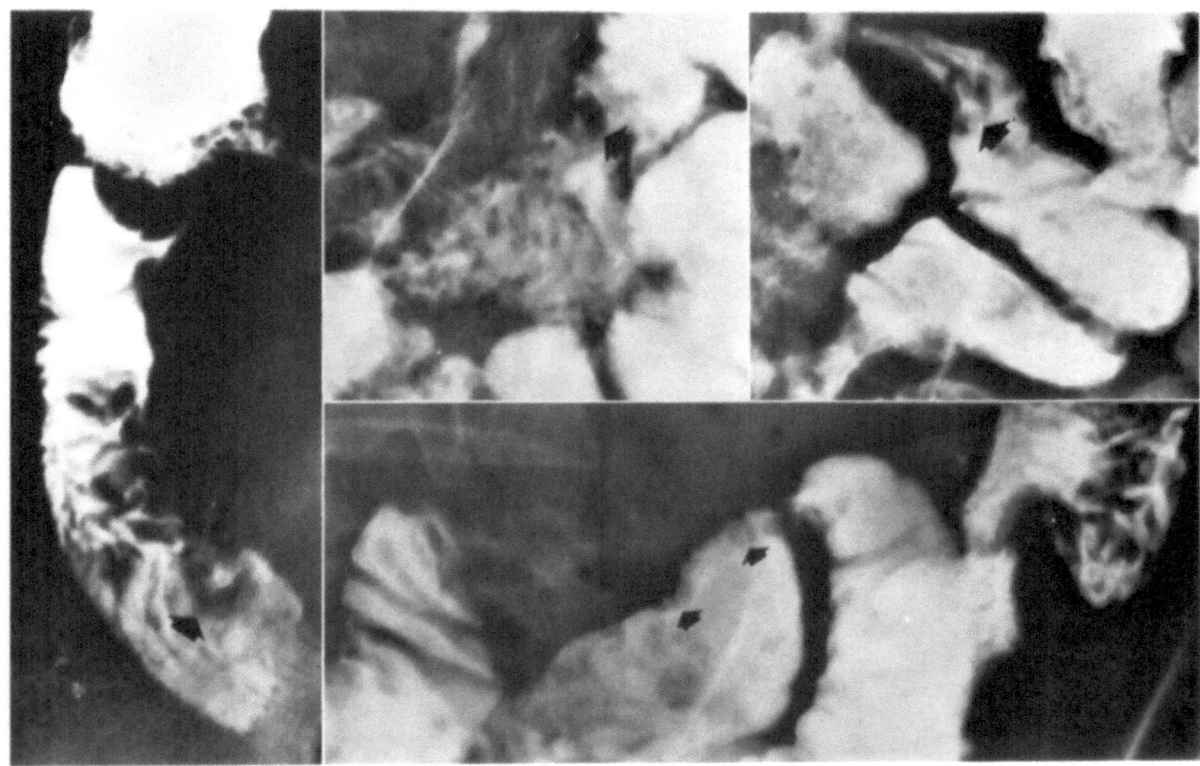

*Fig. 9.22*A. Four cases of granulomas with a central ulcer crater in Crohn's disease. The mucosa in such an area can show highly divergent abnormalities, but also sometimes none at all.

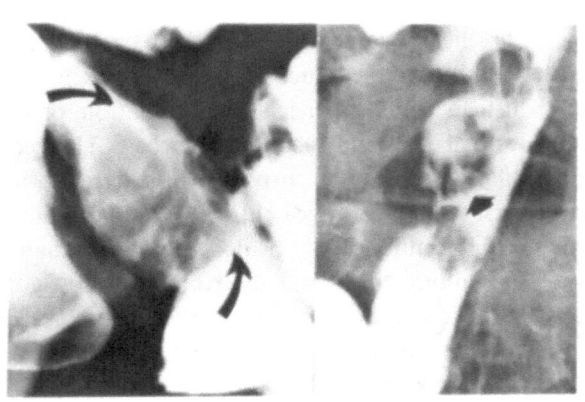

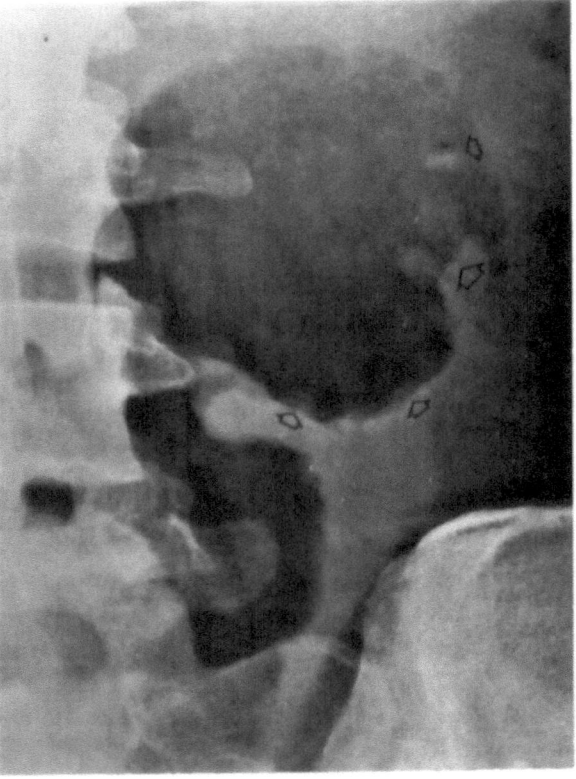

*Fig. 9.22*B. Longitudinal ulcer and aphthoid ulceration in the same patient (Crohn's disease).

Fig. 9.23. Under favorable conditions, solitary granulomas or cobblestones in Crohn's disease are sometimes visible on a survey film of the abdomen.

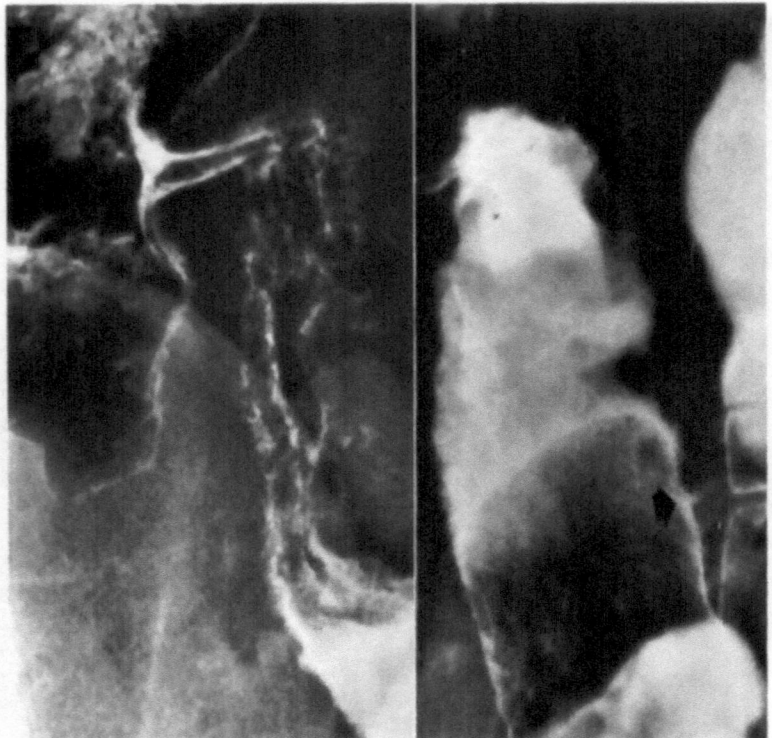

Fig. 9.24. Ulcerative colitis with superficial reflux ileitis in the distal ileum. Rather shriveled cecum and wide-open Bauhin's valve.

blood and mucus. Colic and a palpable resistance are not encountered in ulcerative colitis, nor are there fistulas, fissures, or abscesses around the anus.

It is, however, fortunate that differentiation of a reflux ileitis in ulcerative colitis localized in the cecum from a Crohn's disease is usually obvious on the roentgenograms. In ulcerative colitis, Bauhin's valve is, as a rule, wide open and the cecum is often shriveled. The distal ileum is moderately dilated, and the wall appears smooth over 15–20 cm since ileitis in ulcerative colitis is so superficial that it usually cannot be visualized roentgenologically (fig. 9.24). In Crohn's disease, Bauhin's valve is often somewhat constricted and in many cases there is no shriveling of the cecum (fig. 9.25). In a classic case the irregularly defined mucosal abnormalities that bulge out into the lumen cause the distal ileum also to appear narrower on the x-ray instead of dilated (fig. 9.26). Pronounced shriveling of Bauhin's valve can cause a stenosis that may give rise to an ileus (fig. 9.27).

In contrast, differentiation between a single occurrence of ulcerative colitis with reflux ileitis and a cured Crohn's disease involving the colon and the distal ileum is often exceedingly difficult. This is particularly true if:

1) The patient's history is not really typical or can no longer be determined with accuracy.
2) The entire colon has atrophied and the distal ileum is not longer than about 20 cm.
3) Bauhin's valve is wide open and the cecum has obviously shriveled (fig. 9.28).

A totally atrophied distal ileum and an open Bauhin's valve are also encountered in patients who chronically use laxatives. In these cases, there is an atrophy of the mucosa and the muscular layers instead of a superficial inflammation of the intestinal wall and secondary fibrosis. The cecum is dilated rather than shriveled. Furthermore, in contrast to an ulcerative colitis, these abnormalities are more pronounced in the ileocecal region than in the descending colon and the rectosigmoid (fig. 9.29). Rectoscopic examination of these patients, almost always females, reveals the typical so-called pseudomelanosis aspect.

In exceptional cases, Crohn's disease may appear as

215

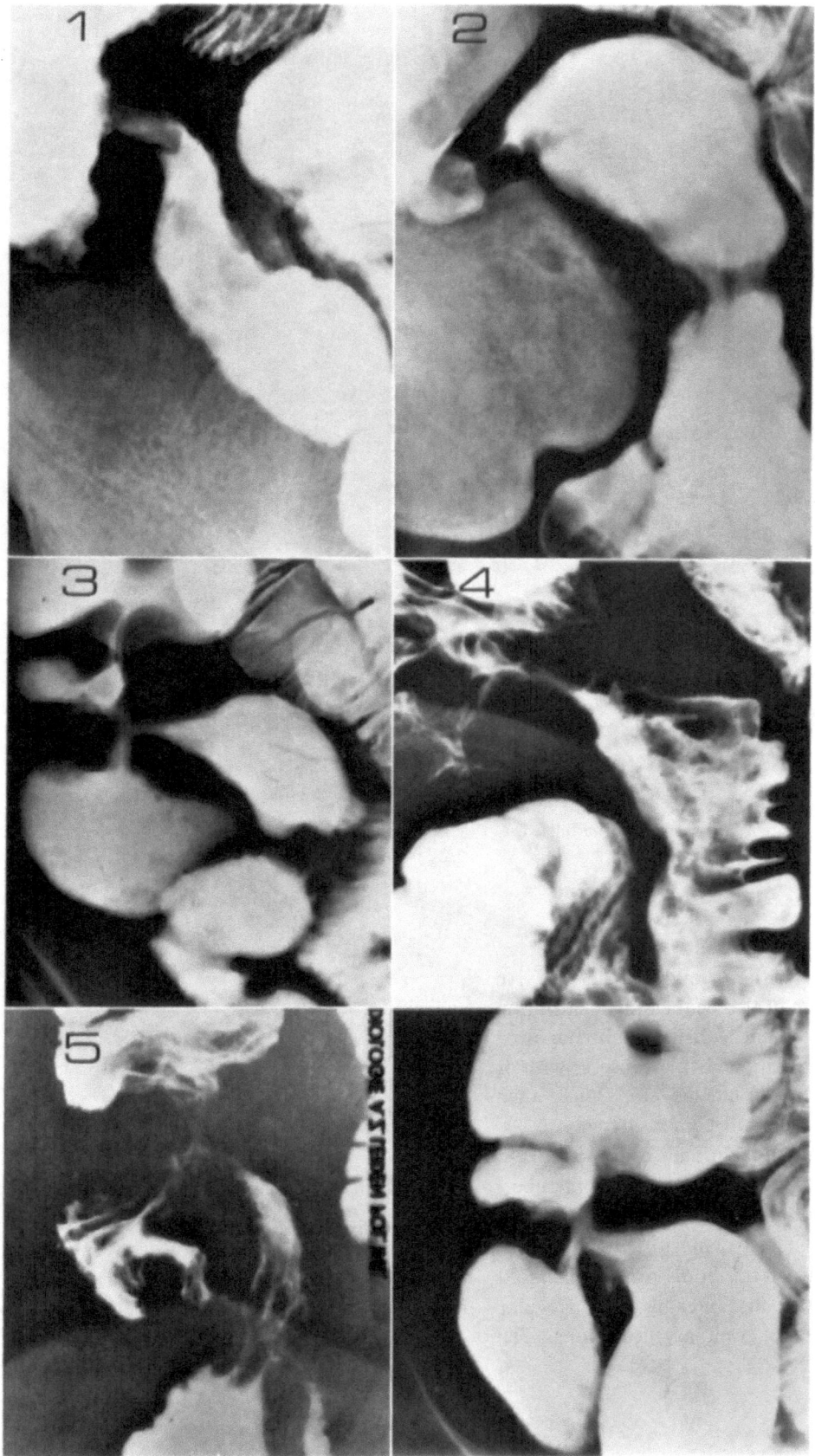

Fig. 9.25. Five cases of Crohn's disease involving Bauhin's valve and the ileocecal region. More pronounced mucosal abnormalities in the distal ileum and frequently an obvious constriction in the region of Bauhin's valve. Shriveling of the cecum depends upon the stage and the spread of the disease.

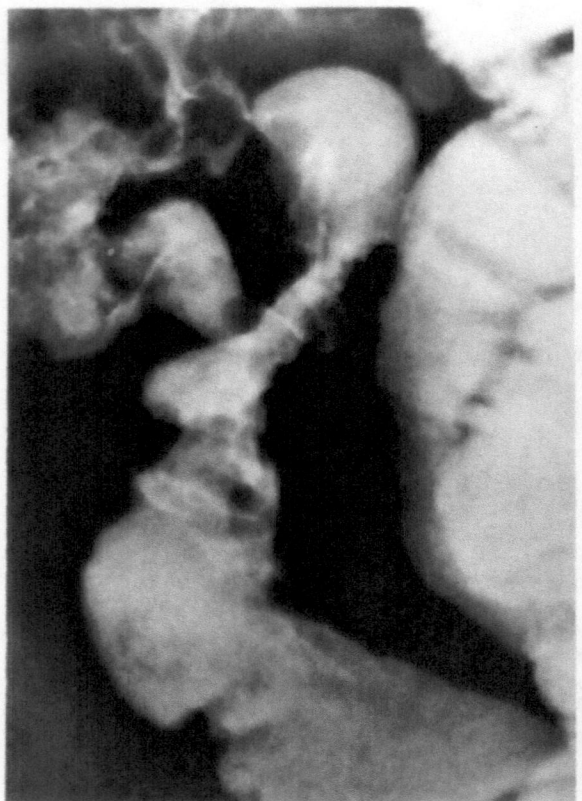

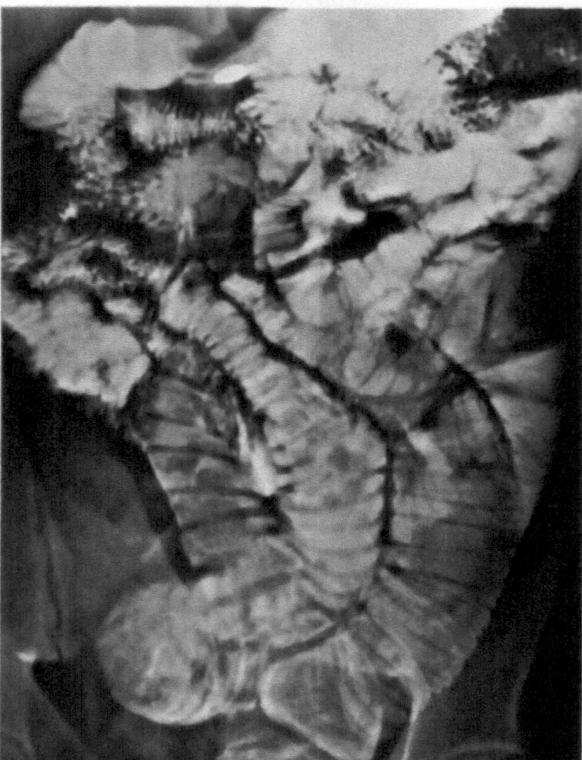

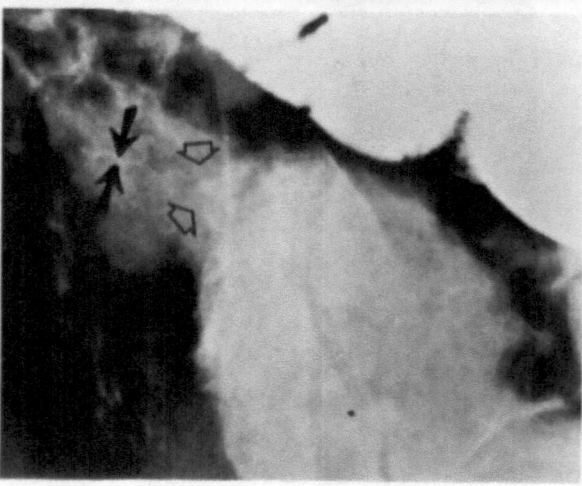

Fig. 9.26. Since the inflammatory process penetrates into all layers of the wall deeper in Crohn's disease than in ulcerative colitis, the distal ileum is often narrower instead of dilated.

an 'acute abdomen' without muscular defense. An inflamed appendix may also be the only localization of the – at the moment – usually unrecognized Crohn's disease. If an appendicular abscess with or without fistulization should develop later, then Crohn's disease should still be considered.

Roentgenologically it is difficult or impossible to differentiate Crohn's disease not only from tuberculosis (fig. 9.30) but also from ischemic abnormalities and eosinophilic gastroenteritis. Both of these diseases may be characterized only by a swollen fold relief in the early stage and later by more irregular changes in the wall as well as ulcerations. The

Fig. 9.27. Marked shriveling of Bauhin's valve can cause an ileus.

totally different history, however, indicates the diagnosis in most cases; in addition there is always marked eosinophilia in the blood in cases of eosinophilic infiltration.

become colic-like and borborygmus may become pronounced. In exceptional cases the disease can have such a mild course during the active phase that these symptoms, suggesting obstruction, may be the patient's first complaint.

Especially if the inflammatory process was fairly superficial, the tendency to form strictures will be less, and fibrous plaques will be seen at the sites of the destroyed mucosa. The mucosal folds that have remained intact are visible inbetween the plaques as round, oval, or elongated ridges (fig. 9.33, page 224).

The differentiation between skip lesions that have become fibrotic and other ulcers in the small bowel that have healed with shriveling and formed stenoses can cause difficulty.

However, the history of a patient with celiac disease or ulcers due to ischemia differs completely from that of a patient with Crohn's disease. Particularly when the stenosis is located in the distal ileum, the differentiation between postischemia and a cured Crohn's disease can be impossible. In both diseases, an asymmetric shriveling produces the same 'Shell sign' (figs. 9.34 and 9.35).

Also a very marked atrophy of the mucosa in the ileocecal region, sometimes fairly irregular in nature with strictures of various sizes, can be due to an ischemia of the intestinal wall (fig. 9.36) and mimic Crohn's disease (cf. fig. 9.28). Therefore it is imperative to obtain relevant information concerning the history of the patient.

Crohn's strictures in the jejunum cannot always be differentiated from those caused by corrosion or localized vasculitis after ingestion of enteric-coated tablets containing potassium or other drugs. This is in particular the case if the ulcers are short, generally circular, and the rest of the jejunal mucosal relief appears to be completely intact (fig. 9.37). When there is a lymphosarcoma stricture, considerable diagnostic evidence is also provided by the accompanying signs. In this disease, we are often confronted with extensive and disordered mucosal destruction. Furthermore, there are several clearly defined areas in which the loops of the intestine are separated from one another. Also multiple com-

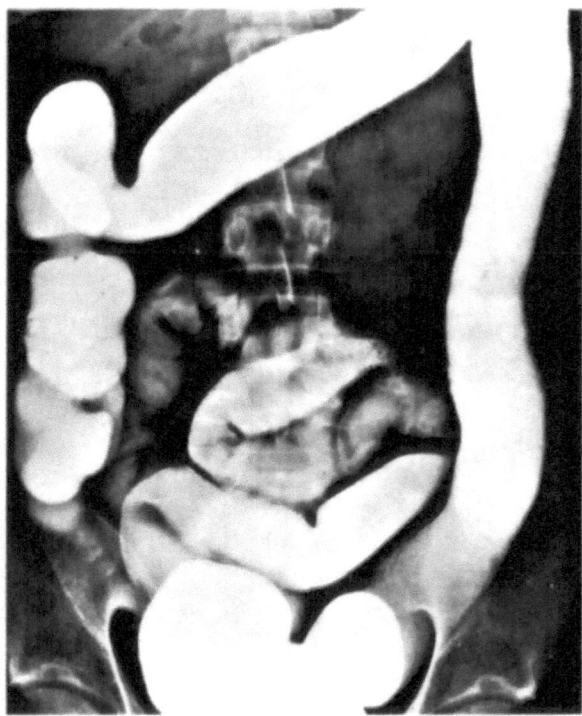

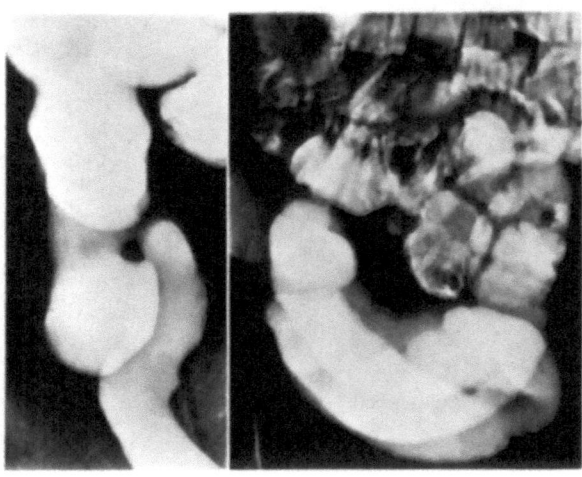

Fig. 9.28. Remission of Crohn's disease of the colon and the last 50–60 cm of the ileum. Here the cecum has shriveled and Bauhin's valve is wide open. The only complaint was a gradually increasing diarrhea of seven years' duration.

As we have already seen, ulcerations in Crohn's disease heal with pronounced fibrosis and later also shriveling (fig. 9.31). As a result of the stenoses that may then develop (fig. 9.32), abdominal pain can

218

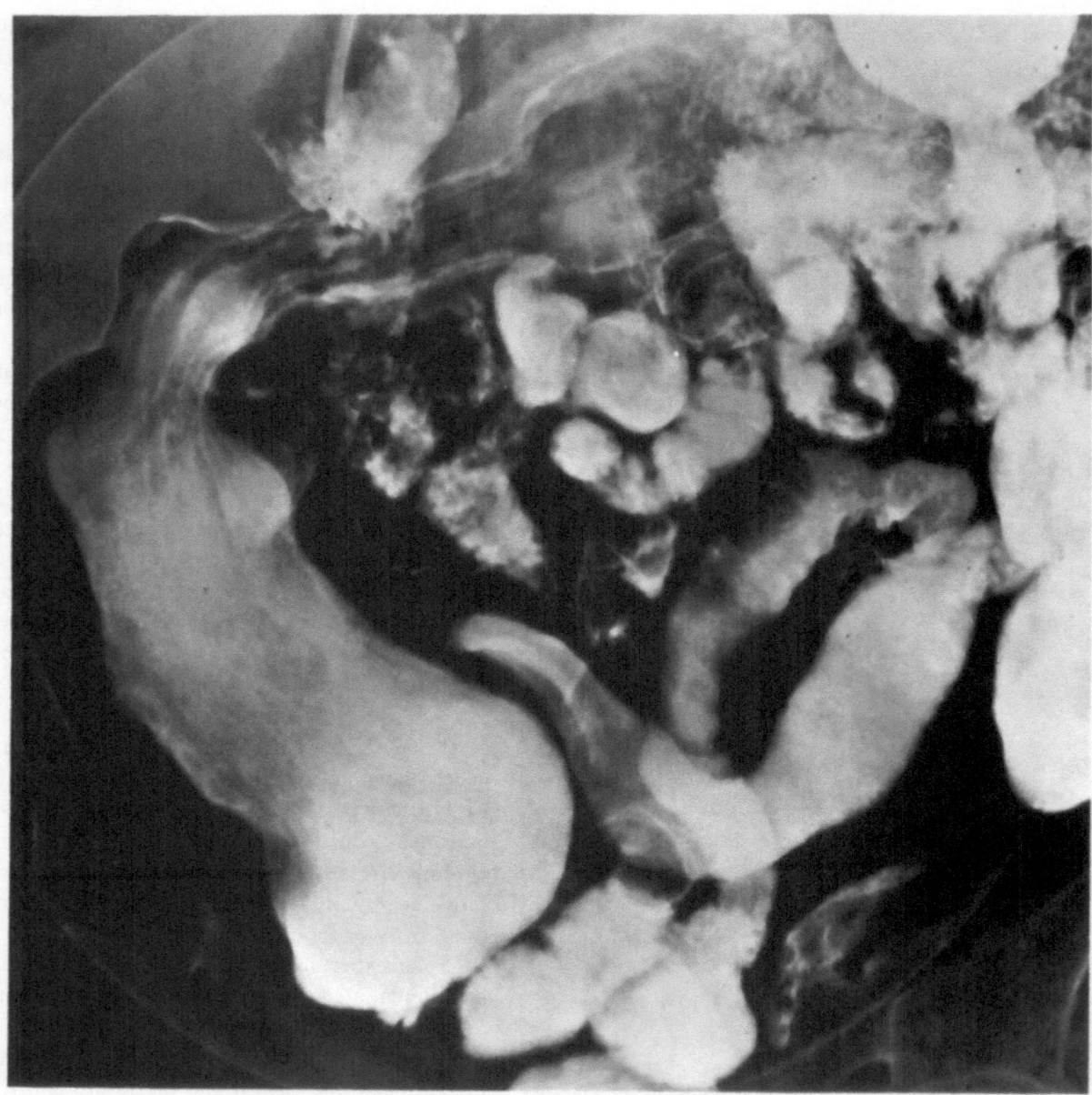

Fig. 9.29. Atrophy of the mucosa in the colon and the distal ileum as a result of the chronic use of laxatives. In such cases the cecum is often dilated instead of narrower.

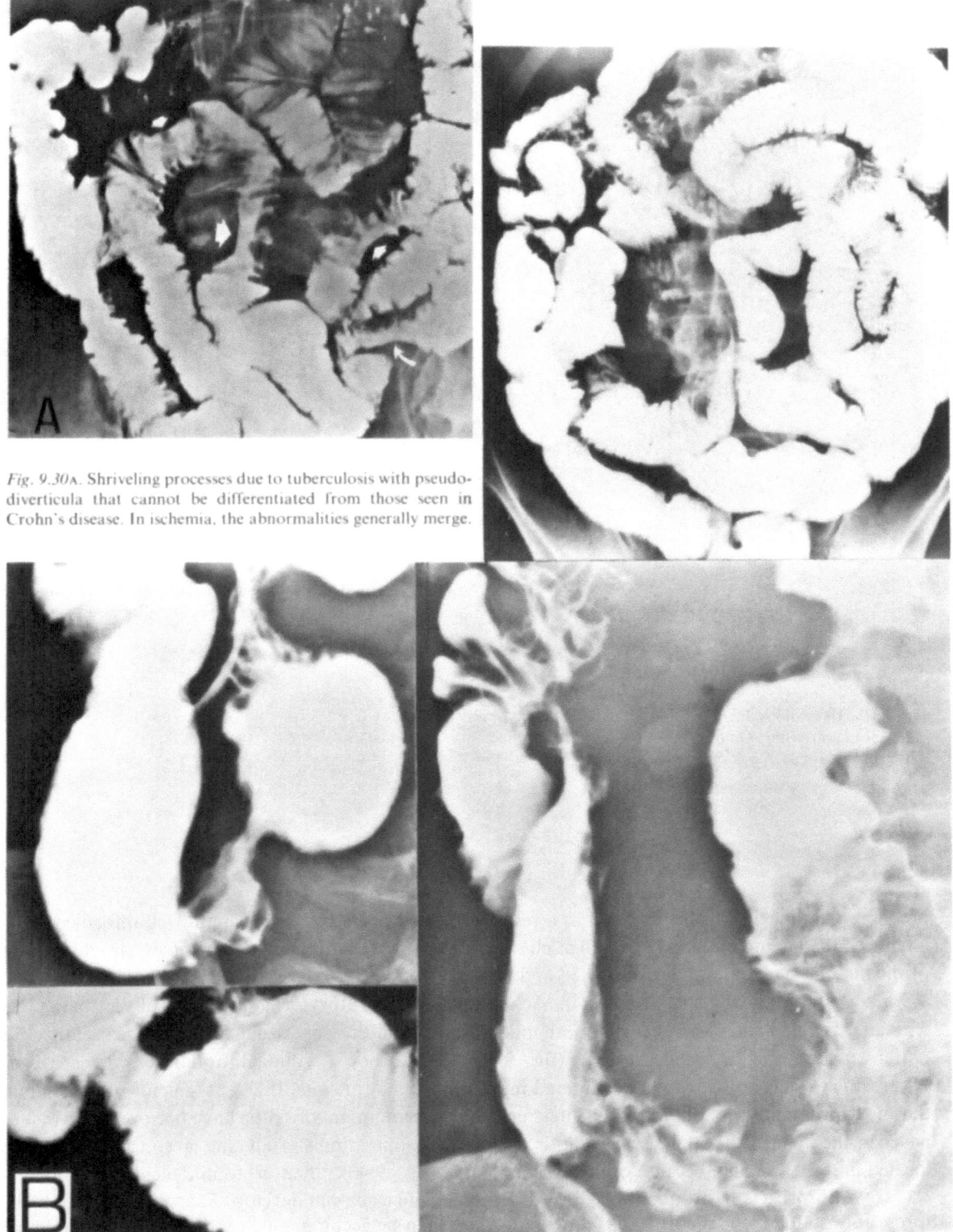

*Fig. 9.30*A. Shriveling processes due to tuberculosis with pseudo-diverticula that cannot be differentiated from those seen in Crohn's disease. In ischemia, the abnormalities generally merge.

*Fig. 9.30*B. These x-rays, showing multiple stenoses with prestenotic dilatations, were taken after an intestinal resection as a result of a traffic accident. It appeared, however, that the stenoses were not due to vascular abnormalities, but to tuberculosis.

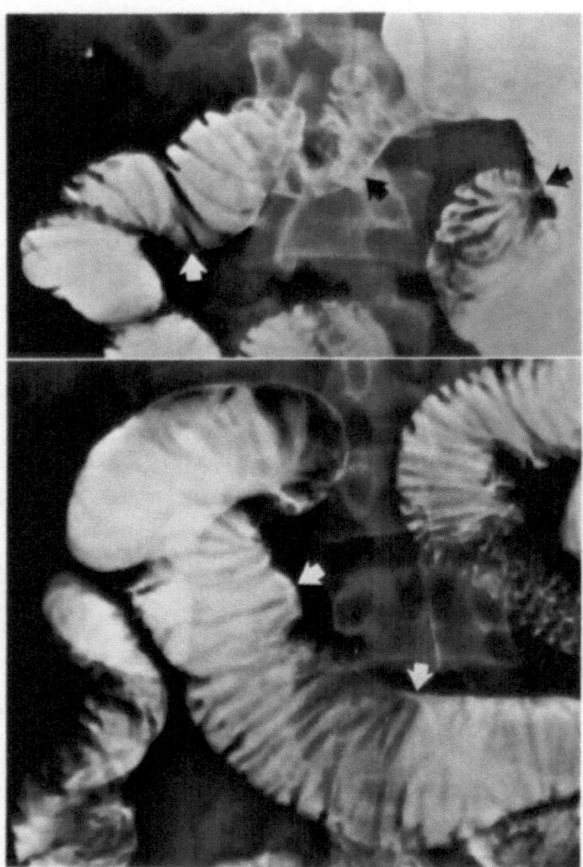

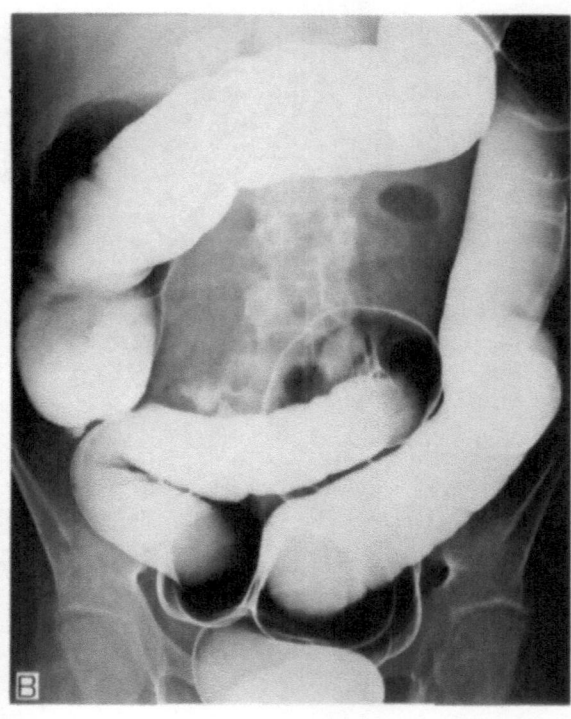

*Fig. 9.31*ʙ. Ileocolic Crohn's disease with smooth intestinal wall and loss of haustration in the colon. (See also page 221.)

*Fig. 9.31*ᴀ. Ulcerations due to Crohn's disease that have healed with fibrotic shriveling. On one side of the intestine the mucosal pattern has disappeared completely.

pression phenomena can be observed as a result of advanced thickening of the wall as well as clustering of the mesenteric lymph nodes (figs. 9.38 and 8.20).

Finally, strictures of a spastic origin in a jejunum with an atrophied and more or less smooth mucosal pattern may occur in celiac disease (fig. 9.39). Ulcers due to celiac disease are encountered in only the most proximal part of the small intestine and never in the ileum. Although a carcinoid is usually located in the ileum and, because of the concomitant excessive fibrosis, is easily identified by the strictures and sudden changes in the course of the intestine (so-called 'kinking'), these lesions sometimes occur as scattered strictures that cannot be distinguished from skip lesions or tumors (fig.

8.40ʟ). If, however, we are well informed as to the patient's complaints, diagnosis should not prove difficult.

Laboratory examination of a patient with Crohn's disease usually reveals a markedly elevated erythrocyte sedimentation rate with an iron deficiency anemia. If large segments of the jejunum or ileum are involved or have been resected in a series of operations producing a so-called short bowel (fig. 9.40), then a folinic acid or vitamin B_{12} deficiency can develop. Exacerbation of the disease can be accompanied by pronounced protein loss in the intestine, and as a result of a hypoalbuminemia, edema of the ankles will be seen. There have been cases in which these symptoms were the first in-

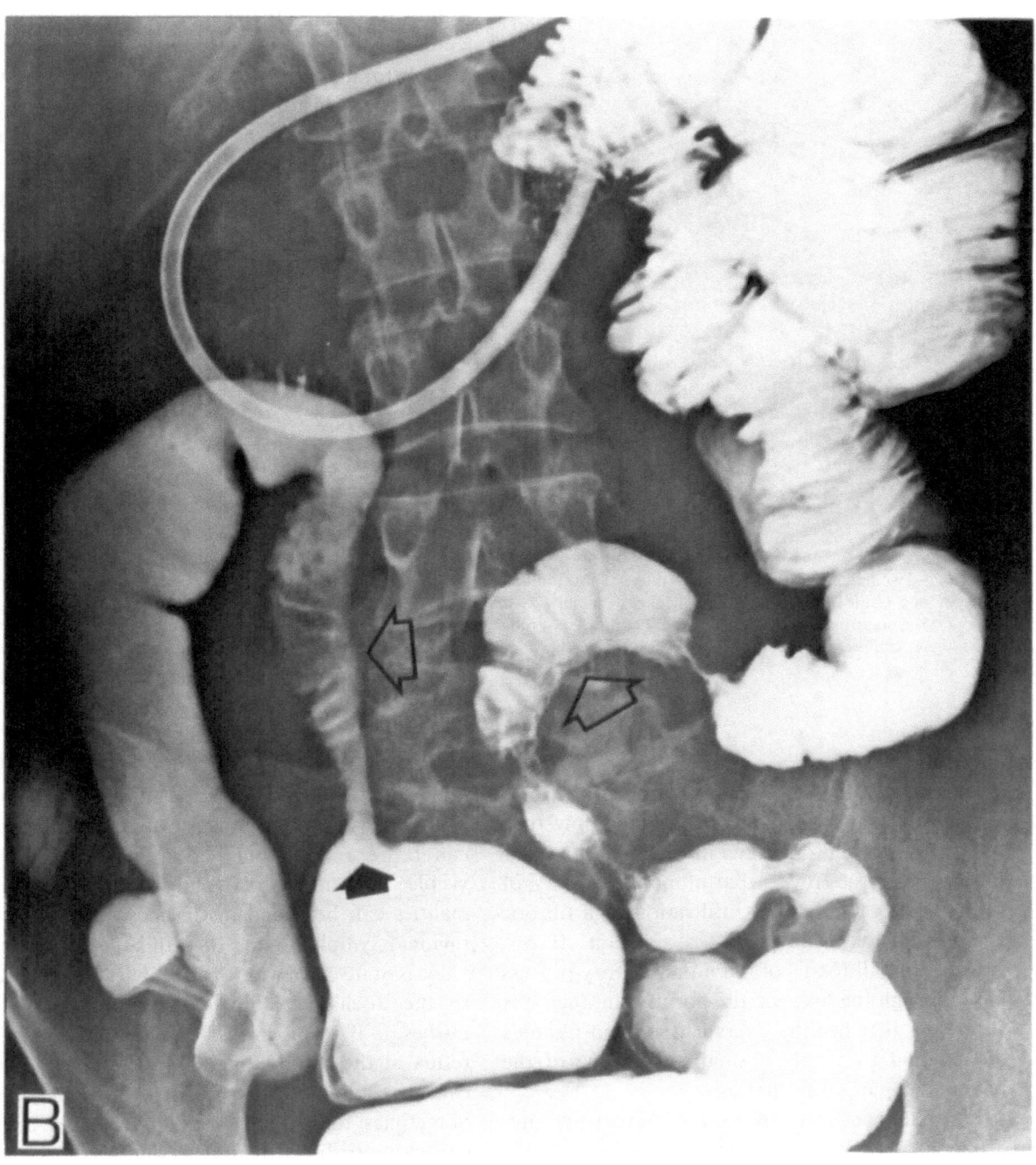

*Fig. 9.31*B. There are shriveled longitudinal ulcers (open arrows) in the ileum and a clear prestenotic dilatation (solid arrow). Past history includes several resection. (See also page 220.)

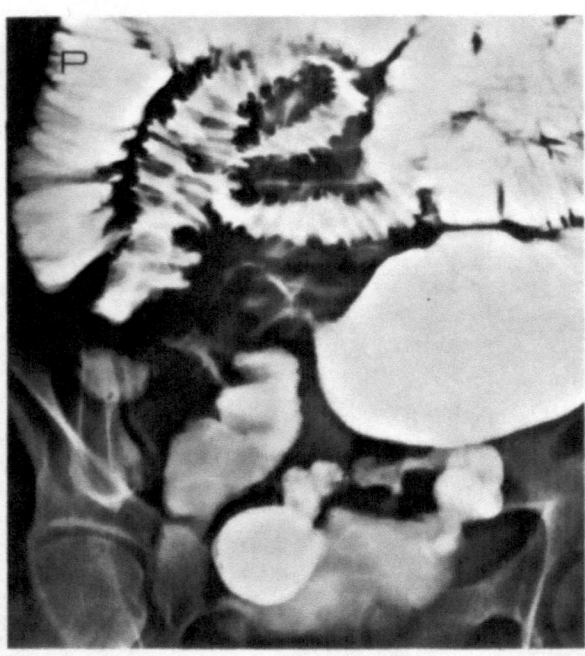

*Fig. 9.32*P. Two patients (PQ) with Crohn's disease show multiple stenoses as a result of ulcers that have healed with fibrosis. In patient Q the abnormalities could be seen only on the spot films taken under compression! (See also page 223.)

dication of Crohn's disease or sometimes a chronic lymphoreticular malignancy in the small intestine.

Liver function is disturbed in 25% of the patients but renal biopsies reveal that in more than 50% of the patients there is fatty infiltration or a fibrotic and lymphocytic inflammatory reaction. If one realizes that all toxins of the inflammatory process pass through the liver via the portal vein, then it is surprising that healthy livers can exist in Crohn's disease and that only a small percentage of the patients acquire liver cirrhosis.

In about one out of every 25 patients, hydronephrosis will develop later as a result of fibrosis in the retroperitoneal region or the minor pelvis.

That one out of every 12 patients with Crohn's disease ultimately dies as either a direct or an indirect result of this disease must be attributed not only to the above-mentioned complications but also

to the increased risk of malignancy. As in ulcerative colitis, there is a greater chance that an adenocarcinoma will develop if a patient has had Crohn's disease for more than 15 years. If a new patient with a fairly short history shows a mucosal pattern with either multiple stenoses or obliterated mucosa suggestive of a tumor, then of course a reticulosis or a lymphosarcoma, respectively, should be considered first and not a malignancy in conjunction with Crohn's disease. If these abnormalities are found in the ileocecal region, then a carcinoma of the cecum is also possible.

3. Reflux ileitis

In 10%–20% of the cases of ulcerative colitis involving the cecum, a so-called reflux ileitis of the most distal 10 or 20 cm of the ileum will occur. In most cases this ileitis can be distinguished quite easily in several respects from the ileitis in Crohn's disease. It is neither hypertrophic nor granulomatous; furthermore, the wall is not thickened but is instead very thin. The mucous membrane is smooth and there are only small superficial ulcers and abscesses in the crypts of Lieberkühn that never lead to the formation of fistulous tracts (fig. 9.41). On the films, an ileum without folds appears rather tube-like. The transition to the mucosa of the normal ileum can be recognized only because folds are again visible. In contrast to Crohn's disease, no abnormalities can be found in the mesentery or in the regional lymph nodes. In reflux ileitis, Bauhin's valve is quite often wide open and lies perpendicular to the diseased cecum. Every time the patient pushes as if to move his bowels, there is marked reflux of the colon contents into the distal ileum, causing radiolucencies on the contrast column. Sometimes these dingy-looking lucencies are incorrectly attributed to mucus and secretion products due to the ileitis. They therefore appear to be more serious than they are. It is necessary to force the colon contents out of the ileum by increasing the amount of contrast medium administered. In this manner the ileum is flushed clean so

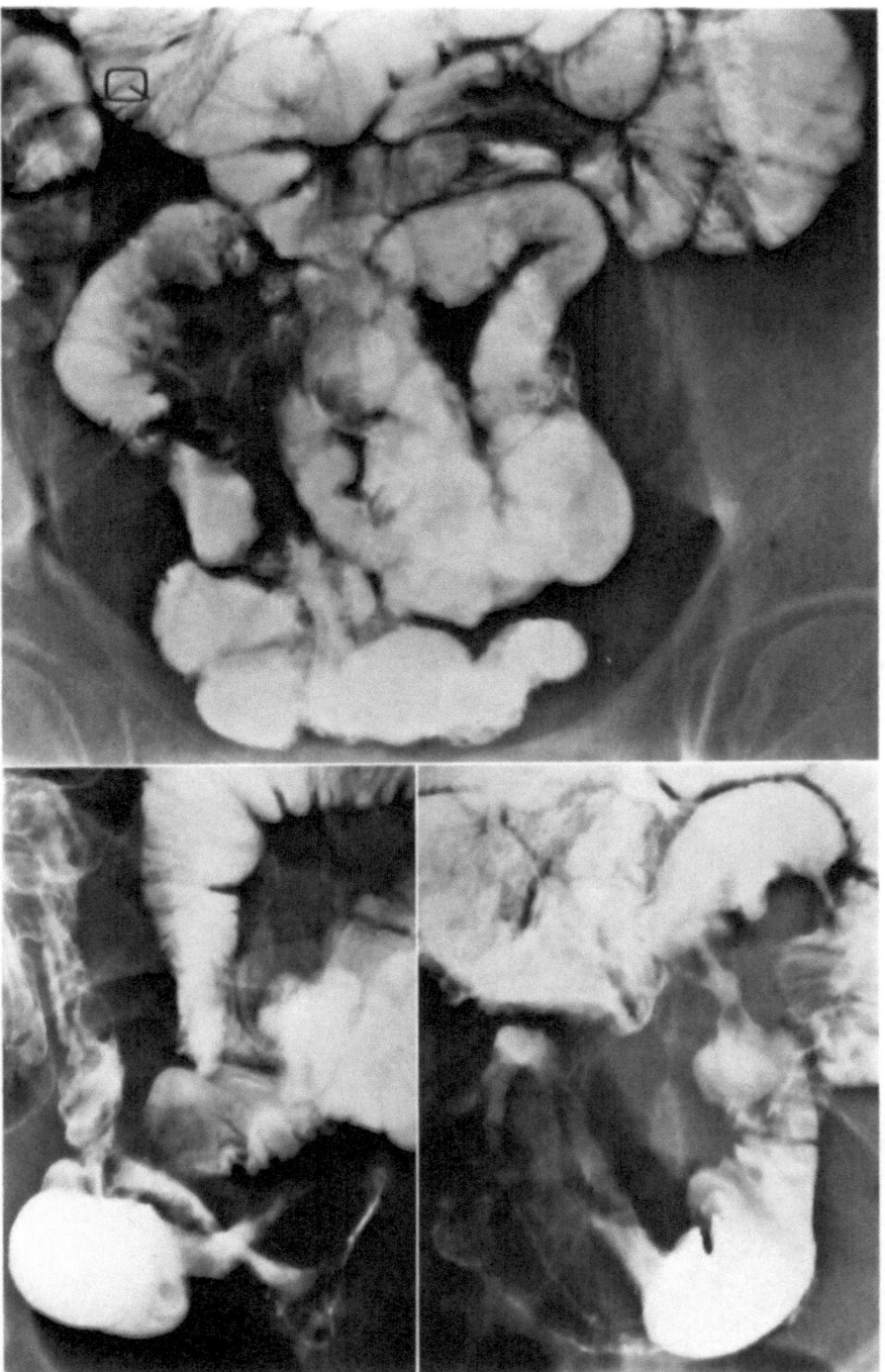

*Fig. 9.32*Q. Two patients (PQ) with Crohn's disease show multiple stenoses as a result of ulcers that have healed with fibrosis. In patient Q the abnormalities could be seen only on the spot films taken under compression! (See also page 222.)

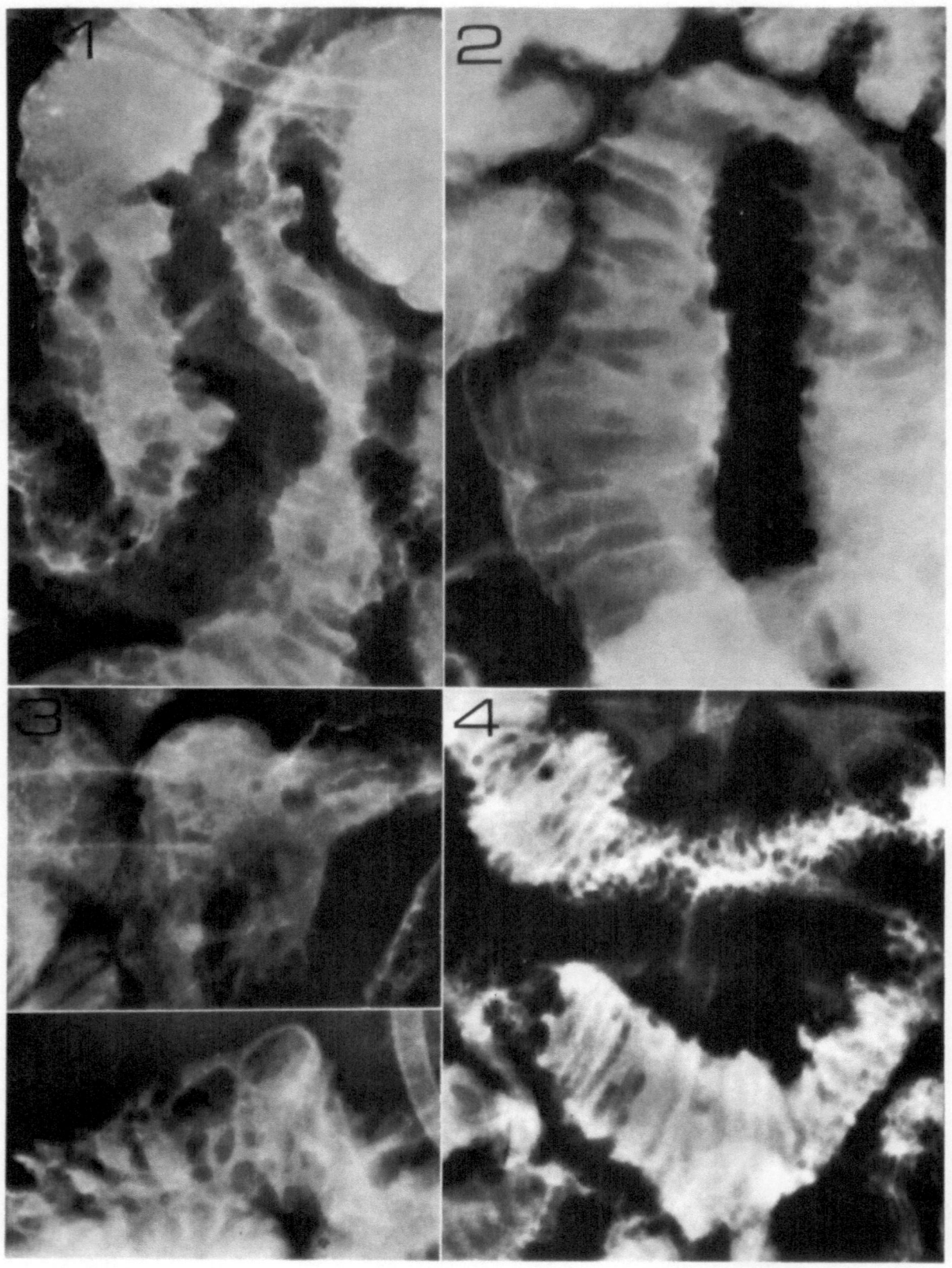

Fig. 9.33. Spot films of four patients with fibrotic plaques that have developed as a result of local destruction of the mucosa. The remaining intact mucosal folds can be seen as round, oval, or elongated rather broad indentations in the barium column.

Fig. 9.34. Emblem of the Shell Oil Company.

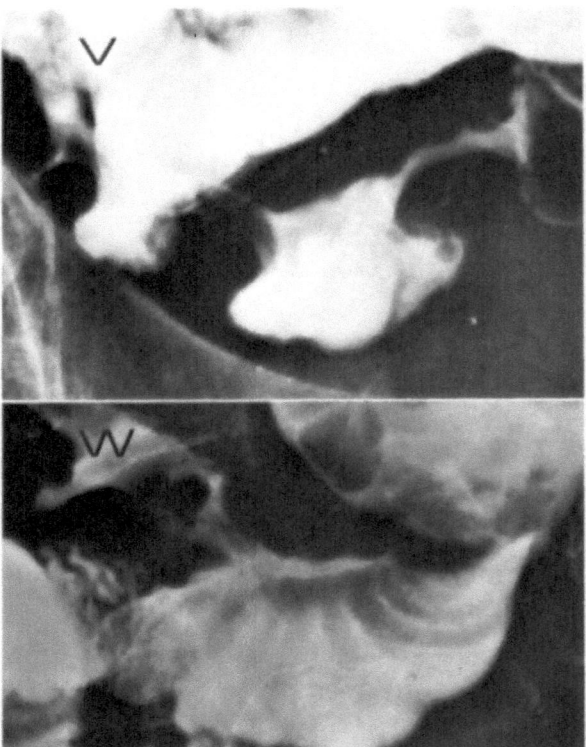

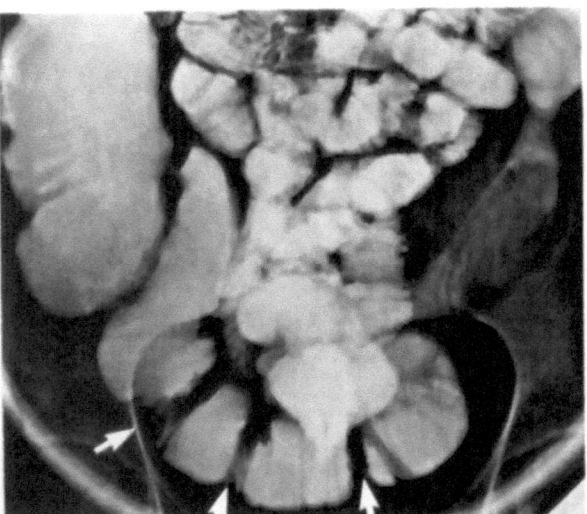

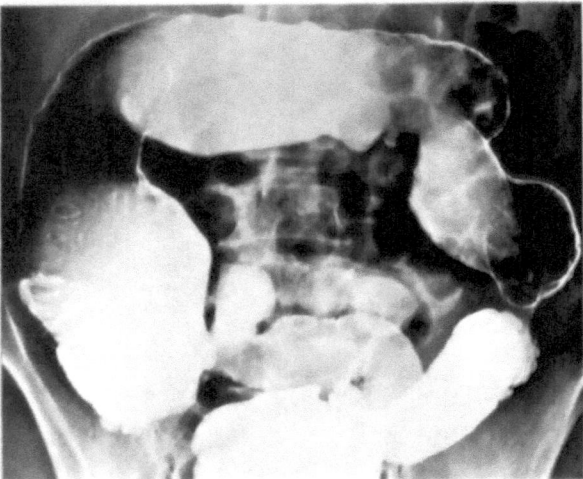

Fig. 9.36 Two cases of so-called ischemic colitis. In one of the patients, the strictures were constantly visible in the distal ileum.

Fig. 9.35. Asymmetric shriveling of ulcerations in the intestinal wall causes the mucosal folds to assume a radial course directed toward the ulcer; this pattern closely resembles the emblem of the Shell Oil Company (the Shell sign). Differentiation between old ulcers in Crohn's disease, ischemia, and tuberculosis is impossible: (v) ischemia; (w) Crohn's disease after 14 years of remission.

226

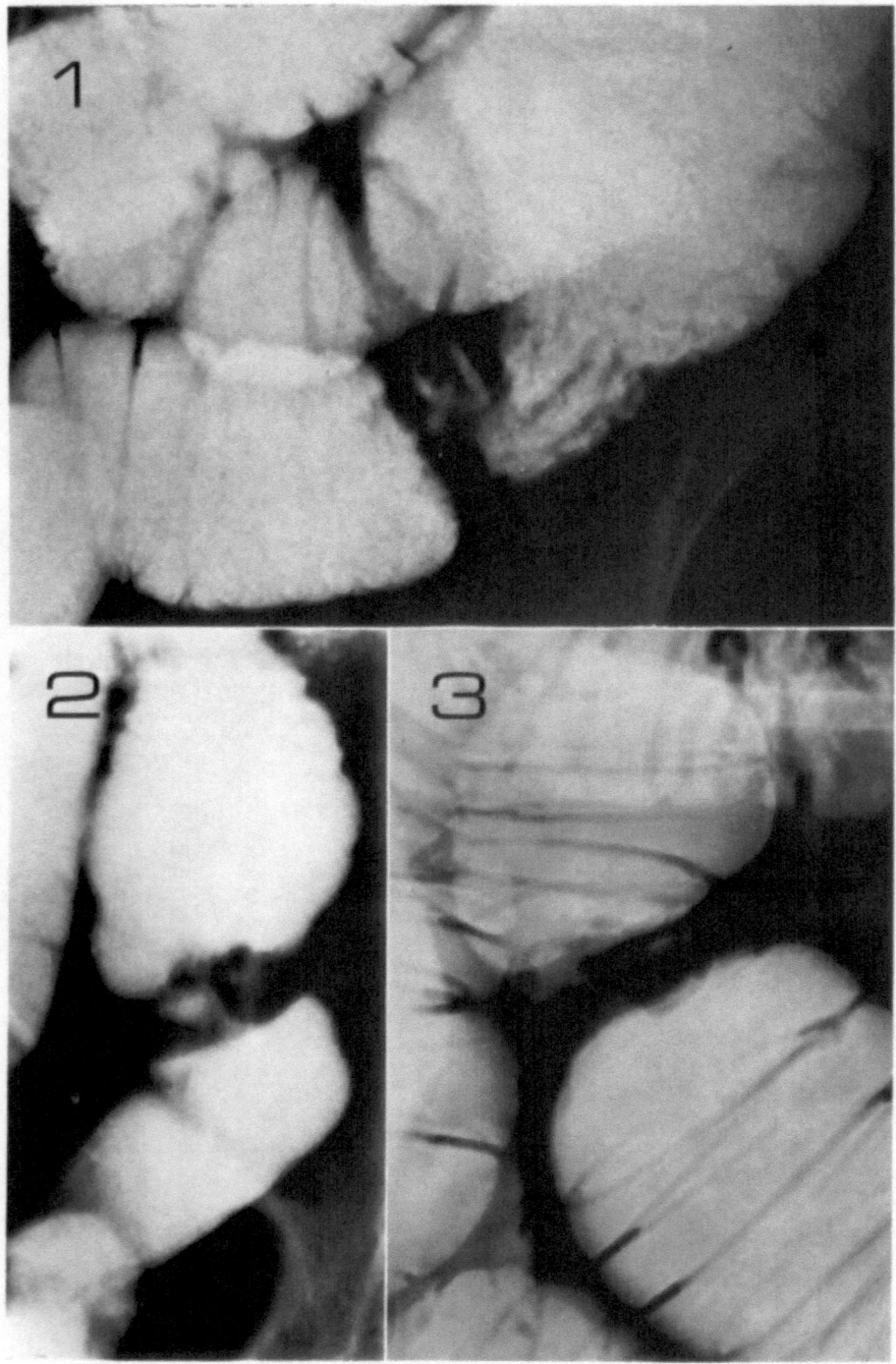

*Fig. 9.37*A. Three patients with short constricting ulcerations of aspecific origin in the small intestine. For patients 1 and 3, ingestion of enteric-coated KCl tablets could be established from the history.

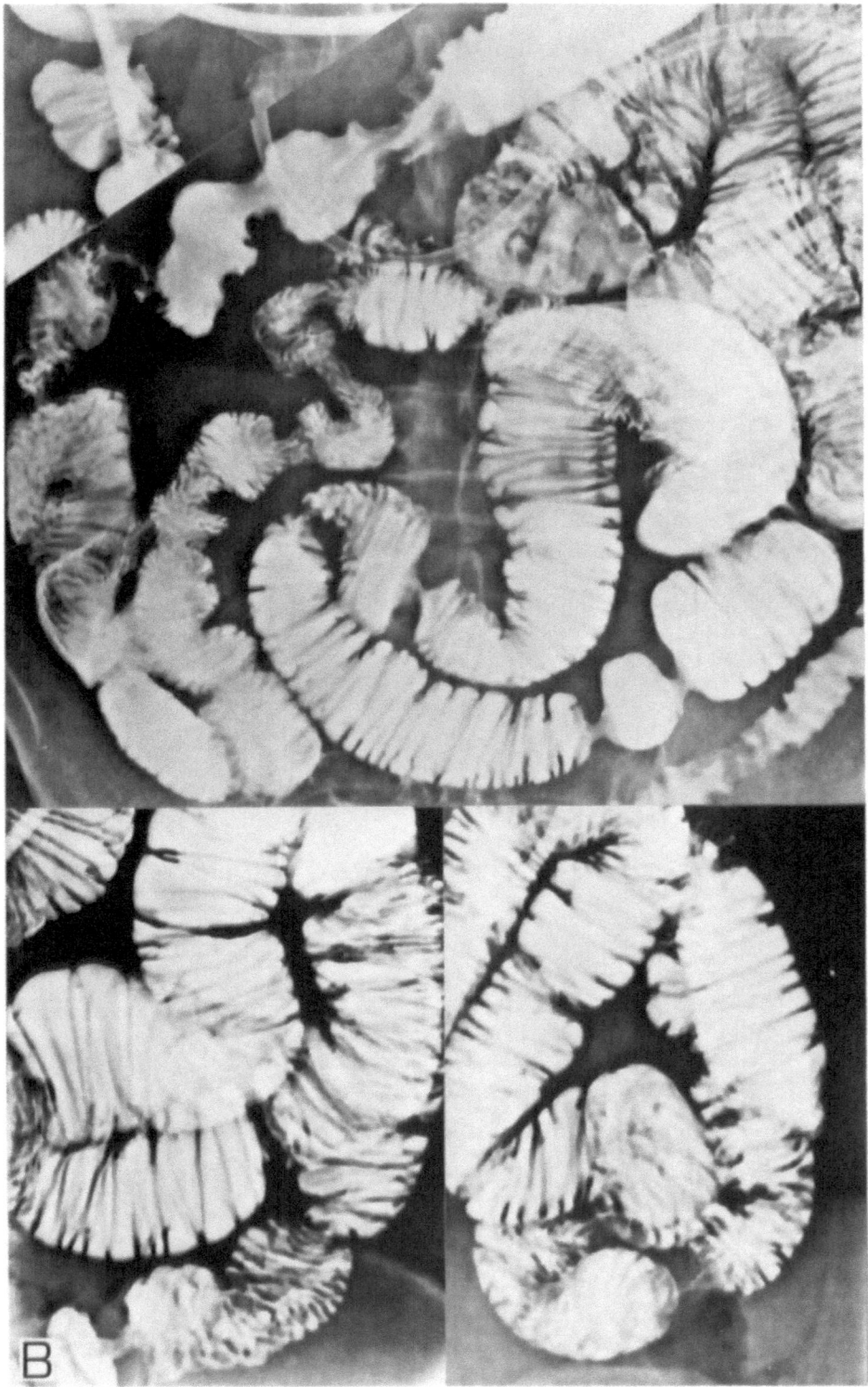

*Fig. 9.37*B. Multiple very short strictures, mainly in the duodenum and jejunum, without further abnormalities of the mucosa. Although quite unusual in Crohn's disease, pathological examination indicated that these abnormalities could indeed be attributed to this illness.

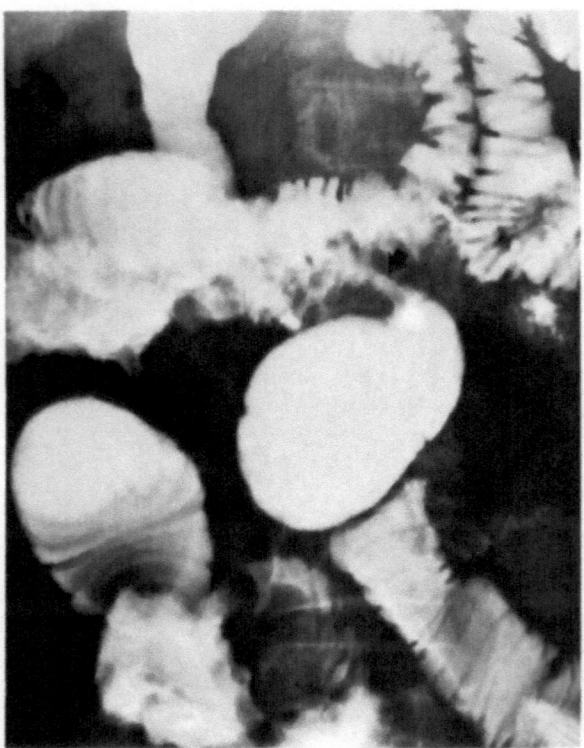

Fig. 9.38. Stenosis (arrow) in the small intestine as a result of lymphosarcoma resembles a skip lesion. However, erratically enlarged spaces between the intestinal loops, compression phenomena, and areas of extensive mucosal destruction can also be seen.

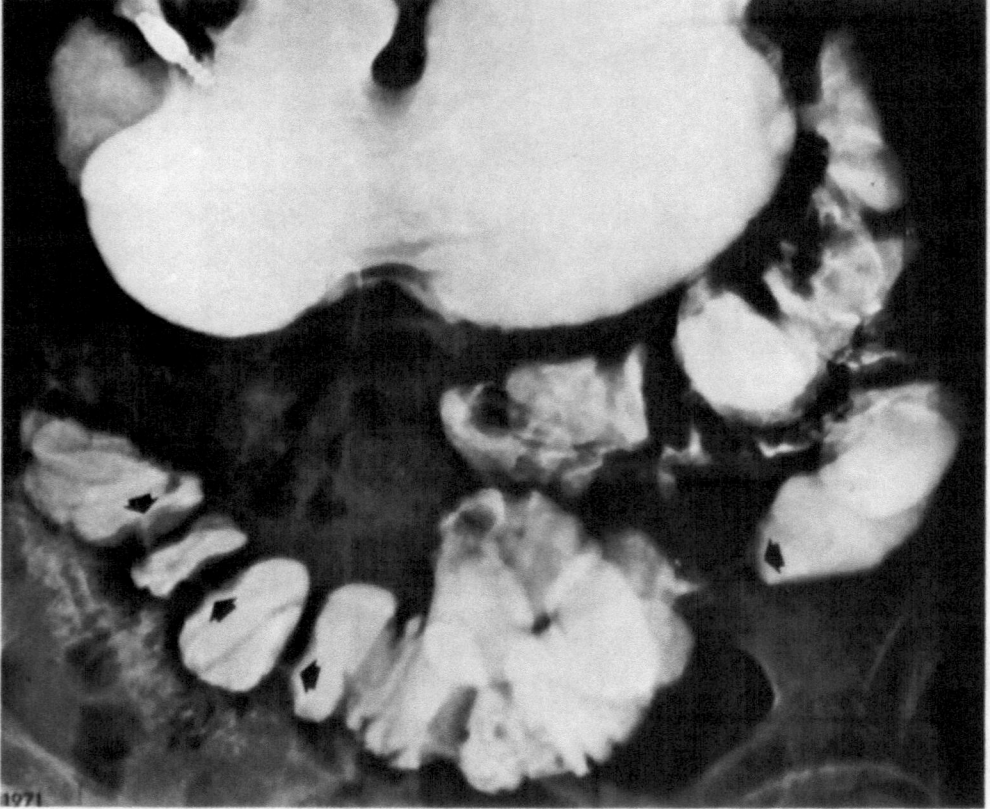

Fig. 9.39. Stenotic areas in the jejunum of a patient with celiac disease. During surgery it was found that the constrictions were located at ulcer sites and were partly due to spasms. Angiographic examination showed that the blood vessels in the small intestine were very fragile.

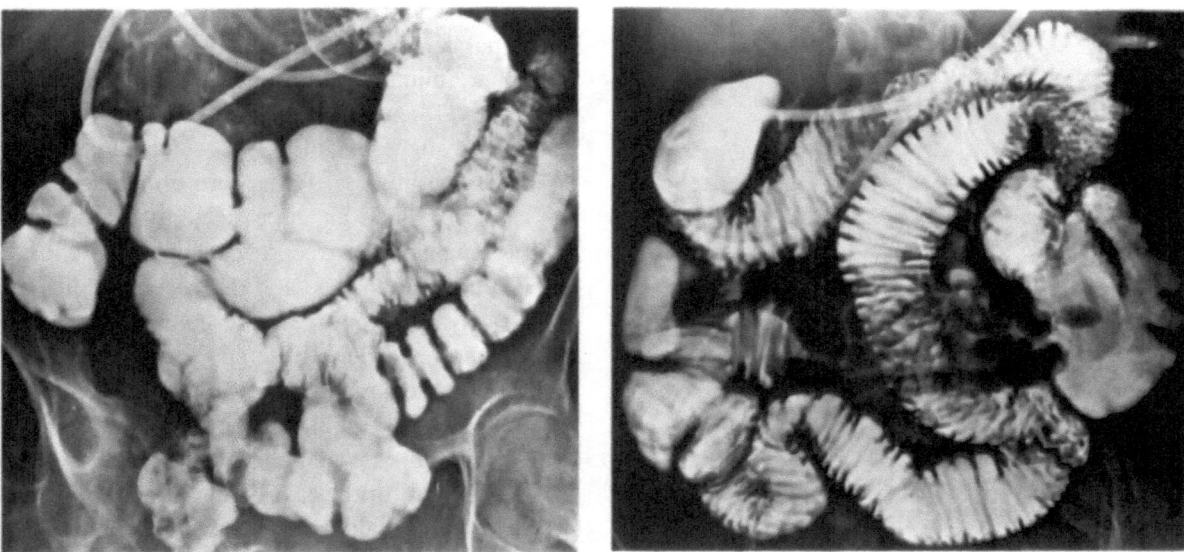

Fig. 9.40. Two examples of a so-called 'short-bowel': after multiple resections the small intestine is at the most 1 m long. Left: 23-year-old patient. Right: recurring stenosis ±10 cm long in the region of the anastomosis with the remaining segment of the colon.

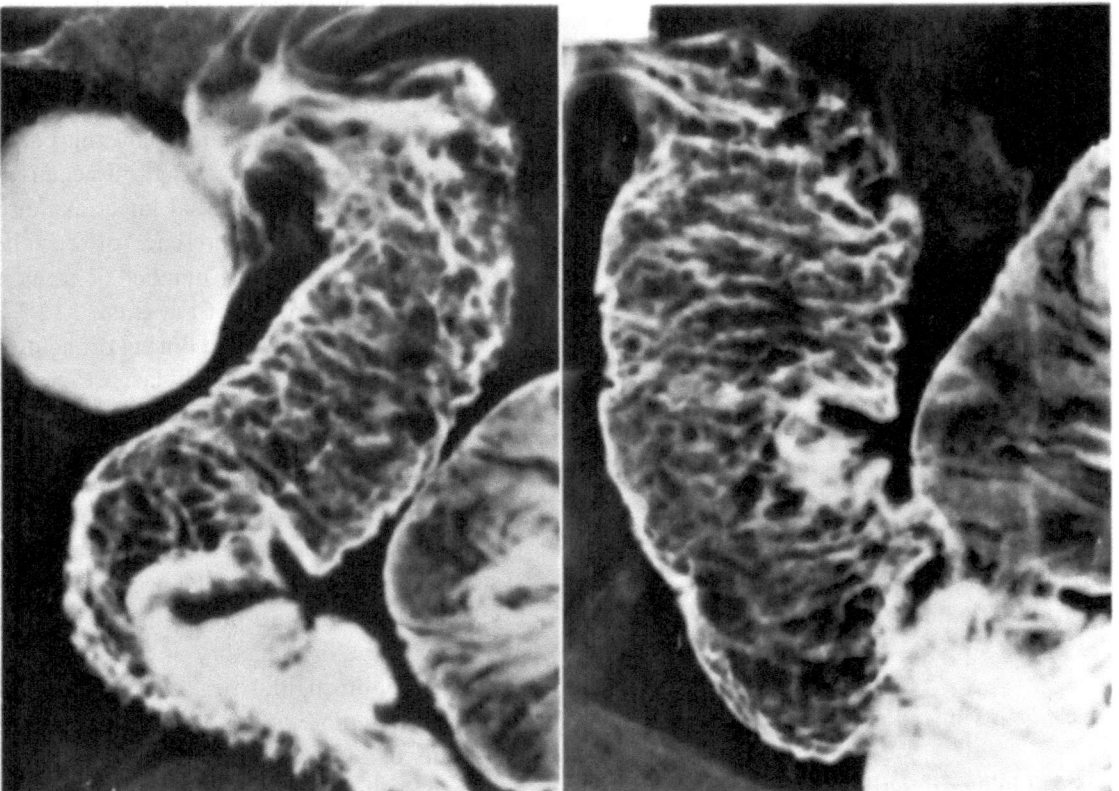

Fig. 9.41. Granular appearance of mucosal surface and very superficial, transversely directed ulcerative grooves in the distal ileum as a result of reflux ileitis in ulcerative colitis. A transverse course of ulcerations in the distal ileum is probably a result of a rather superficial edematous swelling of the mucosa. In Crohn's disease the edema is much more pronounced, which necessarily leads to a predominantly longitudinal folding of the inner surface of those parts of the bowel that are only scarcely provided with mucosal folds.

230

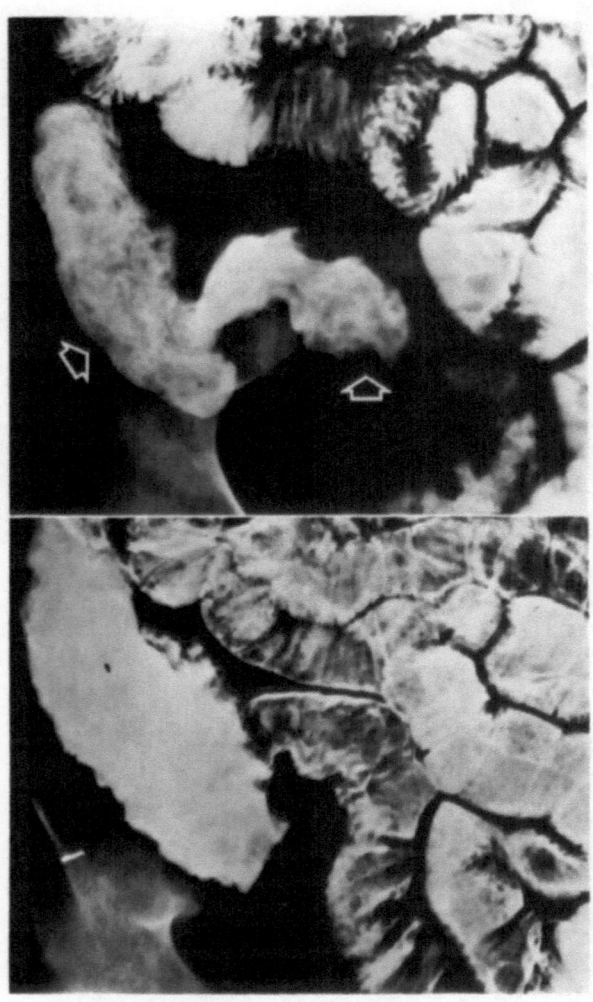

Fig. 9.42. A reflux ileitis sometimes is incorrectly presumed to be worse than it really is if the distal ileum remains contaminated. The intestine must be flushed clean.

that the abnormalities can be seen in their true proportions (fig. 9.42).

4. *Yersinia EC* infections

In 1945, Golden described a disease of the small intestine that he differentiated from the regional ileitis found in Crohn's disease. His patients were women 10–30 years of age who complained of pain in the lower right quadrant similar to that en-

countered in acute appendicitis. The painful terminal ileum was palpable in some cases. Radiological examination showed mucosal changes in the terminal centimeters of the ileum. Round filling defects suggestive of polyps were seen, and in some cases the mucosal folds were broadened. In those cases in which an appendectomy was performed, the appendix proved to be normal but the distal ileum was thickened and there were swollen mesenteric lymph nodes. In the course of a follow-up study over a period of ten years, Crohn's disease was not demonstrated in any of these patients. In other cases, the symptoms were suggestive of Crohn's disease and the patients were referred to the internist or the gastroenterologist. In such cases, there was usually a brief history of cramp-like pain in the lower abdomen, sometimes associated with diarrhea and pyrexia.

Between 1950 and 1962, analogous patients were described by Prevot and others. They were all unable to identify the cause of this infection and believed that the mucosal abnormalities found resulted from hyperplasia of the lymphoid tissue.

Today we know that *Yersinia enterocolitica* is the causative agent in these infections of the terminal loop of ileum. In veterinary medicine this bacterium has long been known as the gram-negative Pasteurella X, which causes lethal infectious diseases. Serological tests for the presence of *Yersinia EC* proved to be positive in a number of cases in the above-mentioned groups of patients.

The titers become elevated during the acute phase of this infection, which usually lasts several weeks, and then gradually during recovery return to normal values.

The clinical manifestations of this disease do not always resemble those of a common gastroenteritis or appendicitis. In rare cases they can mimic a systemic sepsis or they can be accompanied by an erythema nodosum or a polyarthritis. The cardinal symptoms are a brief history of cramp-like pain in the lower abdomen, diarrhea, and pyrexia. Because there are often more or less acute exacerbations, the possibility of a Crohn's disease is considered and as a rule a radiological examination is then done. When the symptoms are suggestive of acute appendicitis, the situation is more difficult. When it seems likely that surgery will be necessary in the near future, a radiological examination of the small

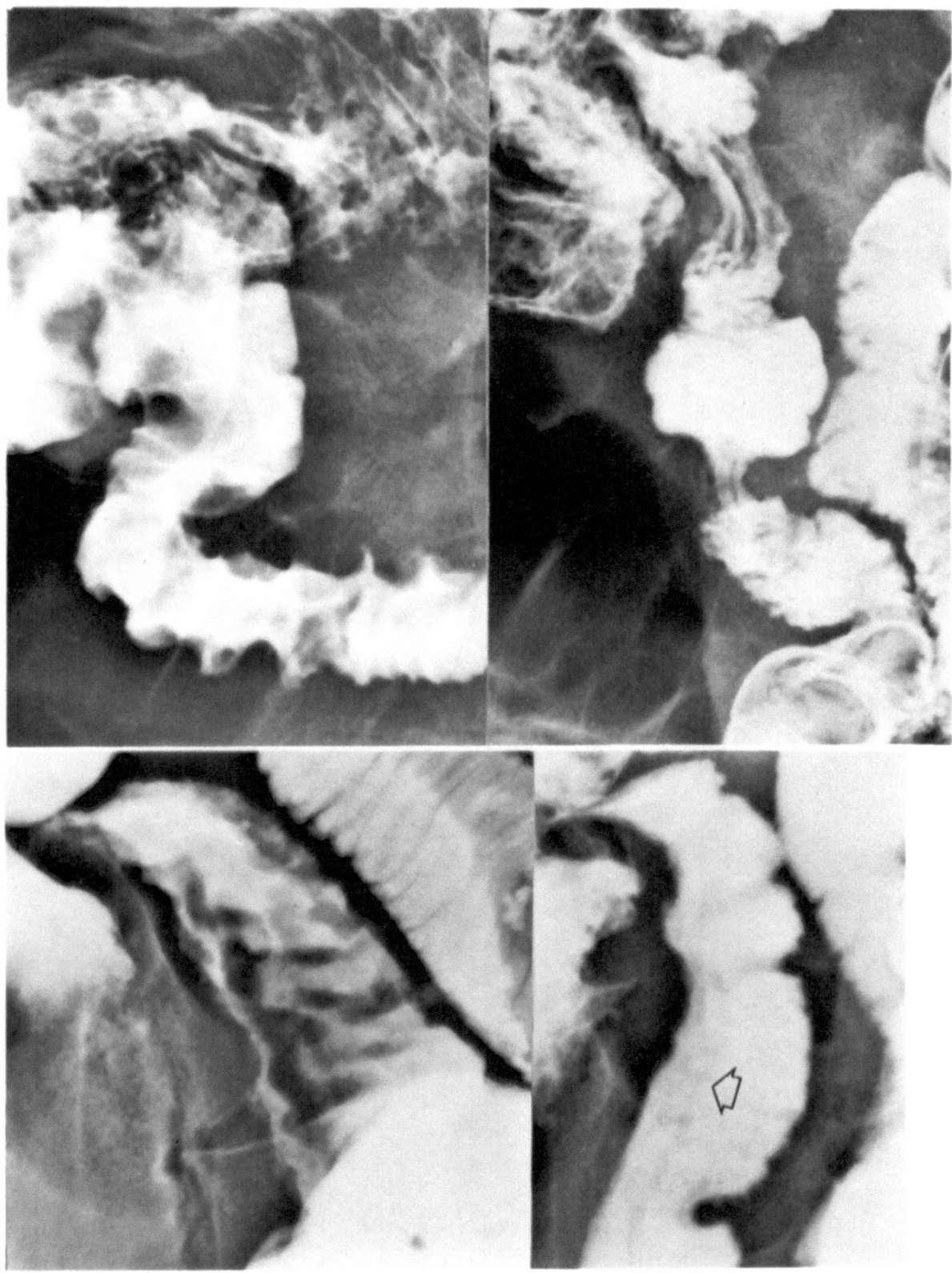

Fig. 9.43. Voluminous nodular defects (top) and thick mucosal folds (bottom) in the distal ileum due to a *Yersinia enterocolitica* infection (left) that disappeared after treatment (right).

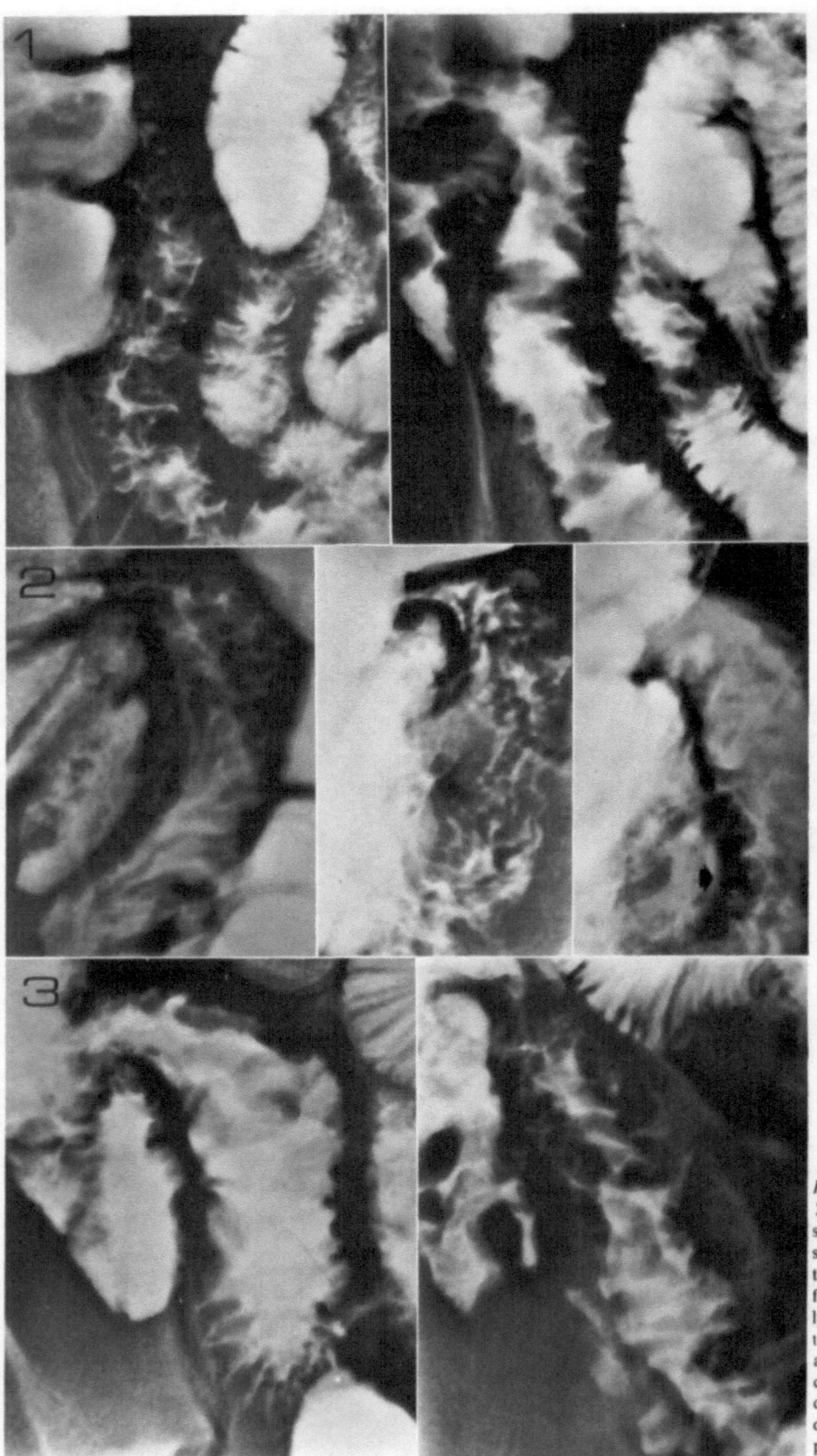

*Fig. 9.44*A. Three patients with *Yersinia EC* infection in the small intestine. In a 10–20 cm segment of the distal ileum there are more or less round filling defects that resemble lymph follicles or inflammatory granulomas. There are also greatly broadened mucosal folds that follow an undulating course. Some filling defects contain a barium deposit (arrow) that is suggestive of a central ulcer crater.

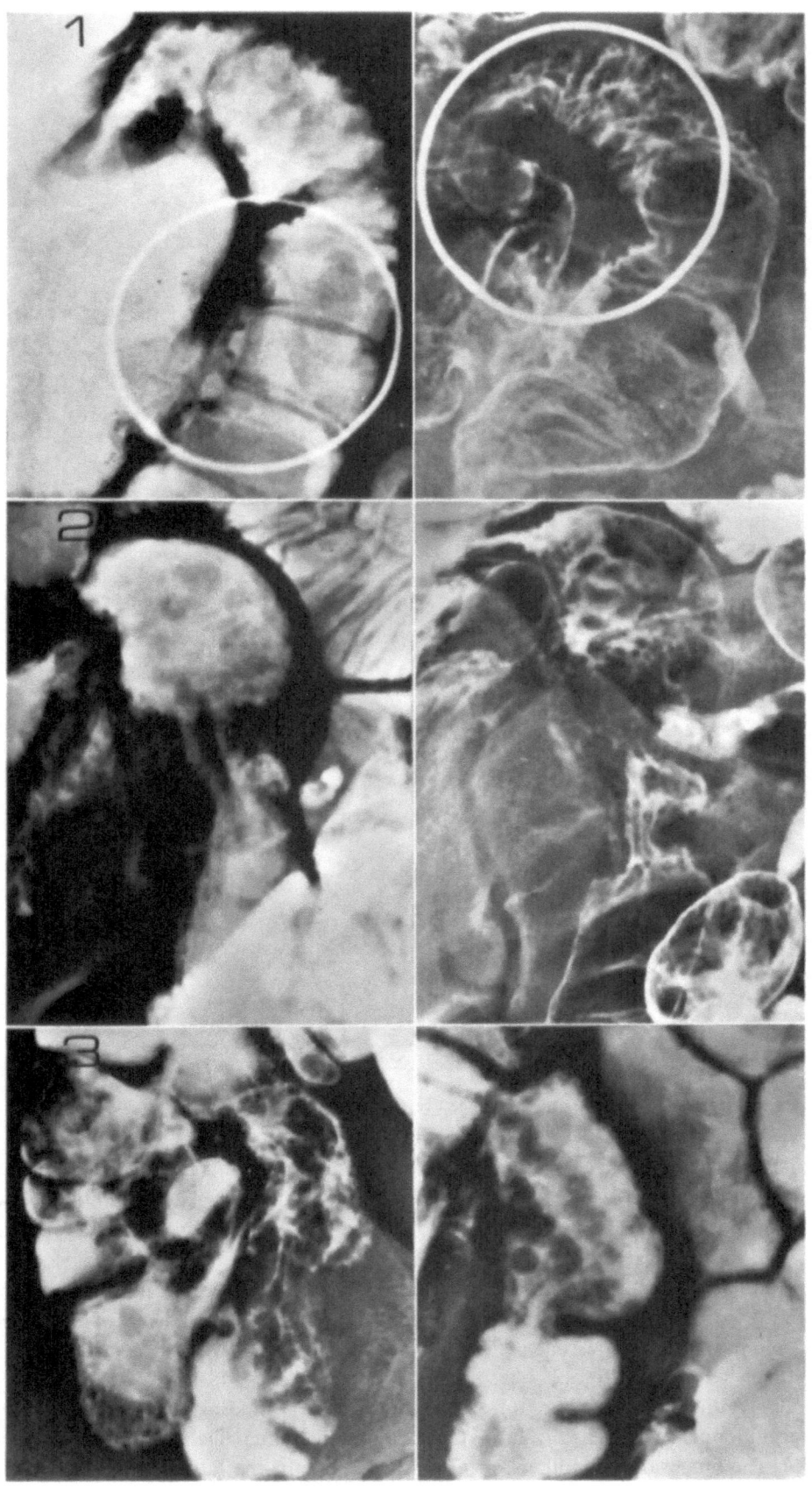

233

*Fig. 9.44*B. The same patients as those seen in fig. 9.44A, 2–3 months later. The abnormalities have clearly diminished in all cases; they have not spread as would be expected for example in Crohn's disease.

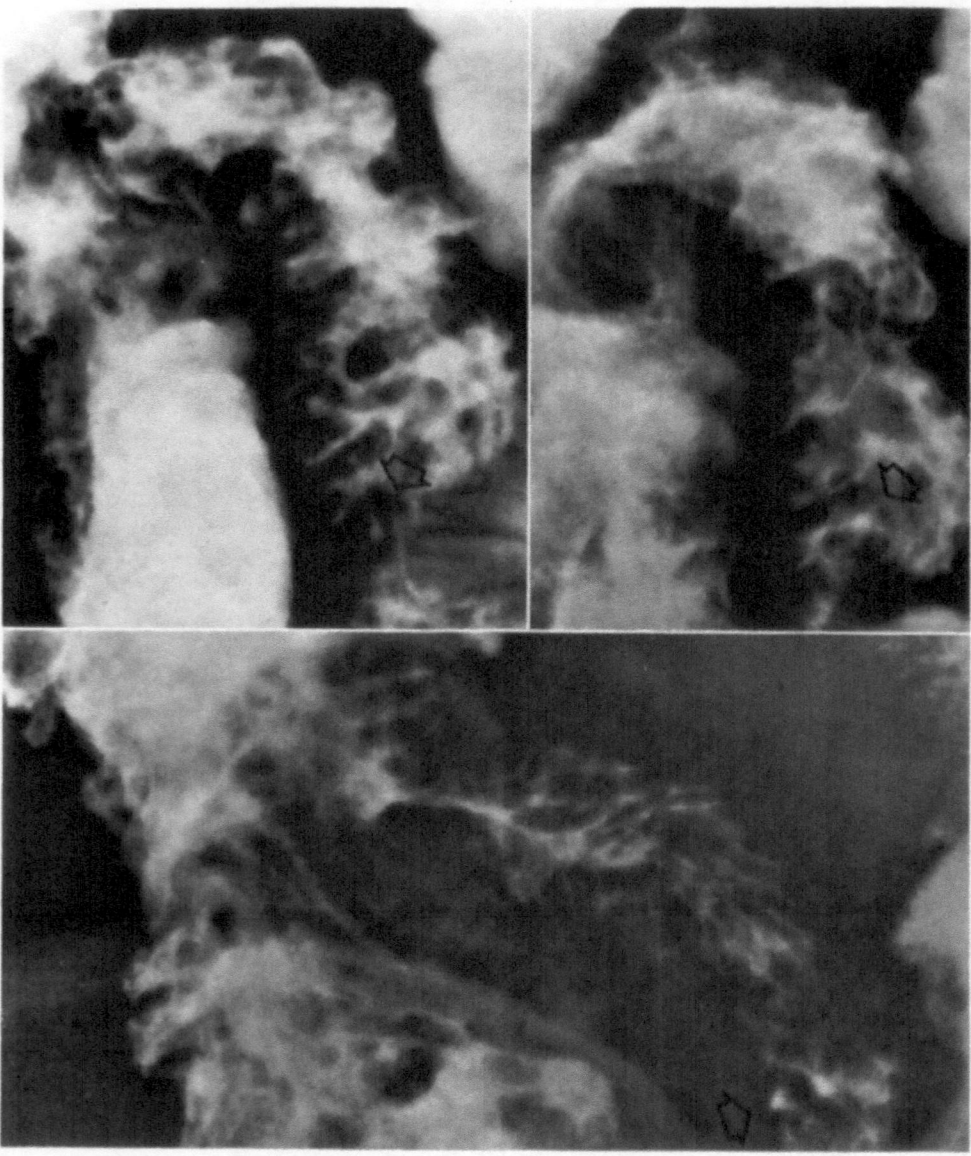

Fig. 9.45. Yersinia EC infection in the distal ileum; pattern is suggestive of aphthous ulcers (arrows).

intestine is not recommended. In such cases, the patient can be spared the inconvenience of an operation by performing the serological and bacteriological tests first. The radiological changes observed only last for several weeks or 2–3 months at the most (figs. 9.43 and 9.44) and are limited to the terminal 20 cm of the ileum. In this area, we can see filling defects, sometimes reminiscent of cobblestones, that are probably due to hyperplasia of lymphoid tissue or granulomas with centrally located ulcers (fig. 9.45). The mucosal folds follow a tortuous course, are increased in number, and unmistakably broadened. The separation between the distal ileum and the adjacent cecal loops can be increased (fig. 9.44A). The broad folds and the increased distance between the intestinal loops are the result of inflammatory edema of the mucosal folds and the intestinal wall, respectively.

These radiological findings are slightly different from those encountered in the initial stages of Crohn's disease. In the latter, the number of mu-

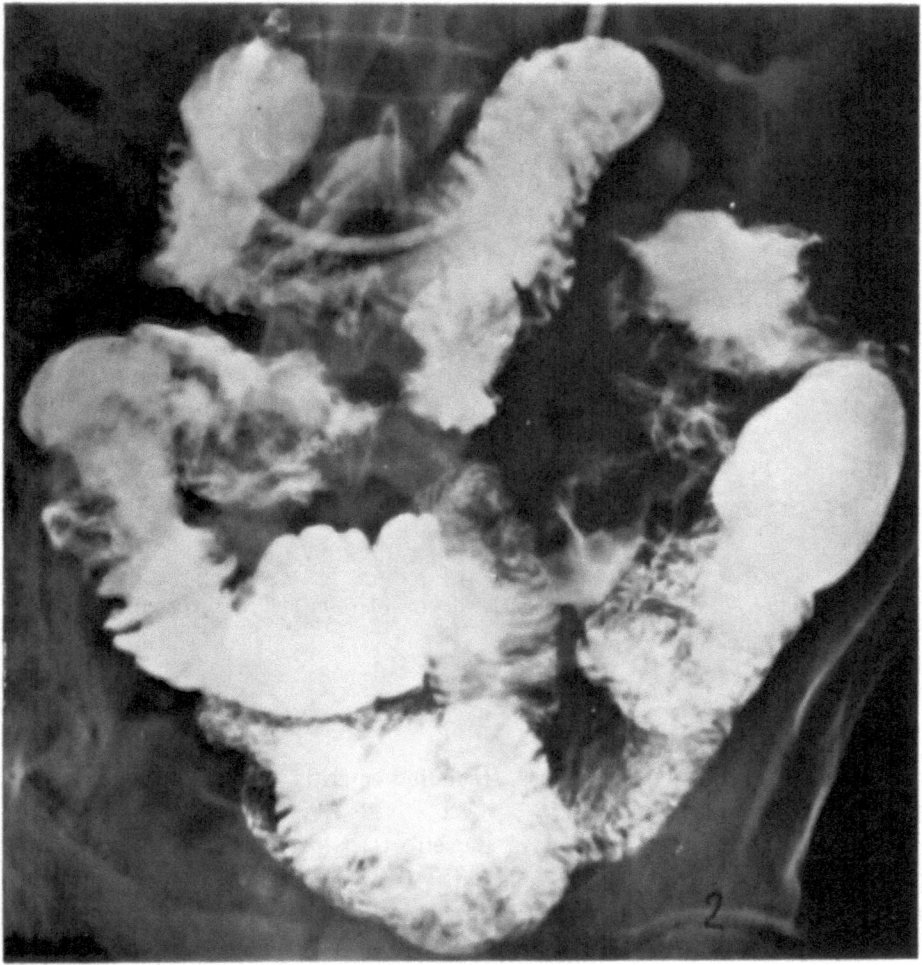

Fig. 9.46. Eosinophilic gastroenteritis, with large infiltrates and extensive destruction so that differentiation from a lymphosarcoma (fig. 9.47) on the basis of radiological criteria is not possible.

cosal folds does not increase and the filling defects causing the typical cobblestone appearance are more pronounced and more oval in shape. In more advanced cases of Crohn's disease, the margins of the intestine are vaguely defined due to the numerous ulcerations that may be present. In comparison with the normal terminal loop of the ileum, the abundance of mucosal folds is the most striking feature and has proved to be a valid criterium for diagnosis of *Yersinia EC* infection.

The radiological features of nodular lymphoid hyperplasia, as observed especially in children and not to be regarded as pathological, are readily distinguishable from the radiological findings in *Yersinia EC* infections. In lymphoid hyperplasia, the

filling defects are regularly arranged and rarely exceed a diameter of 1–3 mm.

5. Eosinophilic gastroenteritis

This recurrent disease, which is also often self-limiting, develops in patients with an allergic diathesis and should not be considered a true inflammatory process. Histologically it is characterized by extensive eosinophilic infiltration throughout all layers of the intestinal wall, particularly the mucosa and the lamina propria of the submucosa. The main localizations are the jejunum and the pars antralis of the stomach as well as, although less common, the duodenum and the proximal ileum. In

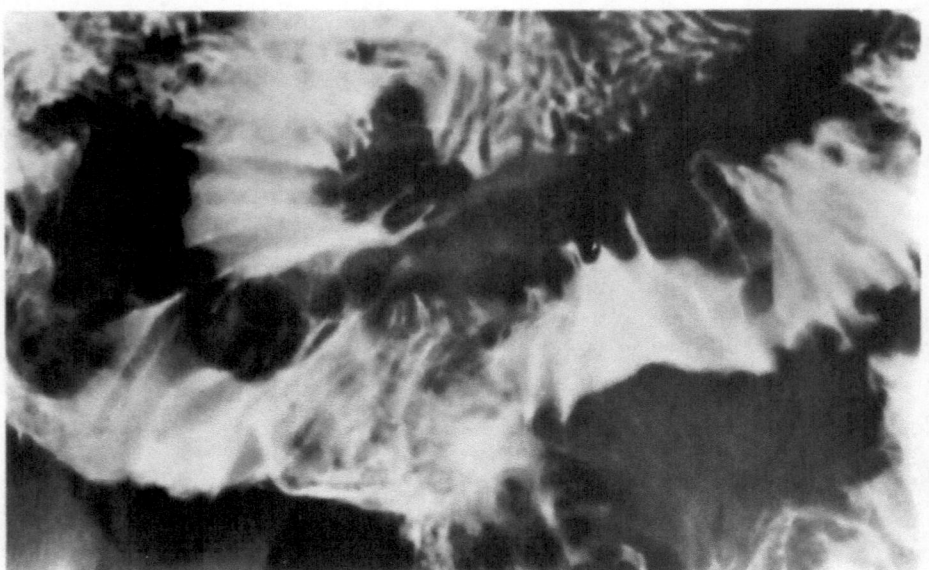

Fig. 9.47. Lymphosarcoma that cannot be differentiated from the highly destructive eosinophilic gastroenteritis in fig. 9.46.

addition to abdominal pain and malabsorption accompanied by diarrhea, there can also be such a marked loss of protein in the digestive tract that edema of the ankles occurs. In addition to a hypoproteinemia there will also be a blood eosinophilia that may even reach values of 80%. On the films, the infiltrates that bulge out into the intestinal lumen appear as polypous growths of various sizes. The mucosal folds show pronounced thickening and follow a tortuous course. The lumen of the involved intestinal loops is usually decreased. If the eosinophilic infiltration has damaged the muscular layers, the lumen may also be dilated locally. Because of the thickened intestinal walls and the edematous swelling of the mesentery, the distance between adjacent intestinal loops is obviously increased on the roentgenograms (fig. 9.46). Ulcerations and fistulas are not seen as a rule, but if they do occur then a lymphosarcoma can be difficult to distinguish from an eosinophilic gastroenteritis (fig. 9.47). Differentiation from a Crohn's disease localized in the proximal intestine as well as a mild case of Whipple's disease can also cause problems. In Whipple's disease, however, the jejunal loops are dilated rather than narrowed and there is no increase in the separation between intestinal loops.

6. Radiation enteritis

In the effort to increase chances of survival for patients with malignant tumors by using radiotherapy, one must be aware of the possibility of permanent damage to adjacent tissues.

Irradiation of tumors in the abdomen implies damage to the digestive tract in particular. In 1931, Desjardins showed that in the digestive tract of animals the small intestine is the most sensitive to roentgen rays. If the small intestine was less mobile, then abnormalities could be expected in the small bowel of all patients treated with a therapeutic dose of radiation. Vulnerability increases from the duodenum toward the ileum; the sensitivity of the transverse colon, sigmoid, rectum, and stomach is, however, less pronounced. Roswitt and his associates believe that the maximum therapeutic dosage is determined by the vulnerability of the small intestine and the kidneys.

The ileum is damaged by irradiation much more frequently than the jejunum since the ileum is more or less fixed in the minor pelvis and is therefore much less mobile than the jejunum. If adhesion has also occurred, then radiotherapy of the reproductive organs can sometimes cause an acute radiation enteritis of the ileum. Reports of radiation enteritis are fairly scarce in the journals of radiology. In part this can be attributed to the mucosal patterns obtained during the conventional follow-through examination. In such cases they usually cannot be evaluated. We now know that these vague patterns are often caused by an increase in the motility and mucus secretion in the irradiated field. As a result there is a pronounced tendency toward flocculation of the barium suspension in this region.

A radiological examination of the small intestine before irradiation of the abdomen is certainly worthwhile. In this manner, adhesion and fusion of ileal loops in the minor pelvis can be discovered, and irradiation can then be performed with the patient in the Trendelenburg position. If the bladder is full and rectal air insufflation is used, the ileal loops can be forced back into the abdominal cavity as far as possible. This considerably reduces the chance of radiation enteritis.

The histological changes characterizing radiation enteritis consist mainly of ulcerations and signs of sclerosis, either isolated, multiple, or in combination (Warren and Friedman, 1942). Both the ulcerations and the fibrosis can lead to the formation of strictures. The ulcerations can be deep-seated but may also develop as only superficial erosions. In addition there can be numerous changes that generally occur secondary to an inflammatory process such as perforations, fistulas, and adhesions. There is almost always a more or less extensive necrosis; in extreme cases, an entire intestinal loop may be gangrenous.

In the early stages, the changes consist of edema and fibrinous exudation. As a result of the deposit of albumin, there is a hyalinization of the collagenous tissue. This occurs especially in the connective tissue of the mucosa and the submucosa as well as in the walls of the vessels in the intestinal wall and the mesentery. The walls of both the intestine and the vessels become thicker, initially as a result of the edema and hyalinization but later also because of the eventual hypertrophy of the muscular tissue. Although the mucosa sometimes appears completely normal without any signs of ulceration, it is in fact atrophied and fixed to the submucosa. Not only arteries but also veins are involved. Histologically they are characteristic of an endarteritis obliterans with endothelial proliferation, medionecrosis, and thrombosis. Moreover, there can also be hyaline degeneration in the walls of the lymph vessels as well as a thickening of the endothelial layer. These lymphatic channels are also often ectatically dilated. Bosniak et al. (1969) clearly demonstrated these changes in the vessel in an experiment with rabbits. They irradiated a 3-cm exposed segment of the small intestine prepared surgically. They then evaluated the circulation immediately after irradiation (1500 and 3000 r) and periodically for five weeks by using angiography. They observed the following:

1) Striking vascular spasms two days after irradiation: reacted favorably to antispasmodics.
2) Five days after irradiation: a deep hemorrhagic ulcer in the irradiated field.
3) Two weeks after irradiation: vascular constriction that could no longer be relieved with papaverine and therefore was caused by an organic change. In this stage there was a chronic inflammation in the intestinal wall.

Macroscopically an intestine that has been damaged by a radiation overdose (5000–6000 r) usually shows edematous swelling along a fairly large segment and appears indurated. The intestine is coated with an opaque serous membrane that is highly telangiectatic, particularly where the intestine is attached to the mesentery.

The intestinal abnormalities resulting from irradiation are due largely to damaged blood vessels in the intestinal wall or the mesentery. The occurrence of vasculitis with thrombosis and perivascular fibrosis disturbs the circulation in the wall of the loops in the irradiated field and sometimes in loops that are clearly beyond the field. In their histological description, Warren and Friedman also noted abnormalities beyond the irradiated field.

The frequencies given in the literature for the occurrence of the clinical symptoms of radiation enteritis vary greatly. The values range from 0.6% to 17% for patients who have undergone abdominal irradiation (Aldridge; Colcock and Braatsch). Most authors indicate that the complaints develop within two years after radiotherapy (De Cosse et al. and

238

Graundins). Numerous exceptions are, however, known – complaints have even developed 30 years after irradiation. Neumeister and Pfeiffer found that intestinal adhesions as a result of surgery greatly increase the chance of lesions in the small intestine because of the decreased mobility. The 30 patients studied by Mason et al. included 24 surgical patients. The most severe abnormalities were localized in the immobile loops.

Since a specific dose causes abnormalities in the small intestine in one patient but not in another, it would seem that the sensitivity varies per individual. There have for instance been cases with a fatal outcome after only a few days of irradiation with a minimum dosage – the so-called x-ray intoxication (Todd). In 1973, Pekka Nummi described two patients with severe diarrhea and a diffuse ulceration in the jejunum and the ileum after irradiation with 1500 rads.

The symptoms of a radiation enteritis can be separated into an acute and a chronic syndrome. The acute symptoms usually include severe pain in the abdomen, nausea, vomiting, and bloody diarrhea. Examination reveals a distended abdomen with a palpable tumor-like mass that is often mistaken for a recurrent tumor. Acute therapeutic measures, such as direct decompression by using a Miller-Abbot tube, are often necessary since the course of the disease may otherwise become catastrophic within a short period. This is, however, often insufficient and then a laparotomy is necessary. Unfortunately the postoperative course is often severely complicated by a peritonitis that frequently results in death (Roswitt and Malsky).

Most patients have a chronic radiation enteritis that develops one to twelve years after radiotherapy (Chau and Fletcher). Intermittent attacks of colic, obstipation, anorexia, vomiting, diarrhea, fatigue and loss of weight, sometimes even cachexia (nutritional cripple), are the usual complaints.

Out of a group of 3000 patients who underwent radiotherapy, Duncan and Leonard saw six with a malabsorption syndrome that consisted of diarrhea, alternating in some cases with obstipation, megaloblastic anemia, and osteomalacia. Before their publication (1965), only five cases of radiation enteritis had been reported. The malabsorption is due to destruction of the mucosal epithelium so that resorption in the intestine is disturbed. We have

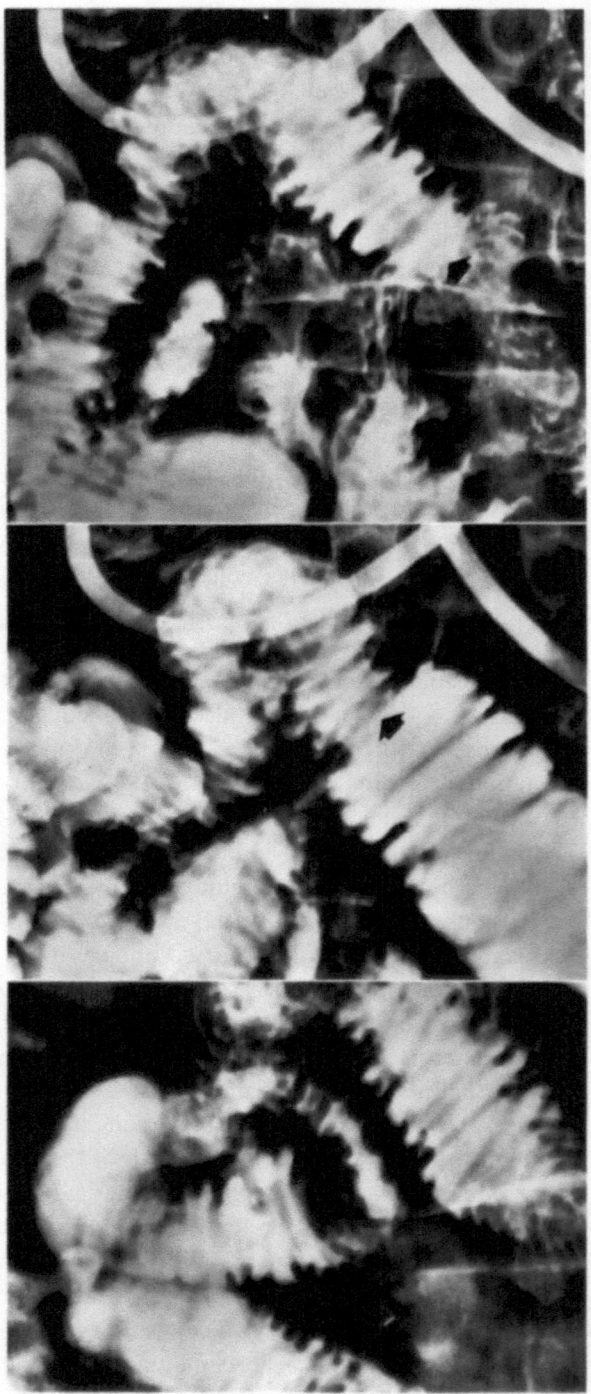

Fig. 9.48A. Radiation enteritis with edematous mucosa. Between the highly swollen mucosal folds are narrow spaces filled with barium that resemble a coarsely toothed saw. The transition to the normal intestinal segments is very abrupt (arrows).

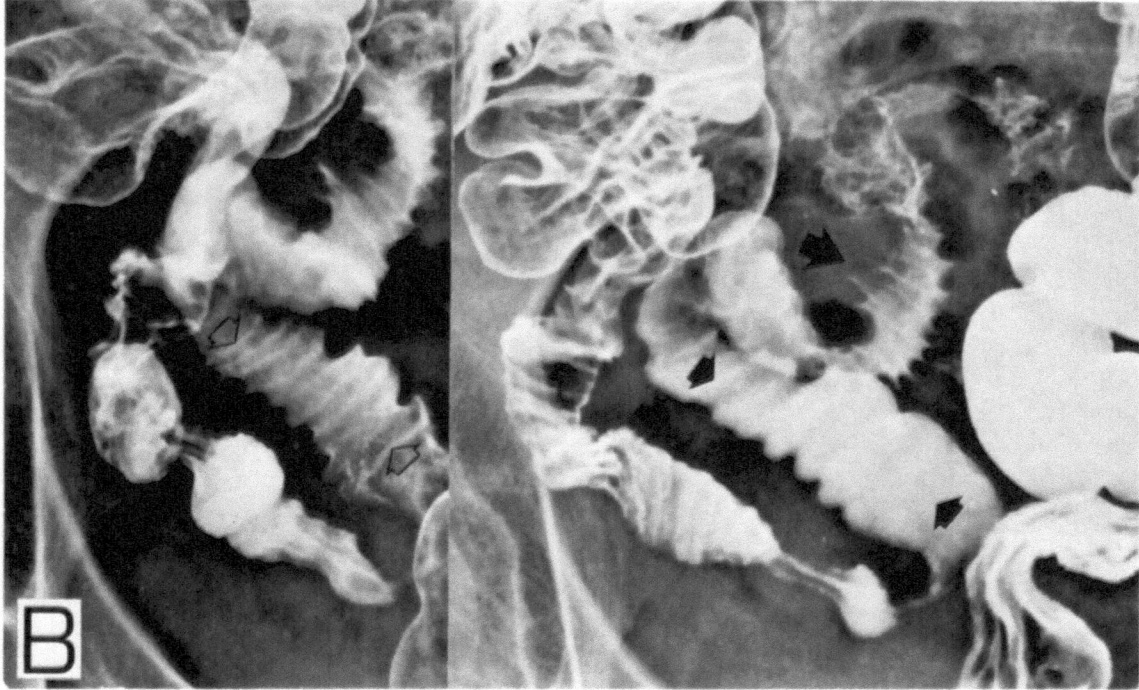

*Fig. 9.48*B. Thickened mucosal folds in the ileum as a result of radiation enteritis after irradiation of the genital tract. The edema is best visible when the bowel is only moderately filled with contrast fluid (open arrows). This examination of the colon was part of a routine checkup. The patient had no complaints whatsoever.

also found that radiological abnormalities as a result of small intestine irradiation can sometimes be observed within several weeks, even if the patient has few or no complaints. This agrees completely with the experiments of Bosniak et al.

The wall of the intestine damaged by an overdose of roentgen rays shows hyperemia and edema. The edema is localized mainly in the submucosa. This is seen on the x-rays as a clear broadening of the mucosal folds with very thin, fairly pointed spaces inbetween (spikes). As a result of the thicker intestinal wall, the distance between adjacent intestinal loops is also obviously increased (figs. 9.48A and 9.49). These abnormalities are probably due to a local anoxia of the intestinal wall and are similar to those seen in cases of hypermotility (fig. 8.59). The edema probably develops only when the anoxia is rather prolonged or is irreversible. As in ischemia, a fibrinous coating develops on the outside of the intestinal loops that causes multiple adhesions with adjacent loops (fig. 9.49). Moreover, ulcerations and necrosis can develop that may lead to bleeding, perforation, and fistulas to nearby organs. Usually

it is the bladder, sigmoid, or rectum. Because of the rigidity and the absence of peristaltic movements, the average diameter of the intestinal lumen can be somewhat greater. The relief of the thickened folds is regular at first but often becomes more disorderly in a later stage.

After a period of months, sometimes years, the scars or fibrotic tissue can lead to obstruction (fig. 9.50). If these local shriveling processes are localized in the mesentery, then 'kinking' is observed just as it does with a carcinoid lesion. In later stages of radiation enteritis, the space between the intestinal loops remains enlarged, partly as a result of the thicker intestinal wall and also because shriveling causes the mesentery to become shorter. In this stage, however, the thickening of the intestinal wall is not because of edema in the submucosa, but usually due to a fibrosis involving all layers.

If the roentgen damage to the small intestine is limited and there are neither ulcerations nor necrosis, the fibrous shriveling will not be extensive and will be more diffuse in nature. In that case, stenoses

240

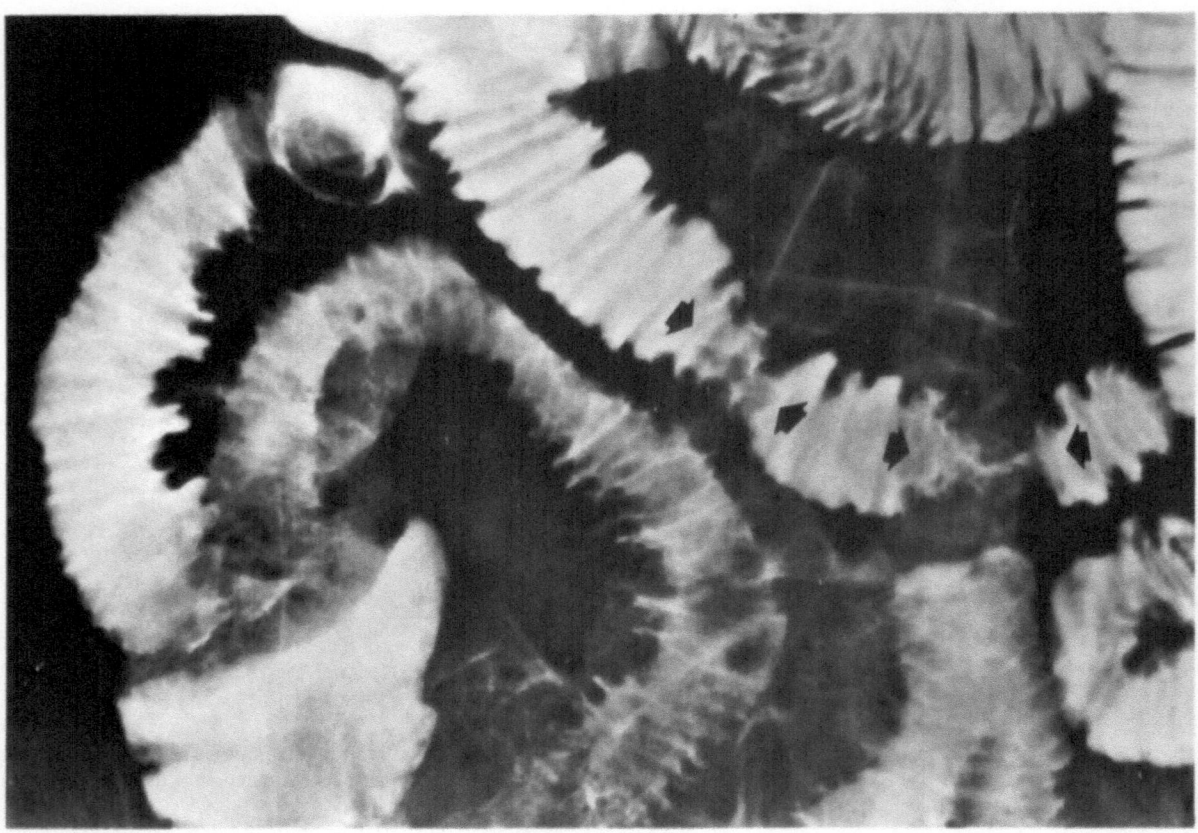

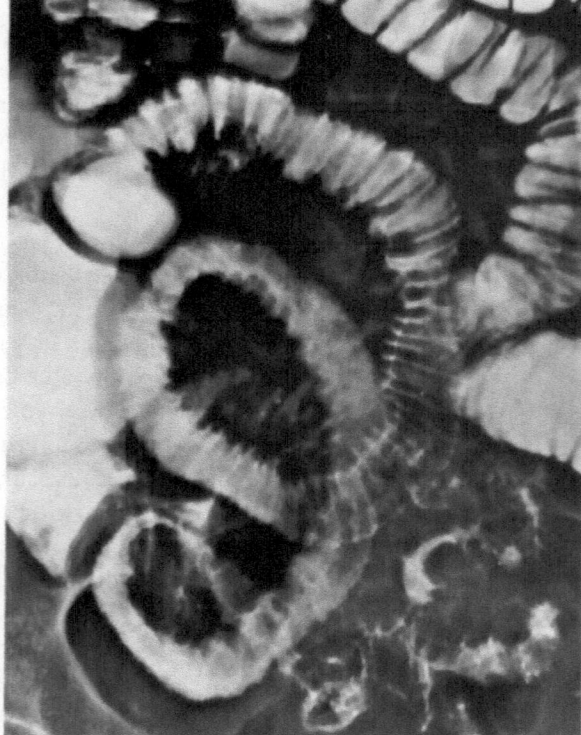

Fig. 9.49. Adhesion of intestinal loops in radiation enteritis; irregular mucosal surface and multiple small ulcerations. Thickened intestinal wall is due mainly to fibrosis instead of edema. Areas resembling skip lesions are indicated by arrows.

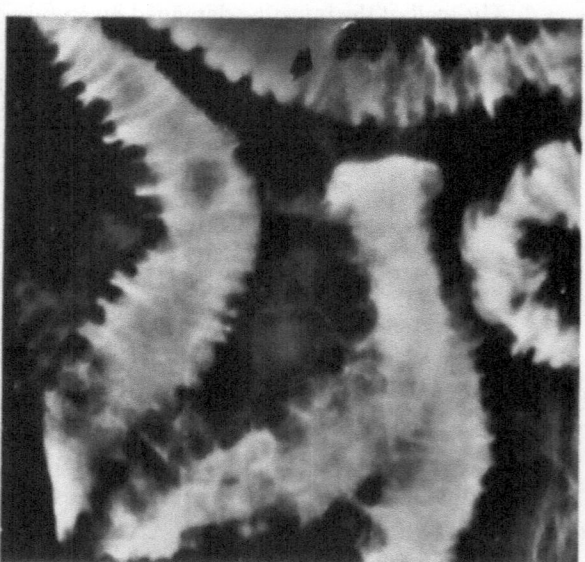

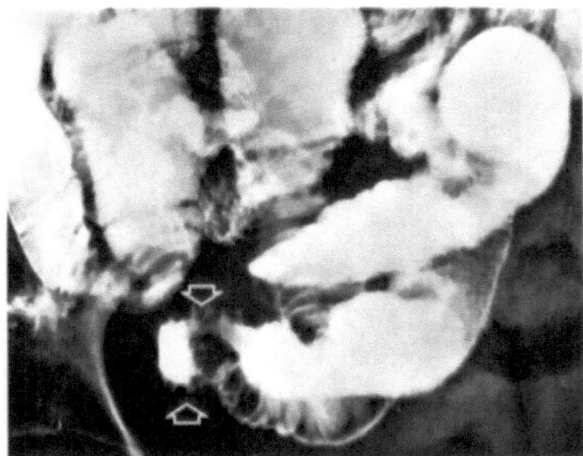

Fig. 9.50. Stenotic area in the intestine due to fibrosis in radiation enteritis.

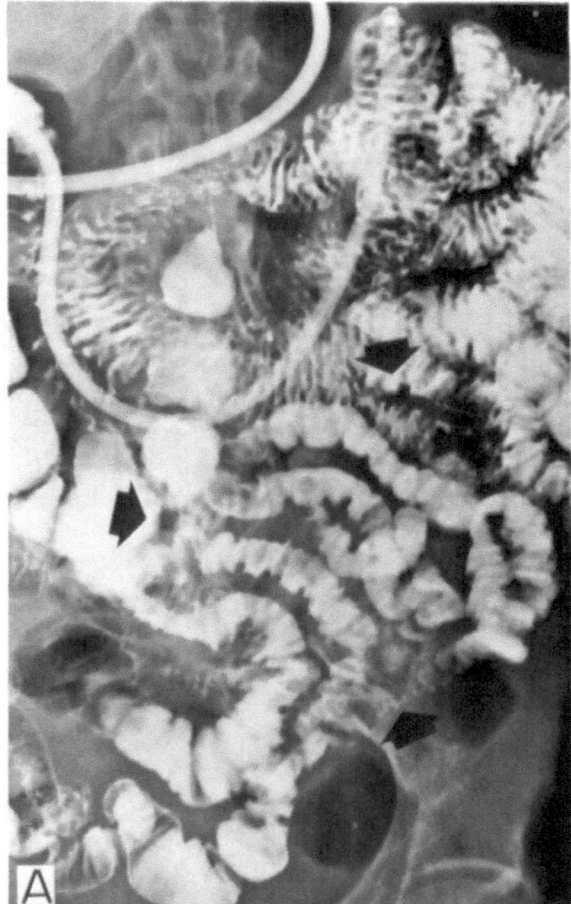

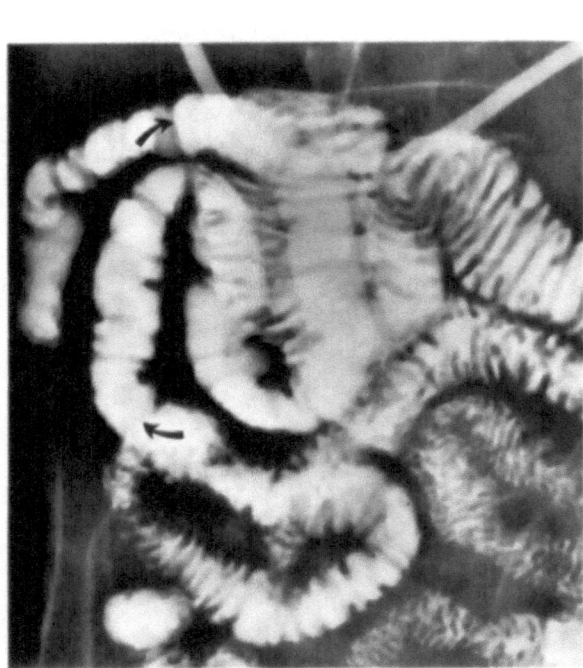

*Fig. 9.51*B. Radiation enteritis with atrophy of the mucosal folds and a decrease in the caliber of the intestine, presumably as a result of fibrosis.

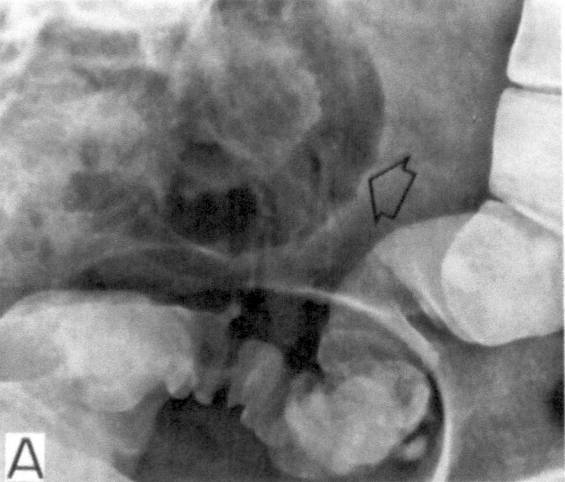

*Fig. 9.51*A. Our attention was drawn to a tube-like air-filled small intestinal loop on a colon examination from elsewhere (bottom). On the enteroclysis examination (top), there seemed to be a radiation enteritis in the proximal ileum. The caliber is decreased and the intestinal wall is thickened. There is a loss of mucosal folds with thickening of the remaining folds.

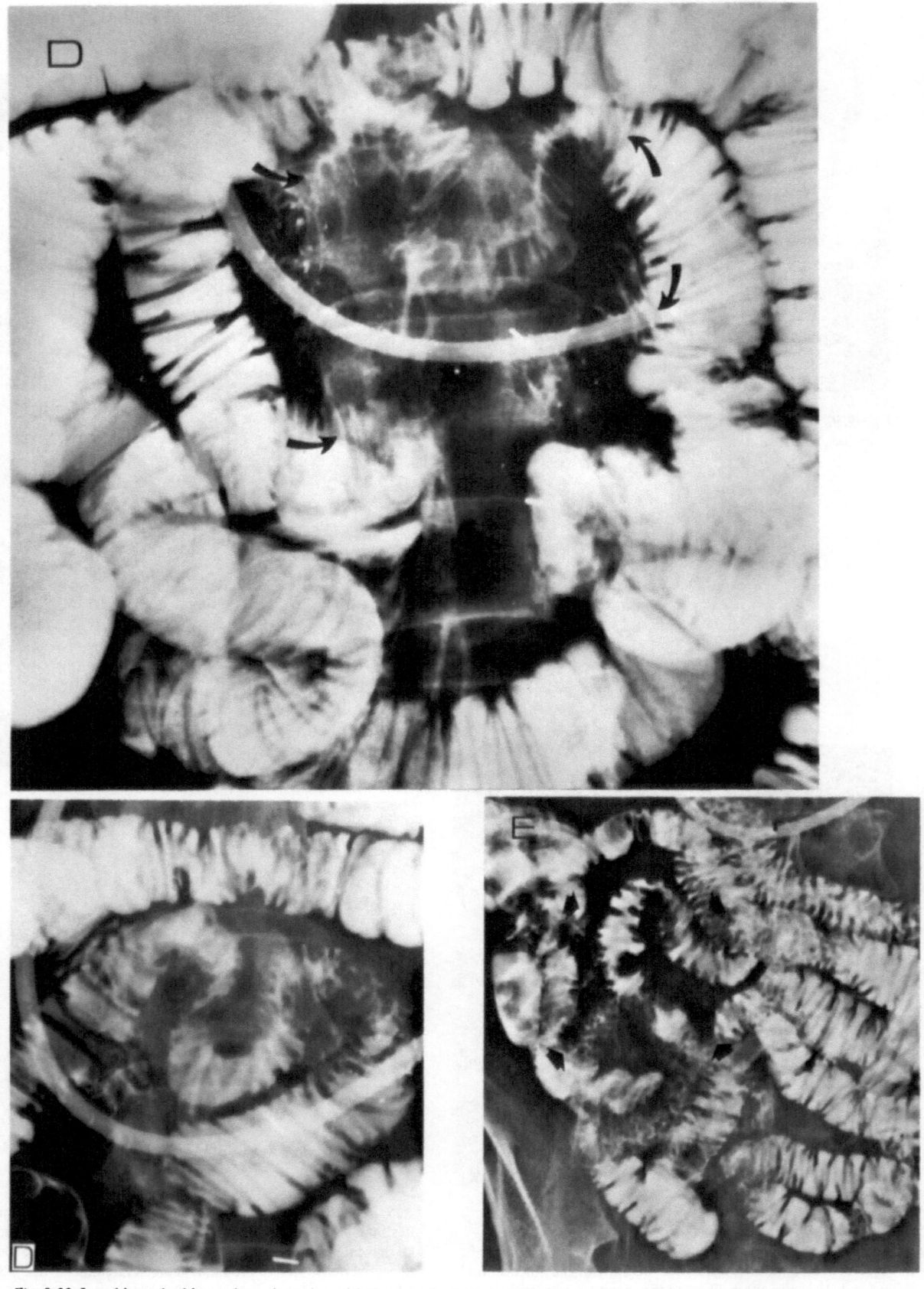

Fig. 9.52. Local intestinal hurry in an intestine with decreased caliber in radiation enteritis. The abnormalities are due to an ischemia and can therefore be found within (D) as well as beyond (E) the irradiated field.

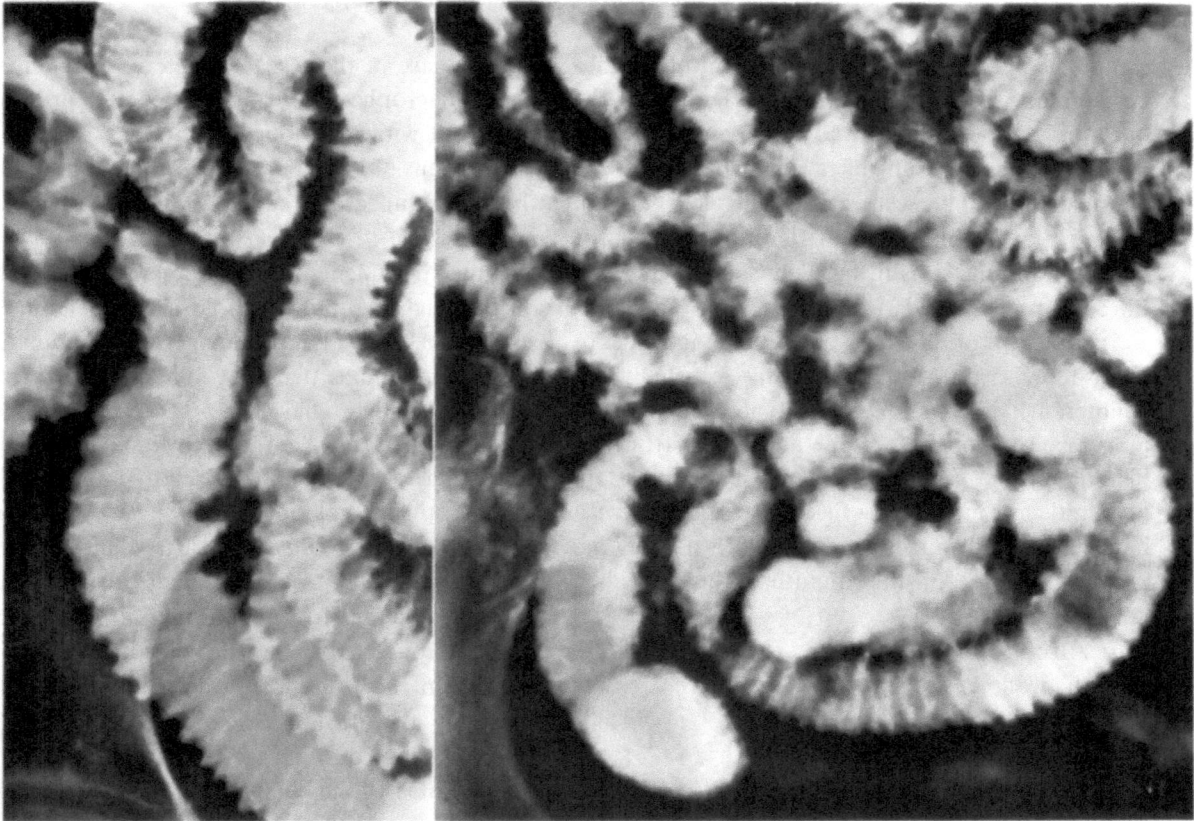

Fig. 9.53. Lymphedema of the entire small intestine as a result of a disturbed lymphatic flow in the center near the spinal column after irradiation. Due to the absence of fibrosis, the intestinal wall here is not as thick as that in fig. 9.49 and the regular arrangement of the mucosa is retained.

will not develop in the small intestine; instead, atrophy of the mucosa will be the predominant feature. As in a colon or stomach damaged by roentgen rays, we will see only a smooth mucosal surface without many folds (fig. 9.51). In the mucosa the epithelium is the most sensitive to roentgen rays. The initial reaction of the more resistant muscularis propria to radiation is as a rule a pronounced hypertonicity. During the radiological examination therefore a marked 'intestinal hurry' is observed in the irradiated field and it is exceedingly difficult to achieve adequate filling of the contracted intestinal loops (fig. 9.52).

In terms of the various findings, the radiological abnormalities in radiation enteritis can be listed as follows:

1) Spasms, recognized by the variation in the caliber of the intestinal lumen and the inability of the intestine to achieve total dilatation. The spasms are due to a moderate ischemia of the intestine and react favorably to antispasmodics.

2) Thickening of the intestinal wall due to fibrosis

or edema, mainly in the submucosa.

3) Rigidity or stiffness of the intestinal wall, also due to edematous or fibrotic changes in the intestinal wall. These are easily recognized because the peristaltic movements have obviously decreased in number and particularly in intensity.

The edema as well as the fibrosis may develop only locally, depending mainly on where the blood or lymph vessels are (or were) occluded. If there is a pure edema of the mucosa, then the mucosal folds often have a cobblestone aspect and cause round or oval bulges in the margins of the contrast column. If there is an edema of the submucosa, the folds are also broadened, but because the mucous membrane is completely intact, the regular arrangement is retained. In such cases the grooves between the folds that extend in parallel become exceedingly thin so that the so-called 'spiking' phenomenon (Mason and Clemett) is observed along the margins of the contrast column.

4) Ulcerations can be deep, leading to stenoses and fistulas, but they can also be very superficial. In the latter case they are difficult to demonstrate

radiologically. The regular arrangement of the mucosal folds is also retained when rigidity of the intestine is due only to a lymphedema that has developed as a result of a disturbance of the lymphatic flow in the center near the spinal column. In these cases, thickening of the intestinal wall is not as pronounced as in fig. 9.49 since there is no fibrosis at all (fig. 9.53).

5) Adhesion of the loops of the small intestine to other loops or surrounding organs is usually encountered in the minor pelvis. The loops can no longer be separated from one another or from the bladder or the cecum by means of compression. Peristaltic movements in a fused intestine can give a highly stretched mucosal pattern with a spiky aspect; sometimes in the literature this is called 'tacking down'.

6) Atrophy of the mucosa, recognized by the smooth wall; mucosal folds are more or less missing.

7. Whipple's disease

This fairly rare disease, which is sometimes hereditary, is occasionally also called – incorrectly – lipodystrophy. Although more is known since Whipple's first description in 1907, this disease remains shrouded in mystery because of its unknown etiology.

The complaints of these patients, predominantly middle-aged men, include abdominal pain, steatorrhea, weight loss, fatigue, and recurrent shifting pain in the joints. Physical examination shows a generalized lymphadenopathy, enlarged liver and spleen, and polyserositis. The skin is often pigmented as in Addison's disease. Hematological determinations reveal a low Hb and decreased protein and calcium concentrations; in addition, the resorption of various food substances is clearly disturbed.

Postmortem studies and pathological examinations of surgical material have shown that the lymph nodes and the lamina propria of the obviously thickened intestinal wall are filled with deposits of fat and fatty acids called 'lipogranulomas'. These deposits contain large foamy macrophages filled with a glycoprotein. Electron-microscopic studies have established that, during the active phase of the disease, bacteria conglomerate in the macrophages but disappear after prolonged treatment with antibiotics.

By means of lymph node biopsies and biopsies of the jejunal mucosa obtained via duodenoscopy, it is now possible to establish the diagnosis and begin adequate treatment and avoid laparotomy. The villi on the thickened mucosal folds in the jejunum are so swollen due to lymphedema and accumulations of lipogranulomas that they sometimes are visible to the naked eye. They then appear on the films as small nodules (fig. 9.54). The radiological abnormalities are further characterized by moderate dilatation of the jejunal loops and a slightly accelerated passage (fig. 9.56). There is a clear tendency toward flocculation or dilution of the contrast fluid so that the time available for making useful films is rather short. It appears that the marked coarsening of the mucosa in the jejunum, always mentioned in the literature and demonstrated on roentgenograms, can be attributed to a large extent to disintegration of the contrast fluid. As far as we have been able to discover, it is less pronounced than is generally assumed. This is clearly demonstrated by comparing the x-rays of a conventional examination (fig. 9.55A) with those obtained during an enteroclysis examination (fig. 9.55B). The films were taken of the same patient two weeks apart. It is stated in the literature that the radiological abnormalities characteristic of celiac disease can closely resemble those of Whipple's disease, but with the enteroclysis examination technique this is not true at all.

Although the abnormalities in celiac disease are also localized mainly in the jejunum, the folds are atrophied rather than broadened. They sometimes are greatly reduced in number or even completely missing. Both the dilatation of the loops and the motility can be much more pronounced and may involve a much larger segment in celiac disease than in Whipple's disease. Strictly speaking the same moderate changes in the mucosal folds and the micronodular villous structure seen in Whipple's disease can also be demonstrated radiologically in lipoproteinemia. Clinically, however, the differentiation between these two diseases is not difficult.

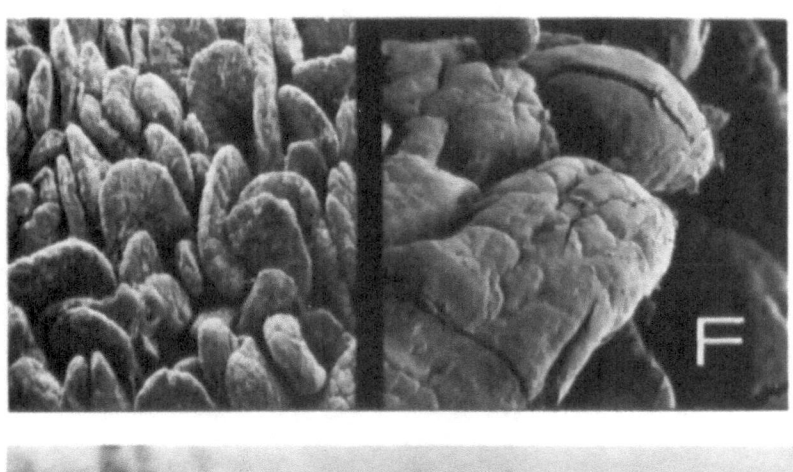

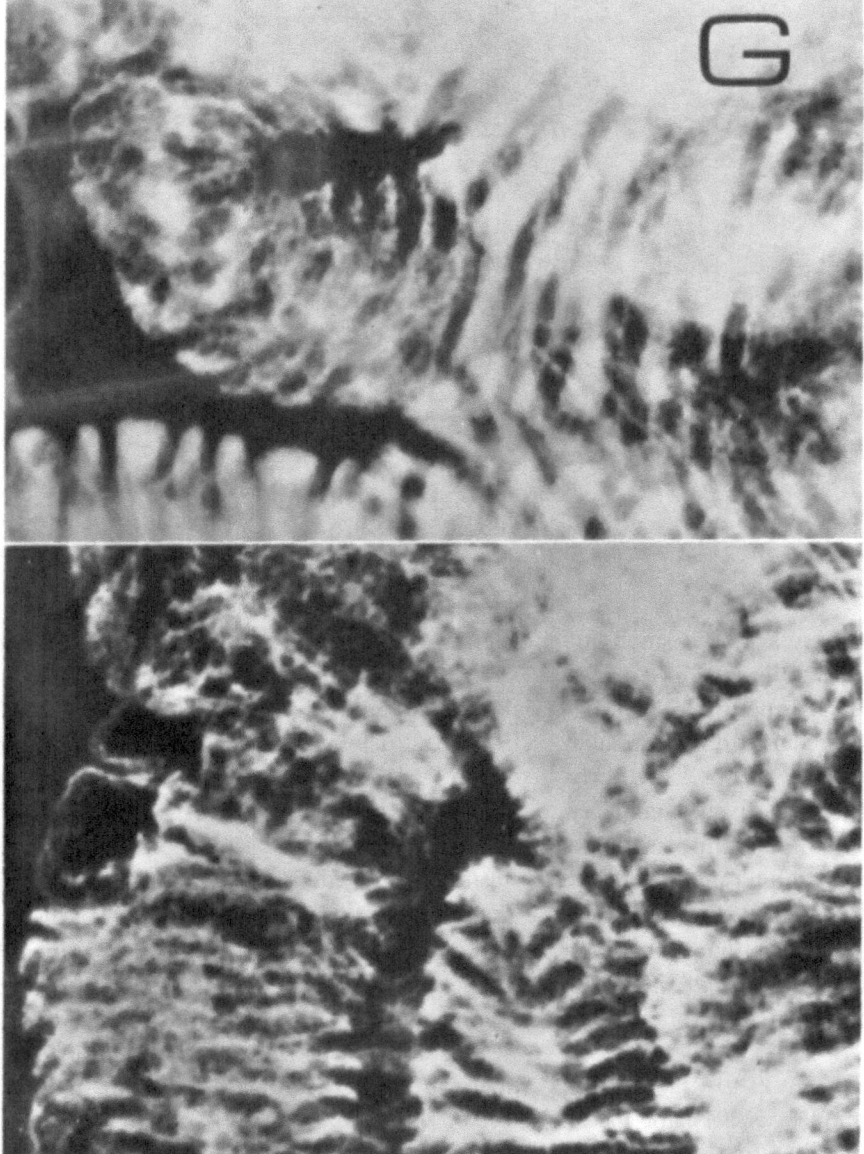

Fig. 9.54. In Whipple's disease the villi can be so swollen that they are ±0.5 mm in size; they then can be seen with the naked eye during endoscopic examination (F); on the roentgenograms (G) these villi are difficult to differentiate from foaming of the contrast fluid (H). The bubble-like villi, however, interrupt the contours of the intestinal wall. (See also page 246.)

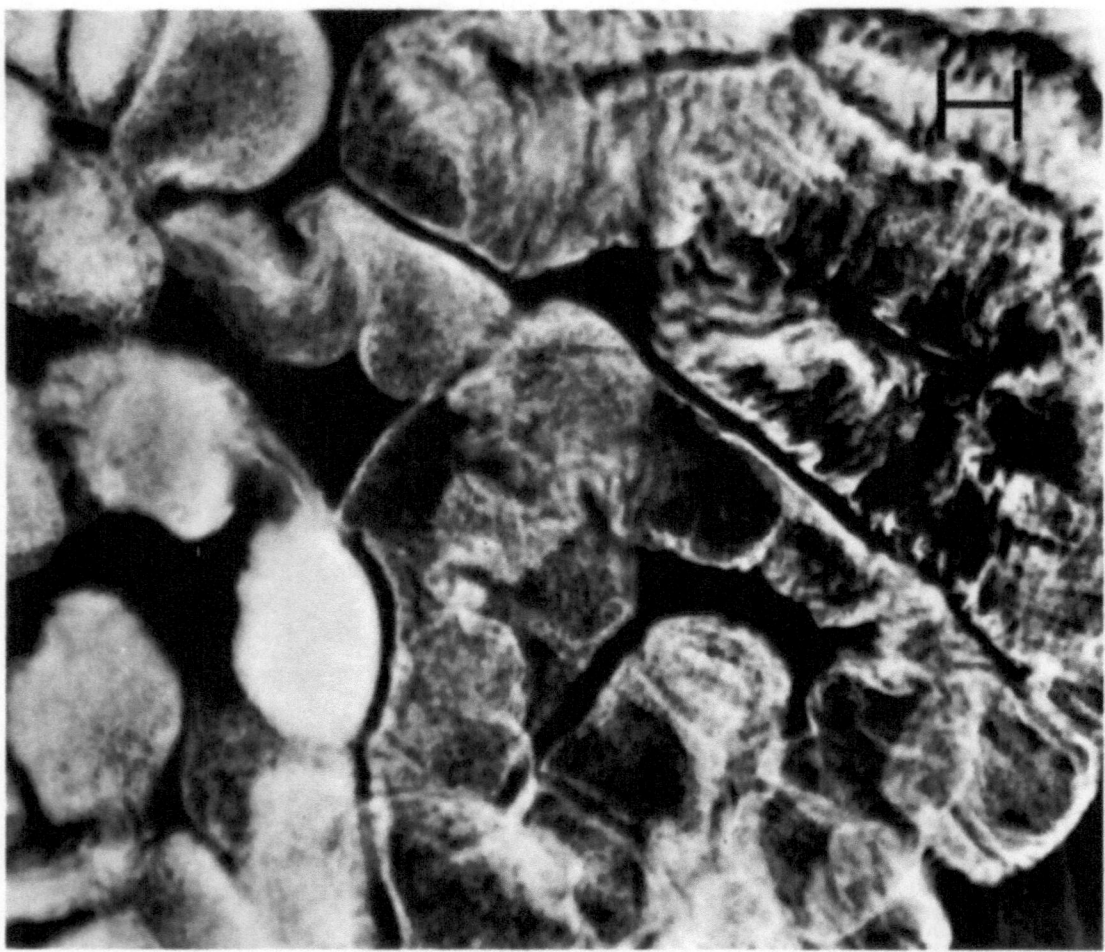

*Fig. 9.54*ʜ. See legend on page 245.

8. Aspecific ulcers

Not all circumscribed strictures in the small intestine can be attributed to skip lesions in Crohn's disease that heal with the formation of fibrous tissue and shriveling. In the ileum and in particular the jejunum, solitary or multiple stenoses are fairly common. They often contain a relatively small ulcer that usually is not visualized on the films. In a large number of cases, the ulcer is annular and is located in the center of the stenotic segment. In other cases it is a normal crater-shaped ulcer that sometimes penetrates quite deep into the intestinal wall. The latter is markedly thickened at the ulcer site due to edema and fibrosis.

There is no general agreement as to what should be identified as an ulcus simplex or aspecific ulcer. Some believe that all ulcerations for which a cau-sative agent cannot be demonstrated belong to this group. Others, including ourselves, feel that this criterium depends too much on the diagnostic experience and capability of different clinics, their laboratories, and medical staff. According to Evert (1948), the aspecific ulcer is small and generally solitary, and is not accompanied by pathological changes elsewhere in the digestive tract.

The frequency of the aspecific ulcer in the small intestine as indicated in the literature is of limited value. It is, however, striking that none of the values listed are very high so that in any case it must be a relatively rare phenomenon. It is interesting that the earliest mention of an aspecific ulcer in the small intestine dates from 1805 (Baillie), and in 1922 the American Richardson described the first jejunal ulcer of this type.

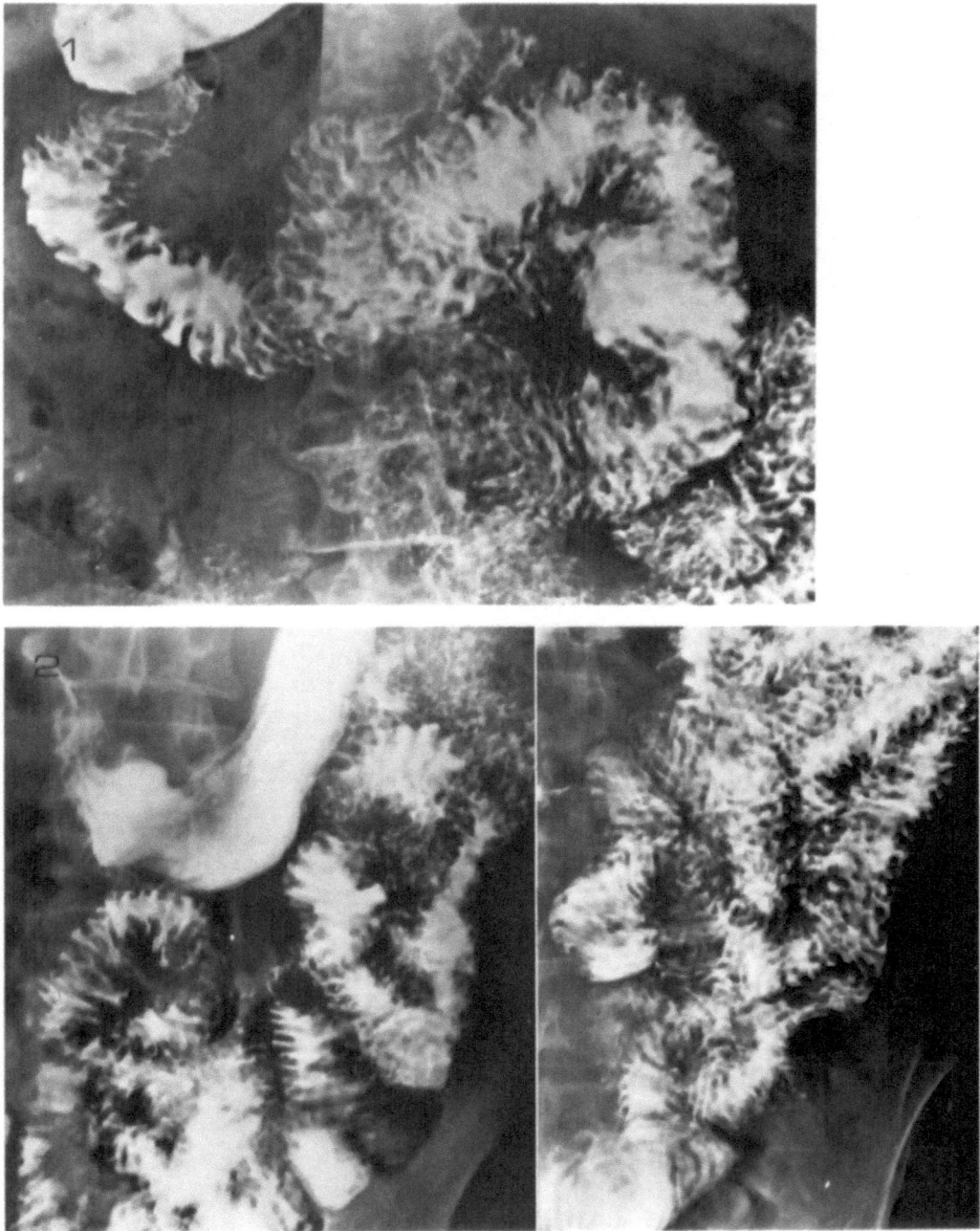

Fig. 9.55A. Conventional transit examination of the small intestine of two patients with Whipple's disease. In both patients a coarse mucosal pattern, dilated jejunal loops, and rapid flocculation of the barium suspension were observed.

8.1. Etiology

There are several causative agents for this type of ulcer. It may be an inflammatory process in the small intestine such as, for instance, a bacillary dysentery, or injury of the mucosa by foreign bodies or the presence of ectopic mucosa from the stomach. Some believe that infections that are not enteral in origin can also cause an enteral ulcus simplex. Thus, for example, pneumococci were cultured from an ulcer in the small intestine of a patient with a pneumococcal infection in the upper respiratory tract. In another patient with furunculosis, an ulcus simplex recurred with each exacerbation of the disease (Ebeling). Rosenow induced

248

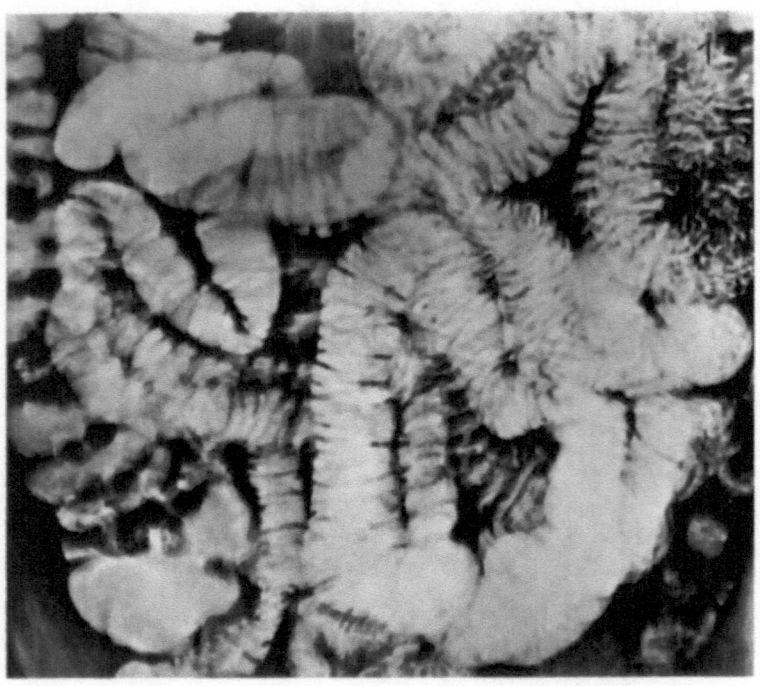

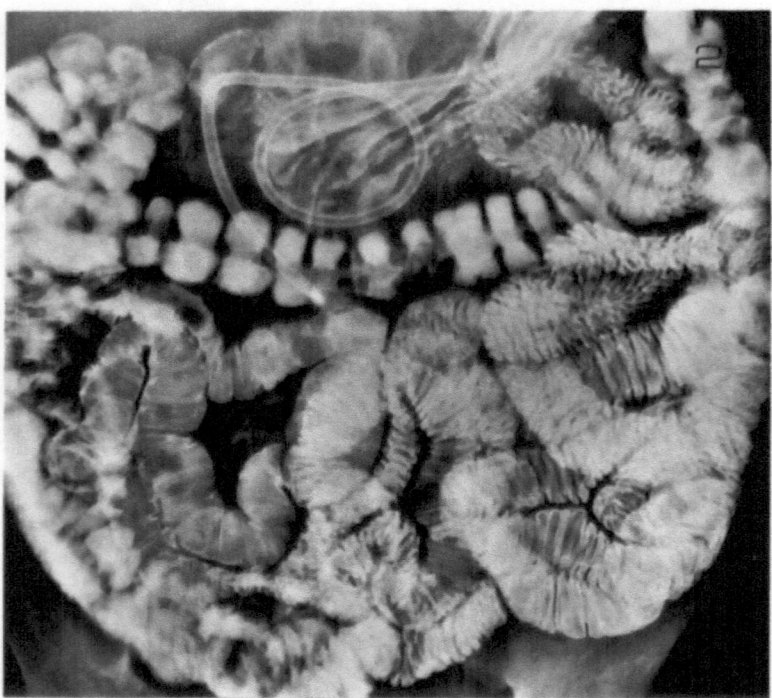

*Fig. 9.55*ʙ. The same patients as seen in fig. 9.55ᴀ, examined by using the enteroclysis method. The mucosal folds now appear normal. Although patient 2 had been treated for this disease during the interim period and patient 1 had not, we have not been able to establish on the basis of our experience that the mucosal pattern will change significantly as a result of therapy.

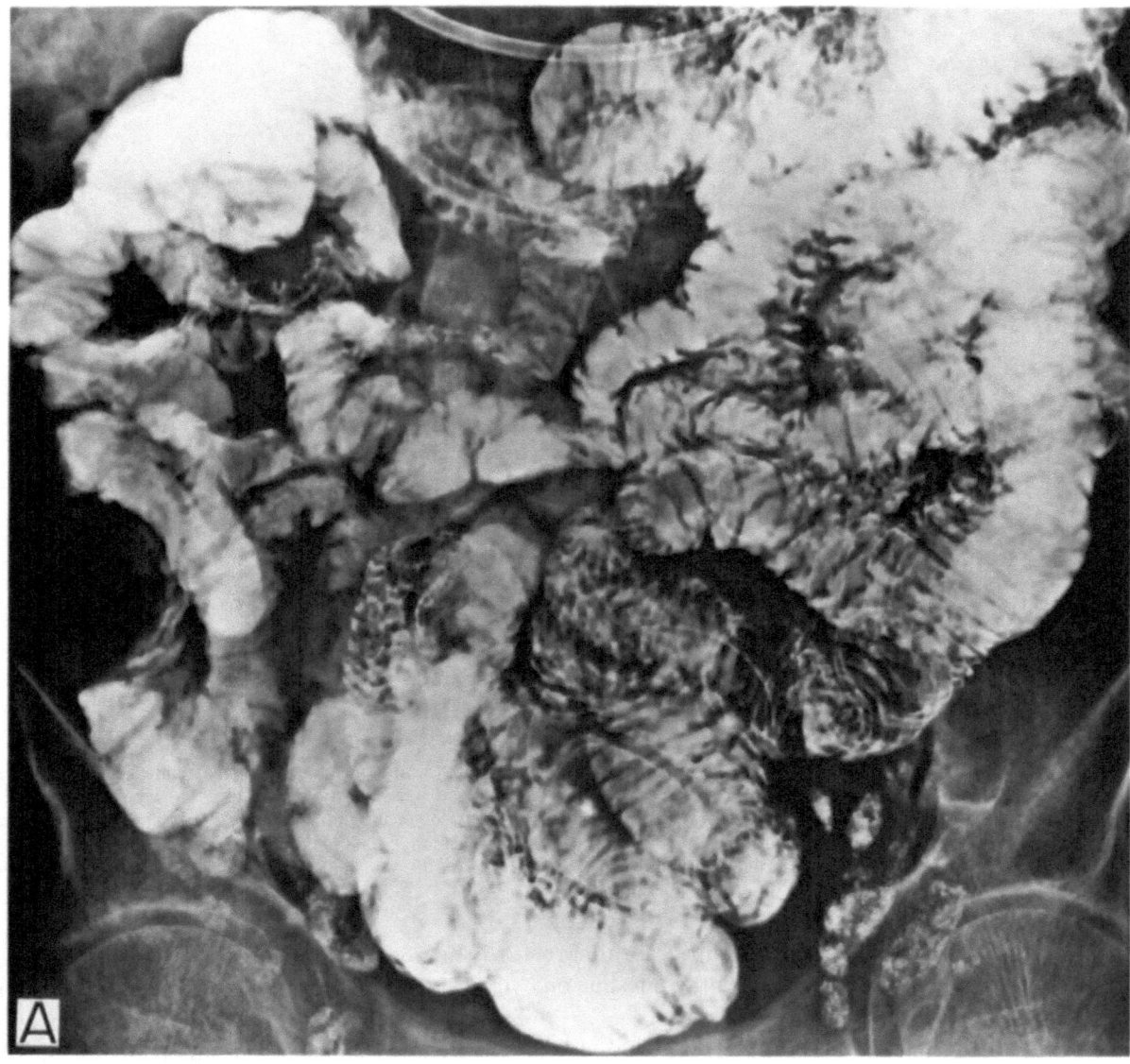

Fig. 9.56. Whipple's disease with increased caliber in the jejunum as the only sign; normal motility and mucosal relief. The probable diagnosis was established on the basis of the roentgen examination. Because motility is normal, the caliber does not increase in the ileum and the barium suspension does not flocculate. Drug-induced atony and celiac disease were considered unlikely.

experimental ulcers with a specific species of streptococcus (Ebeling).

In the proximal part of the intestine, ulcers can develop as a result of a Zollinger-Ellison syndrome, although in that case the cause is generally easily recognized. Strangely enough a marked increase and subsequent decrease in the frequency of the aspecific ulcer, also called the ulcus simplex, has been noted since 1964. This increase in frequency appears to be the result of treatment with enteric-coated KCl tablets, irrespective of the use of diuretics from the thiazide series (Lindenholmer). It is not known precisely how or why these tablets induce ulcers. Presumably the locally enhanced KCl concentration causes vascular lesions, and the ulcerations must be considered ischemic necroses. The possibility that the ulcers develop secondary to caustic injury of the mucosa that then heals with the formation of fibrous tissue can, however, not be ignored entirely. The stenoses are only 0.5–1.0 cm

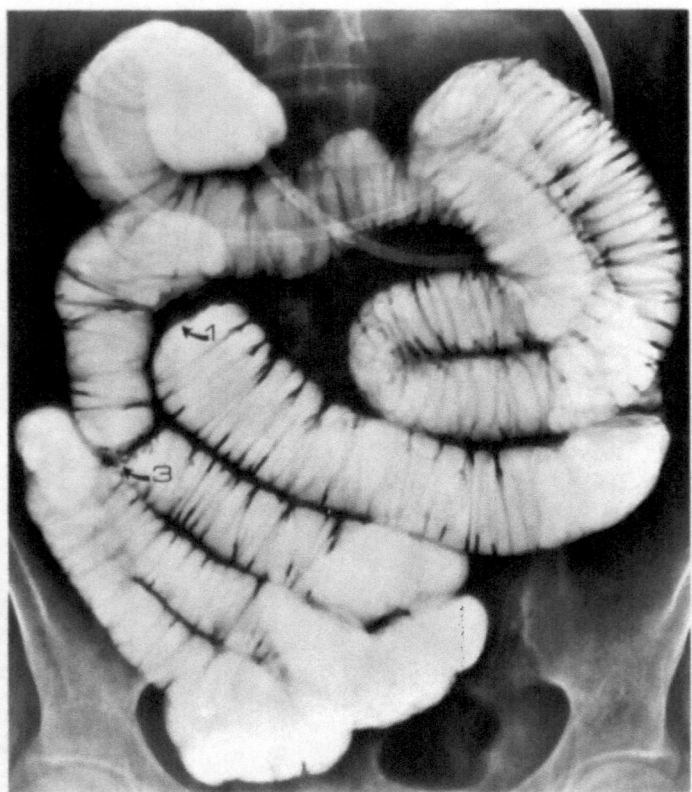

Fig. 9.57. Survey films of a patient who had complained of colic-like pain in the abdomen for years. Dilated intestinal loops with two short annular strictures (1 and 3). The spot films revealed, however, that there were in fact three stenoses that were clearly visible only when the loops were well filled. The dilatation of the loops on the distal side of the third stenosis siggests that more constrictions probably exist further on: this was confirmed at surgery. None of the conventional examinations had ever revealed any abnormalities. This patient had been considered an unconfirmed Crohn's disease case for 20 years and was scheduled for an ileocecal resection. It is obvious that Crohn's disease is not involved at all (see also page 251).

long; they are smooth with an abrupt transition to the more or less funnel-shaped healthy intestine on either side.

Although experiments with rats, dogs, and monkeys have proven that KCl causes ulcers in the small intestine, Jordan believes that there must also be other reasons for this increase in frequency. KCl had been in use many years before 1964 and the decrease in the frequency was noted even before the use of enteric-coated KCl tablets was restricted. Such drug-induced ulcerations satisfy the criterium of Evert and are considered an ulcus simplex by Sturges and Krone. Flendrig, Lubbers, and Van Tongeren believe otherwise. Other medications that can induce ulcers in the small intestine are chlorpromazine, digitalis, and adrenocortical hormones.

Quite often the etiology of these solitary, but sometimes also multiple, ulcerations can no longer be determined.

The most common cause of ulcerations characterized by the formation of fibrotic rings and stenoses that lead to obstruction is probably a disturbance in the blood supply to the involved intestinal segment. Stenoses due to ischemia can be either solitary or multiple. They are generally 2–3 cm long, longer therefore than those caused by other factors.

The vascular anomaly may be the result of an embolus or a thrombosis, a vasculitis, or a pronounced stenosis of the major branches of the celiac trunk and the superior mesenteric artery. The most common cause of vascular insufficiency is arteriosclerosis. A congenital vascular anomaly or an insufficiency due to atrophy of the mucosa, as in celiac disease, is fairly rare.

A somewhat divergent point of view is postulated by Ravdin and Litwin who suggest autodigestion after ischemia. Mecheles considers vascular spasms

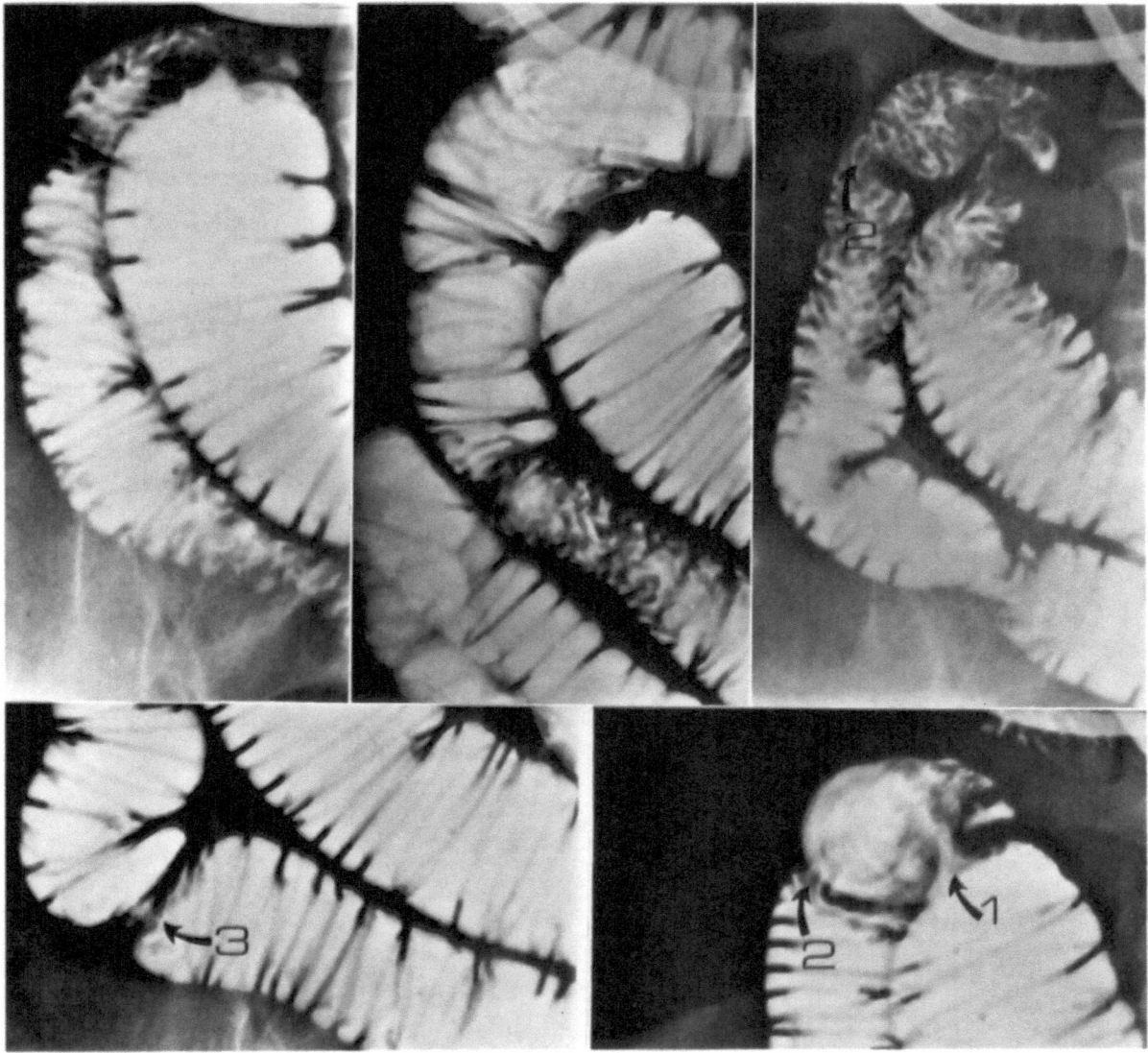

Fig. 9.57. See legend on page 250.

as the causative factor. The observations of Delavierre, Teicher, and Morin support the theory
that the origin is vascular in nature; they noted the
microscopic changes of an endarteritis obliterans.
Goehrs and his associates demonstrated the presence of multiple tiny emboli in the submucosa.

In rats, acute ulcers can be induced by oral or
parenteral administration of a dose of indomethacin equal to 5–80 times that given to man. Here,
too, microscopic local changes in the vessels and
thrombosis were observed. In man, the ulcer will
develop three months to five years after therapy is
initiated. Often, however, no vascular anomalies

can be found at all and if they are observed then it is
difficult or impossible to determine whether they
are primary or secondary.

8.2. Pathology

In about two-thirds of the cases, the ulcus simplex
develops in the ileum (Goehrs and Evert), usually
within 80 cm of the duodenal flexure or within 60
cm of the ileocecal valve (Evert). Delavierre and
Ebeling point out that a second ulcer can often be
found in the stomach, duodenum, ileum, or rectum.
The aspecific ulcer is frequently multiple; it may
even occur in groups of two or three, sometimes

252

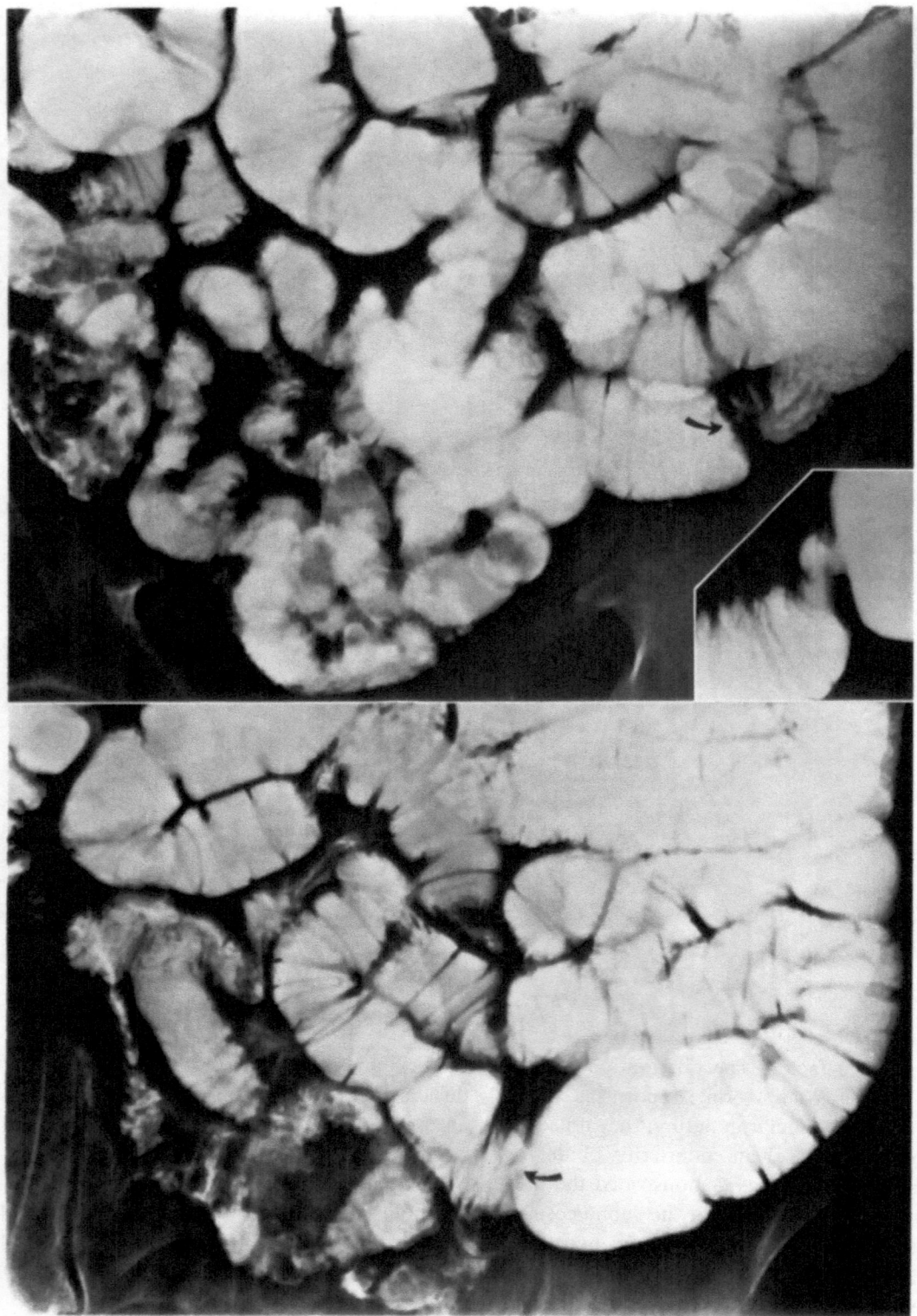

Fig. 9.58. Solitary ulcer with pronounced prestenotic dilatation in the lower left quadrant. The patient had complained of attacks of abdominal pain for many years although abnormalities had never been demonstrated. Because of a prestenotic dilatation on one of the x-rays not shown here, it was assumed that there might be one more ulcer in the upper right quadrant; the surgeon, however, found six!

even more (Holtzwessig). If several ulcers are found, then the various stages of healing can also be observed. According to some authors (Litwin and Dowdle), the ulcus simplex is usually located opposite the mesentery. Others (Watson and Evert) believe that this relationship, which implies a vascular lesion, is not clearly evident. Dockerty described a number of cases in which a thrombosis of the small mesenteric arteries could be demonstrated. Aspecific ulcerations are small and clearly circumscribed; they penetrate deep into the mucosa and the underlying layers, and there is little or no inflammatory reaction in the surrounding areas. If a stricture is evident, then fibrosis in the submucosa has advanced out of all proportion to the size of the ulcer. In such a case, some edema of the submucosa may be seen on the proximal side of the ulcer.

Microscopically the ulcus simplex resembles the peptic ulcer in the stomach or duodenum. The ulcer floor, which is smooth, is covered with a thin layer of fibrin and leucocytes. The surrounding epithelium is not involved and the rim of the ulcer is sharply defined. The surface area of the damaged mucosa is greater than that of the underlying layers, thus the margins of the ulcer decrease stepwise with the depth. In the event of perforation, the opening in the serosa is often as small as the head of a pin (Ebeling). The ulcer floor itself consists of granulation tissue with lymphocytic and plasmacellular infiltrates. The inflammatory reaction involves all layers and spreads beyond the ulcer. Beneath the granulation tissue is the collagenous connective tissue that will ultimately cause the stenosis.

8.3. Symptomology

In contrast to the pathology, the symptomology of the ulcus simplex is not straightforward. In some cases the aspecific ulcer mimics a duodenal ulcer, but in other cases there are practically no complaints. The ulcer is found predominantly in patients between 30 and 50 years of age, although it has been reported in patients from 0 to 83 years of age (Ravdin). In men under 50 years of age, the ulcers generally are localized in the terminal segment of the ileum. The ulcus simplex occurs in men more often than in women with a frequency of 2:1 (Dowdle) or 3:1 (Evert, Dockery, Watson, and Ebeling). The complaints can vary greatly and are unreliable for diagnosis. They are determined main-

ly by the localization of the lesion as well as the occurrence of complications such as strictures, bleeding, and perforations. If the ulcer is in the ileum, there will be few or no complaints. If the ulcer lies in the jejunum, the complaints will resemble those for a duodenal ulcer; this becomes more pronounced as the distance from Treitz's ligament decreases (Litwin). There is then a gnawing postprandial pain, often around the navel, that occurs later with respect to a meal than that of a duodenal ulcer.

Formerly, bleeding and perforation of these deep ulcers led to a high mortality of about 50%. The symptoms of these complications, especially the frequently occurring obstruction, should therefore be considered important. The patient complains of colic-like pains, sometimes accompanied by vomiting, diarrhea, and eventually loss of weight. A partial obstruction need not always cause clinical phenomena; on the other hand, sometimes even a swollen intestinal loop can be palpated (Sturges).

Occasionally there will be hemorrhage, but usually only the fecal benzidine reactions are positive (Evert) and anemia may develop. The symptoms of a perforation are similar to those of a perforating gastric ulcer, although the initial pain may be localized lower in the abdomen.

According to many authors (Ebeling, Goehrs and Ravdin), the duration of the complaints can vary greatly – from a few weeks to many years if perforation does not occur. A perforation incidentally can occur quite suddenly without any previous indications that such a possibility exists. According to the literature, the perforation is sometimes so minute that it is not discovered during surgery (Litwin).

In 1927, Ravdin pointed out that in the event of obstruction or perforation in the digestive tract, it is essential to consider the small intestine as well. If a gastric or duodenal ulcer cannot be located during surgery, then the jejunum and ileum should be inspected carefully. Sturges emphasizes that in connection with the increasing aggressive use of drugs, complications in the small intestine must be considered in every case of an acute abdomen. In order to prevent these complications, an early diagnosis is very important. It has been seen in the past that the rarity of this disorder and the divergent symptomology make a preoperative diagnosis of a prim-

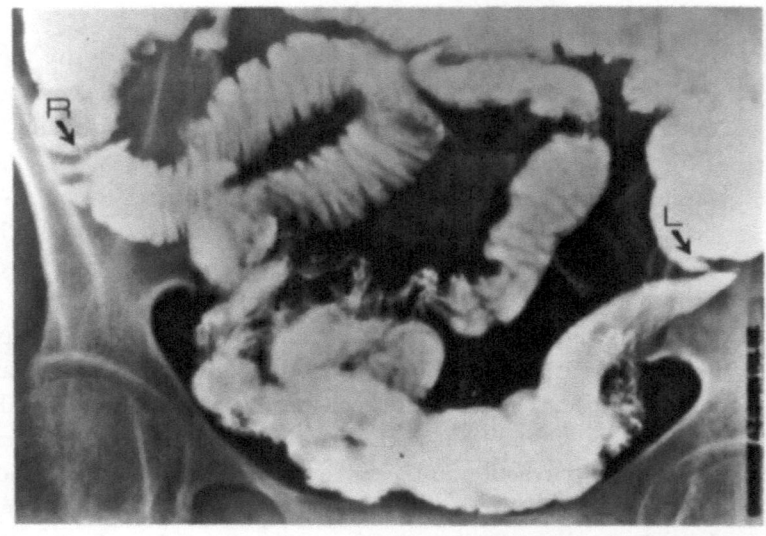

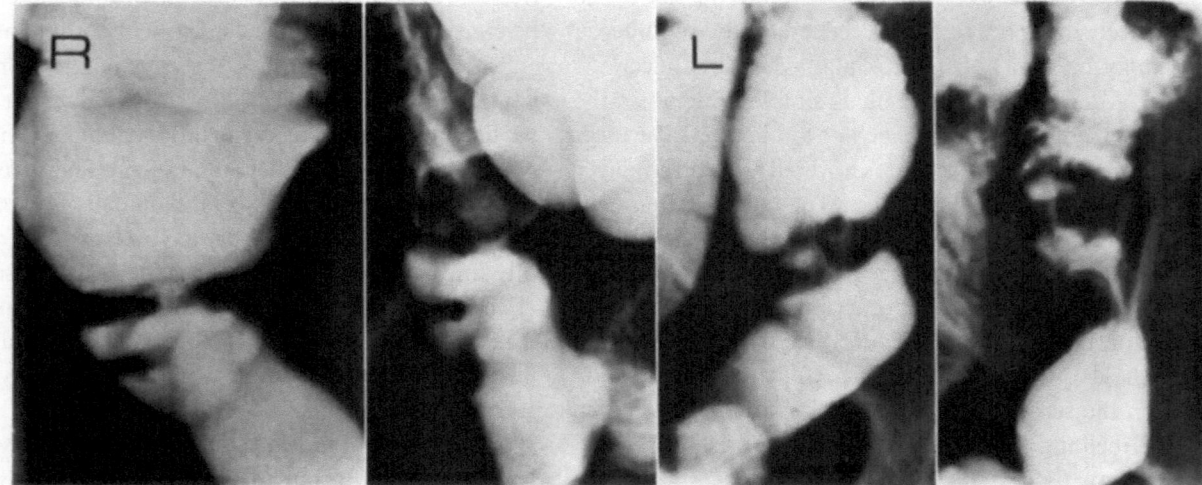

Fig. 9.59. A patient who complained of colic in the upper abdomen several times a week. The survey films showed a constant prestenotic dilatation on both sides. They appeared from the spot films to be due to short constricting aspecific ulcers. Strangely enough the intestinal mucosa on the distal side of the left-hand stenosis in particular is atrophied so that a primary vascular disease or damage due to corrosion involving a larger segment than normal is possible. There are neither radiological nor clinical indications of Crohn's disease. Because of a (too) low gastric acid concentration, the patient had taken pep-acid tablets over a prolonged period in the past.

ary ulcer of the small intestine exceedingly difficult.

As a result of the greatly improved examination techniques of the past few years, these aspecific ulcers are being found with ever-increasing frequency before the patient goes to the operating table, so the mortality has become quite low. It is sometimes noted during surgery that the stenosis may have been caused in part by a pronounced muscular spasm. Pathological-anatomical studies show that in these cases there is an active ulcer and a marked hypertrophy of the prestenotic muscles. Although the patient's complaints, colic-like pain and eventually also vomiting after meals, clearly indicate an obstruction, experience has shown that

this diagnosis has often not even been considered.

An ulcus simplex should be considered in the following cases:

1) Complaints resembling those of a duodenal ulcer without roentgenological abnormalities in the stomach or duodenum.
2) Gastrointestinal hemorrhage without abnormalities in the esophagus, stomach, duodenum, or colon.
3) Gastrointestinal bleeding or intermittent partial obstruction with attacks of colic-like abdominal pain or decreased peristalsis and dilatation of the intestinal loops.

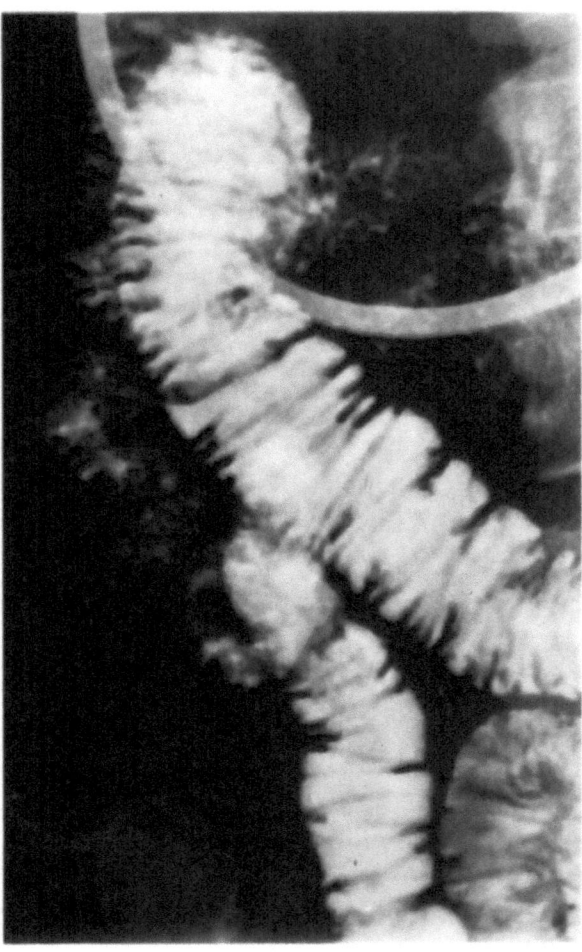

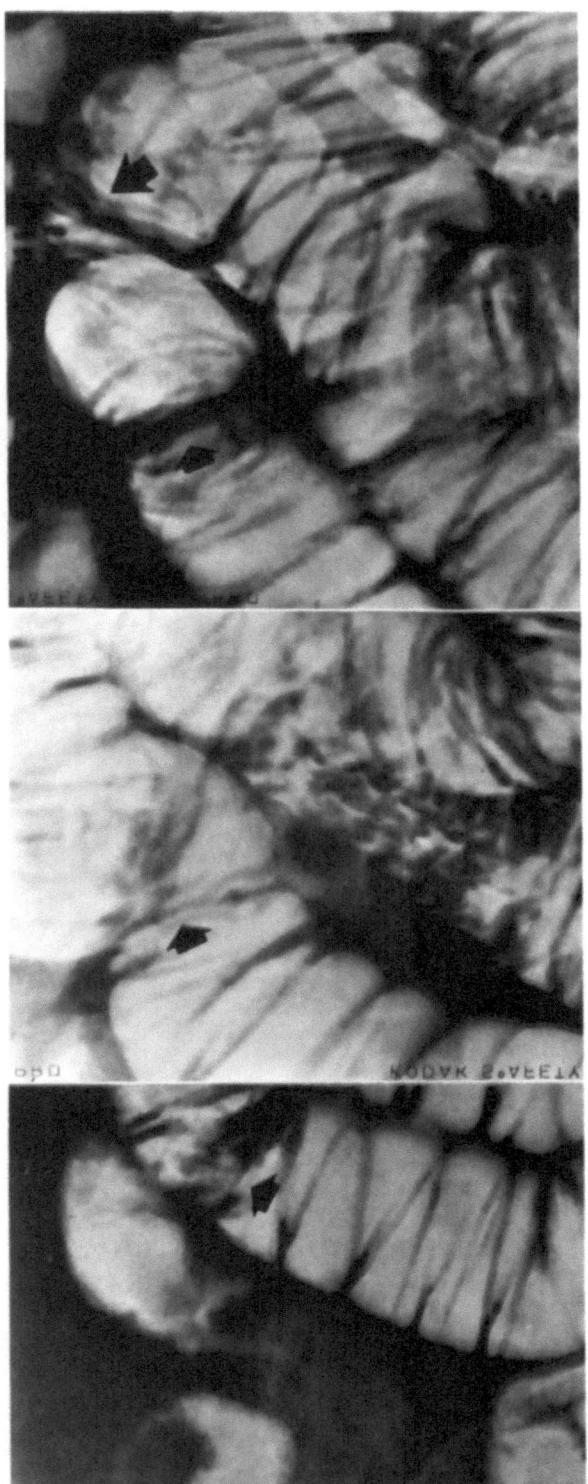

Fig. 9.60. The patient had suffered from colic-like attacks of pain in the abdomen during the past year. Seven years ago, diuretics had been prescribed. In the upper right quadrant is a solitary stricture, and possibly there is a second one on the proximal side ±3 cm further on. The stricture was not observed during the examination itself so that no spot films of this region were made. Unfortunately, subsequent developments are unknown.

4) Peritonitis due to perforation although no perforated ulcer can be found.

8.4. Radiodiagnosis

If a roentgenological examination is carried out according to the enteroclysis method, it is not difficult to establish the diagnosis (figs. 9.57–9.60). With this method the fluid is forced into the intestinal loops and striking prestenotic dilatations will develop. If this dilatation is overlooked during

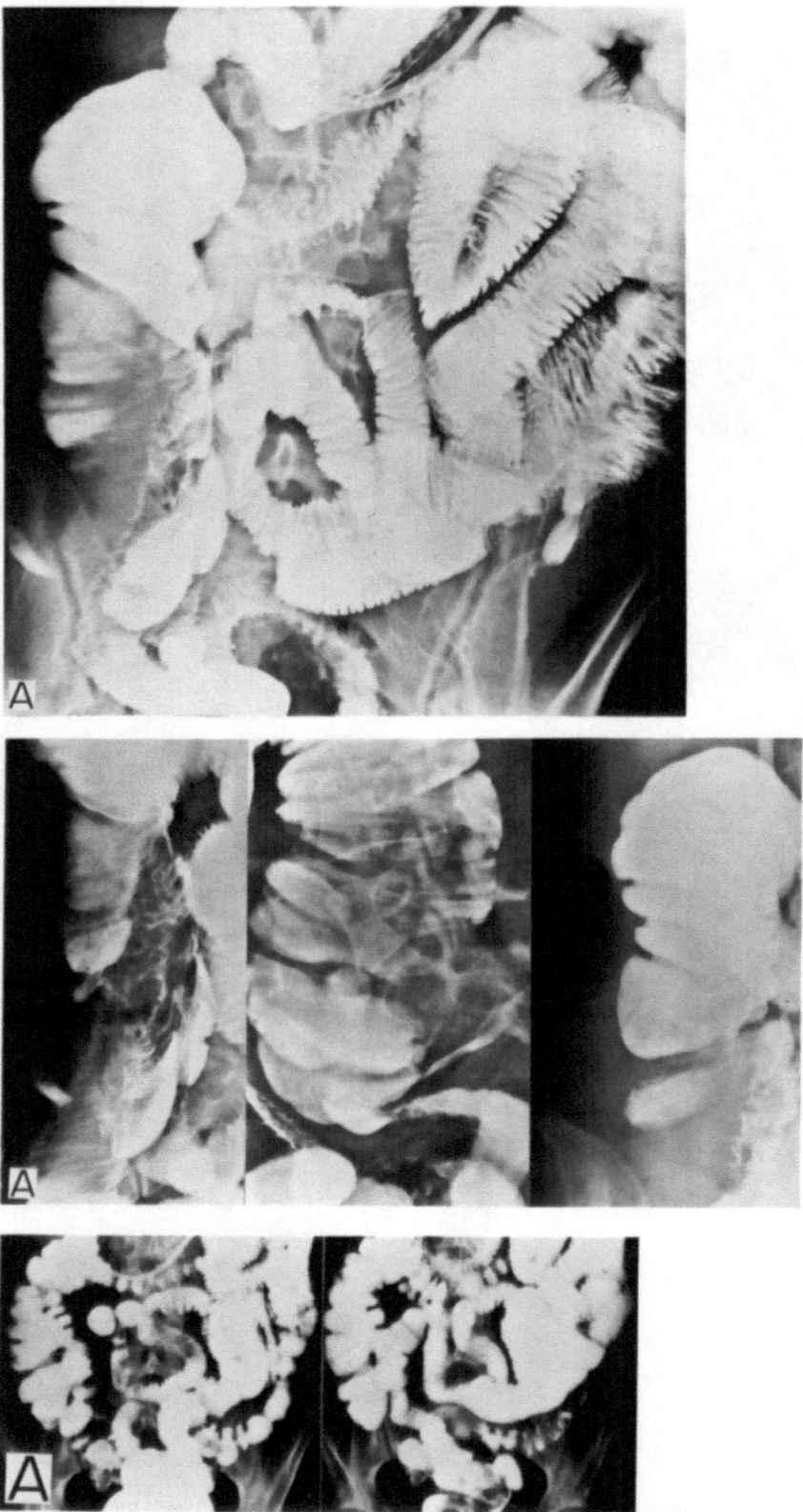

*Fig. 9.61*A. A very sick middle-aged woman. The clinical signs indicated an inflammatory process. On the plain film, the process appears to be localized predominantly in the cecal region with pronounced spread into the mesentery in the lower left quadrant as well as in the middle of the abdomen (top). There are no signs of destruction. Since the appendix is displaced but appears otherwise normal (middle), an appendicular infiltrate can be excluded. To the right of the ascending colon is an air configuration indicative of an abscess (middle right). Conservative treatment led to rapid recovery. A subsequent follow-up examination showed that all abnormalities had disappeared (bottom). According to the results of a laparotomy à froid, the abnormalities could be attributed to an ovariocele abscess. (Courtesy of G.N. Hardy – Sittard.)

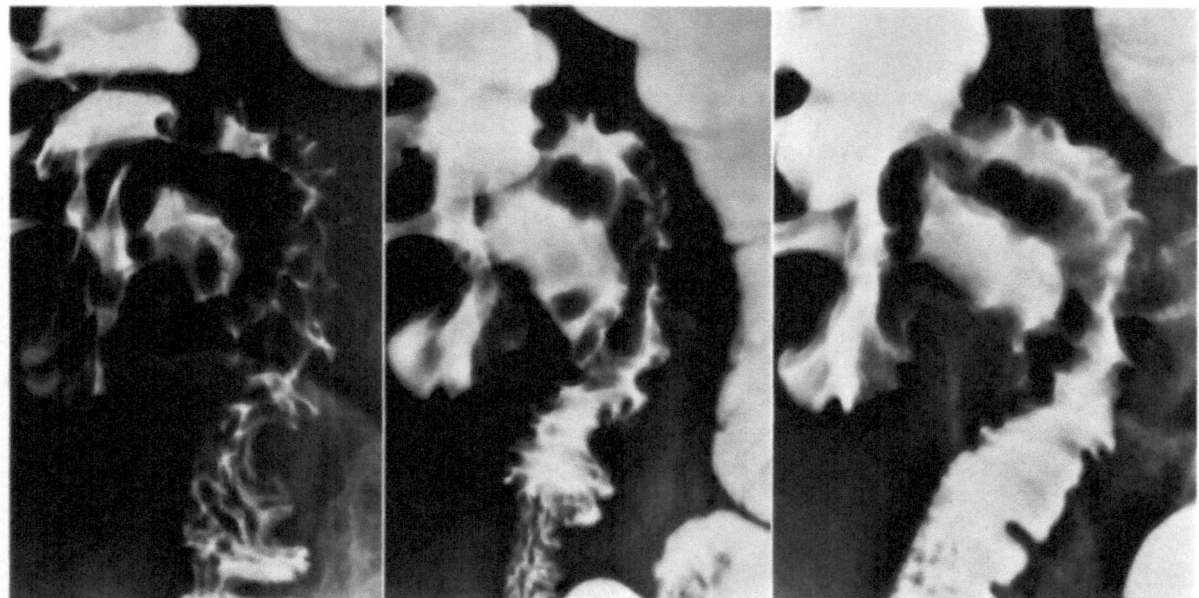

*Fig. 9.61*B. Infiltrate of unknown origin in ileocecal region. Surgery revealed that the large oval accumulation of contrast medium was an ulcer crater. No indications of appendicitis or Crohn's disease.

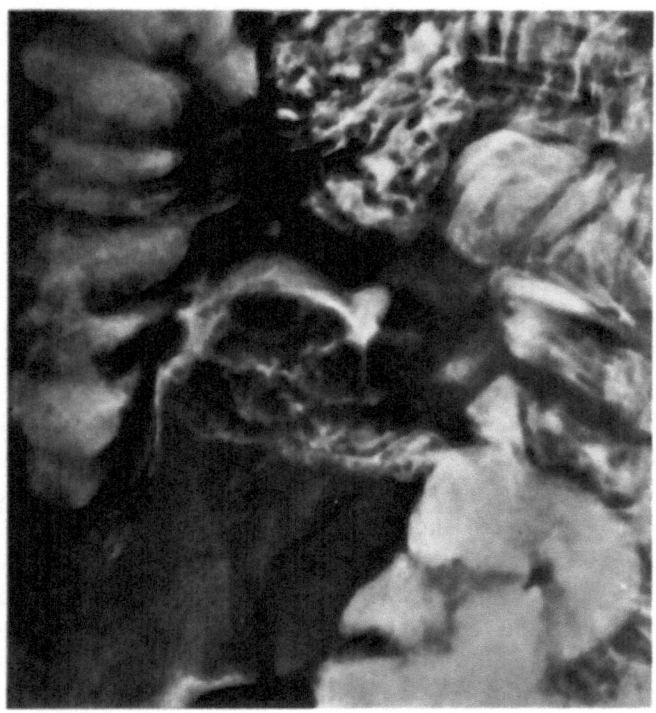

Fig. 9.62. Infiltrate in ileocecal region due to inflamed Meckel's diverticulum. The correct diagnosis was not established radiologically.

the examination and is discovered later during careful reexamination of the films, a new examination should be carried out in order to obtain further information concerning the nature of the stenosis.

A proximal stenosis is sometimes so pronounced that the barium suspension can barely pass through it; as a result, the identification of more distal stenoses is severely hampered. It may then be necessary to perform a retrograde enteroclysis examination via the colon. It is important to remember that even if only one prestenotic dilatation can be seen, several strictures may be present. The dilatation may be visible only at the most proximal stenosis or the most constricting of the existing stenoses. Since fluid flow has already been reduced by a more proximal stenosis, it will pass easily through the distal stenoses. Therefore it is necessary

258

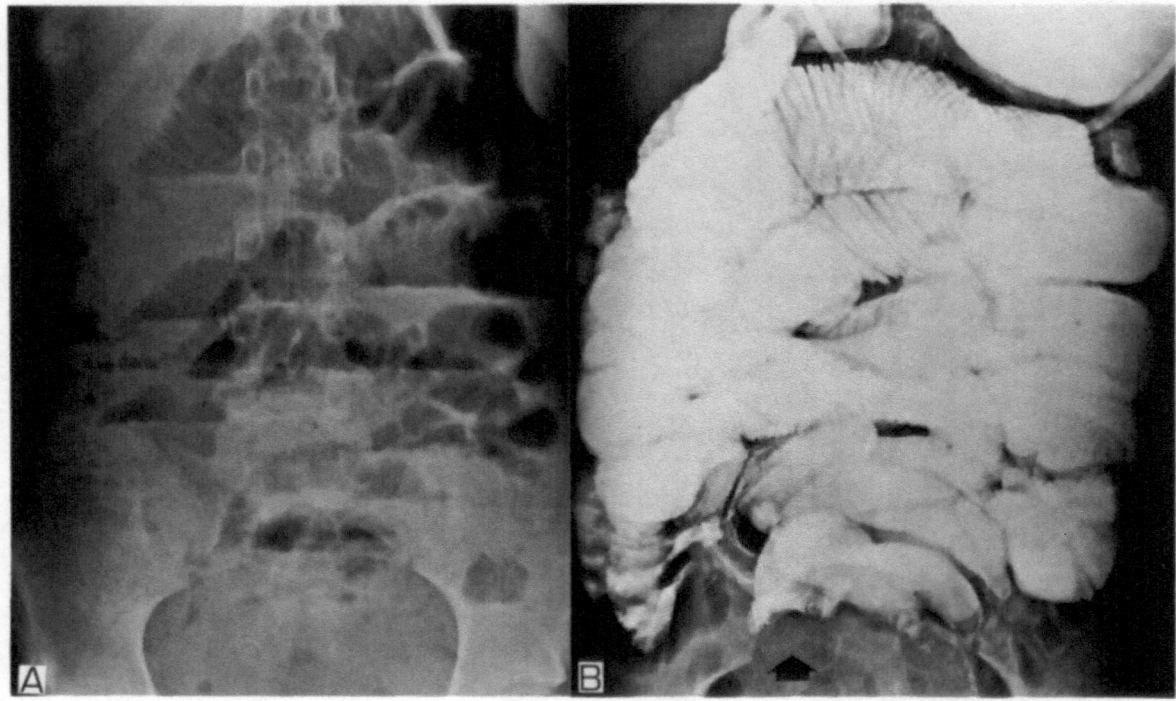

*Fig. 9.63*A–C. Ileus as a result of an appendicular infiltrate. The patient received 800 ml of barium suspension, s.g. 1.3; 800 ml barium suspension, s.g. 1.2; and 800 ml of water. Examination lasted 45 min. Conservative treatment resulted in complete recovery. (See also page 259.)

that the surgeon examine the entire small intestine carefully during the operation. If he does not do so, there is considerable chance that one or more stenoses will be left behind. The patient's complaints will continue or recur within a short period of time. A new roentgenological examination will then show a prestenotic dilatation at another location.

Aspecific stenoses and ulcerations in the jejunum or ileum are usually very short and can therefore be distinguished from those caused by tumors and those due to Crohn's disease. In the case of a tumor, the margins are usually irregular and a space-occupying process can be seen. Crohn's disease usually involves much longer and irregularly defined segments and often similar ulcerations and stenoses are localized elsewhere.

9. Appendicular infiltrates

This term refers not only to the infiltrates that originate in the appendix. It is also used in the broader sense to indicate all infiltrative processes in the right lower quadrant that must be included in the differential diagnosis, such as those originating from the ovaries (fig. 9.61A). After all, inflammatory processes do develop in the lower right quadrant of the abdomen that cannot be explained (fig. 9.61B). Obviously in such cases a process originating in the appendix or in a Meckel's diverticulum should be considered first (fig. 9.62). Although these assumptions frequently turn out to be correct (figs. 9.63 and 9.64), it is not always true. In the course of several weeks, sometimes even months, the infiltration process heals with or without conservative or symptomatic therapy. Often it disappears on its own without significant persistent abnormalities. The radiologically visible abnormalities are usually localized in the last 10–15 cm of the ileum and the medial wall of the cecum (fig. 9.65). If there is a definite space-occupying infiltrate, the abnormalities are more pronounced. The entire lower end of the cecum may then be involved and the deformation of the distal ileum can be so marked that the normal anatomy of this part of the

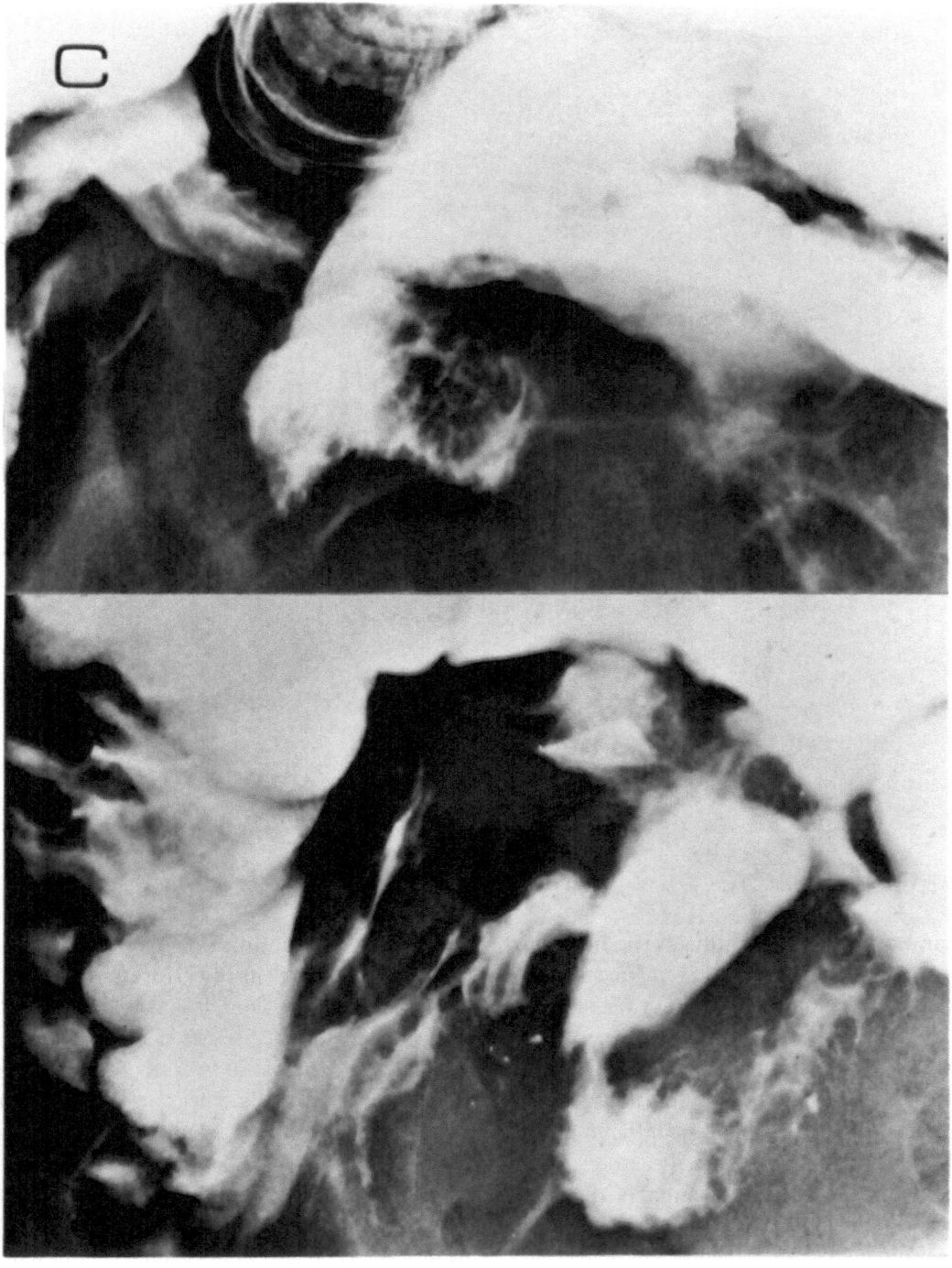

*Fig. 9.63*C. See legend on page 258.

260

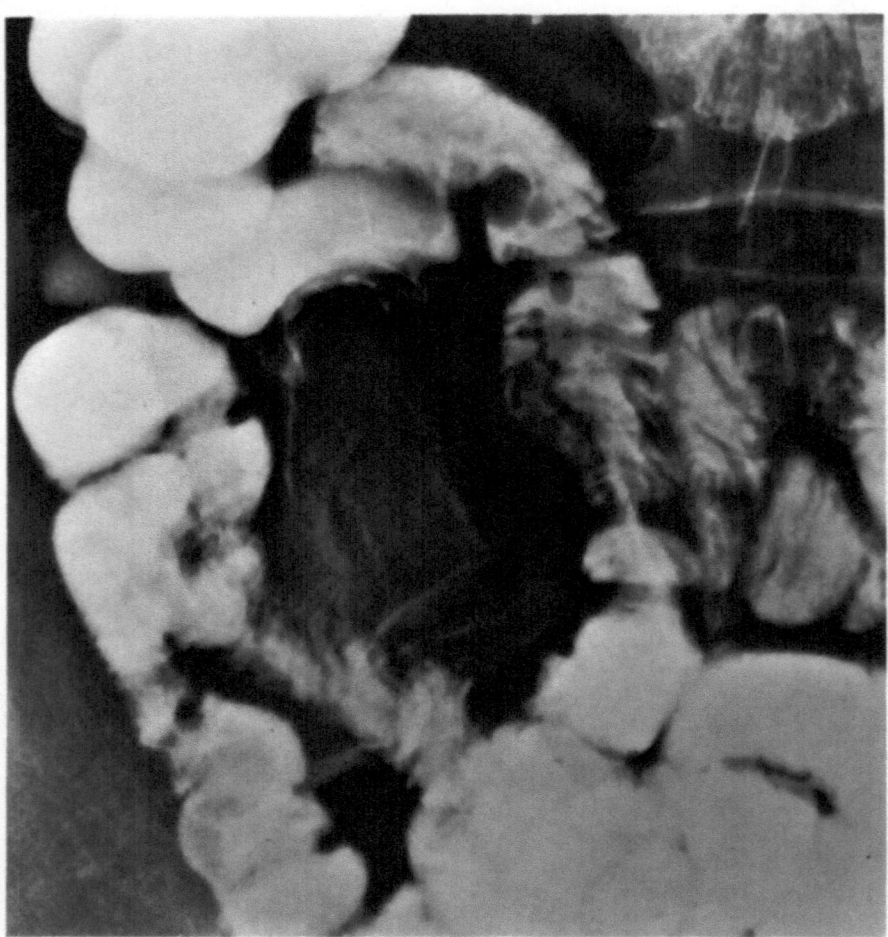

*Fig. 9.63*D. Appendicular infiltrate that can be diagnosed with little difficulty.

intestine can no longer be identified. The mucosal folds in the distal ileum, however, remain more or less unchanged; they may show only a stretched appearance. When there is a disease of the distal ileum itself, then in particular the mucosa shows clear abnormalities but there is no deformity of the ileum. A misleading factor is that the inflammatory process can be localized elsewhere. It can occur in the upper abdomen, if the appendix is directed upward, and in the lateral flank if the cecum is mobile and is directed toward the median plane (fig. 9.66).

Frequently an impression of the spread of the process can be obtained from the normal survey film of the abdomen. This is either because the gas in the intestinal lumen can be used to visualize the margins of that lumen or because a space-occupying soft tissue shadow contains no gas or appears abnormal (fig. 9.67R).

Of course the infiltration abnormalities can sometimes cause an ileus or perforation into the free abdominal cavity or Douglas' pouch (fig. 9.67s).

Infiltrations or abcesses as a result of an amebiasis are rare, at least in western European countries. However, if the patient is a so-called migrant worker from one of the Mediterranean or South American countries or has had an abdominal infection during a stay in the tropics, this possibility should be considered (fig. 9.68). Another phenomenon that is observed almost exclusively in patients from Dutch harbor towns along the North Sea, where the herring catch is brought in and prepared for consumption, are the extensive infiltrates with fistulization caused by the herringworm (fig. 9.69). Today, salting of the herring, which kills the worms, is mandatory so that this delicacy can be consumed without fear of complications.

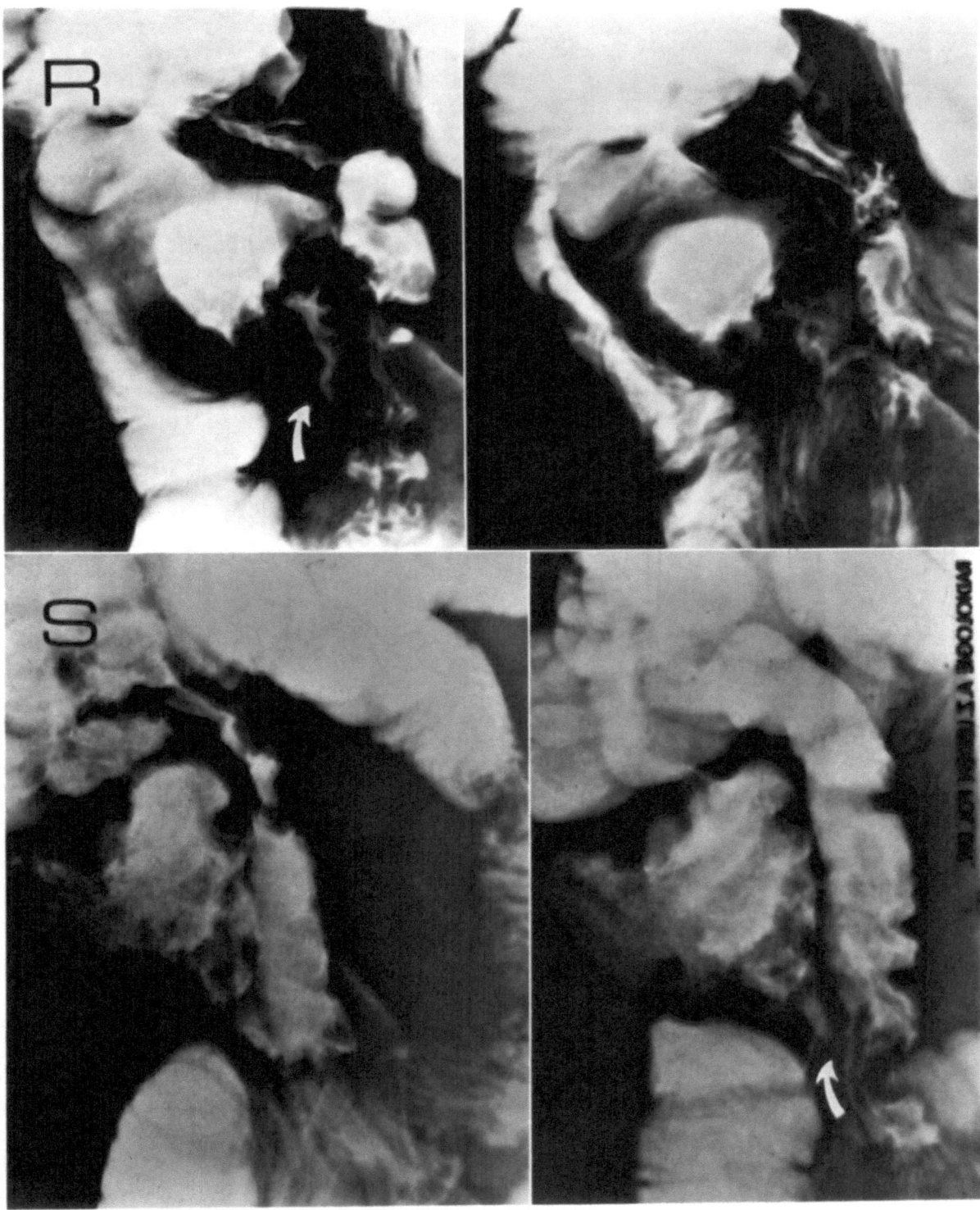

Fig. 9.64. (R) Infiltrate in ileocecal region with a large deposit of contrast medium, similar to that seen in fig. 9.61. This presumably is a sacculation in the cecum with an ileal loop coiled around it. Short irregular filling of the appendix. (S) Two months later the infiltrate has disappeared and the filling of the appendix, although not longer, is more regular. Ileal loop is fused with lowest part of the cecum.

262

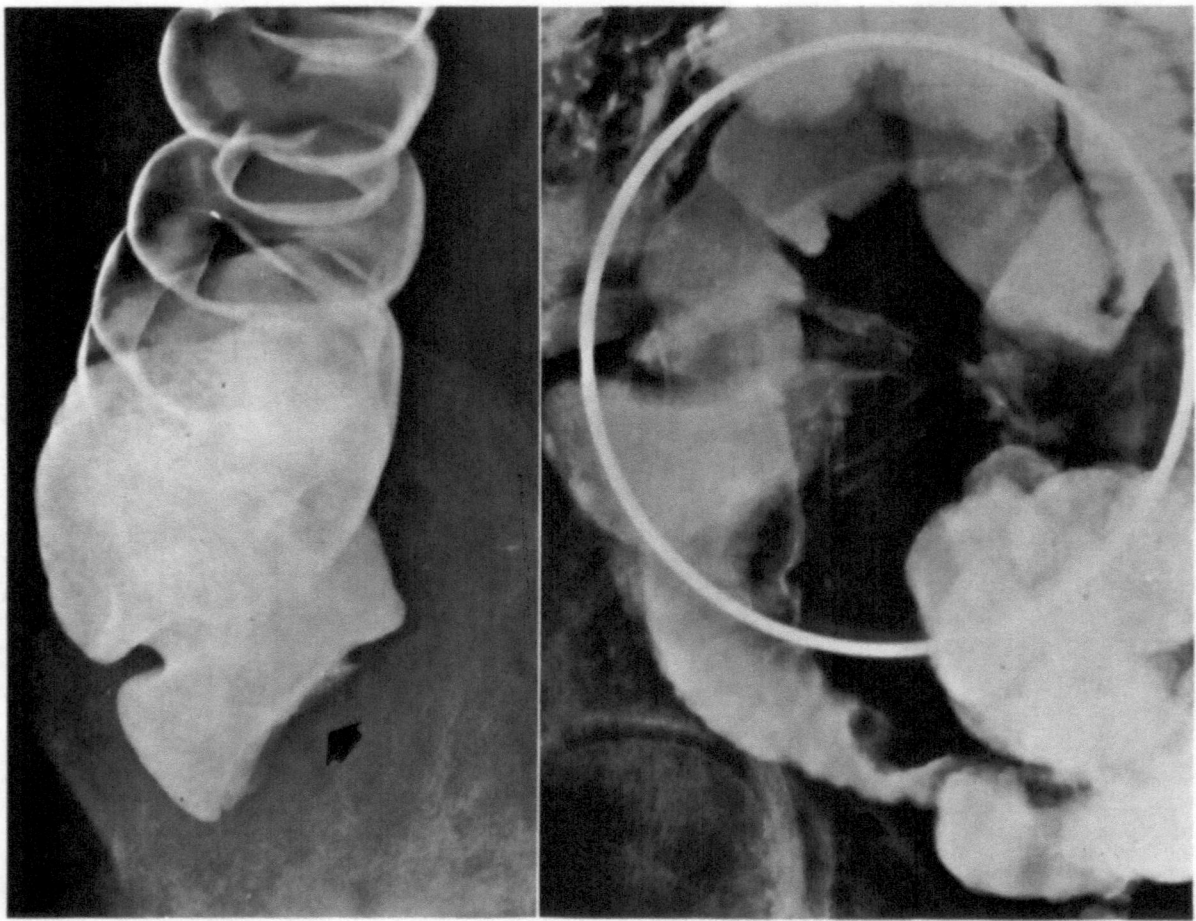

*Fig. 9.65*A. Large appendicular infiltrate, causing impressions on the medial site of the cecum and the ileal loops in the lower right quadrant, that led to a moderate obstruction of the small intestine. Appendix is not filled here but may be visible over a short distance in other cases. A tumor must also be included in the differential diagnosis.

10. Zollinger-Ellison disease

In Zollinger-Ellison's disease, solitary or multiple adenomas or slow-growth carcinomas involving the gastrin-secreting cells in the pancreatic islands of Langerhans cause markedly increased secretion of gastric acid.

The mucous membrane in the various parts of the digestive tract cannot withstand this large quantity of gastric acid. Therefore, the mucosal folds are broadened in the jejunum as well as the stomach and the duodenum. This disease should be considered a chemical enteritis. Ulcers with secondary stenosis can be found in the jejunum and the distal

half of the duodenum similar to those that develop as a result of the action of gastric acid on esophageal mucosa. Because of the high acidity in the duodenum the enzymes for the digestion of fats and proteins are inactivated and steatorrhea develops. In other cases there is only 'intestinal hurry' and a watery diarrhea. During the radiological examination, the unusually strong tendency toward flocculation of the contrast fluid is striking. In some cases the loops of the small intestine are highly dilated (figs. 9.70 and 9.71). The cause of this dilatation is not clear. It is questionable whether the increased fluid secretion to neutralize the excess acid and the increase in bulk resulting from dis-

263

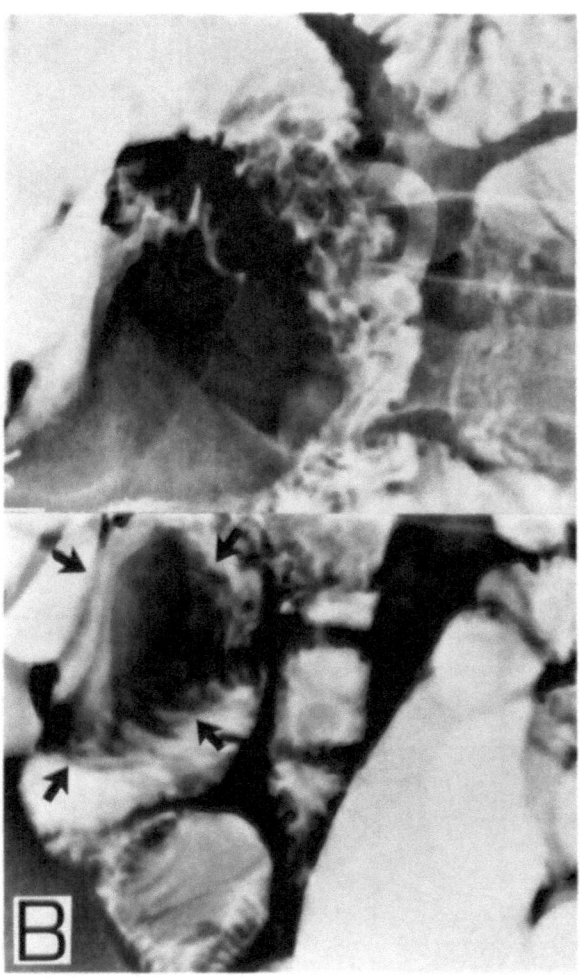

*Fig. 9.65*B. Oval empty spaces in the middle of the lower pole of the cecum. Since the appendix does not contain contrast medium, an appendicular infiltrate was considered. In the course of several months no clinical evidence could be found to support this finding; eventually the diagnosis was confirmed surgically.

turbed digestion provide a complete explanation. The exceedingly small gastrin-secreting cell groups are usually multiple, and in addition metastases to the liver or other glands occur. These can be demonstrated during the examination in more than half of the cases. Local excision is impossible and gastric resection is the only possible therapy.

11. Radiological manifestations of serum protein disorders

11.1. Protein-losing enteropathy

Edema of the ankles and a hypoalbuminemia, with or without diarrhea, are sometimes the first symptoms indicating a disease of the small intestine. Since hypoalbuminemia is often accompanied by an edematous swelling of the mucosal folds in the jejunum, it is important to be able to recognize this radiological sign (fig. 9.72).

Some protein loss through transudation of tissue fluid is a physiological phenomenon in the digestive tract. As a rule, however, these proteins are also resorbed. Loss of proteins from the digestive tract can be caused by a disturbed protein synthesis or pronounced leakage of proteins, due to various processes inside as well as outside the digestive tract. The resorption is either incomplete or the liver cannot handle the increased supply.

Protein loss can, when synthesis is unimpaired, also be congenital. Then the discharge of lymph in the mesentry is disturbed because of hypoplasia of the lymphatic channels. Such a hypoplasia is also accompanied by underdeveloped lymphatic channels in the extremities. In contrast the lymphatic channels in the intestinal mucosa are clearly dilated. On the roentgenogram it is noted that the mucosal folds are broadened, the intestinal loops are slightly dilated, and the spaces between the loops are somewhat larger due to the thicker intestinal wall (see fig. 8.8). In most cases, protein loss is acquired as a result of various inflammatory processes in the small intestine, Whipple's disease, or diverse tumors. Portal hypertension, disturbed liver function, cardiac insufficiency, or disturbed kidney function can also lead to an elevated protein loss.

11.2. Immunoglobulin deficiency

Much less common than albumin loss is a disturbed gamma globulin synthesis. Gamma globulins seem to play an important role in the immunologically determined humoral immunity against numerous, sometimes definitely malignant, diseases. Humeral immunity must be distinguished from cellular immunity. The former is connected with the so-called immunoglobulins, several types of which have now been identified as IgA, IgM, IgG, etc. A deficiency of these three types of gamma globulins can occur

264

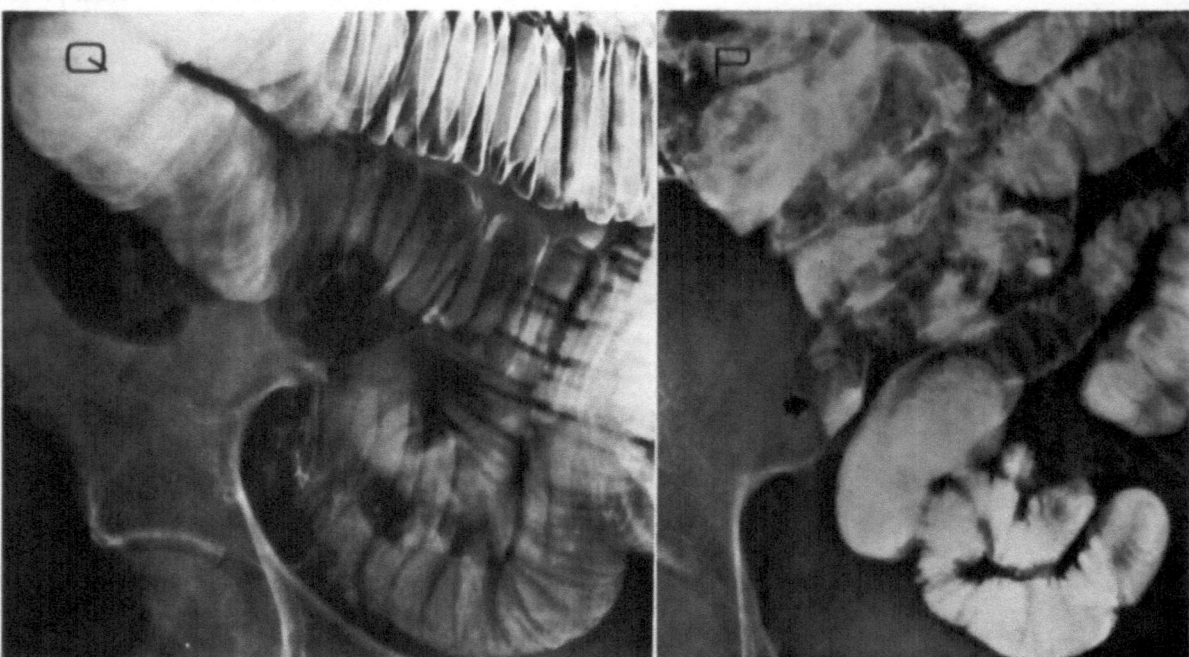

Fig. 9.66. (Q) Ileus as a result of an obstructing infiltrate in the lower right quadrant. (P) Three months later there is a partial dilatation or a extravazation of a perforated appendix visible (arrow). Surgery: retrocecal appendicular infiltrate + abscess.

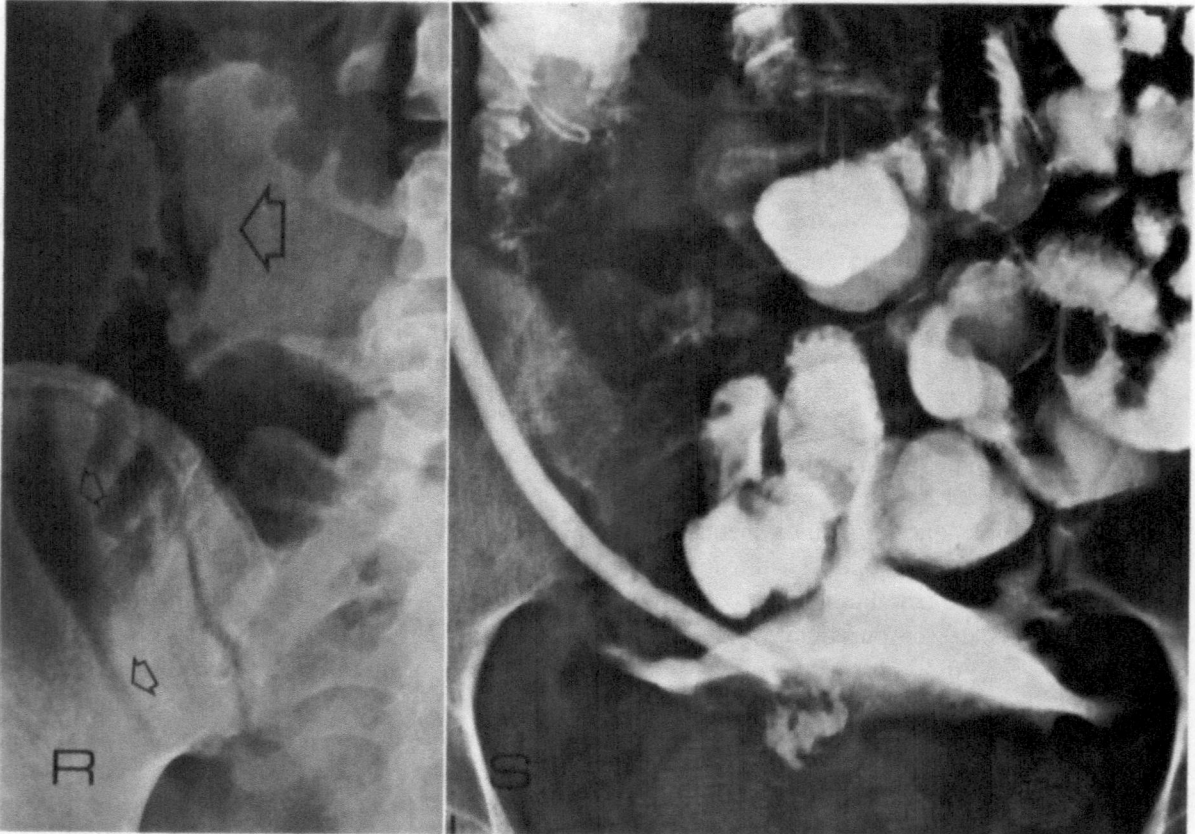

Fig. 9.67. (R) Pathological gas configurations in the ascending colon and lateral abdominal wall due to a high appendicular infiltrate with perforation to the retroperitoneal space. (s) In the postoperative phase there was also perforation into Douglas' pouch.

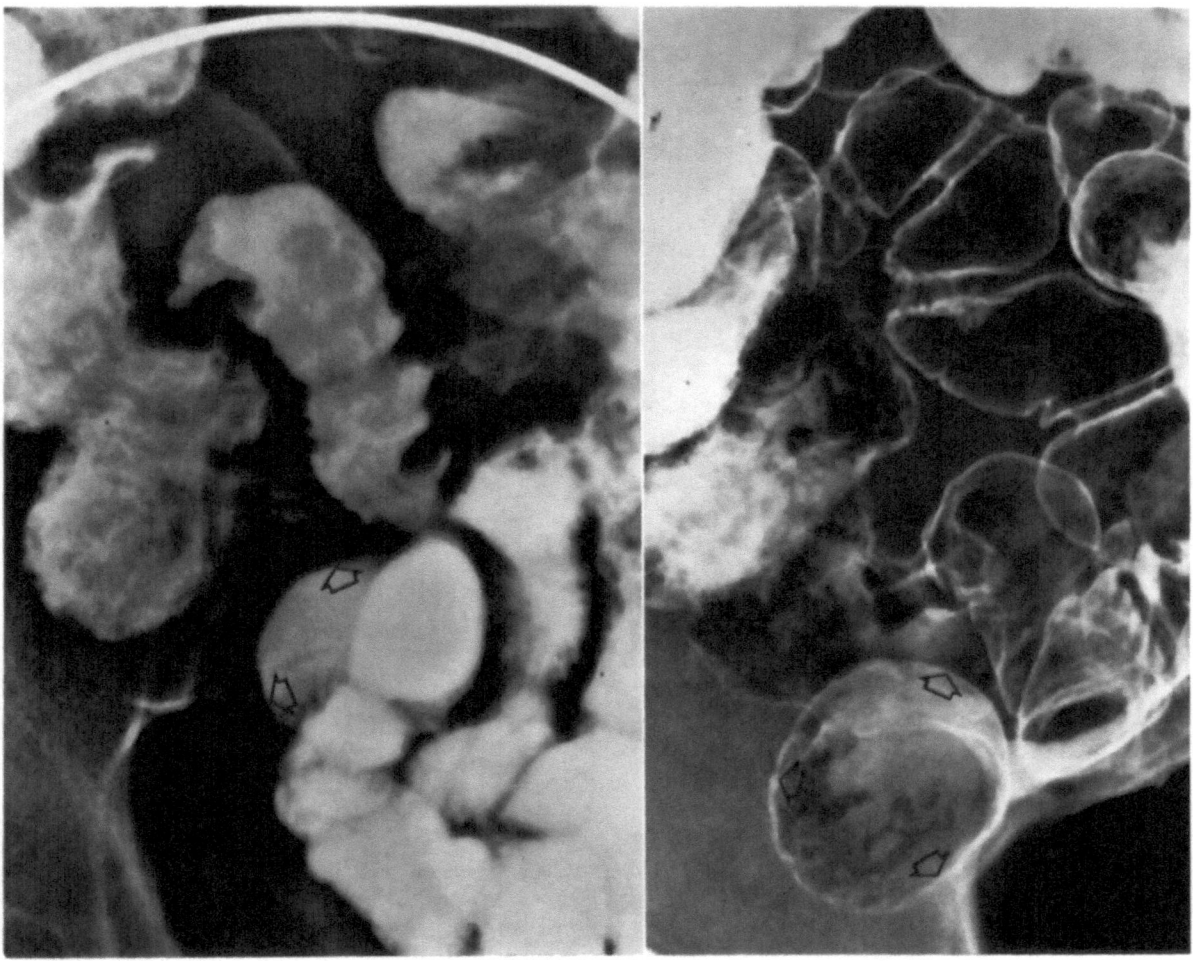

Fig. 9.68. Amebic abscess at lowest end of cecum.

selectively, or in combination as well as in various degrees, and produce an agammaglobulinemia or a hypogammaglobulinemia. A disproportion of these immunoglobulins is called dysgammaglobulinemia.

An abnormally low level of immunoglobulins can be either congenital or acquired; the latter is probably more common. In agammaglobulinemia, hypogammaglobulinemia, or dysgammaglobulinemia, the albumin level usually remains normal so that the total protein concentration is barely reduced and edema does not occur. However, patients with a disturbed gammaglobulin synthesis are highly susceptible to infectious diseases such as lambliasis that can lead to a reduced albumin concentration and swollen mucosal folds

(fig. 9.73B). Several diseases that involve a disturbance of the immunoglobulin pattern are celiac disease, pernicious anemia, atrophic gastritis, and benign and malignant lymphoma (alpha chain disease), Waldenströms macroglobulinemia and primary amyloidosis.

It has been found that these diseases have a greater incidence of malignancy, particularly in the digestive tract. The benign lymphoma is especially treacherous since it can suddenly turn into a malignant lymphoma after many years (fig. 9.76).

The clinical symptoms and laboratory findings for diseases accompanied by an immunoglobulin deficiency can vary widely. Several of the most common symptoms are:

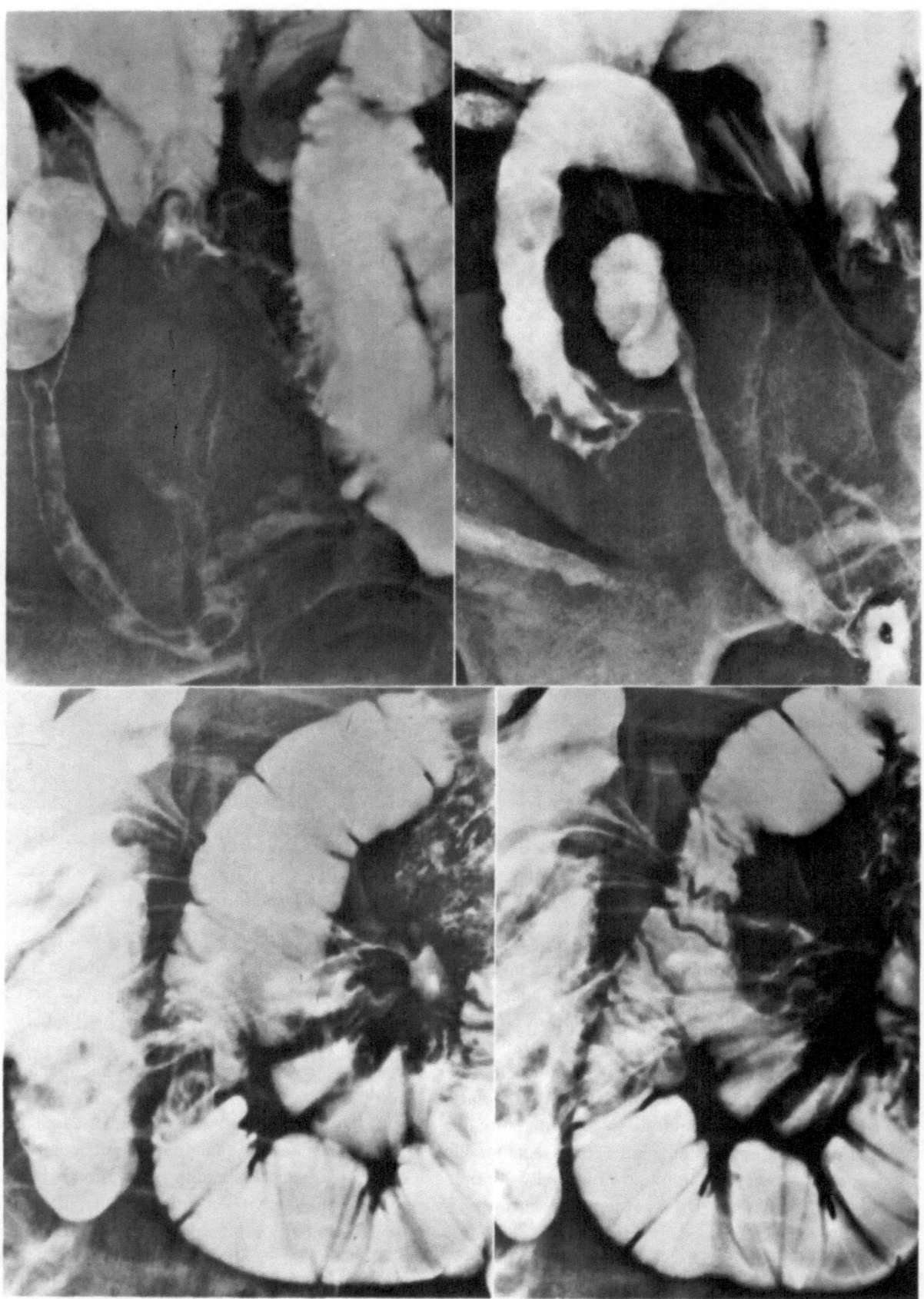

Fig. 9.69. Infiltration phenomena in the lower right quadrant due to herringworm disease. Multiple adhesions, fistulous tracts, and stenotic intestinal loops. Differentiation from Crohn's disease is difficult; in this case, however, normal filling of the appendix indicates that it is not an appendicular infiltrate.

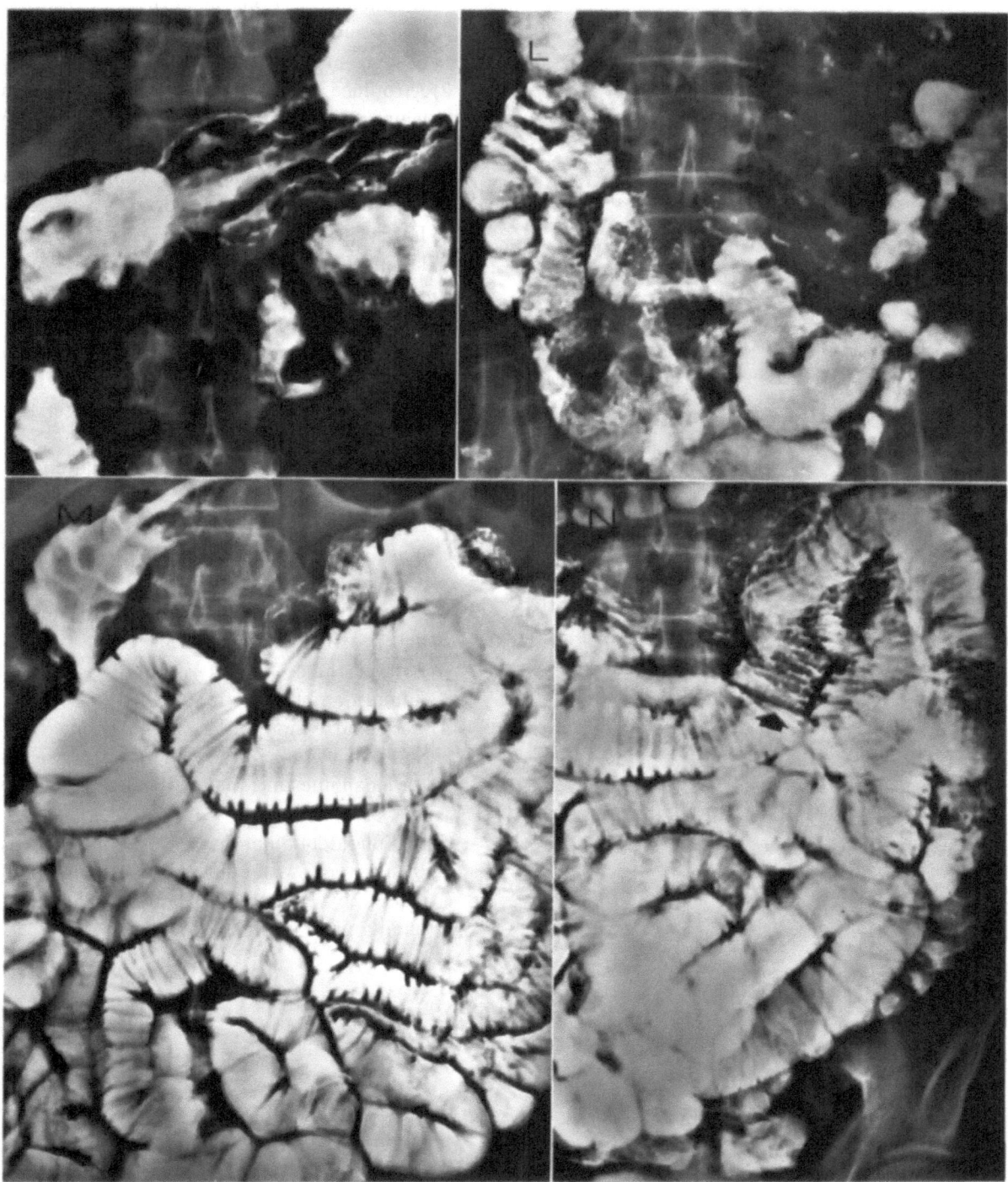

Fig. 9.70. Zollinger-Ellison disease. (KL) Conventional examination: coarse mucosal folds and highly disintegrated contrast fluid. (MN) Enteroclysis: moderately dilated intestinal loops both in the ileum and in the jejunum. Normal motility. Mucosal folds normal; only in the proximal duodenum are they obviously too coarse. In spite of the administration of large quantities of contrast fluid in order to withstand the damaging fluids as much as possible, flocculation developed immediately after termination of the infusion (N).

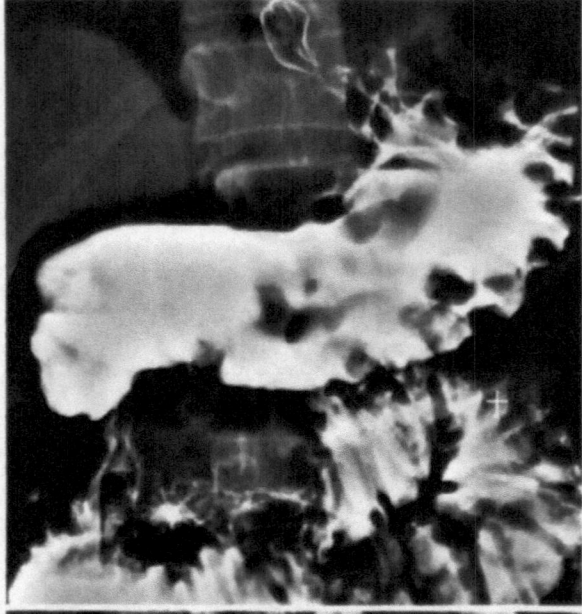

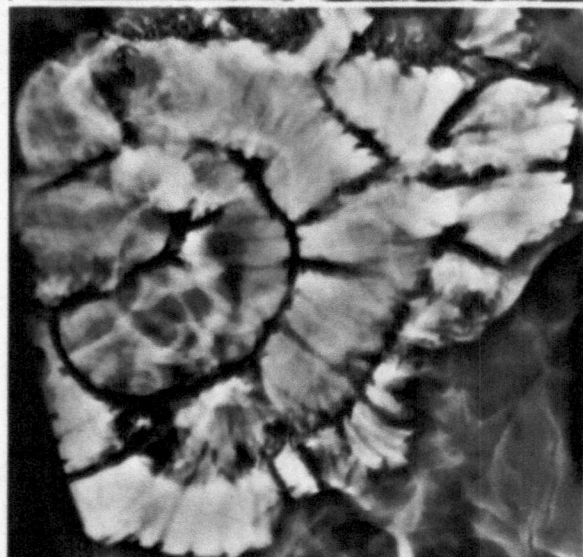

1) Malabsorption, diarrhea and steatorrhea, due to secondary infections, achlorhydria, gluten-sensitivity and disturbed resorption as a result of changes in the intestinal wall.
2) Atrophied villi in the duodenum and proximal jejunum, sometimes accompanied by a gluten sensitivity.
3) Atrophied mucous membrane, sometimes in conjunction with an achlorhydria.
4) Either no plasma cells, or very many, in the lamina propria of the intestinal wall.
5) An agammaglobulinemia, hypogammaglobulinemia, or dysgammaglobulinemia.
6) Increased susceptibility to intestinal infections.

Radiologically the following can be observed:

1) Greater tendency toward flocculation of the contrast fluid; this can be established by taking one or two residual exposures after the examination is completed (fig. 9.77, top left).
2) Absence of mucosal folds on the side of greater curvature (atrophic gastritis) or in the duodenum and proximal jejunum (celiac disease).
3) Irritable mucosal patterns in the proximal jejunum (lambliasis) (fig. 9.73A).
4) Very coarse more or less irregular mucosal folds and a thickening of the wall in a large segment of the small intestine, mainly the ileum (lymphoma) (fig. 9.74).
5) Lymphoid nodular hyperplasia; the mucosa is then covered with numerous 2- to 4-mm nodules caused by hyperplastic lymph follicles in the lamina propria (figs. 9.75–9.77).

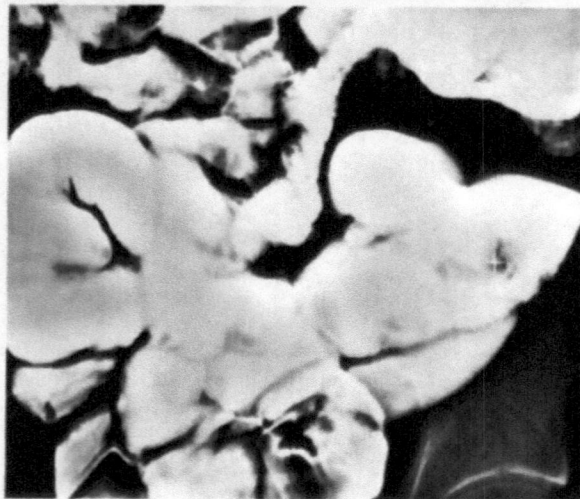

Fig. 9.71. Zollinger-Ellison disease. Very coarse mucosal folds in the stomach, duodenum, and jejunum with pronounced dilatation of the loops in the jejunum and the ileum.

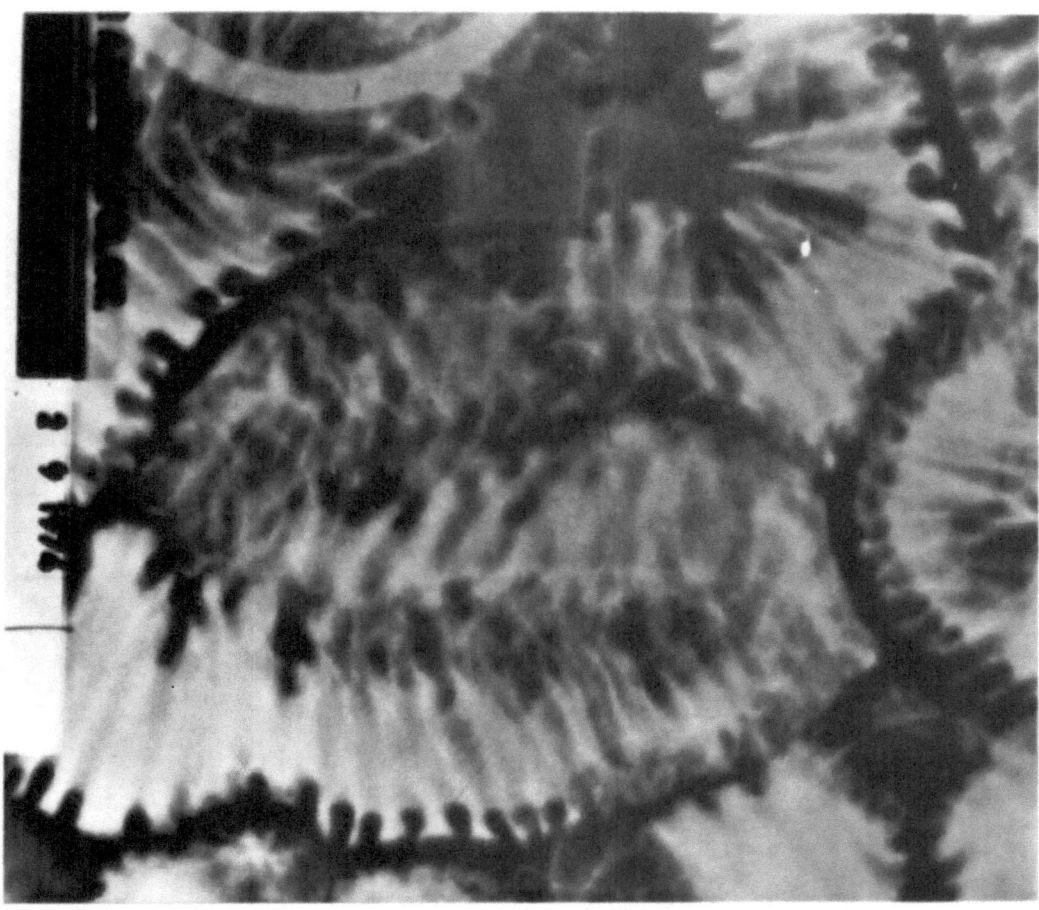

Fig. 9.72. Omega-shaped edematous swelling of the mucosal folds in a patient with protein loss in the small intestine as a result of an ulcerative colitis.

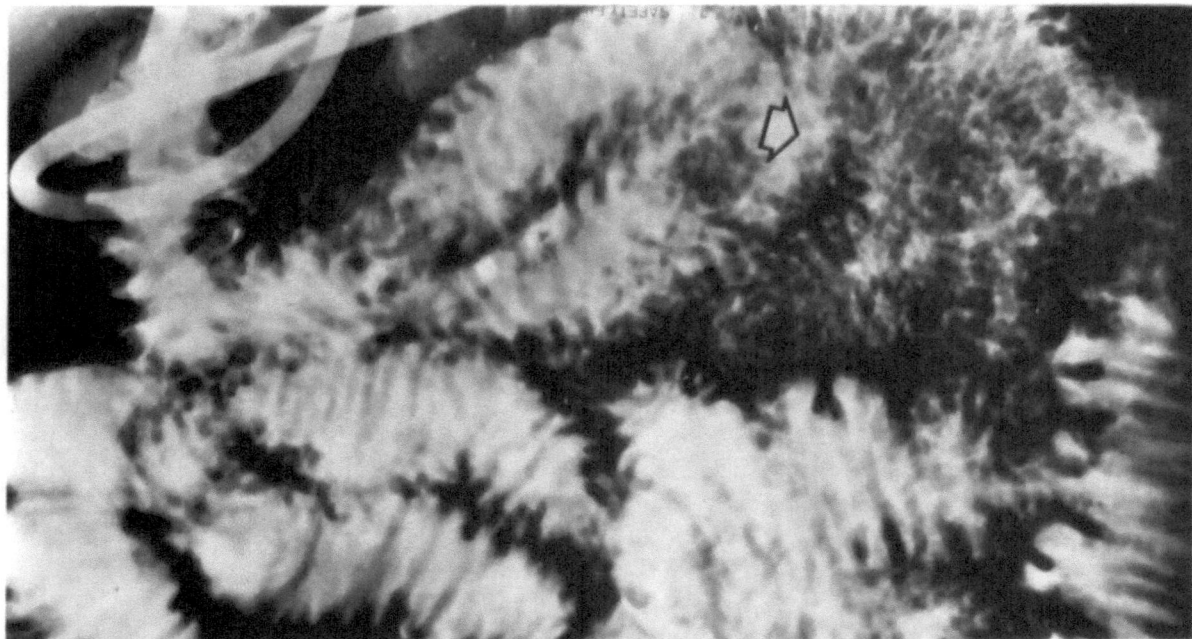

*Fig. 9.73*A. Irritability of the jejunum in a case of lambliasis. Rapid disintegration of the contrast fluid (arrow), probably due to hypersecretion.

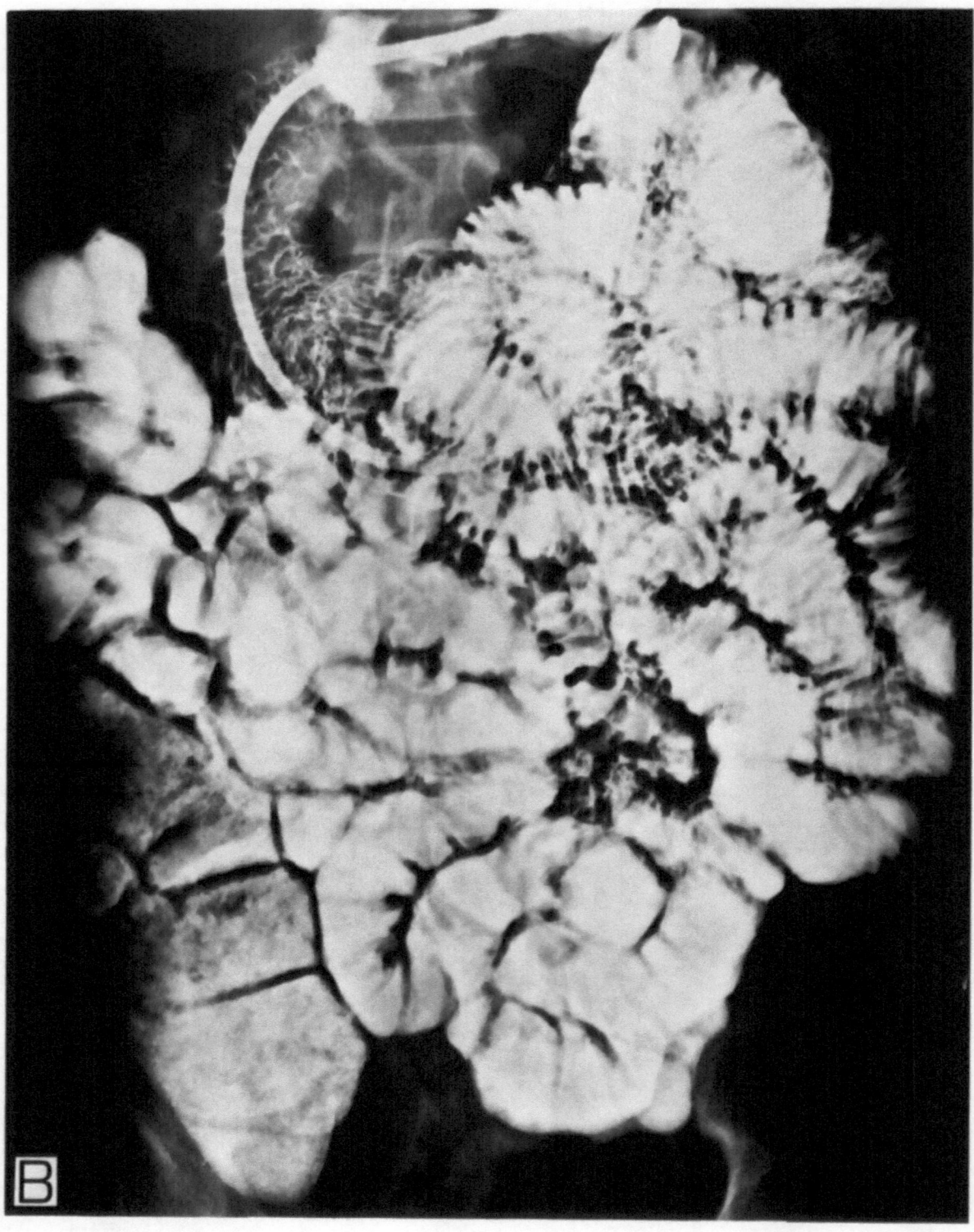

*Fig. 9.73*B. Patient with agammaglobulinemia and signs of severe malabsorption leading to the loss of 15 kg in three months. The mucosal folds are obviously thickened here. Undigested food remnants in the colon.

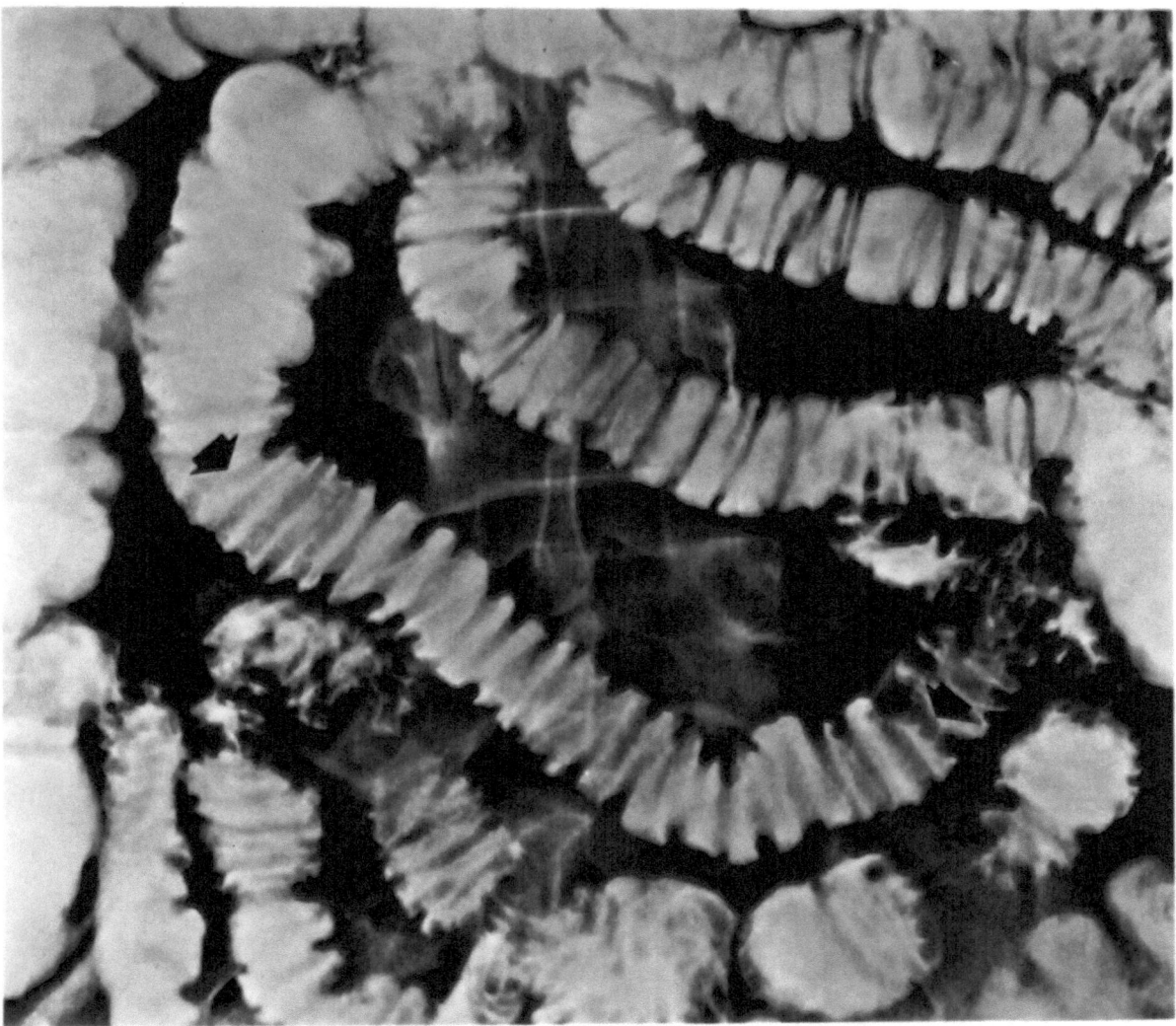

*Fig. 9.74*v. Mucosal folds are obviously too coarse along several decimeters in the proximal ileum. This middle-aged patient had lost considerable weight in the last six months, and a malabsorption and a slowly increasing diarrhea had developed. For these abnormalities of the mucosa, the following must be considered: (1) superficial lymphoma, (2) ischemia, (3) Crohn's disease.

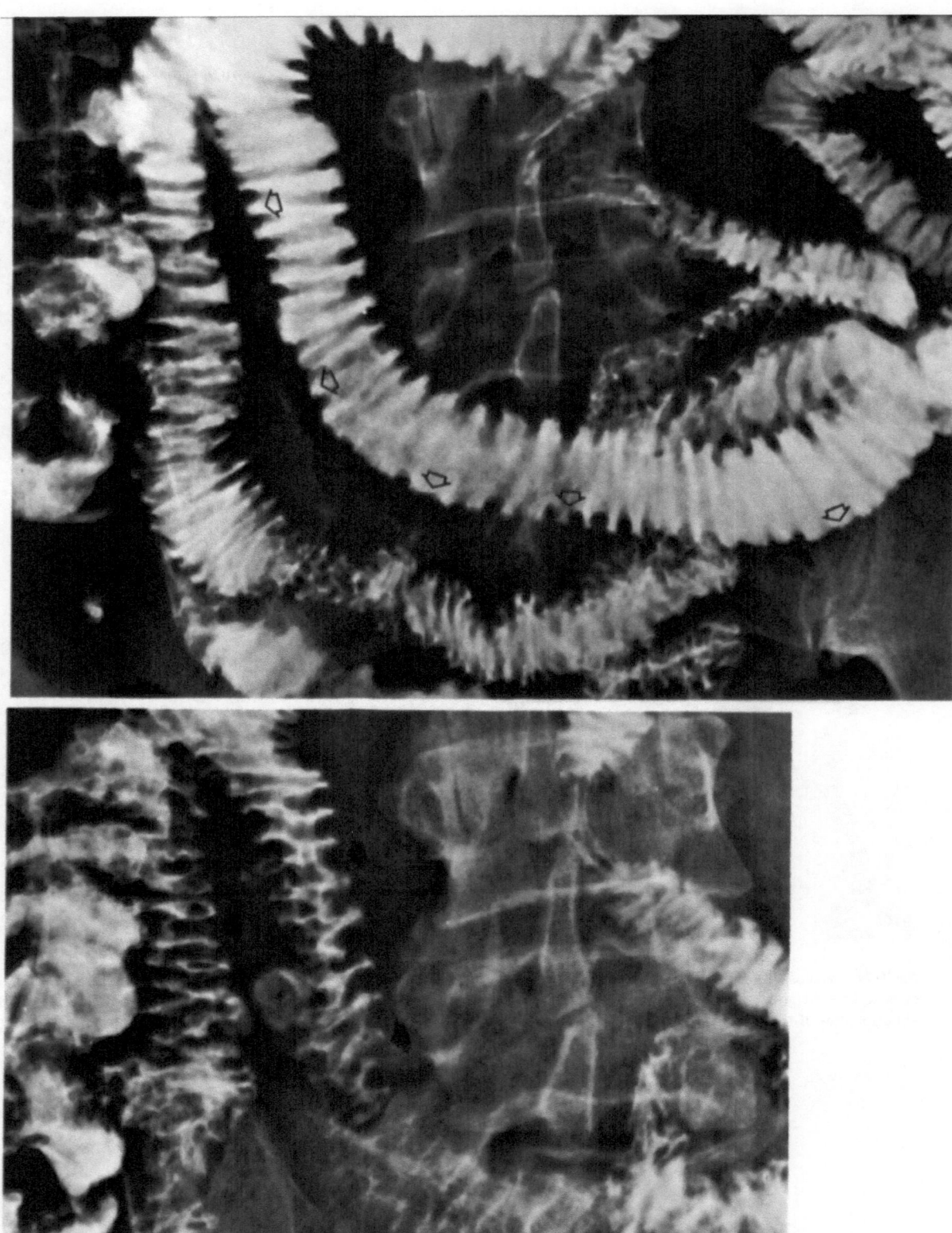

*Fig. 9.74*w. Three months later a repeat examination revealed that the abnormalities had spread and increased slightly in severity. The mucosal surface has fairly irregular margins, possibly as a result of superficial ulcerations. On the basis of the course of the disease during this period and other examinations, ischemia and Crohn's disease can probably be excluded and a lymphoma must be seriously considered. Experience has shown that these abnormalities can suddenly, but also very gradually, develop into a malignant lymphoma. Follow-up of this patient was not possible since he refused further treatment. The biopsy revealed multiple deposits of plasma cells in the lamina propria.

273

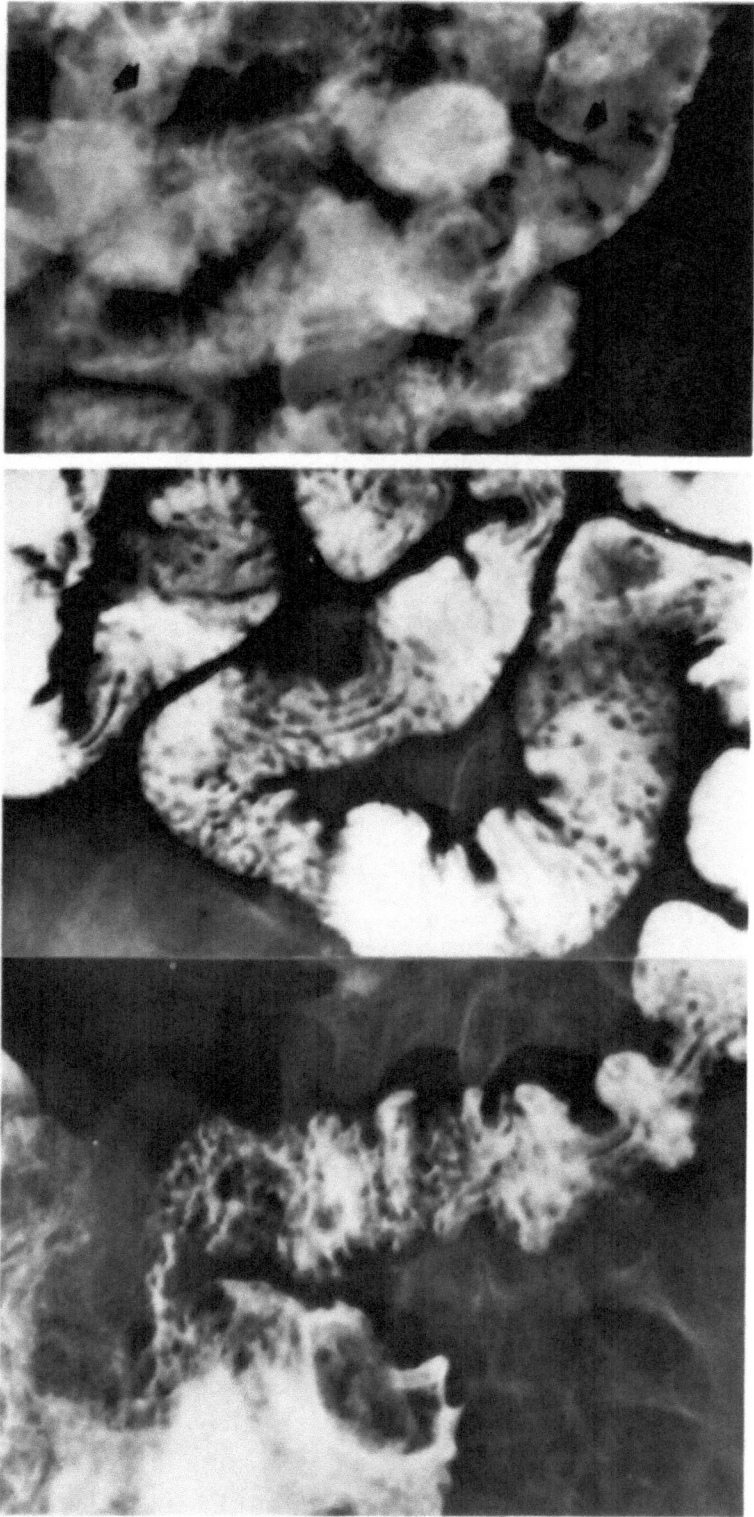

Fig. 9.75. Lymphoid nodular hyperplasia in case of immunoglobulin deficiency, covering more than 50 cm of the distal ileum. During contraction, the lymph follicles can be seen with difficulty or not at all (bottom).

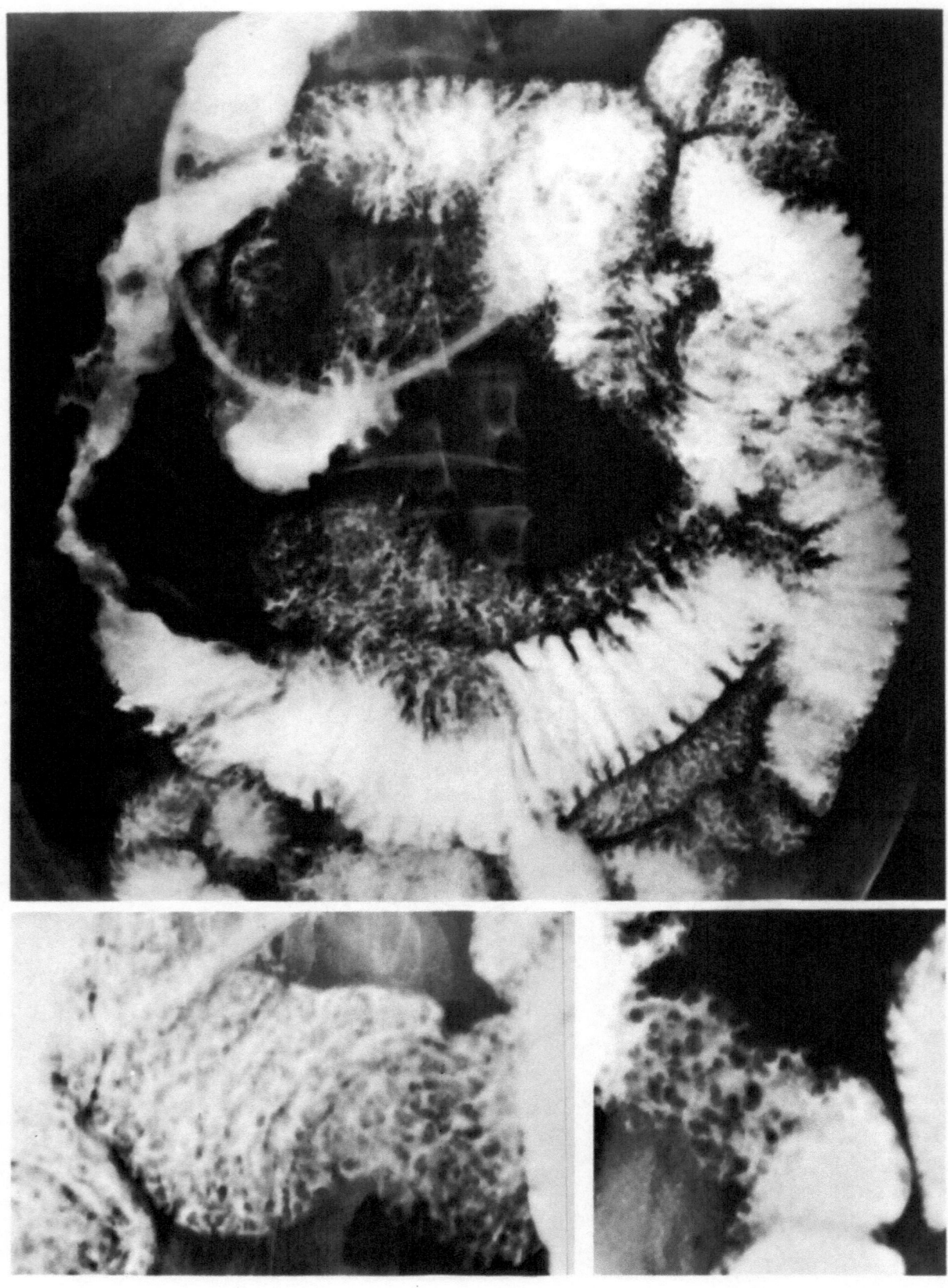

Fig. 9.76. Hypoglobulinemia with an extensive lymphoid hyperplasia of the small intestine and a lymphosarcoma in the jejunum. Details of the jejunum (bottom left) and the ileum (bottom right).

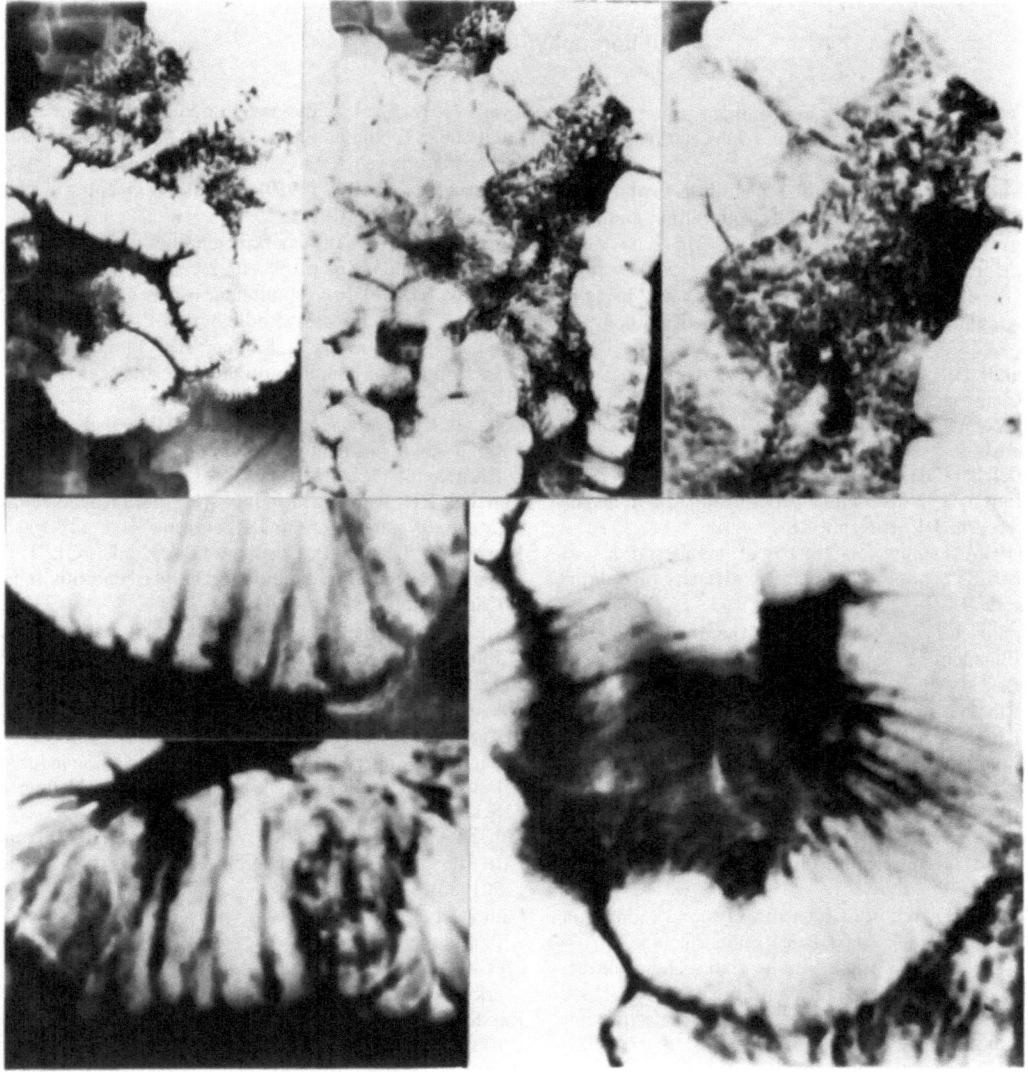

Fig. 9.77. Extensive lymphonodular hyperplasia in a patient with a known immunoglobulin deficiency. Note the irritability in the jejunum, which is apparent by the marked tendency to flocculate the barium suspension. In this patient, there were no signs of lambliasis, which causes a similar pattern (see fig. 9.73).

Bibliography: chapter 9

Aldridge AH (1942) Intestinal injuries resulting from irradiation treatment of uterine carcinoma. Am J Obstet Gynecol 44: 833–857.

Ament ME, Rubin CE (1972) Relation of giardiasis to abnormal intestinal structure and function in gastrointestinal immuno-deficiency syndromes. Gastroenterology 62: 216–226.

Bosniak MA, Hardy MA, Quint J, Ghossein NA (1969) Demonstration of the effect of irradiation on canine bowel using in vivo photographic magnification angiography. Radiology 93: 1361–1368.

Bucker J, Feindt HR (1951) Pseudopolyposis lymphatica ilei. Fortschr Roentgenstr 74: 59–65.

Carrera GF, Young S, Lewicki AM (1976) Intestinal tuberculosis. Gastrointest Radiol 1: 147–155.

Chau PM, Fletcher GH, Rutledge FN, Dodd GD Jr (1962) Complications in high dose whole pelvis irradiation in female pelvic cancer. Am J Roentgenol 87: 22–40.

Clemett A (1968) Lecture on 'Intestinal manifestations of systemic disease'. School of Medicine, University of California, March 1968.

Colock BP, Braatsch JW (1968) Surgery of the small intestine in the adult. Philadelphia: Saunders, 161–165.

Davis TJ, Berk RN (1977) Immunoglobulin deficiency diseases of the intestine. Gastrointest Radiol 2: 7–11.

De Cosse JJ, Rhodes RS, Wentz WB, Reagan JW, Dworken HJ, Holden WD (1969) The natural history and management of radiation induced injury of the gastrointestinal tract. Ann Surg 170: 369–384.

Delavierre Ph, Levasseur J-C, Kron B, Ruault P, Bastian et Tran van B (1973) Les ulcères primitifs du grêle. Sem Hop Paris 49: 2052.

Desjardins AU (1931) Action of roentgen rays and radium on the gastrointestinal tract. Am J Roentgenol 26: 145.

Dowdle E (1942) Multiple primary nonspecific jejunal ulcers, with chronic duodenal dilatation. Ann Surg 166: 348.

Duncan W, Leonard J (1965) The malabsorption syndrome following radiotherapy. Q J Med 34.

Ebeling W (1933) Primary jejunal ulcer. Ann Surg 97: 857.

Ekberg O (1977) Crohn's disease of the small bowel examined by double contrast technique: a comparison with oral technique. Gastrointest Radiol 1: 355–359.

Evert JA, Black BM, Dockerty MB (1948) Primary nonspecific ulcers of the small intestine. Surgery 23: 185.

Friedman WB (1955) Pathogenesis of intestinal ulcus following irradiation. AMA Arch Pathol 59: 2–4.

Goehrs HR, Morlock CG, Dockerty MB (1957) Primary non-specific ulcers of the small intestine. Proc Mayo Clin 32: 351.

Goldberg HI, O'Kieffe D, Jenis EH, Boyce HW (1973) Diffuse eosinophilic gastroenteritis. Am J Roentgenol 119: 342–351.

Graundins J (1969) Über Strahlenspätschäden am Dünndarm. Langenbecks Arch Klin Chir 324: 120–130.

Gryboski JD, Self TW, Clemett A, et al. (1968) Selective immunoglobulin A deficiency and intestinal nodular lymphoid hyperplasia: correction of diarrhea with antibiotics and plasma. Pediatrics 42: 833–837.

Hodgson JR, Hoffman HN II, Huizenga KA (1967) Roentgenologic features of lymphoid hyperplasia of the small intestine associated with dysgammaglobulinemia. Radiology 88: 883–888.

Khilnani MT, Keller RJ, Cuttner J (1969) Macroglobulinemia and steatorrhea: roentgen and pathologic findings in the intestinal tract. Radiol Clin North Am 7: 43—55.

Kyle J (1972) Crohn's disease. London: Heinemann.

Lindholmer B, Nijman E, Raf L (1964) Nonspecific ulceration of the small bowel. Acta Chir Scand 128: 310.

Litwin MS, Crane C (1960) Primary nonpeptic ulcer of the jejunum. Ann Surg 151: 594.

Marina-Fiol C (1962) Bemerkungen über die Ileitis follicularis. Gastroenterologia (Basel) 98: 19–29.

Marshak RH (1975) Granulomatous disease of the intestinal tract (Crohn's disease). Radiology 114: 3–22.

Marshak RH, Hazzi Ch, Lindner AE, Maklansky D (1974) Small bowel in immunoglobulin deficiency syndromes. Am J Roentgenol 122: 227–240.

Marshak RH, Hazzi Ch, Lindner AE, Maklansky D (1975) The small bowel in immunoglobulin deficiency syndromes. Am J Roentgenol 122: 227–240.

Marshak RH, Ruoff M, Lindner AE (1968) Roentgen manifestations of giardiasis. Am J Roentgenol 104: 557–560.

Mason GR, Dietrich P, Friedland GW, Hankes GE (1970) The radiological findings in radiation induced enteritis and colitis. Clin Radiol 21: 232–247.

Neumeister K, Pfeiffer J (1966) Klinische Analyse der Akuten Intestinalen Strahlenreaktionen bei Röntgen-, Radium- und Telekobaltbestrahlungen. Strahlentherapie 129: 512–519.

Nilehn B, Sjostrom B (1967) Studies on Yersinia enterocolitica. Acta Pathol Microbiol Scand 71: 612–628.

Nummi P, Fritmen J, Mäkönen H (1973) Radiation induced small bowel injury following telecobalt therapy of bladder tumor. Scand. J Urol Nephrol 7: 30–32.

Osborn Anne G, Friedland GW (1973) A radiological approach to the diagnosis of small bowel disease. Clin Radiol 24: 281–301.

Philips RL, Carlson HC (1975) The röntgenographic and clinical findings in Whipple's disease. Am J Roentgenol 123: 268–273.

Prevot R (1950) Röntgendiagnose der entzündlichen Darmerkrankungen. Fortschr Roentgenstr 72: 547–563.

Ravdin IS (1927) Primary ulcer of the jejunum. Ann Surg 85: 873.

Roswitt B, Malsky SJ, Reid CB (1972) Severe radiation injuries of stomach, small intestine, colon and rectum. VA Radist Ther Cent – VA Hospital, Bronx, NY – Am J Roentgenol 14: 460–475.

Rogers LF, Goldstein HM (1977) Röntgen manifestations of radiation injury to the gastrointestinal tract. Gastrointest Radiol 2: 281–291.

Shimkin PM, Waldman TA, Krugman RL (1970) Intestinal lymphangiectasia. Am J Roentgenol 110: 827–841.

Sielaff HJ (1970) Die radiologische Diagnostik der Dünndarmerkrankungen. Therapiewoche 20: 3207–3215.

Simpkins KC (1972) Some aspects of the radiology of Crohn's disease. Br J Surg 59 (10).

Sjostrom B, Nilehn B (1968) Some aspects of the inflammation of the ileocoecal region with special reference to Yersinia enterocolitica. Bull Soc Int Chir (5).

Sturges HF, Krone ChL (1973) Ulceration and structure of the jejunum in a patient on long-term Indomethacin therapy. Am J Gastroenterol 59: 162.

Teicher I, Mueulbauer MA, Allen AC (1963) The clinical-pathological spectrum of primary ulcers of the small intestine. Surg Gynecol Obstet 116: 196.

Todd TF (1938) Rectal ulceration following irradiation treatment of carcinoma of cervix uteri. Surg. Gynecol Obstet 67: 617–631.

Warren J, Friedman N (1942) Pathology and pathologic diagnosis of radiation lesions in gastrointestinal tract. Am J Pathol 18: 499.

Watson MR, Helwig EB (1968) Primary nonspecific ulceration of the small bowel. Arch Surg 87: 600.

Wiechen PJ van (1974) Radiological changes in the distal part of the ileum in association with *Yersinia enterocolitica* infections. Radiol Clin Biol 43: 242–253.

See also the nos. 39, 94, 146, 148 and 199 of the bibliography of pages 187 and following.

10. TUMORS

1. General

Although the small intestine is approximately twice as long as the esophagus, stomach and colon together, tumors of the small bowel are relatively rare. They account for about 25% of all tumors of the digestive tract. The reason for this apparent immunity is a matter of conjecture; it is presumed that the lack of stasis in this part of the digestive tract is significant. In the absolute sense, however, tumors of the small intestine cannot be considered rare. They are found in about 20% of autopsy material. In contrast to the colon and especially the esophagus and stomach, where malignant tumors are more common than benign ones, only one-fifth of all tumors in the small intestine are malignant.

In the past a tumor in the small intestine was seldom demonstrated preoperatively by means of radiological examination. Until recently this diagnosis was established in only about one out of every five cases. This poor result was due in part to the fact that benign tumors are usually asymptomatic until they reach a certain size and recurrent complaints of obstruction occur. In the jejunum, that part of the intestine where peristalsis is the most active, a temporary intussusception will sometimes develop. Malignant tumors, too, are not discovered until growth of the tumor causes obvious stenotic phenomena. The patient then complains of colic-like pains in the abdomen that are usually localized around the navel. Intussusceptions are seldom or never seen in conjunction with malignant tumors. The latter rarely have a pedicle and growth tends to be extraluminal, sometimes with invasion of the surrounding tissue. Abdominal pains, often accompanied by diarrhea and sometimes also by a clinical malabsorption, are encountered in two-thirds of the patients with tumors. These findings are by no means a specific symptom for a tumor of the small intestine. There also can be periods without complaints, which is misleading. The same is true for bleeding in the digestive tract. This is encountered in one-half of the patients and it is often presumed, understandably, that the blood loss originates in the colon or the stomach. It should therefore first be established by means of physical and radiological examinations that there are no abnormalities in these two parts of the digestive tract. Subsequently the possibility of a tumor in the small intestine must be considered and included in the differential diagnosis. Often, however, the correct diagnosis is not discovered until the patient is on the operating table. Frequently he has had complaints for at least a year, and at that stage a palpable mass can be felt in one-third of the cases. From the preceding it will be understandable why tumors found in the small bowel during surgery are predominantly malignant. In contrast, at autopsy most of the tumors of the small intestine appear to be benign. If bleeding is diagnosed and localized, either clinically or angiographically, a laparotomy should follow. Negative findings based solely on external palpation of the intestinal loops are completely worthless; the lumen of the intestine must be inspected by using multiple incisions. If there is even a moderate constriction of the intestinal lumen, an enteroclysis examination can be used to provoke a striking prestenotic dilatation.

Another advantage of the enteroclysis technique is that an obvious increase in the distance between the descending limb of the duodenum and the spinal column may become evident. This is seen during the fluoroscopic monitoring of the position of the tube in the right lateral position (fig. 10.1). This can indicate a tumor of the pancreas, some other retroperitoneal tumorous growth, or metastasis in a lymph node from a primary tumor elsewhere.

280

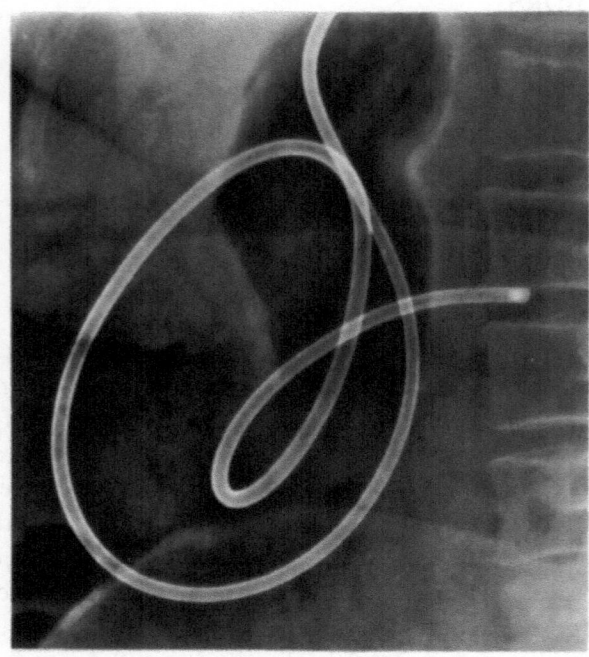

Fig. 10.1. Obvious broadening of the retroperitoneal space by metastases – in this case of a melanoma.

Metastatic growth in particular may not involve at all the mass of intestinal loops so that widening of the prevertebral space may be completely overlooked in the AP projection.

Although these factors have brought about a real improvement in the diagnosis of tumors, the enteroclysis technique alone is not the only important aspect. In addition to the use of this method of examination, the precision with which the clinician scans each separate intestinal loop, using spot films, is essential, just as in the search for a Meckel's diverticulum.

Once good roentgenograms that permitted easy evaluation of the anatomy of the intestinal loops became possible, the need for further spot films became evident. After all, spot films were of little use when the loops were inadequately filled. The enteroclysis technique also stimulated many clinicians to make a greater personal effort, thus producing an increased potential effect of all of these factors. The net result is that one out of every 100 patients who comes to our department for a roentgenological examination of the small intestine is found to have a tumor, either benign, malignant, or metastatic. Not all tumors cause obstructive phenomena. A precise examination of the mucosal

pattern is therefore valuable not only for inflammatory and vascular diseases but also for the detection of a malignant process. Thus an intramural process growing along the length of the intestine that, if peristalsis remains normal, causes only a somewhat coarsened mucosal pattern may be a benign or malignant lymphoma. At a somewhat later stage and especially more distal in the intestine, a lymphoma may only produce a smooth mucosa that appears atrophied. Sometimes there are ulcerative changes, and a barely thickened intestinal wall. Destruction or space-occupying processes, which we would like to see as evidence of tumor growth, may be missing entirely.

Of course an ileum without fold relief and an increase in the space between adjacent intestinal loops can also be caused by primary amyloidosis or Crohn's disease. However, ulcerations rarely develop in amyloidosis and are frequently encountered in Crohn's disease. In Crohn's disease the broadening of the space between the loops can be due to either thickening of the intestinal wall itself or thickening of the layer of fat that surrounds the intestine. Usually in these cases the process is in an active stage. After remission of Crohn's disease or atrophy of the mucosa as a result of the chronic use of laxatives, the inner wall of the intestine is also smooth, but there is no thickening of the wall. Finally, in ischemia the segment without mucosal relief is usually not very long. Sudden, rather erratic changes in the course of the intestinal loop can indicate fibrotic shriveling as a result of a nearby carcinoid. A local intussusception might suggest a polypoid formation that in itself is not visible.

Displacement or compression of intestinal loops, sometimes visible in only the supine, prone, or lateral position, can indicate benign or malignant tumor growth in the retroperitoneal space (fig. 10.2), the abdominal wall, or the mesentery (fig. 10.3).

However, sometimes spread of a retroperitoneal tumor via the mesentery to or around the intestinal lumen can cause changes which give the impression that the tumor originates in the intestinal wall. Broadening of the mesentery then produces large empty spaces between the intestinal loops that suggest a lymphosarcoma (fig. 10.4). Local dilatations of an intestinal loop without a subsequent stenosis can be the result of local injury to nerve

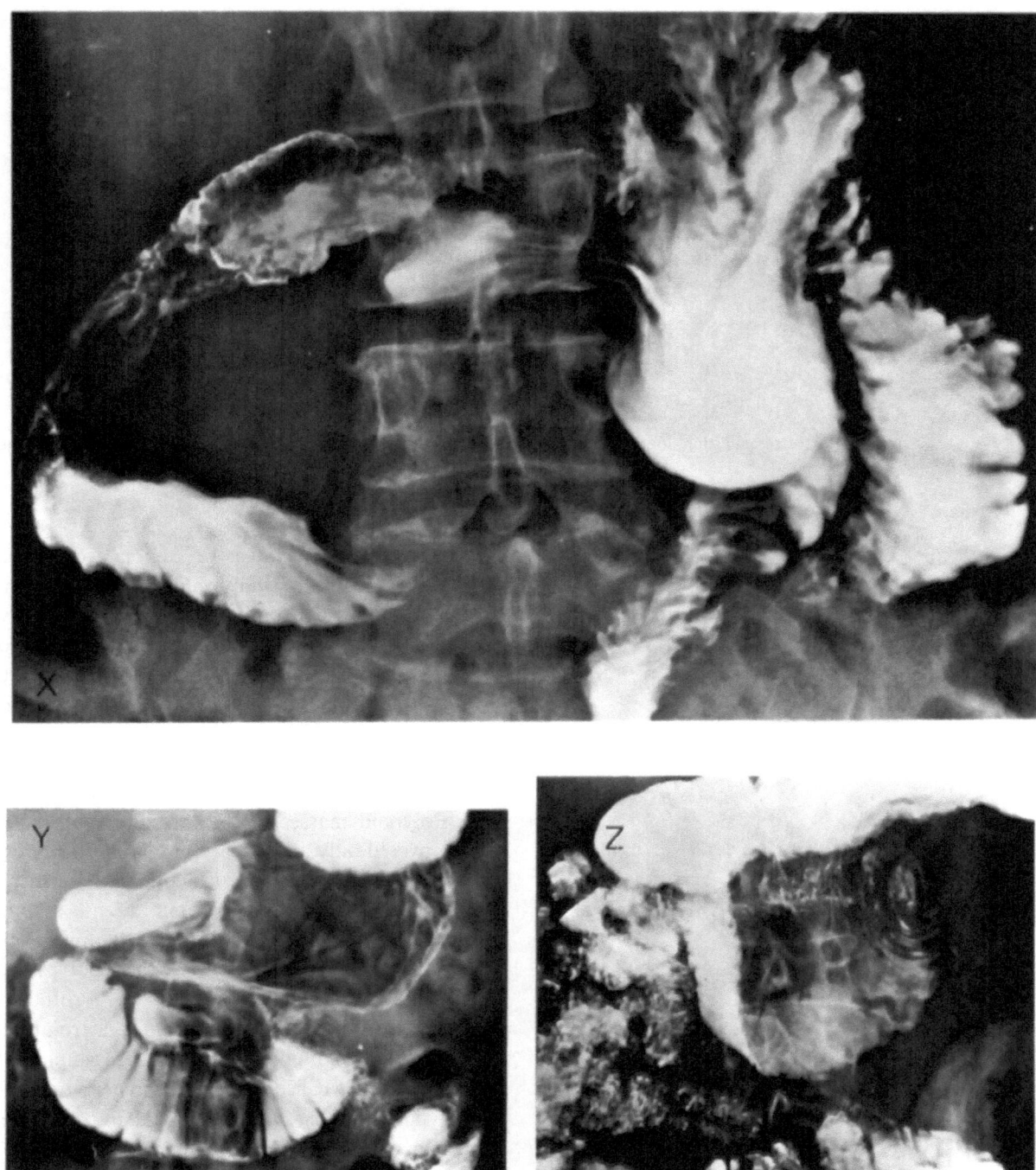

Fig. 10.2. (x) Retroperitoneal lymphoreticular malignancy with marked compression of a fairly long segment of the duodenum. (Y) Compression at the duodenojejunal junction by a tumor in the tail of the pancreas. (z) Compression of the transverse limb of the duodenum by a large retroperitoneal leiomyosarcoma. There is also a developmental anomaly in the intestinal loops; the jejunum lies in the right half of the abdomen.

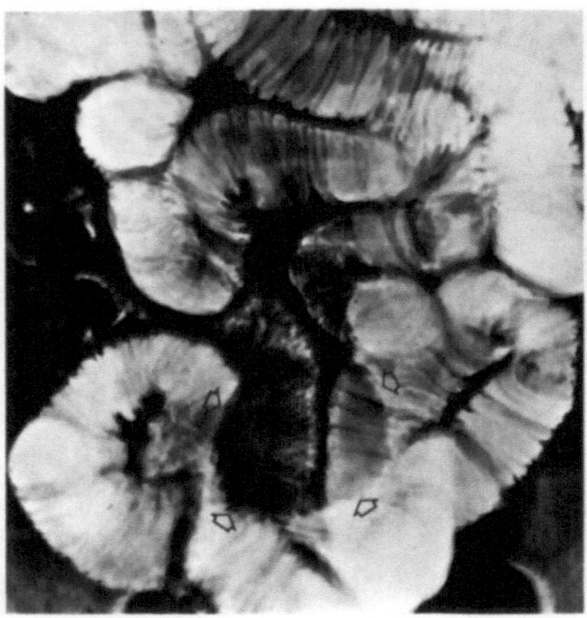

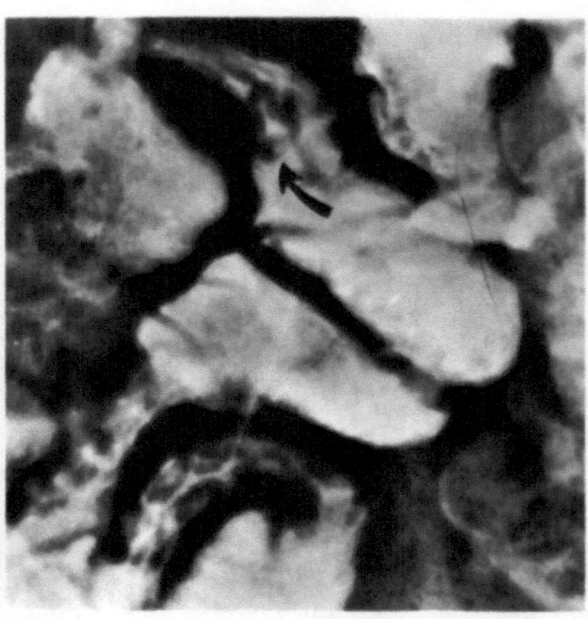

Fig. 10.3. Displacement of the intestinal loops by a mesenteric cyst.

Fig. 10.5. Inflammatory granuloma with central ulcer crater in Crohn's disease.

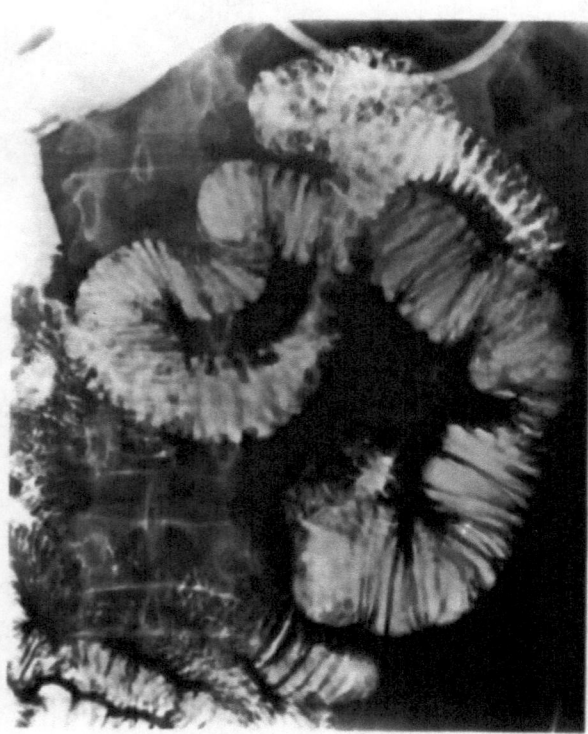

Fig. 10.4. Retroperitoneal liposarcoma that has spread via the mesentery to encircle the intestinal lumen so that, partly because of the empty spaces between the intestinal loops, a lymphosarcoma is suggested.

tissue because of invasive tumor growth as in lymphosarcoma. Usually, however, in these cases there are also concomitant phenomena that reveal the diagnosis. Local stretching of the mucosal folds can be the result of an intramural leiomyoma that causes little or no bulging into the lumen or of a duplication cyst. Compression can cause deceptively similar patterns (fig. 10.8); incorrect evaluation of this technique must therefore be avoided.

Polypoid masses in the intestinal lumen, often discovered only after a careful search of spot films, can be from metastasis of tumors elsewhere, a (sometimes hereditary) systemic disease accompanied by polypoid formations, or lymphoreticular tumor growth. In the latter case these polyps can be very tiny and numerous so that it is difficult or impossible to differentiate it from a gastrointestinal polyposis or lymphoid hyperplasia. Lymphoid hyperplasia, also called lymphatic polyposis or pseudopolyposis lymphatica, accompanies diverse generally benign diseases such as an infection with *Giardia lamblia*. If this hyperplasia of the follicles is restricted to the proximal jejunum or is seen only in the distal ileum of a young patient, there are usually no problems with the differential diagnosis. There can, however, be considerable difficulty when a more or

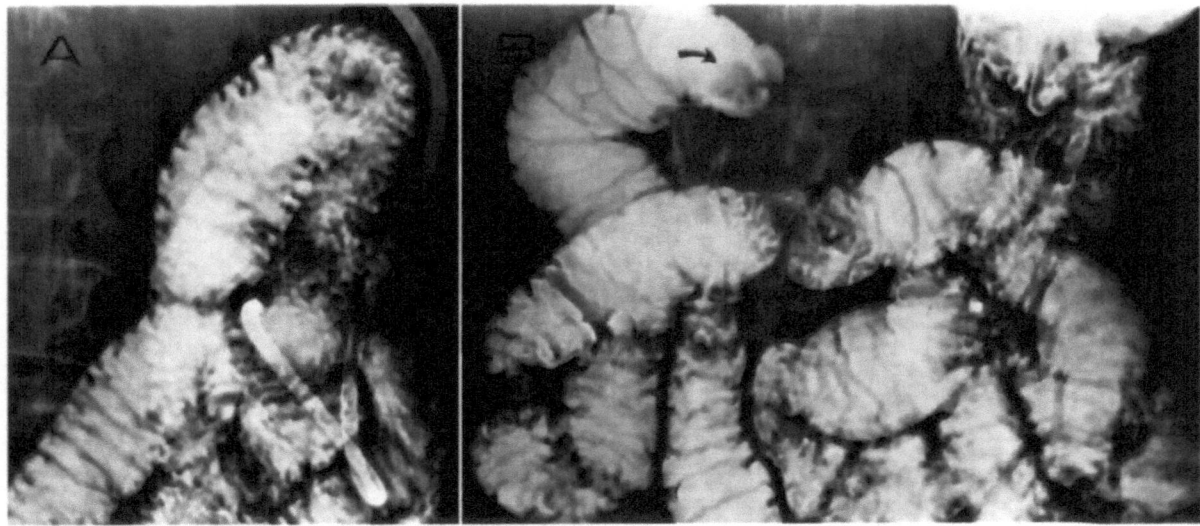

Fig. 10.6. Smoothly defined round bulge in the stump of an afferent loop after a BII resection due to invagination of the suture line. The afferent loop rarely fills spontaneously (A). However, in more than 50% of the cases, filling is obtained after administration of a hypotonic agent (B).

less extensive lymphatic polyposis is found in the distal part of the jejunum or the proximal part of the ileum. This is especially true when there are no signs of hyperplasia in the last decimeters of the ileum where the greatest quantity of lymphatic tissue is found.

Finally when evaluating the films, it should always be remembered that configurations can be seen that suggest tumor growth but are in fact caused by a completely different phenomenon. One example is an inflammatory granuloma with a central ulcer crater that is deceptively similar to a metastasis with central necrosis (fig. 10.5).

The polypoid formation in fig. 10.6B, which is due to the invagination of the end of the afferent loop after a gastrectomy of the BII type, resembles a bulge in the cecum caused by the invagination of an appendical stump of the appendix after removal of that organ. Often it is only possible to fill the afferent loop with contrast medium after peristalsis has been eliminated by administering a hypotonic agent.

Configurations that suggest a tumor are not only caused by real structures of a completely different nature; they may also be due to misleading patterns that generally persist for only a short time. Sometimes these temporary misleading patterns are the result of inadequate filling of the intestine (fig. 10.7) or the use of compression by the clinician (fig. 10.8). Sometimes there is autocompression by adjacent tissue structures such as an intersecting vessel (fig. 10.9). A less common misleading pattern develops when in a specific projection a normally existing structure, often part of the skeleton, appears to enclose a space-occupying process (fig. 10.10).

The easiest way to classify tumors of the small bowel is as follows:

1) generalized gastrointestinal polyposis,
2) benign tumors,
3) semimalignant tumors,
4) malignant tumors,
5) metastasis.

2. Polyposis

A number of diseases occur in the digestive tract that are characterized by a widespread polyposis and a marked familial incidence. In two of these disorders, familial polyposis and Gardner's syndrome, the small polyps are adenomas. They occur

284

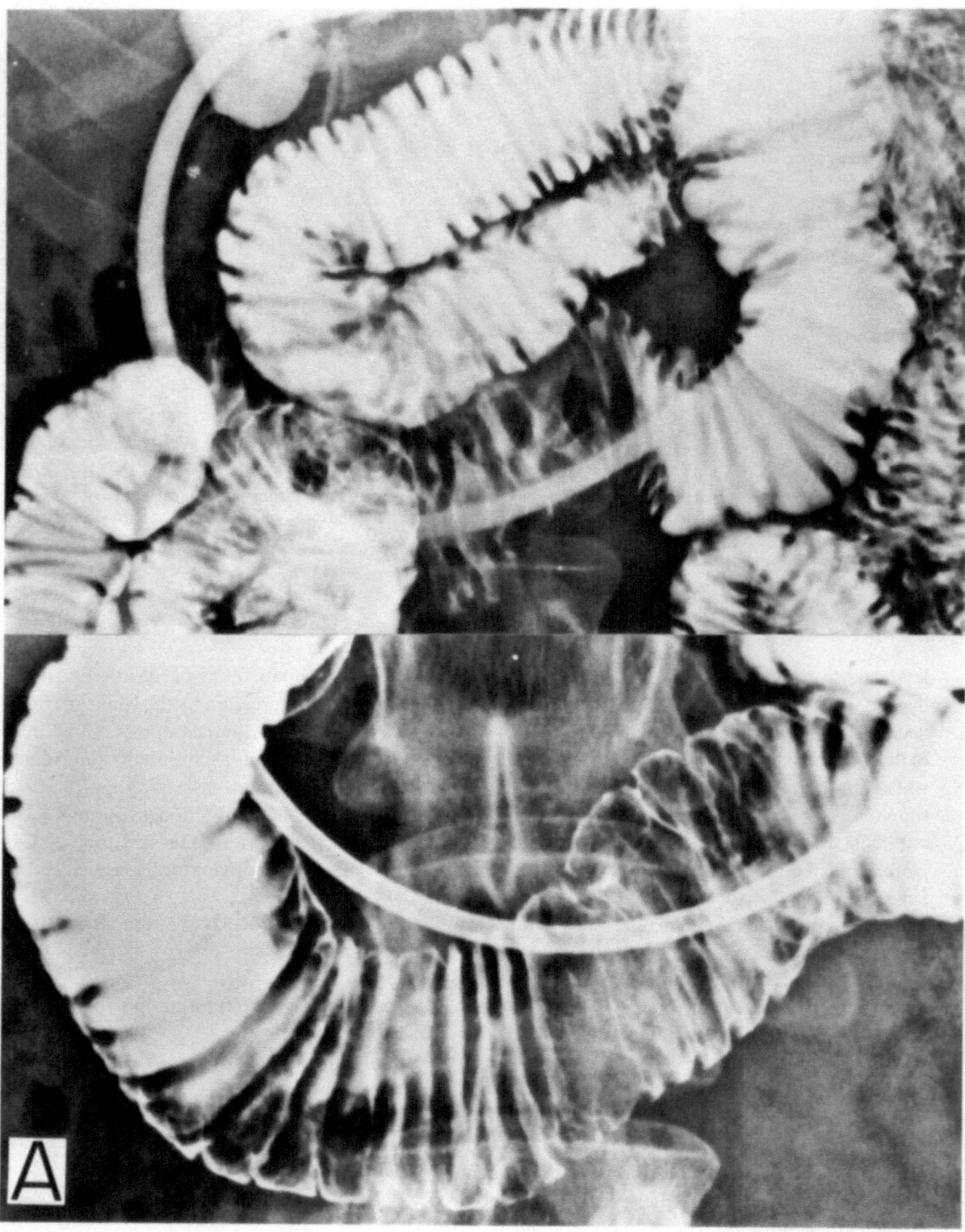

*Fig. 10.7*AB. (A) Irregular mucosal relief in the duodenum at the point where it crosses the aorta (top) which disappears during hypotonic duodenography (bottom). (B) Highly irregular mucosal relief in the duodenum where it crosses the aorta in a patient with complaints of frequent vomiting and a history of atony-inducing drugs. Endoscopic examination revealed a completely normal mucosa. (See also page 285.)

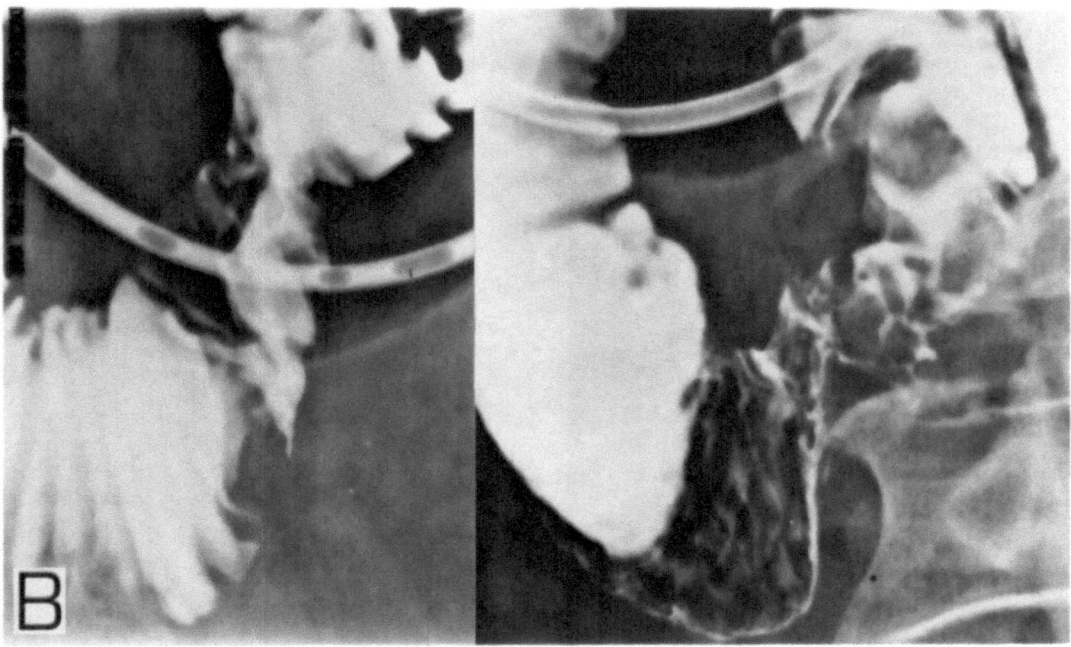

*Fig. 10.7*B. See legend on page 284.

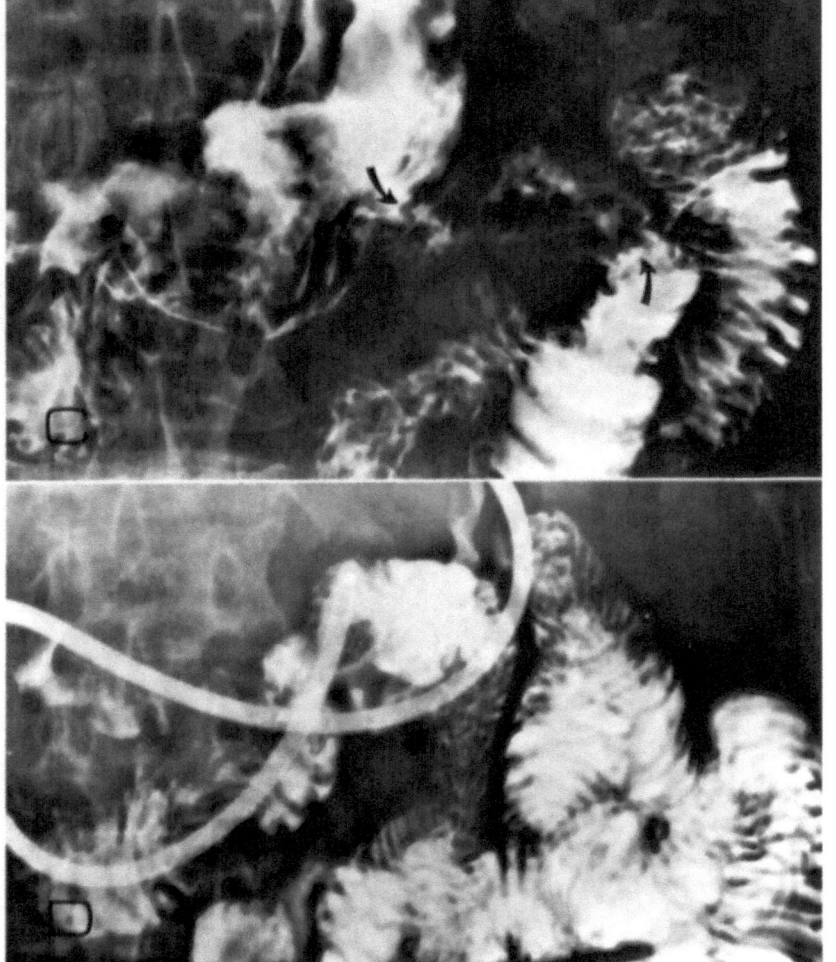

*Fig. 10.7*CD. (C) Irregular mucosal pattern in the proximal part of the jejunum (between the arrows) following gastric examination and due exclusively to inadequate filling of the intestine. Proximal and distal to the suspect region the mucosal relief was normal so that disintegration of the contrast fluid was out of the question. (D) In the course of an enteroclysis examination one week later, this part of the intestine was well filled and no abnormalities could be seen.

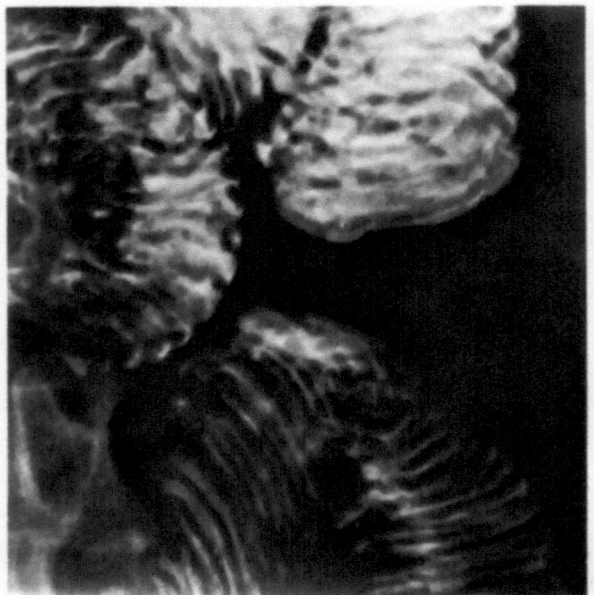

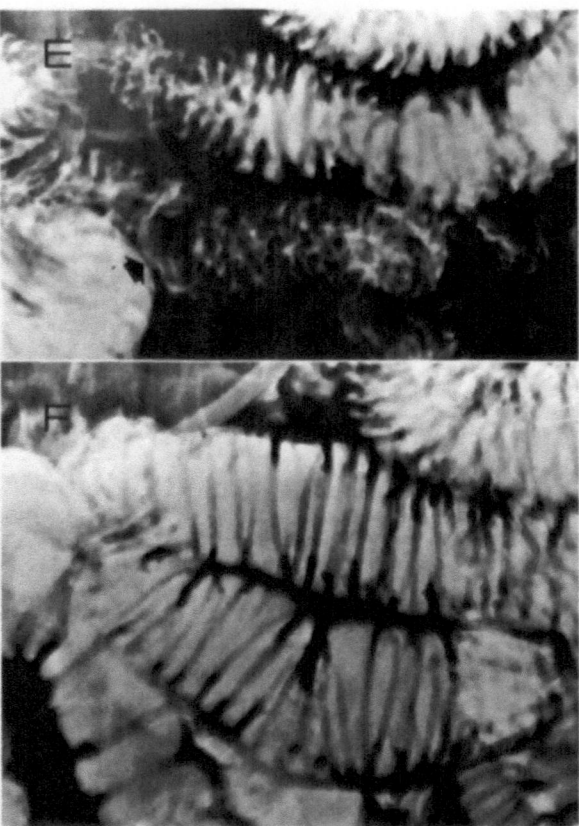

Fig. 10.8. Misleading pattern resembling leiomyoma due to local compression of the intestinal loops.

Fig. 10.9. Configuration resembling a round bulge in the intestinal loop (E) disappears when the intestine is well filled (F).

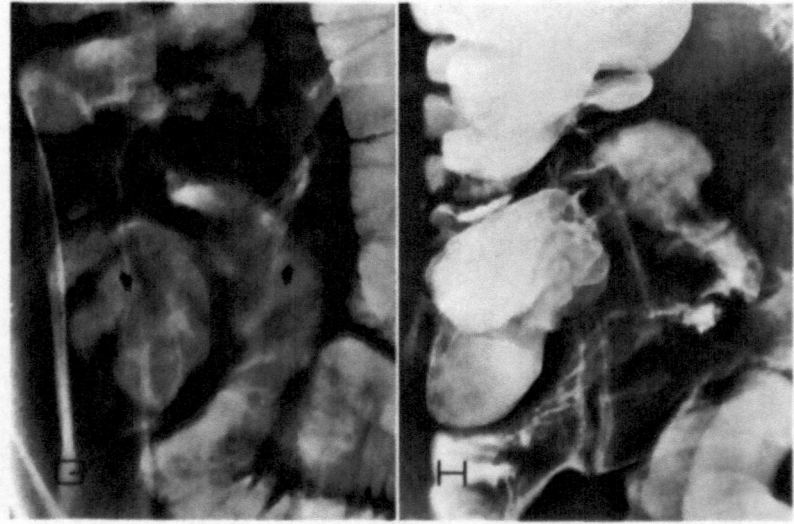

Fig. 10.10. This configuration, caused mainly by bone structures, somewhat resembles a space-occupying process in the region of Bauhin's valve (G). In a different projection the misleading pattern has completely disappeared (H).

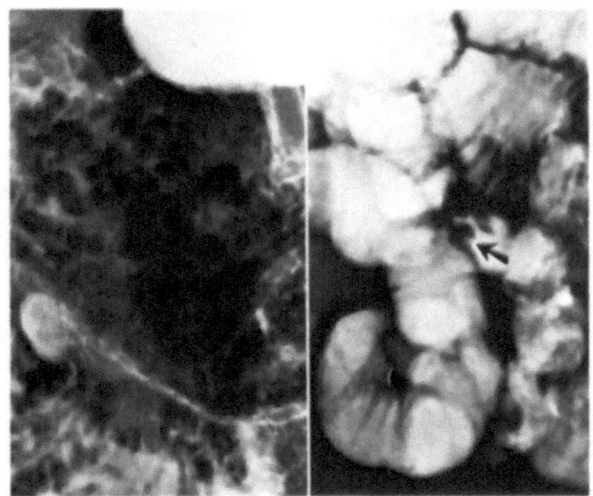

*Fig. 10.11*A. Polyps in the stomach and a few of equal size in the small intestine due to the Peutz-Jeghers syndrome. Polyps were also found in the rectum of this patient.

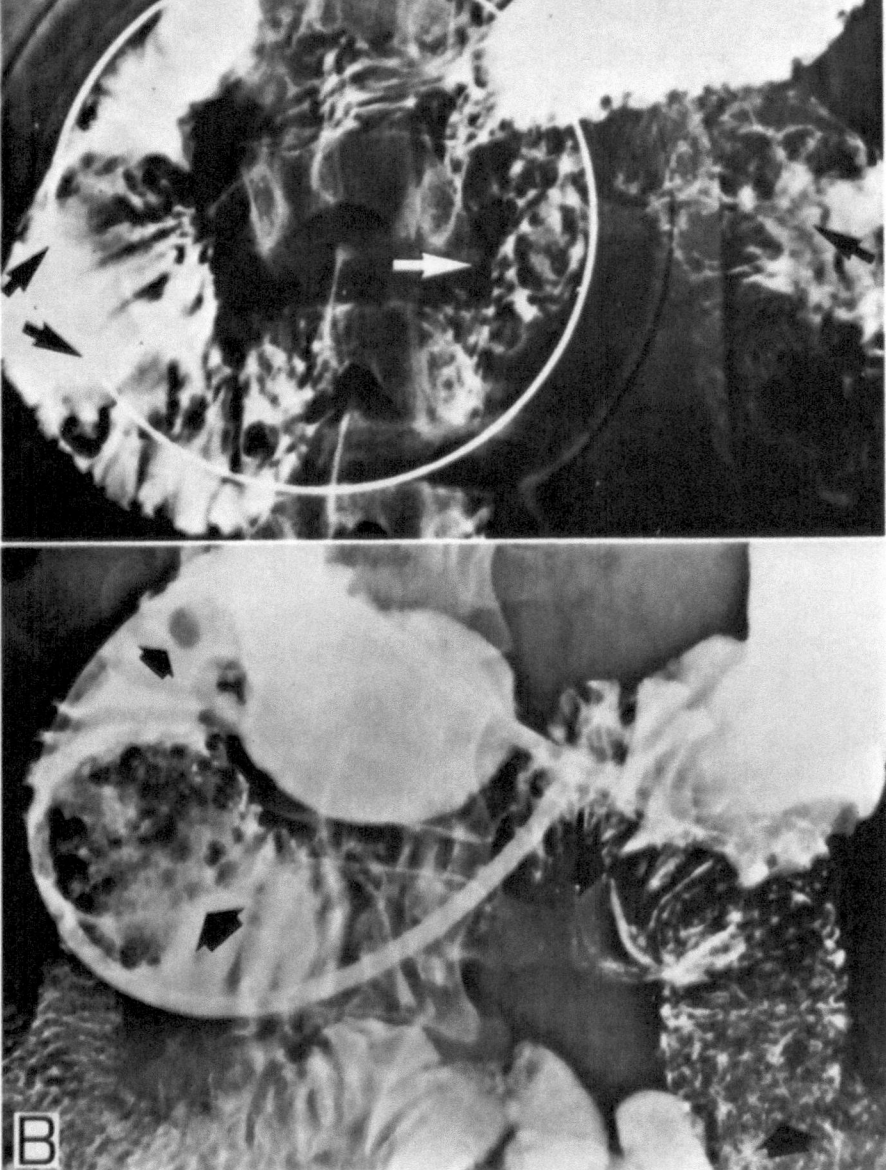

*Fig. 10.11*B. Polyps of different size in the duodenum due to a Peutz-Jeghers syndrome in two different patients.

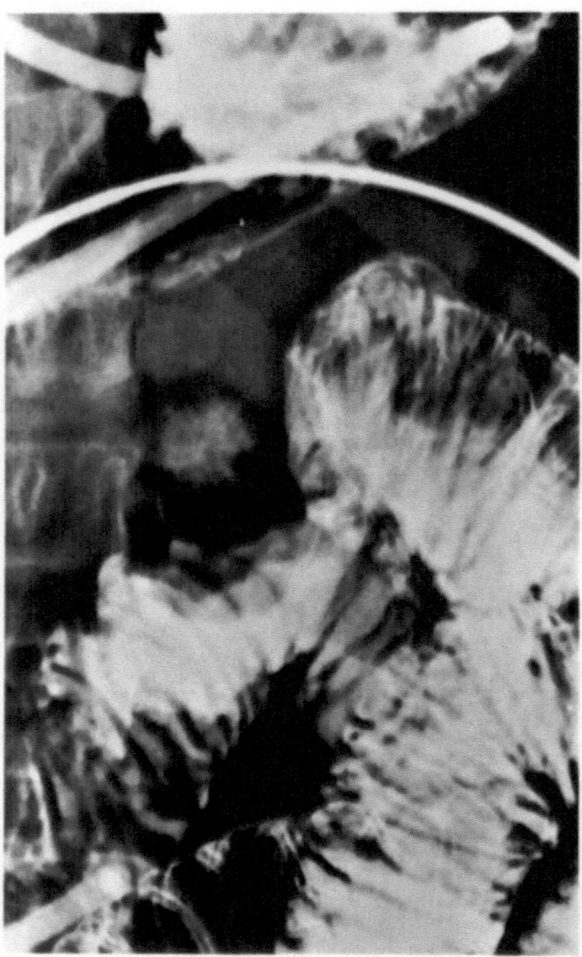

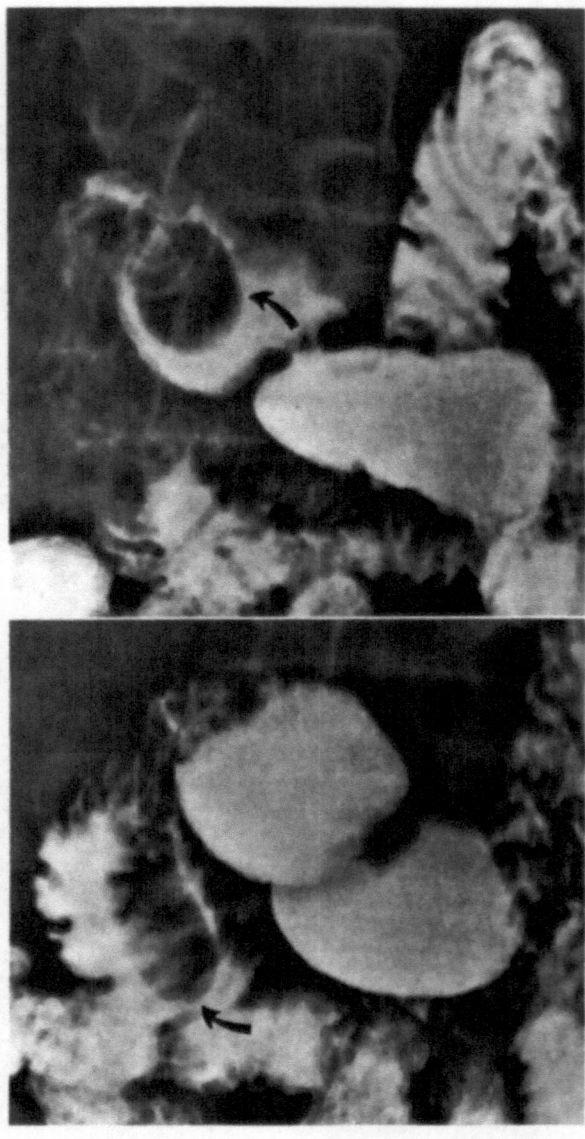

Fig. 10.12A. Leiomyoma of the jejunum with centrally located calcifications. (Courtesy of Prof. A. de Schepper, Antwerp.)

Fig. 10.12B. A characteristic of lipomas is that they are easily deformed.

storage and is somewhat suggestive of Addison's disease. The polyps can be so small that they are invisible or so large that they cause hemorrhage and attacks of pain as a result of recurrent intussusceptions. The polyps can be distributed diffusely or in patches and they are generally more numerous in the jejunum than in the ileum. The Cronkhite-Canada syndrome is much more rare. In addition to the hyperpigmentation, it can also be accompanied by alopecia, dystrophy of the nails, and a severe malabsorption. In this disease, which possibly should be considered a form of generalized juvenile polyposis, the polyps are inflammatory and epi-

thelial in nature and often contain multiple cysts filled with mucin. The Cronkhite-Canada syndrome has a high mortality. It is not hereditary and so far has been found only in adults over 40 years of age.

3. Benign tumors

As previously mentioned, although the benign tumors in the small intestine predominate over the malignant in number, they cause no obstruction – or at least not until quite late. Partly for this reason they are only occasionally diagnosed. At least one-

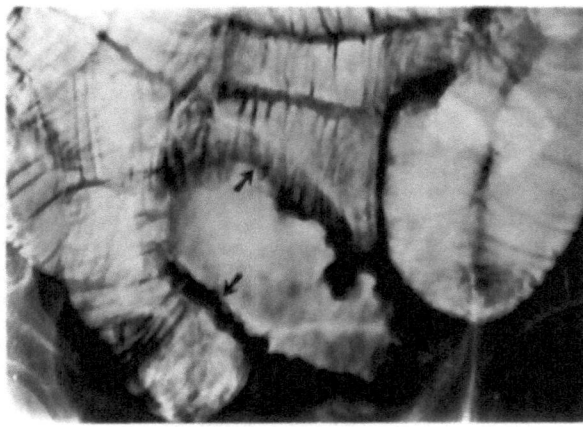

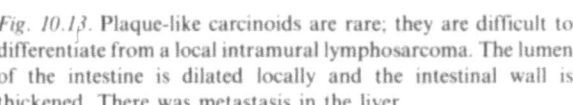

Fig. 10.13. Plaque-like carcinoids are rare; they are difficult to differentiate from a local intramural lymphosarcoma. The lumen of the intestine is dilated locally and the intestinal wall is thickened. There was metastasis in the liver.

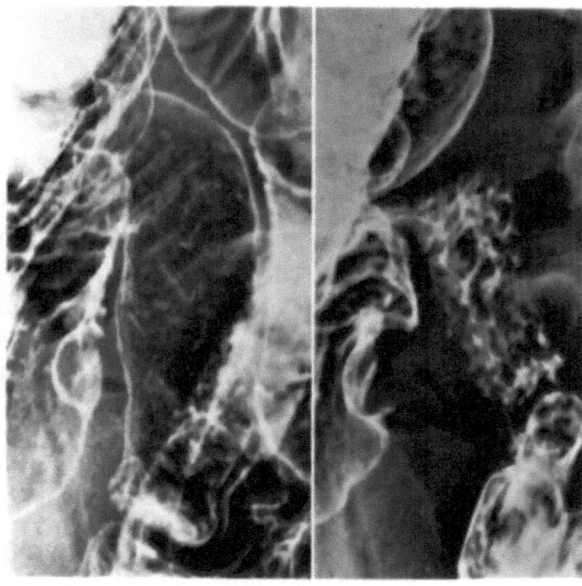

Fig. 10.14. Small carcinoid tumor at the base of the appendix that is almost impossible to distinguish from an invaginated stump after an appendectomy.

third of the benign tumors cause recurrent occult or gross bleeding via the rectum. However, this has not increased the frequency with which this diagnosis is established. In the case of teleangiectasia or hemangiomas, both occurring mainly in the jejunum, the bleeding can even be profuse. Still it is seldom possible to discover the lesion during transit examination of the small intestine. Teleangiectasias are only dilatations of existing vascular structures. The hemangiomas, which originate in the submucosal vascular plexus, can be scattered and quite tiny. If the presence of calcified phleboliths does not indicate the nature of the disease, an angiographic examination will be necessary to determine the diagnosis.

In addition to vascular tumors, we also find solitary adenomatous polyps, myomas, lipomas, and fibromas with approximately equal frequency in the small bowel. Fibromas, like vascular tumors, often develop intramurally or extraluminally and are rarely discovered by means of radiological examination.

Although leiomyomas lie within but mainly outside the small intestinal wall, they are diagnosed more frequently than any of the other benign tumors because of their size. Leiomyomas can occur everywhere in the small intestine, but are most

common in the jejunum. A central necrosis with ulceration, hemorrhage and calcification can develop in leiomyomas even when there is no malignant degeneration (fig. 10.12A). A characteristic of the larger intramural benign tumor is that the folds of the intact mucosa stretch across the growth. It should be mentioned, however, that external compression of the intestinal loops can produce a somewhat similar effect. The compression of intestinal loops resulting from the intraluminal or mesenteric spread of a lymphosarcoma can usually be recognized because of the concomitant stenoses and obliteration of the mucosa.

Lipomas can also be found throughout the small intestine, but generally they are encountered in the most distal part of the ileum. They are usually round or oval, but can sometimes be multipolypoid. In Bauhin's valve they cause sharply defined irregular masses in the contrast column. These masses are quite prominent in the cecum. Because lipomas spread mainly in the submucosa or intraluminally, they lead to intussusceptions and sometimes cause recurring complaints of obstruction. One characteristic of lipomas is their weak structure; as a result they are easily deformed (fig. 10.12B). Differentiation from air bubbles can be difficult unless several films showing the abnormality are available.

4. Semimalignant tumors

Carcinoids are plaque (fig. 10.13) or nodule-like growths in the intestinal mucosa that originate in the serotonin-producing argentaffin cells in the floor of the crypts of Lieberkühn. Carcinoids, solitary and multiple, can be encountered everywhere in the digestive tract but also occur elsewhere in the body such as the biliary ducts, the pancreas, or the bronchial tree. The most common site is the appendix (fig. 10.14), but in almost one-third of the cases they are found in the distal ileum (fig. 10.15). Carcinoids occur predominantly in younger patients. In general they grow very slowly and are therefore regarded as a low-grade malignancy. In at least one-third of the cases there is also metastasis, almost always in the liver but sometimes also in other organs. Metastasis is most common when the carcinoid is localized in the ileum or colon (fig. 10.16), and is exceedingly rare when the primary site is the appendix. When localized in the region of Bauhin's valve, it must be differentiated in particular from hypertrophy, lipomatosis, and lymphoma (fig. 10.28D). If the tumor is eccentric and the distal ileum appears stretched, then of course both a hypertrophic Bauhin's valve and lipomatosis are less likely.

The serotonin produced by the tumor is a protein-like hormone that enhances peristalsis and causes bronchospasms and diarrhea. Normally most of the serotonin produced is metabolized in the liver and only minimal amounts enter the bloodstream. If larger quantities enter the liver or if the serotonin is produced in the liver by the metastases, then it also enters the right site of the heart and causes endothelial growths on the cardiac valves. A pulmonary stenosis, tricuspidal insufficiency, and dilatation of the heart with a right-sided decompensation can result. The filtering action of the pulmonary circulation keeps the left side of the heart free of these complications. If there is metastasis in the liver, bradykinin is also produced. Like serotonin, bradykinin is a protein-like hormone that causes the 'flush syndrome' so characteristic of carcinoid. The flush syndrome lasts 5–10 min and is typified by a pronounced redness and hotness of the

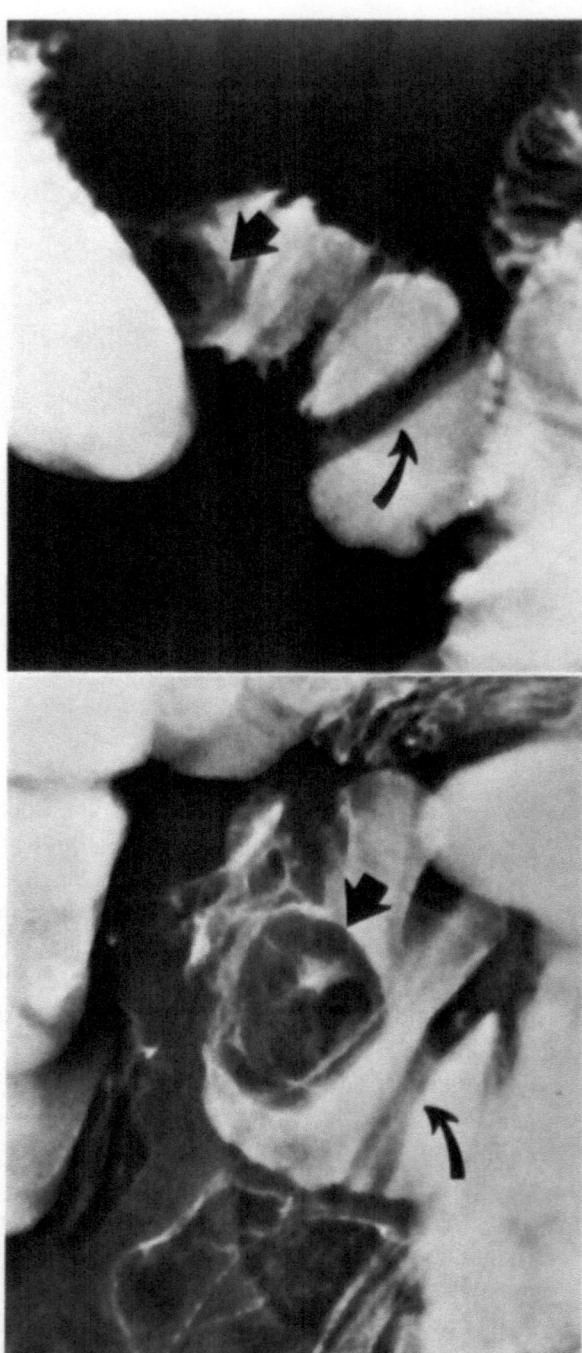

Fig. 10.15. Two cases of intramural carcinoids in the distal ileum (thick arrows). Extensive fibrosis in the intestinal wall and the mesentery causes constrictions of the intestinal lumen; when the intestine is well filled, these constrictions are clearly visible as deep grooves (thin arrows).

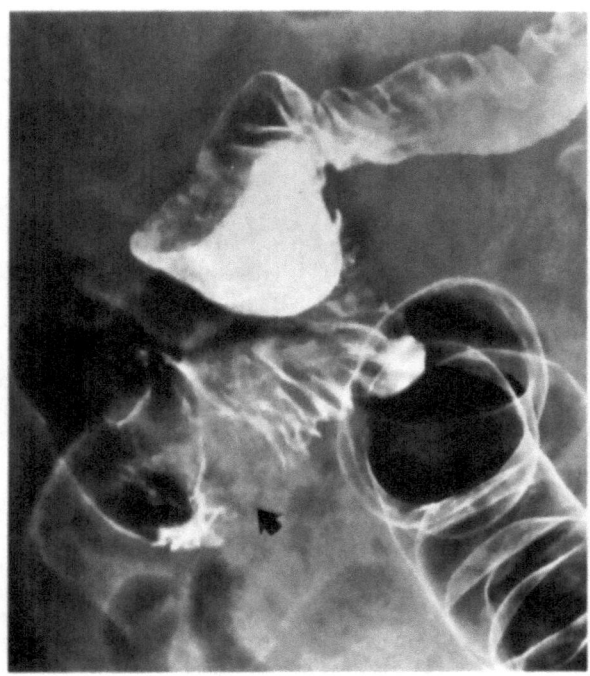

Fig. 10.16A. Extensive carcinoids with more or less smooth polycyloid margins in the cecum. Extensive metastases in the liver.

upper half of the body followed by tachycardia and vasodilatation and ending with cyanosis. Strain or fear, and sometimes consumption of alcohol or cheese, can provoke a flush reaction.

One-third of the patients who were found at autopsy to have had a carcinoid had had no complaints. The diagnosis of carcinoid can be verified biochemically in blood and urine by the increased levels in the breakdown products of serotonin and bradykinin. Radiologically the easiest way to establish the diagnosis is an angiographic examination of the celiac trunk that reveals the highly vascularized metastases. The latter are frequently present and are always much larger than the primary lesion.

In the intestine, carcinoids are often intramural and small so that they cannot be demonstrated. If they are somewhat larger, they cannot be distinguished from any other tumor that bulges out into the lumen and is covered with an intact mucosa (fig. 10.15). In a later stage, there is extensive fibrosis in the area surrounding the carcinoid. As a result of this shriveling, the lumen of the intestine can show annular constriction and pseudodiverticula (fig. 10.17) or will follow an abrupt change in course

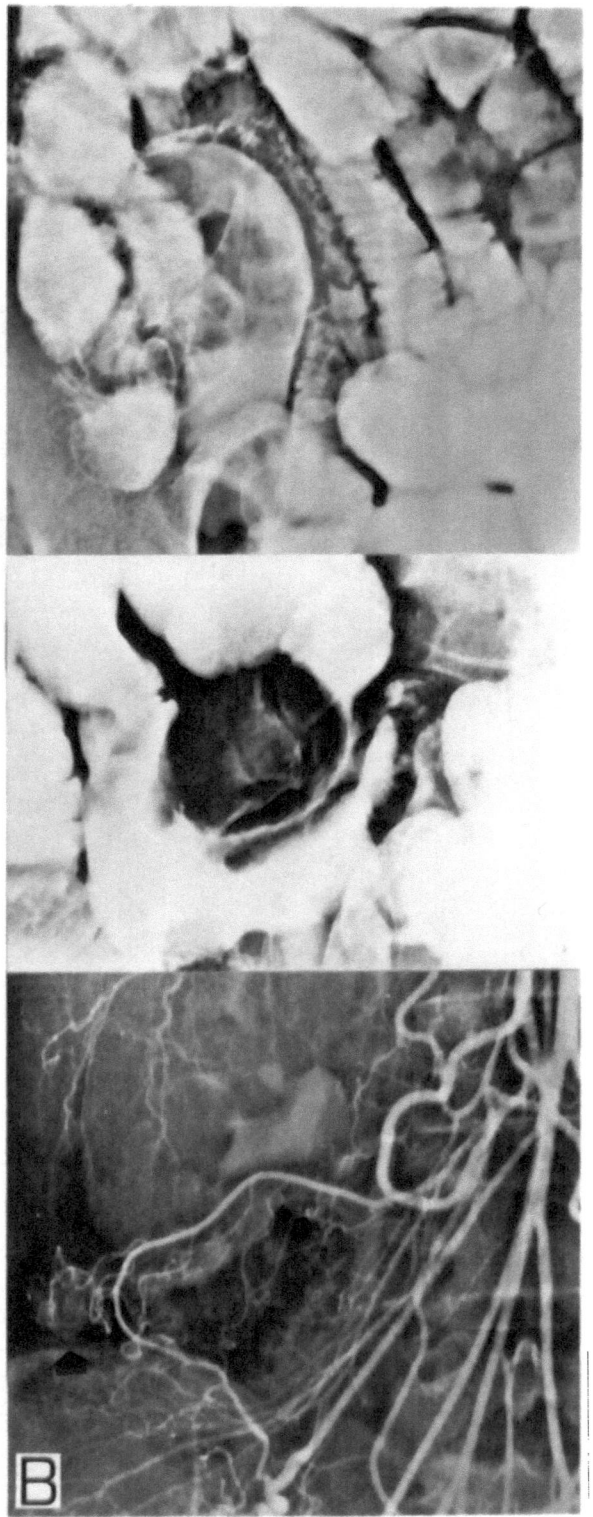

Fig. 10.16B. Carcinoid in Bauhin's valve with stretched distal ileum, almost invisible on the plain film (top), but easily seen on the compression spot film (middle). An angiogram (bottom) revealed not only the carcinoid but also metastases in the liver.

292

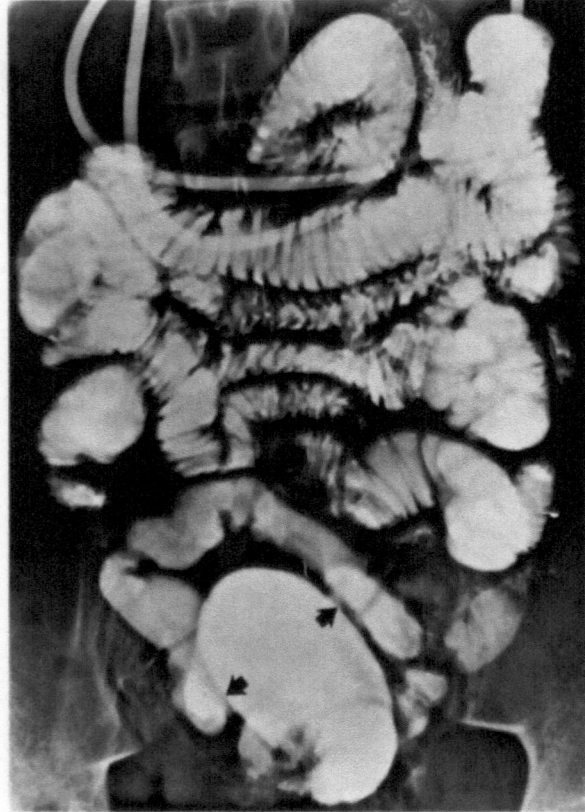

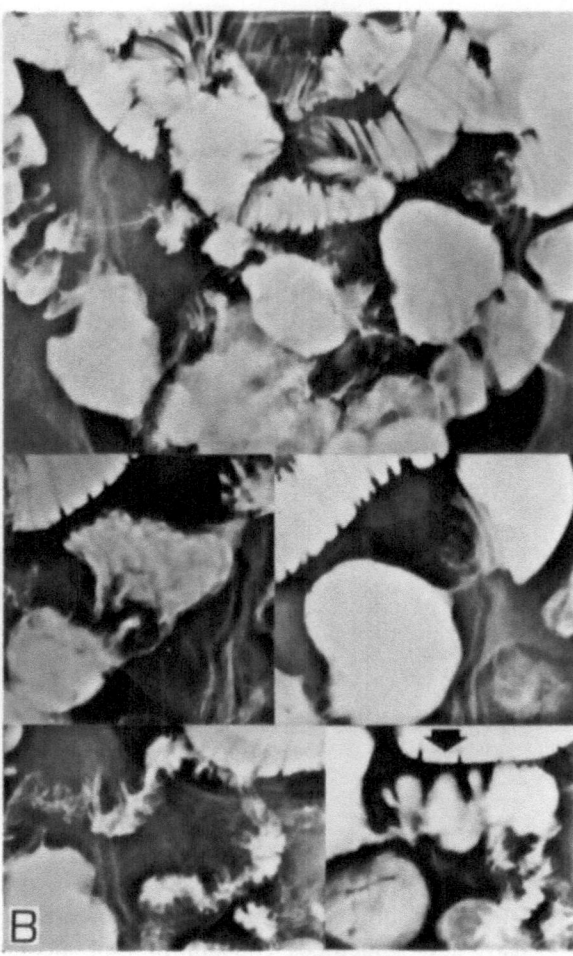

B

*Fig. 10.17*B. A middle-aged woman suffered from sensations of heat that were attributed to menopause; her general practitioner prescribed hormonal therapy. The radiological examination revealed hypermotility of the small intestine with constricting lesions and pseudodiverticula in the ileum due to carcinoids.

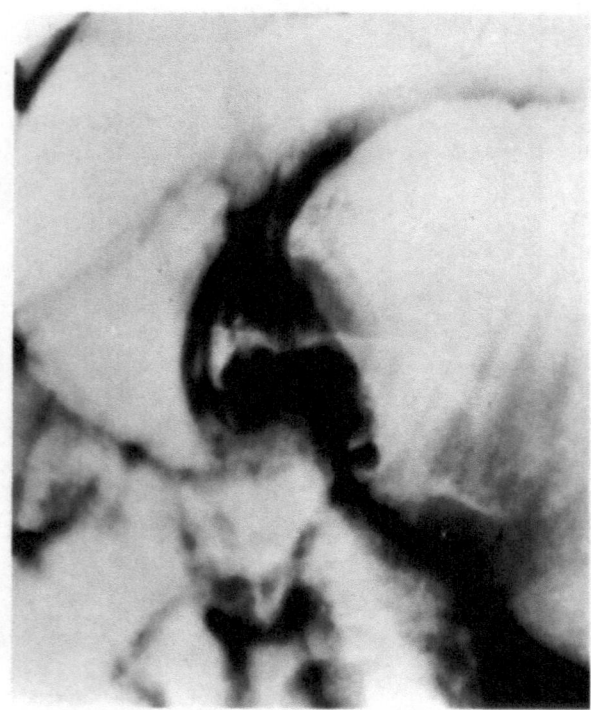

*Fig. 10.17*A. Annular stricture due to small carcinoid tumor with marked shriveling. On the survey film an obvious prestenotic dilatation (arrows) was noted that had to be located in the small intestine since the rectum and sigmoid were not yet filled with contrast medium.

designated as 'kinking' (fig. 10.18). The serotonin secreted by the tumor can cause a pronounced hyperperistalsis and the increased pressure inside the bowel may be the reason of diverticula formation (fig. 10.18A). Possibly due to the compression, hyperperistalsis can be temporary and more or less localized (fig. 10.19). The mucosal pattern is then somewhat feathered, just as in cases of mild anoxia in an intestine with a decreased caliber. When the tumor is extraluminal, a feather-like mucosal pattern can also be seen. As in the case of a leiomyoma, the intestine lies stretched out across the tumor and may therefore be more dilated than normal.

A disease that somewhat resembles carcinoid in many respects but is not in the least malignant is

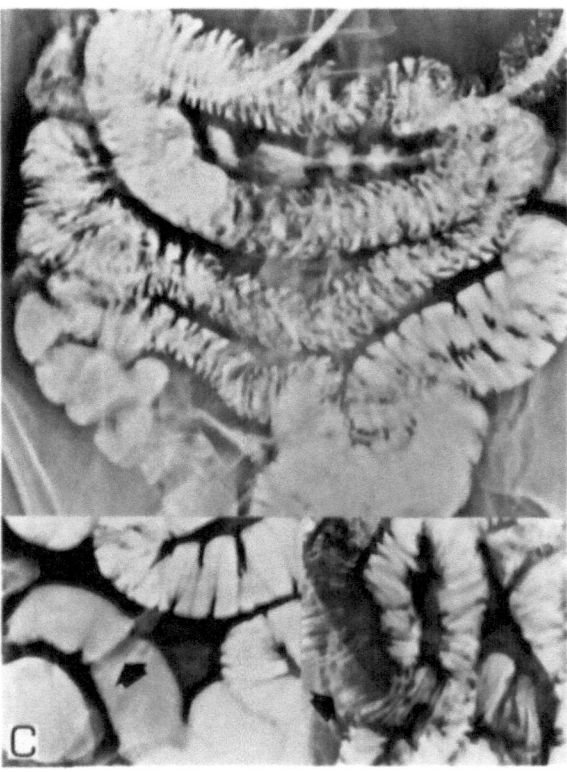

Fig. 10.17C. Patient with hypermotility of the small bowel. Moreover, a very subtle lesion in the distal ileum consisting of an intramural defect in the intestinal wall during the empty phase of the examination and a constriction when the intestine was well filled. Upon surgery, the suspected carcinoid was found.

endometriosis. This is the heterotopic localization of endometrium in women between 30 and 40 years of age, but sometimes younger or older.

Although occurring predominantly in organs and tissues in the minor pelvis and the sigmoid, localizations in the appendix, cecum, and ileum are also occasionally seen. The disease is characterized by a dysmenorrhea and a pain that increases and decreases periodically because the ectopic tissue is totally involved in the menstrual cycle. In endometriosis, too, the tumor, which is absolutely benign, is intramural. It is subserous and seldom grows through the mucosa in the direction of the lumen. Cyclic bleedings usually do not reach the lumen of the intestine so that there is no rectal bleeding. The mucosal pattern remains intact and is lost only when bleeding is so profuse that the stretched mucous membrane becomes nectrotic. The recurrent bleedings lead to widespread fibrosis, annular obstructions, stenoses several centimeters

long, angulation, and kinking that radiologically cannot be distinguished from that due to carcinoid.

5. Malignant tumors

The most important primary malignant tumors in the small intestine are, in order of frequency, lymphoreticular tumors, adenocarcinomas, and leiomyosarcomas. There are, however, numerous references in the literature that state that adenocarcinoma occurs more frequently than lymphosarcoma and reticulosarcoma together.

Leiomyosarcoma is usually discovered fairly late because it is a slow-growing tumor and, since it is extraluminal, does not cause obstruction in the early stages. At the time of diagnosis, the tumor is often quite large and can be felt as a palpable mass. Even more than in leiomyoma, the radiological aspect is characterized by quite pronounced and more or less parallel intestinal mucosal folds (fig. 10.20). In the more advanced stages, invasion and destruction of the intestinal mucosa do occur so that this characteristic pattern disappears (fig. 10.21). Then there are also often clear signs of ulceration and central necrosis. Leiomyosarcomas are encountered everywhere in the small bowel although they seldom occur in the duodenum and retroperitoneal space (fig. 10.22).

The diagnosis is usually not established until quite late, and only surgical intervention can be considered since these highly vascularized tumors barely react to chemotherapy and radiotherapy. In spite of this the five-year survival rate is almost 50%; the prognosis is therefore relatively favorable.

In adenocarcinomas, on the other hand, annular strictures develop rapidly; as a result this disease is discovered much sooner.

Adenocarcinoma occurs more frequently in the proximal part of the small intestine, sometimes in the duodenum (fig. 10.23) and in particular near the duodenojejunal junction (fig. 10.24). A localization in the duodenum gives clinical symptoms that somewhat resemble those of a slightly atypical peptic ulcer. This is deceptive and does not lead to early diagnosis. In general, adenocarcinoma appears as a short, irregularly defined constricting lesion (fig. 10.25). In the duodenum, however, the tumor is sometimes multipolypoid in form, mu-

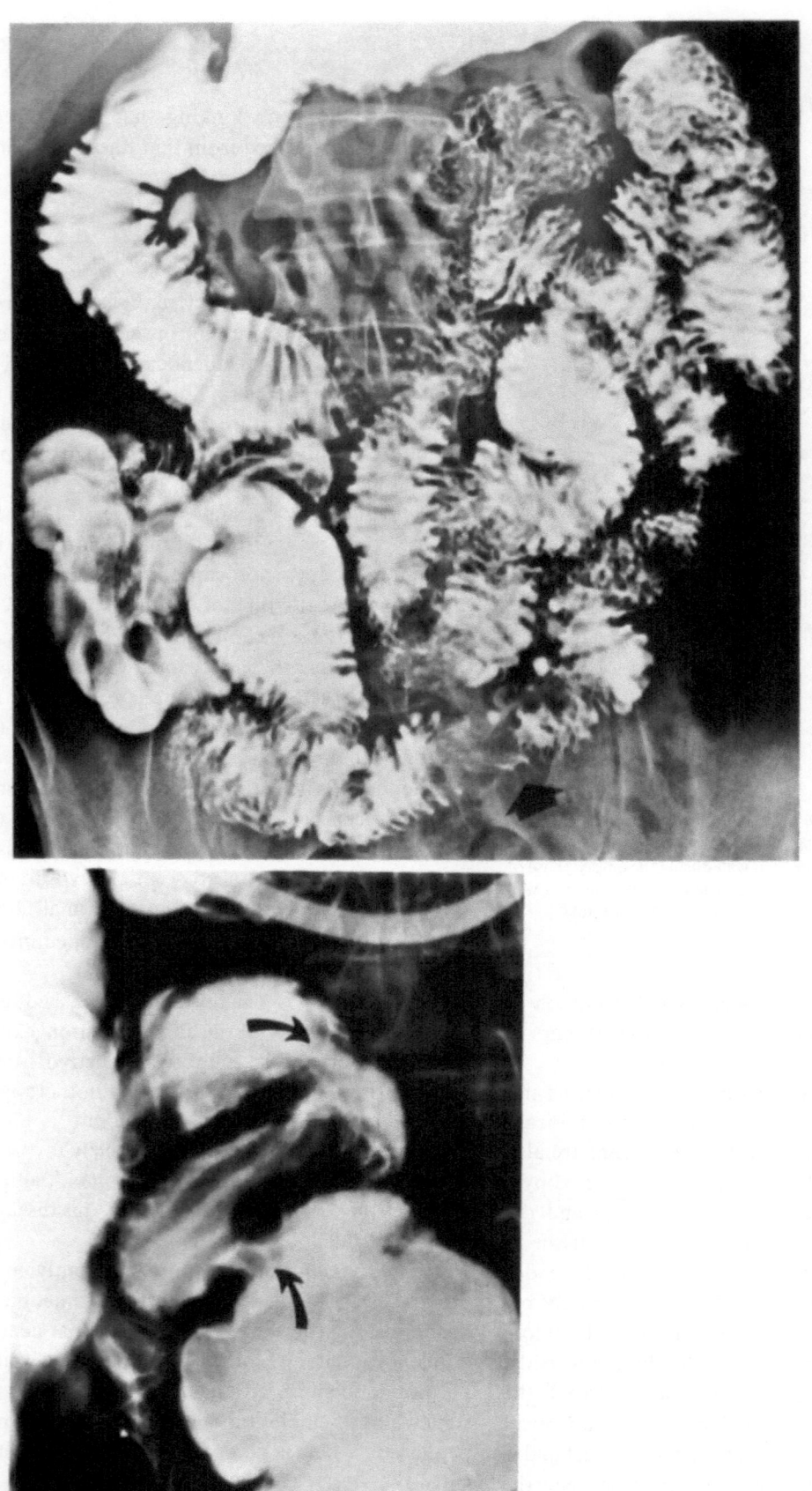

*Fig. 10.18*A. Hypermotility with the formation of diverticula in the ileum (top) and abrupt changes in the course of the intestine (kinking) caused by local shriveling of the mesentery due to a carcinoid (bottom).

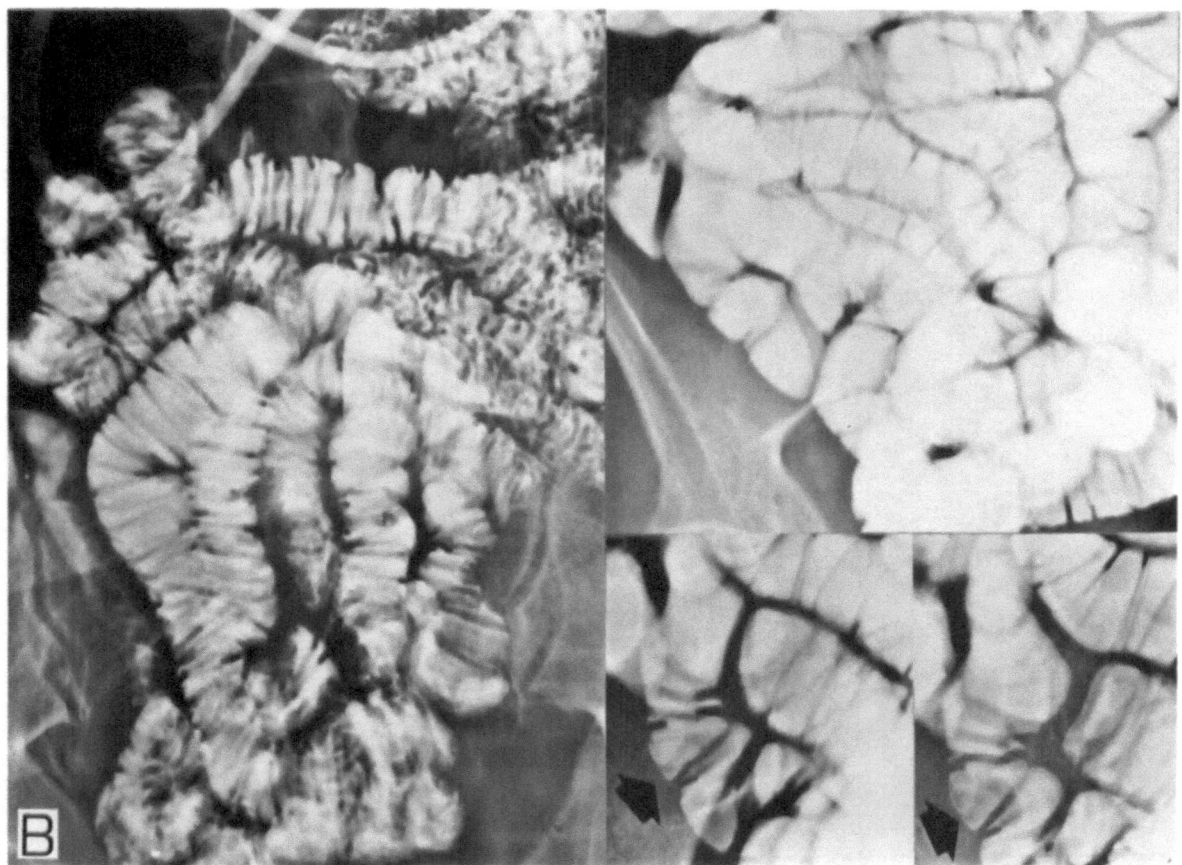

*Fig. 10.18*B. Generalized hypermotility of the intestine. At a rate of flow of 75 ml/s, less than 400 ml contrast medium were needed to reach the cecum – instead of the statistical average of almost 700 ml. Since carcinoids were suspected and such a moderate filling of the intestine prevents proper evaluation of the mucosa, the examination was then continued by increasing the rate of flow to 150 ml/s. This detail of the plain film thus obtained shows that even in the case of hypermotility such a high rate of flow causes paralysis of the intestine. Intramural carcinoids were not found during this phase of the examination; however, the 'kinking sign' in the distal ileum (arrow) can be regarded as a secondary indication of carcinoids. This diagnosis was confirmed at surgery.

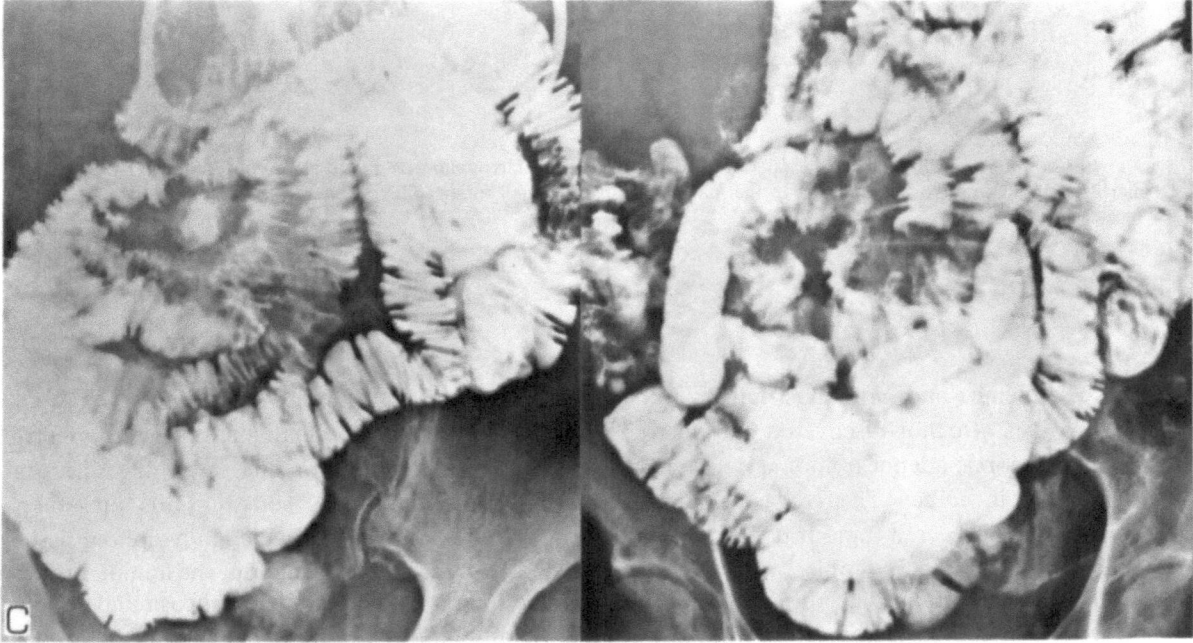

*Fig. 10.19*A. Local hypermotility in a patient with carcinoids and metastases in the liver. The empty spaces in the middle of the convolution of intestinal loops are probably caused by both mesenteric shriveling and the carcinoids themselves.

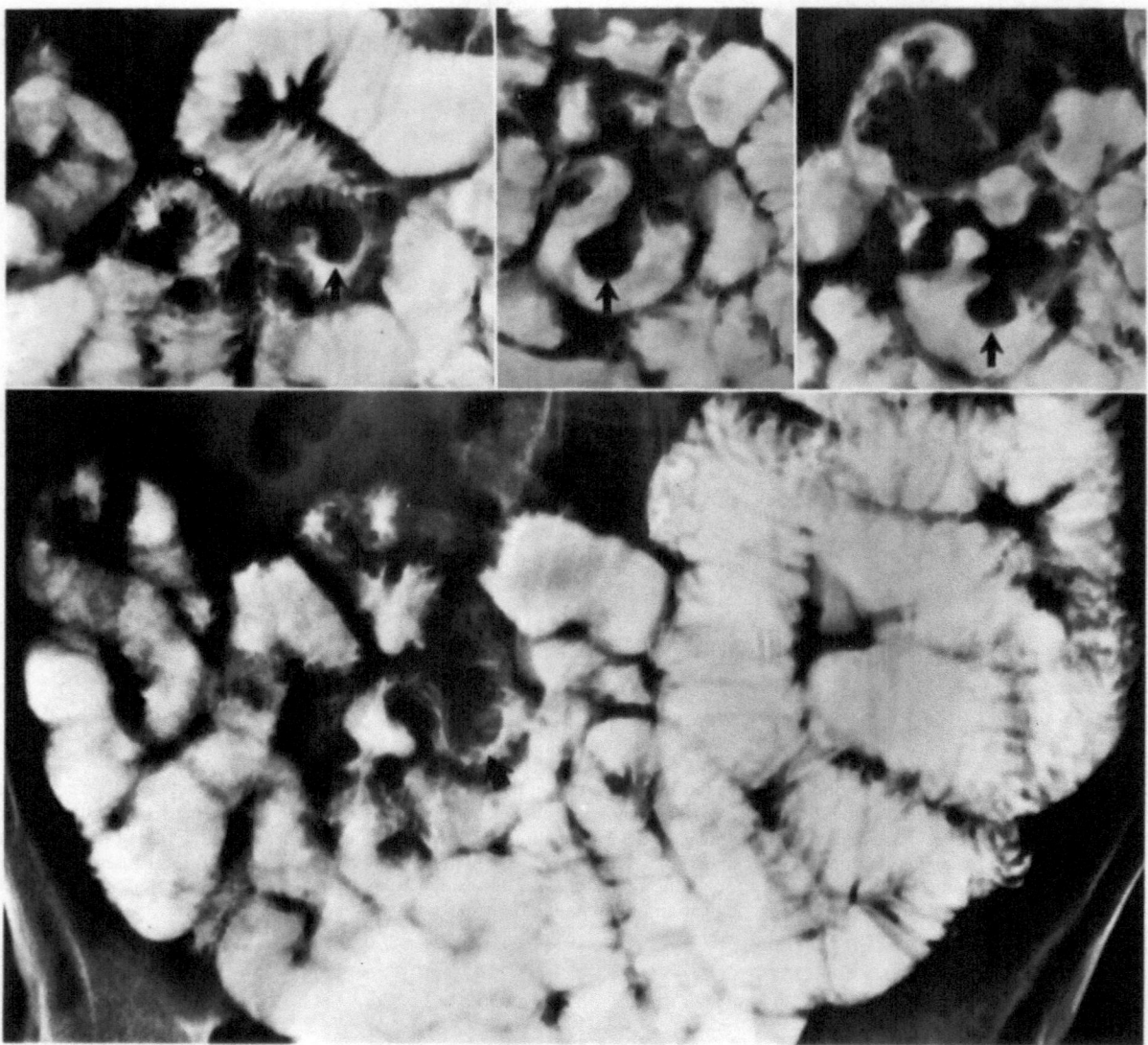

*Fig. 10.19*ʙ. Intestine with very local hypermotility and high tone (narrow lumen) due to serotonin produced by a carcinoid. The marble-sized space (arrows) seen next to the lumen must be the small tumor. There were metastases in the liver.

cous-producing, and not constricting. For these reasons it is also not discovered as quickly. Like leiomyosarcoma, adenocarcinoma is more common in men than in women. The five-year survival rate is about 20%; however, a tumour proximal to Treitz's ligament has a less favorable prognosis than one localized more distally. This difference in prognosis is because a tumor in the distal intestine can be removed by means of a simple resection. A localization proximal to Treitz's ligament requires the more major 'Whipple' operation.

Lymphoreticular malignant growths are probably the most common in the small intestine, and not adenocarcinoma as stated in the literature. The entire small intestine is rich in lymphoid tissue. It is spread diffusely throughout the lamina propria and is found in follicles in the mucosa and submucosa, mainly in the distal ileum. The distal ileum is therefore also the most frequent localization of lymphosarcoma and reticulosarcoma. Other com-

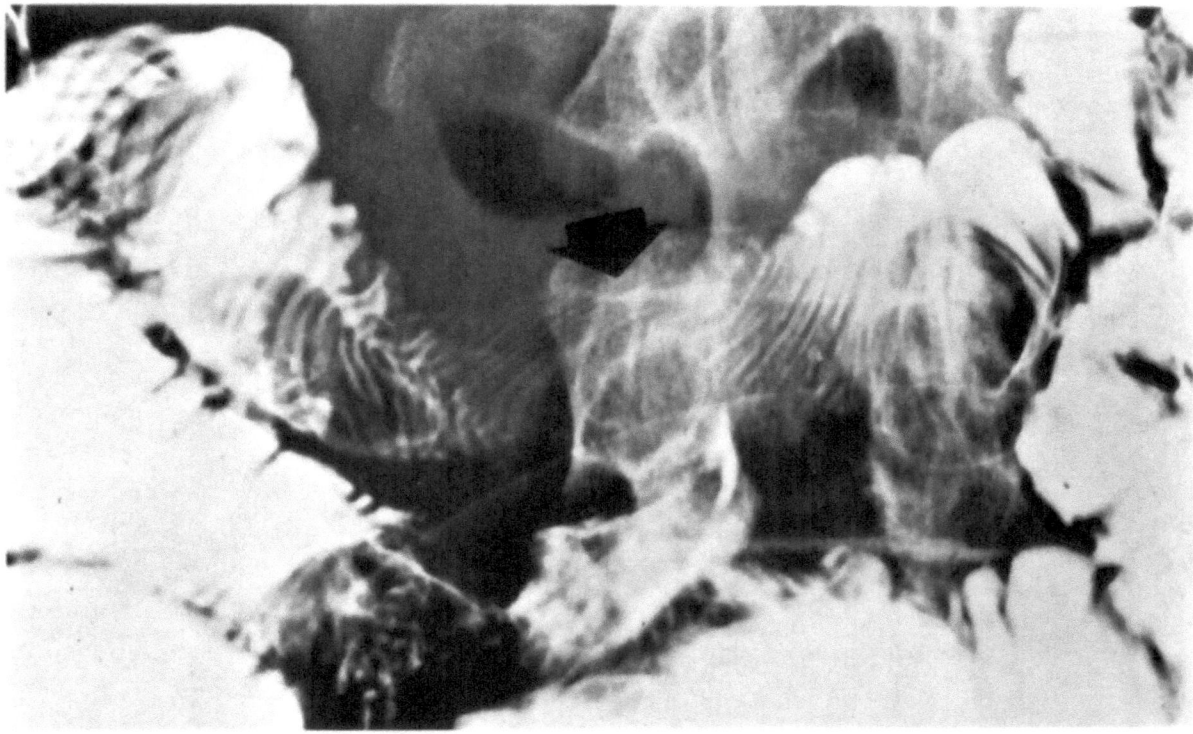

Fig. 10.20. Stretched and more or less parallel mucosal folds in a very long segment (±10 cm) of the small bowel caused by a leiomyosarcoma.

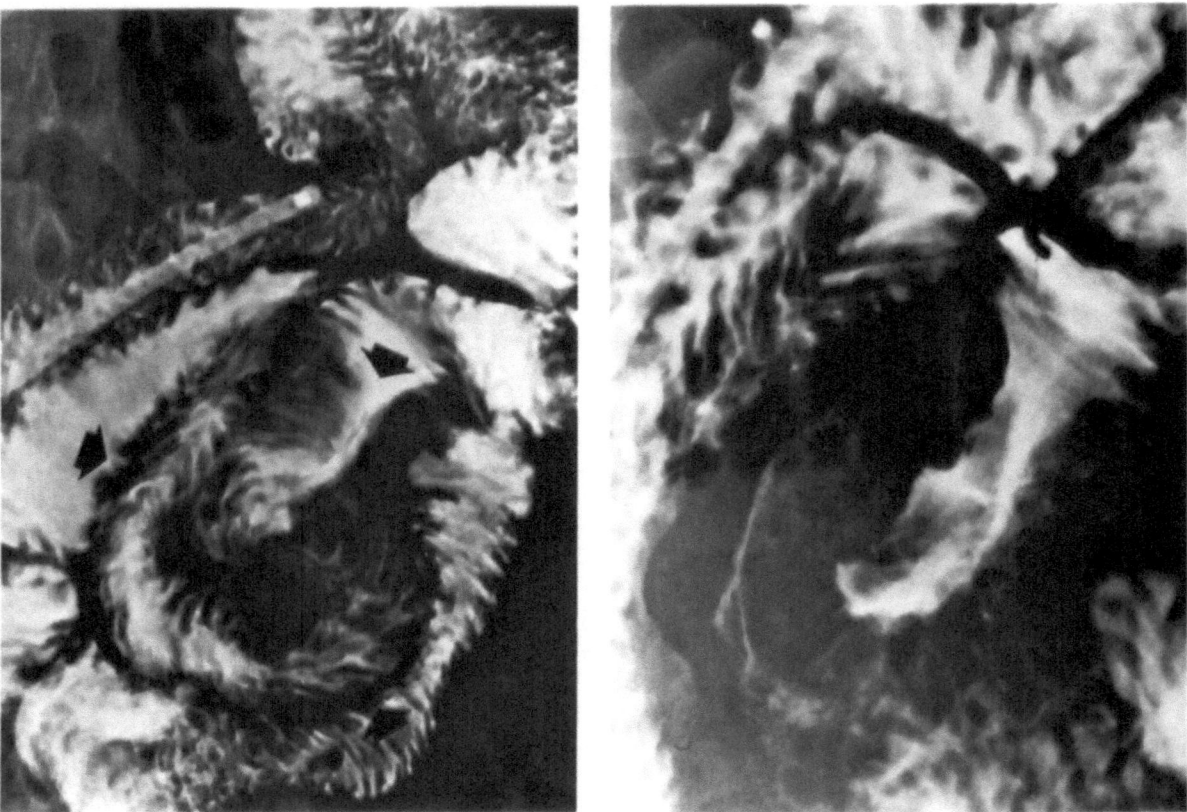

Fig. 10.21. Large leiomyosarcoma that can no longer be differentiated from any other extensive tumorous mass such as the liposarcoma in fig. 10.4 and the lymphosarcoma in fig. 10.28.

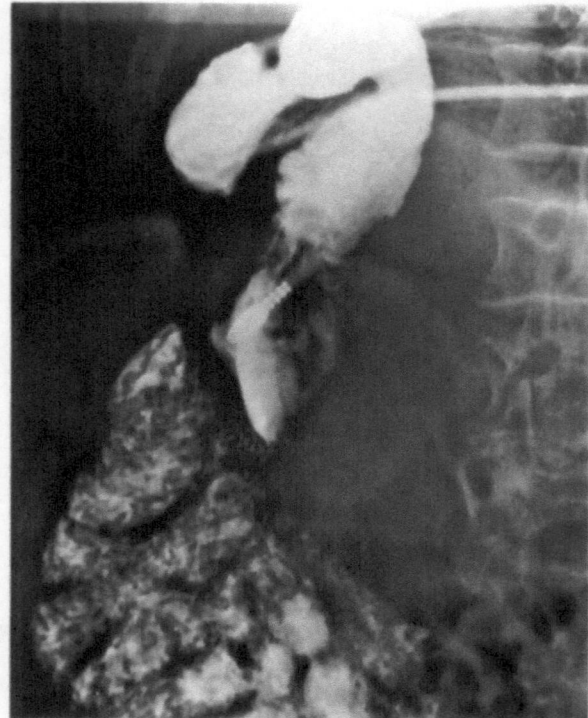

Fig. 10.22. Large leiomyosarcoma, growing in the retroperitoneal space, that probably did not originate in the duodenum. Pronounced displacement of the mass of intestinal loops.

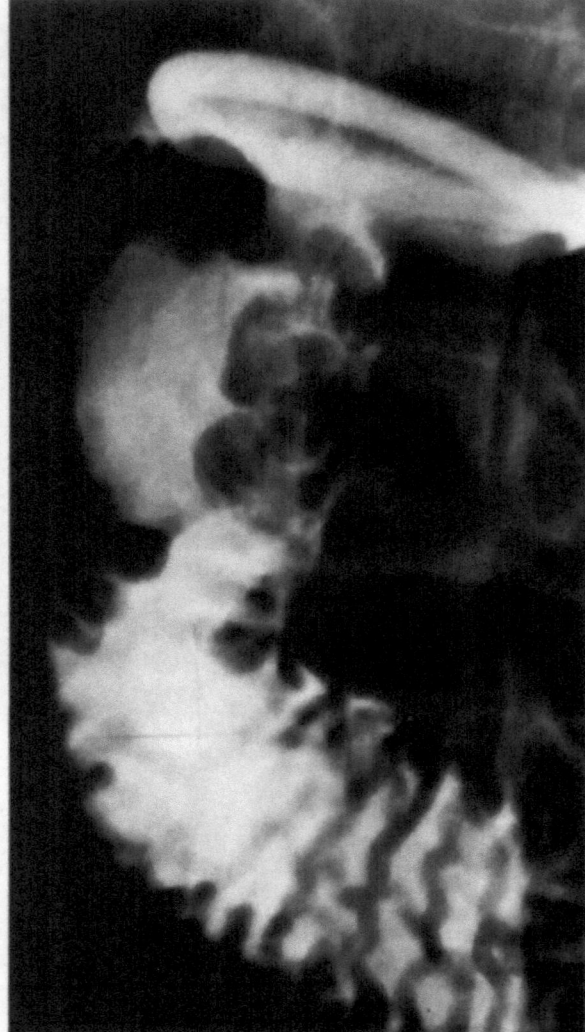

Fig. 10.23A. Large ulcerous adenocarcinoma in the descending limb of the duodenum.

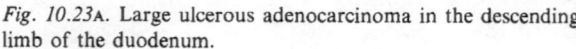

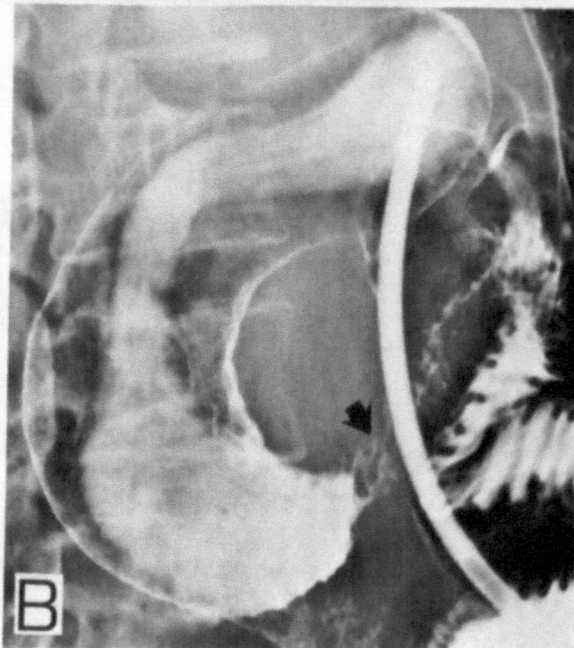

Fig. 10.23B. Adenocarcinoma of the horizontal limb of the duodenum; proximal to this the walls of the duodenum are completely smooth. The latter phenomenon was never explained.

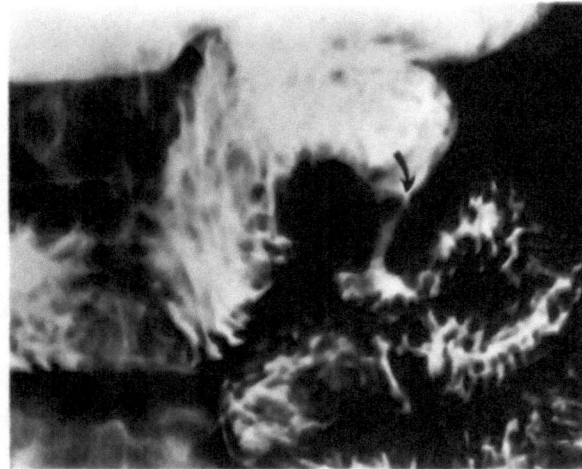

Fig. 10.24. Smooth stenosis, ±3 cm long, in the duodenojejunal junction due to an adenocarcinoma.

mon sites are the duodenum, jejunum, and appendix. Solitary localizations are less common (fig. 10.26). In most cases, however, the sites are multiple and include several segments of the intestines (fig. 10.27м).

Histologically reticulosarcomas differ little from lymphosarcomas except that the lymphocytic infiltrates consist of less mature cells with larger nuclei and there is more reticular tissue. Reticulum cell sarcomas (fig. 10.27) usually grow faster than lymphosarcomas and in most cases growth along the length of the intestine is much less extensive. It seems that the tumor seldom reaches this stage. If five-year survival for lymphosarcoma after surgical, radiotherapeutic, or cytostatic treatment is about 50%, that for reticulum cell sarcoma is 25%, at the most.

Tumors originating in the lymph follicles or the lamina propria are called primary lymphomas. The mesentery and the abdominal lymph nodes can also be involved, but there are no or very few sites in other organs. A generalized lymphoreticular sarcoma or malignant lymphoma can be encountered in the liver, spleen, or skeleton. In one-fourth of these cases, there are also localizations in the small bowel and then it is called secondary lymphoma. In small children, certainly more than 50% show localizations in the small intestine.

A lymphoreticular process in the small intestine can manifest itself in many different ways clinically but especially radiologically. In primary or secon-

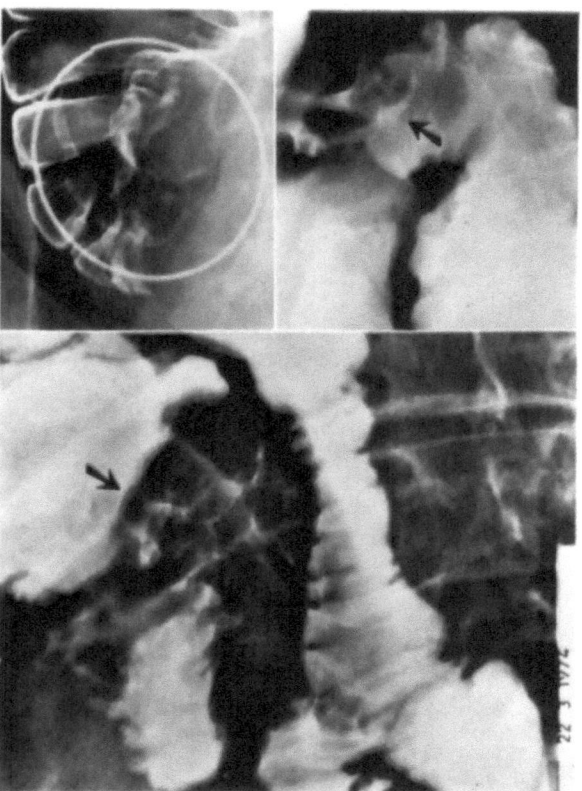

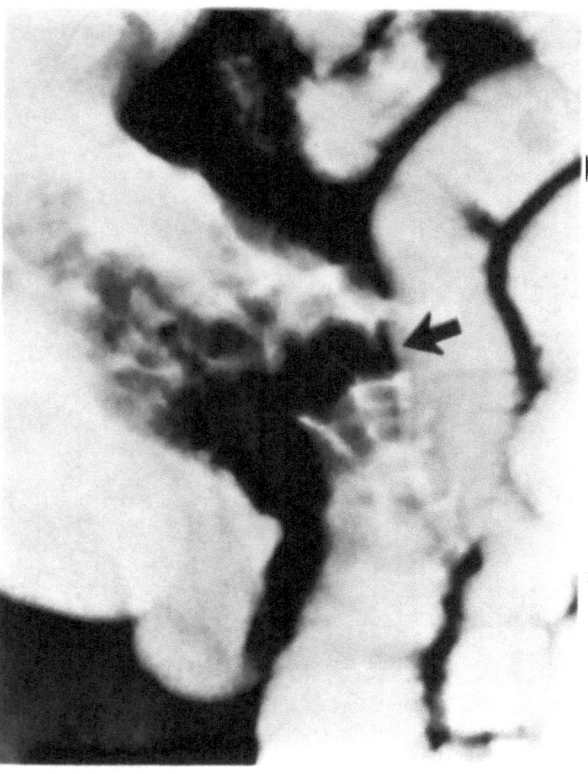

Fig. 10.25. Two cases of short strictures with irregular margins in the ileum caused by adenocarcinoma.

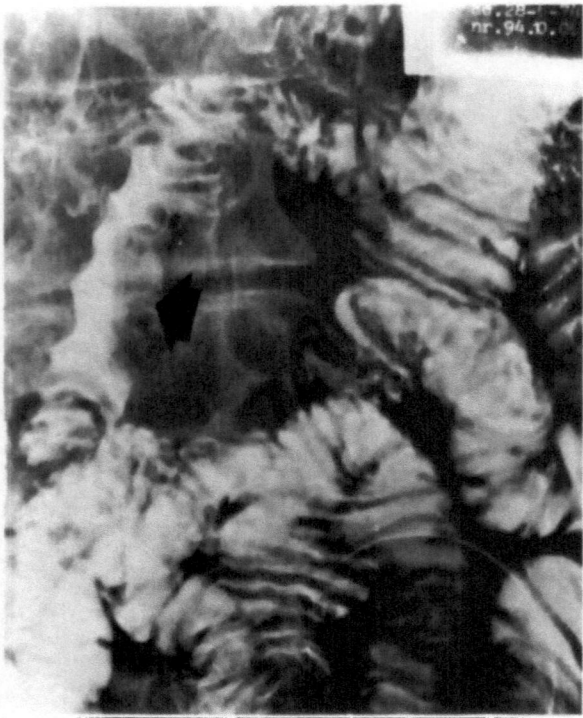

Fig. 10.26. A solitary lymphosarcoma is encountered less frequently. It is presented here as an extended stenosis in the jejunum.

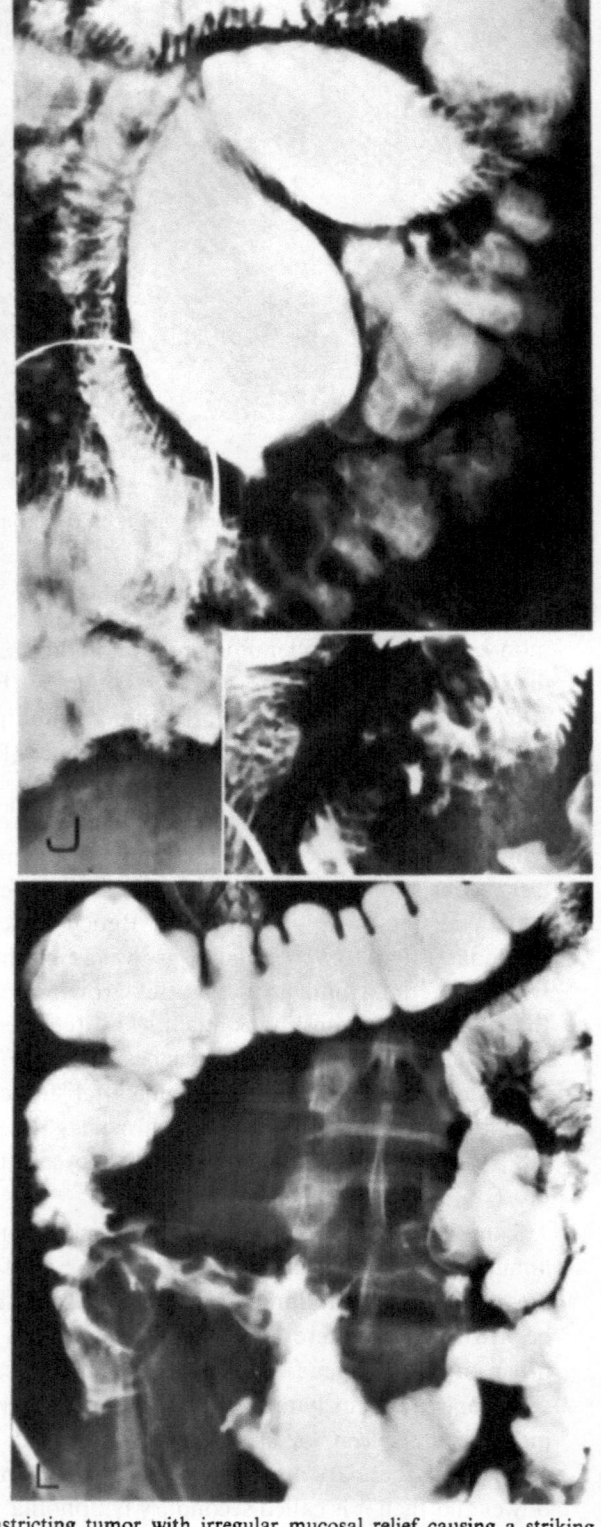

Fig. 10.27. Four cases of reticulum cell sarcoma. (J) Short constricting tumor with irregular mucosal relief causing a striking prestenotic dilatation. Two years later metastases were found. (K) See page 301. (L) Large and rapidly growing retroperitoneal reticulum cell sarcoma in a 23-year-old man that spread to the mesentery and did not cause obstruction until a late stage. There are highly stretched folds with an irregular course in the distal ileum. Initially the process was thought to be an appendicular infiltrate. (M) Reticulum cell sarcoma with predominantly extramural growth and therefore compression-like patterns and stretched mucosal folds at the sites of the lesions. The mucosal relief in the proximal jejunum in the upper left quadrant resembles that of the ileum (top) and becomes strikingly smooth as filling of the lumen increases (bottom). (See also page 302.)

301

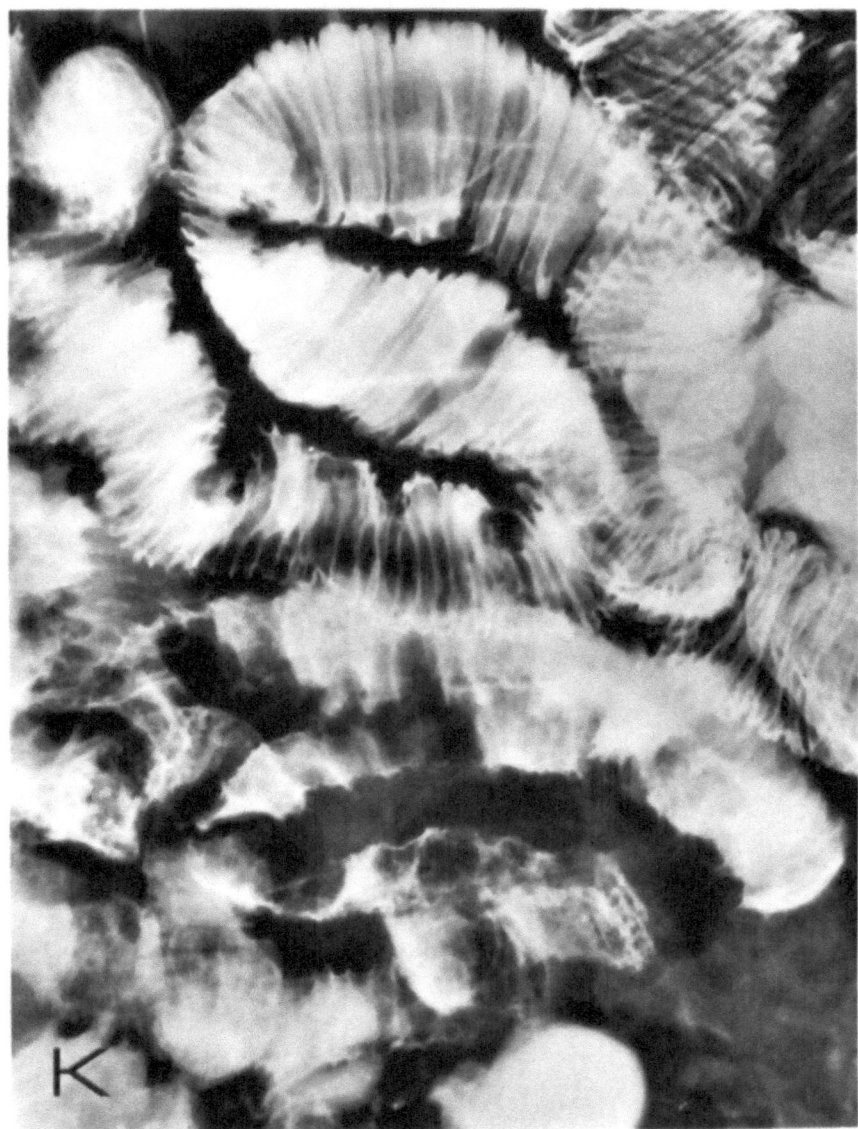

*Fig. 10.27*K. Unusual reticulum cell sarcoma growing along the surface and involving a large segment of the small bowel. This caused the complete disappearance of the mucosal relief in some areas and folds that are infiltrated or thickened by edema in others. The intestinal wall is obviously thickened.

dary lymphoma there may be multiple intramural lesions or polypoid defects bulging out into the contrast column (fig. 10.28A). The lesions can be so small that they are not much bigger than those seen in lymphoid hyperplasia. In other cases they can be quite large, giving rise to intussusception or obstruction. The surface of the nodules may be ulcerous or show clear centralized necrosis as seen in a leiomyo(sarco)ma or a melanoma. Obviously perforations and fistulas may then also develop.

Widespread growth of the tumors into the mesentery or outside the lumen of the intestine occurs. Multiple compression effects and large erratically shaped spaces between the intestinal loops will then

be seen on the x-rays (fig. 10.28B–E). If the tumor lies within Bauhin's valve, there is a chance that it will be diagnosed as hypertrophy or a lipomatosis (fig. 10.28D).

In most cases there is only diffuse infiltrative growth into the lamina propria, mucosa, or submucosa of the intestinal wall. The tumor can start as a small lesion (fig. 10.29A) and then spread extensively and even involve the full length of the small intestine without causing radiologically clear abnormalities (fig. 10.29B). At the same time, clinical symptoms may be entirely absent. They may consist only of nonspecific general complaints such as pain, malaise, anorexia, loss of weight, and

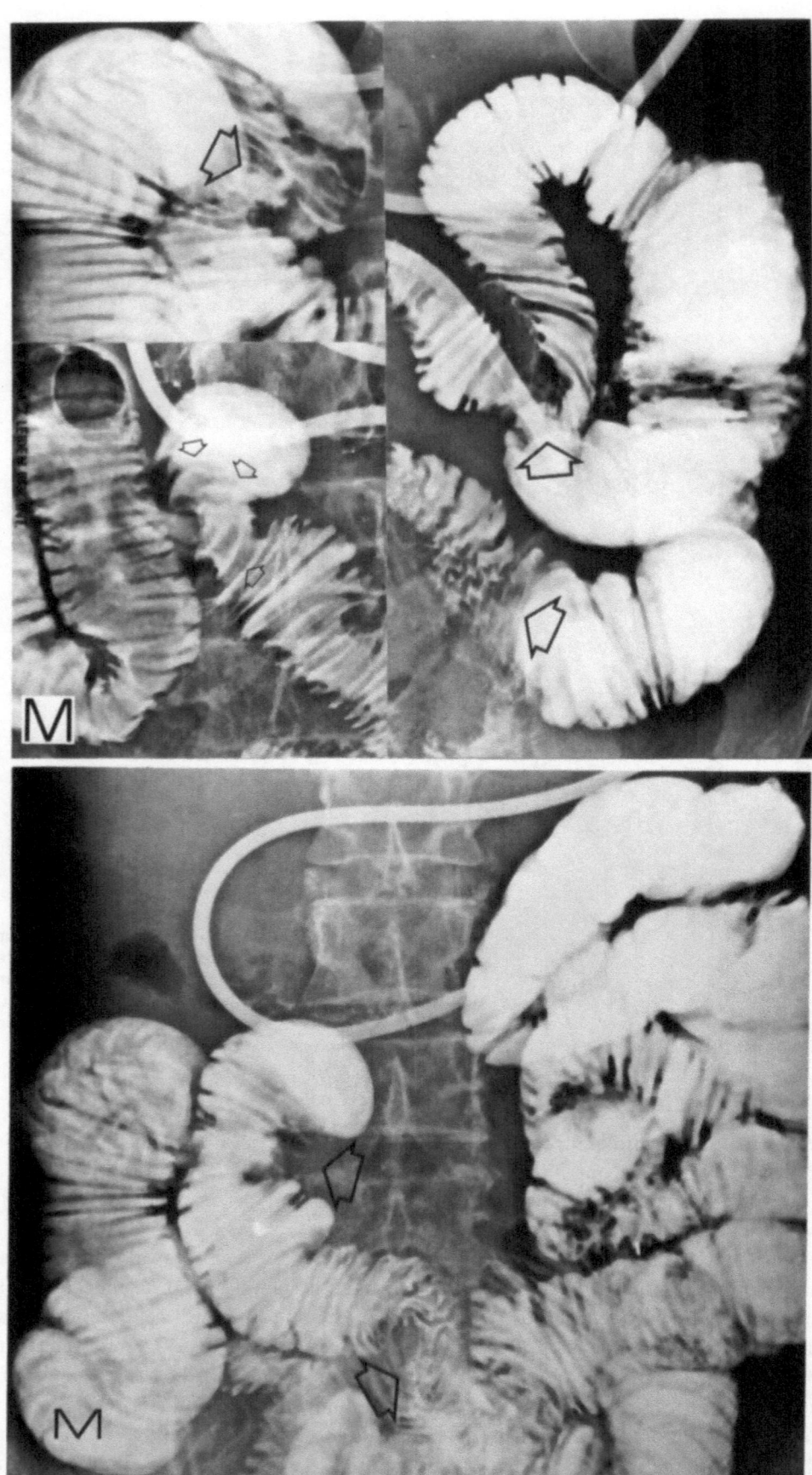

*Fig. 10.27*м. See legend on page 300.

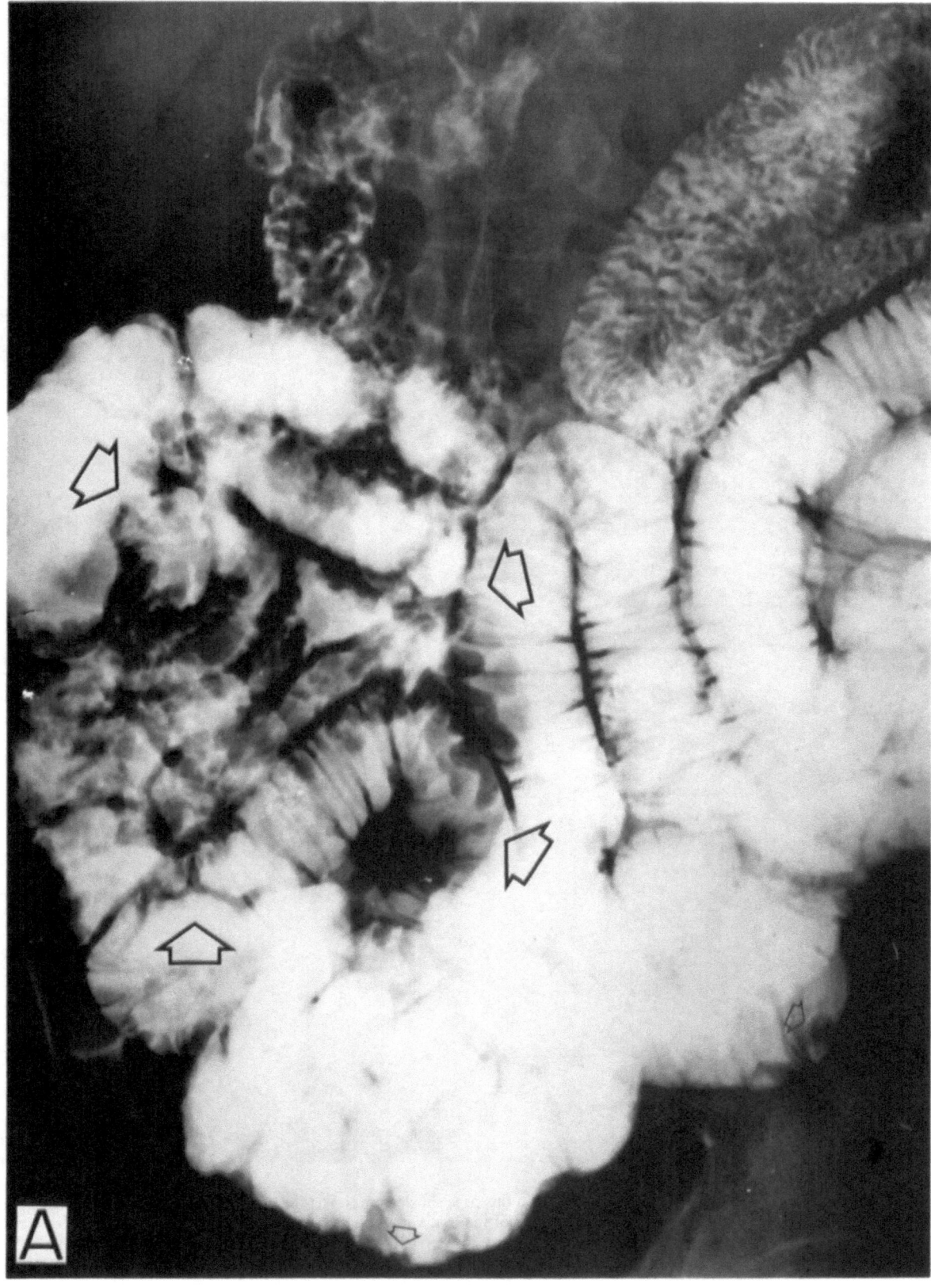

*Fig. 10.28*A. Non-Hodgkin's lymphoma of the digestive tract with numerous scattered sites about 1 cm in diameter. In the small intestine the lesions are visualized best in the right half of the abdomen but they also exist elsewhere.

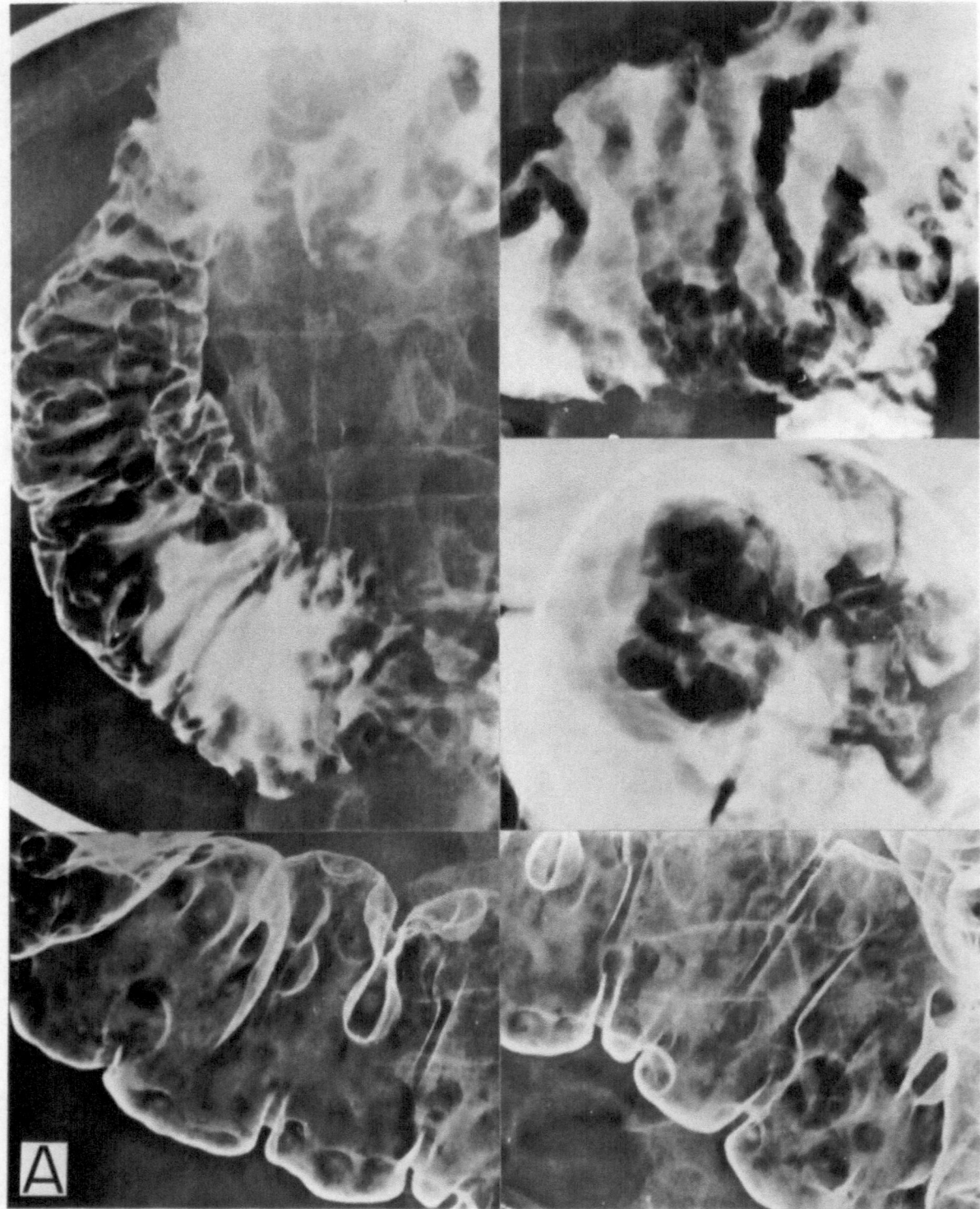

*Fig. 10.28*A. Non-Hodgkin's lymphoma. The figures on this page show, from top left to right, the duodenum, the stomach, and the ileocecal valve below it, and finally (bottom) segments of the transverse colon.

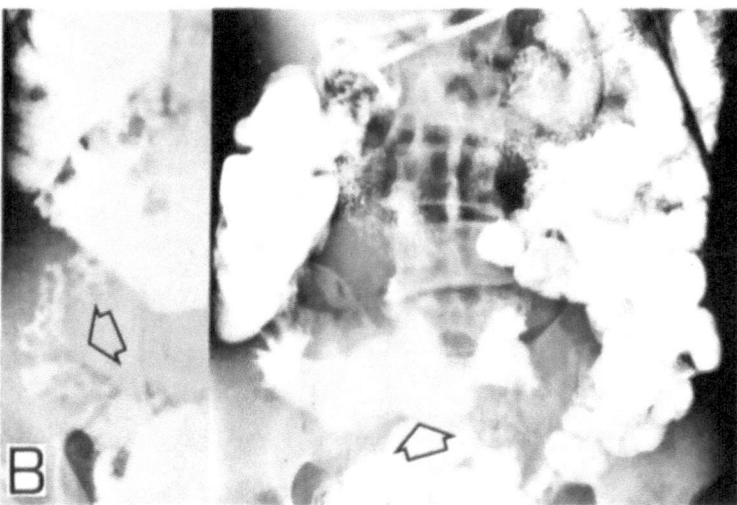

Fig. 10.28B. Lymphosarcoma of the distal ileum with multiple nodules, about 3–5 mm across (left) and a large aneurysmal dilatation (right). Large empty spaces in the mass of intestinal loops are due to invasion of the mesentery.

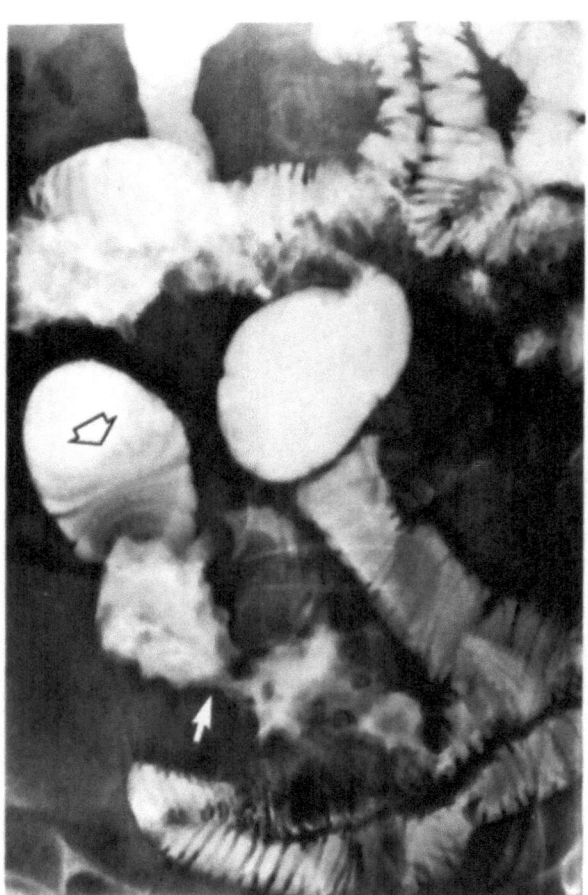

Fig. 10.28C. Extensive lymphosarcoma with diverse localizations in the intestinal wall and the mesentery. Compression effects (open arrow), multiple empty spaces between the intestinal loops, and complete necrosis of the intestinal wall (solid arrow).

anemia. As a rule there are also multiple deficiencies as a result of malabsorption, protein loss, and edema.

A lymphosarcoma often grows rather slowly and does not cause obstructive phenomena until fairly late, if at all.

The few complaints and the subtle radiological abnormalities barely increase; in fact they may even decrease temporarily. However, there may be a sudden marked increase in the rate of growth such that a widespread tumorous mass develops within several months. There is then pronounced widening of the spaces between the intestinal loops on the films and extensive necrosis and destruction of the mucosal membrane (figs. 10.28BCE and 10.30).

It is possible that in the slow initial phase the process is not yet malignant, and that this first stage of growth should be called a 'benign lymphoma'. This first stage is prolonged and there are few clinical and radiological symptoms. Therefore the malignant lymphoma must be considered not only the most insidious tumor in the small intestine, but also the most insidious disease of all the small intestine pathology. Even the histological examination of mucosal biopsies has not changed this situation; it probably has even increased the problems of differential diagnosis. Often no abnormalities at all are found; at most, the number of plasma cells or mature lymphocytes in the lamina propria of the intestinal wall has increased. In other cases

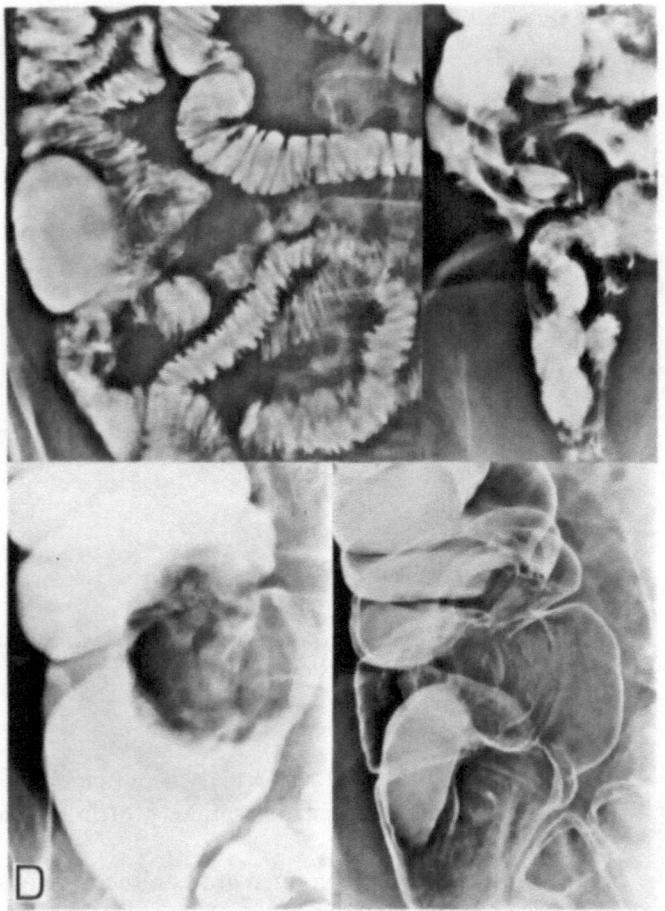

*Fig. 10.28*D. Non-Hodgkin's lymphoma of Bauhin's valve, nonobstructing and visible only on the enteroclysis film (top). A prior colon examination revealed a large Bauhin's valve that was incorrectly attributed to hypertrophy (bottom).

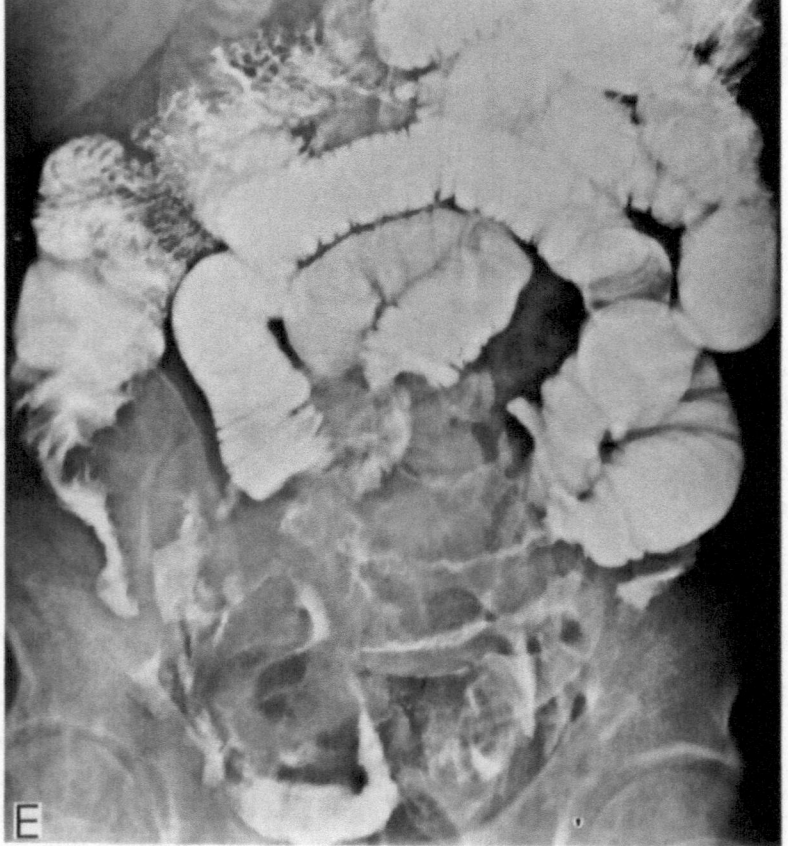

*Fig. 10.28*E. Hodgkin's disease with pronounced involvement of the mesentery leading to erratic stenoses of the intestinal loops in the middle of large 'empty' spaces in the lower abdomen.

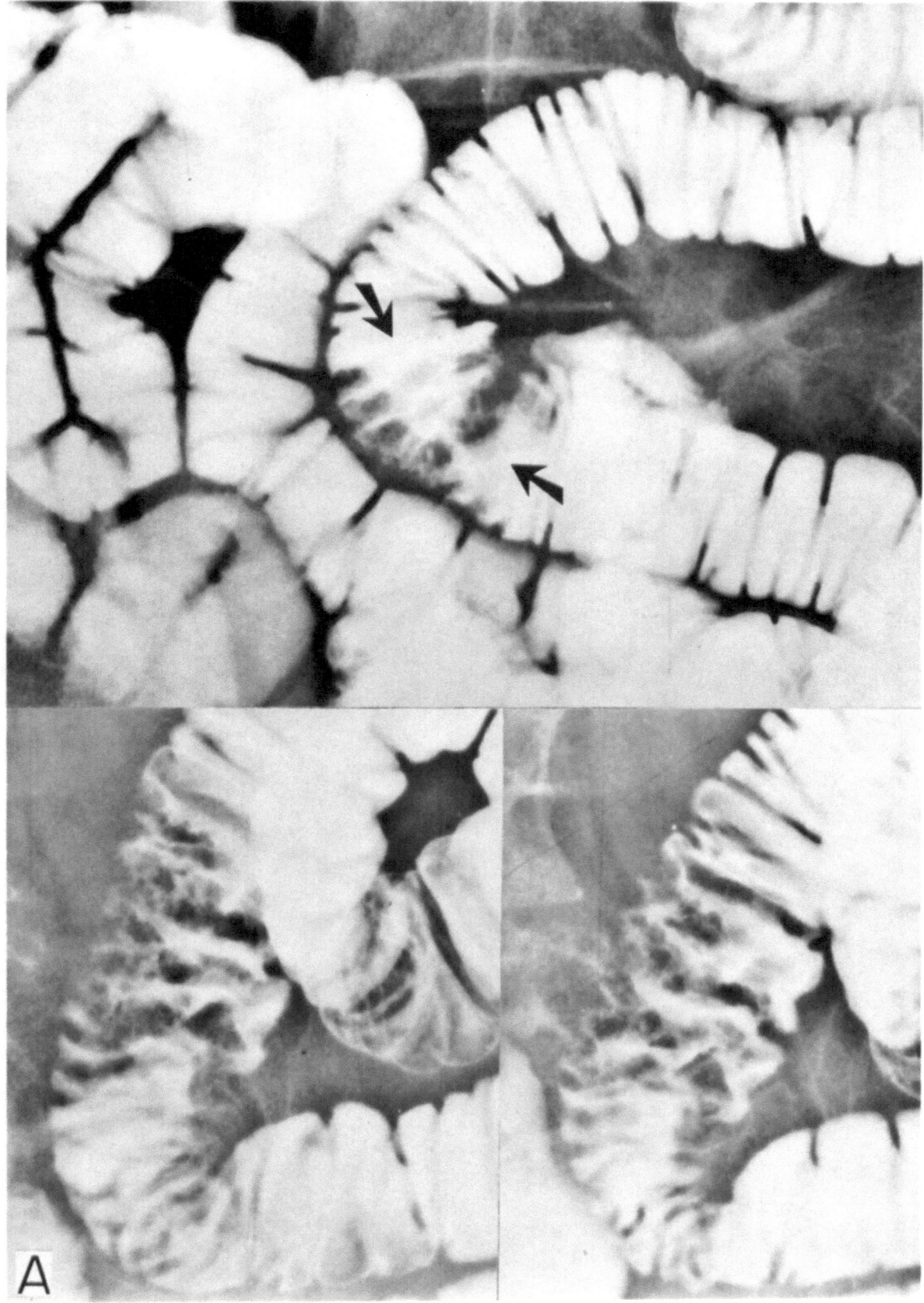

A

*Fig. 10.29*A. In a 40-year-old woman, an accidental finding consisting of five irregularly thickened folds; on the compression spot films (bottom), a conglomeration of lymph follicles is clearly visualized in this region. The distance between the relevant barium column and that of the adjacent loop has not increased so that the intestinal wall itself cannot be thickened. In spite of the radiological report of a suspected very small lymphoreticular malignancy growing within the mucosa, the surgeon was exceedingly reluctant to perform a laparotomy. Eventually the suspected diagnosis was confirmed by the pathologist.

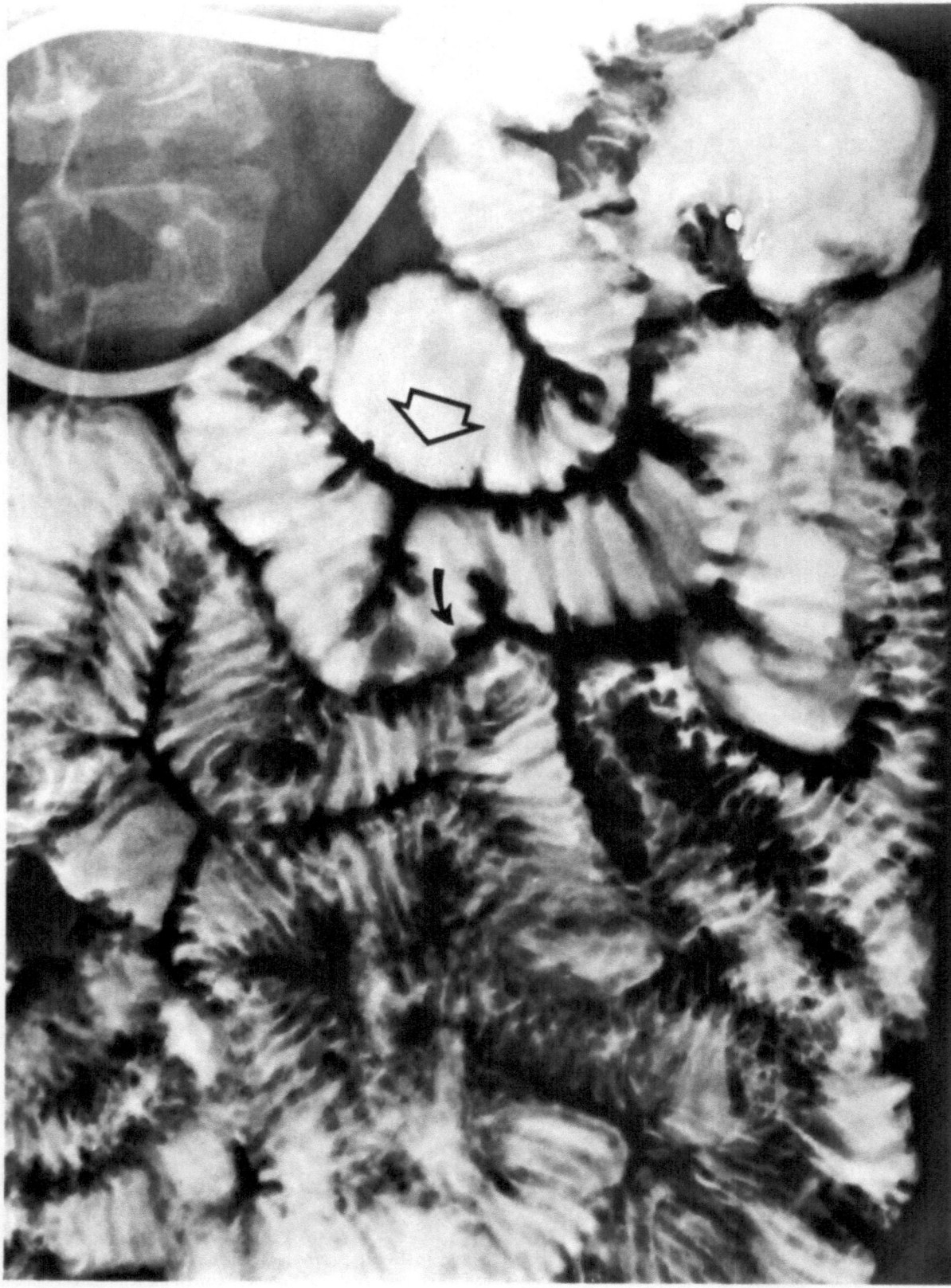

*Fig. 10.29*ʙ. Malignant lymphoma in the jejunum with only slight radiological abnormalities. In the proximal jejunum, the degree of obliteration and broadening of the folds varies (open arrow). There are several nodular defects (solid arrow). In the distal ileum, the folds are only swollen. No abnormalities can be seen in the ileum.

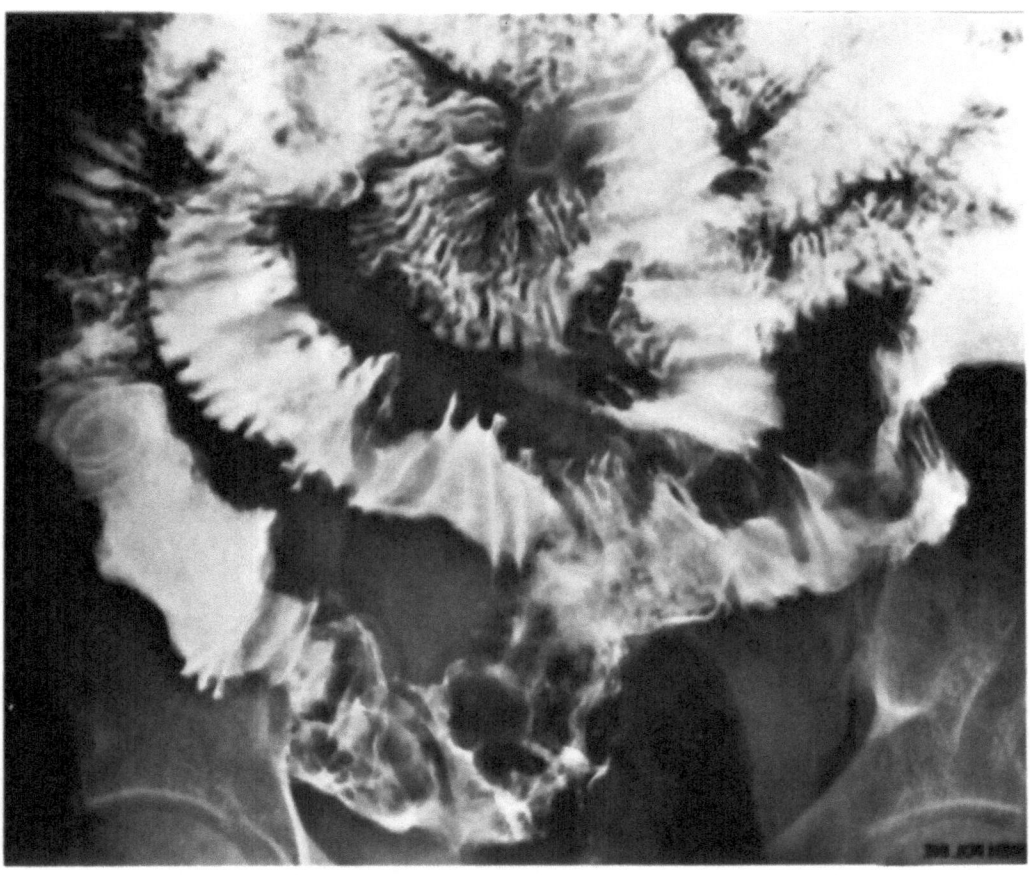

Fig. 10.30. The same patient (20-year-old man) as in fig. 10.29B, about six months later. Now even in the ileum, which presented no abnormalities during the previous examination, an extensive obliteration of the mucosal relief is seen.

the villi appear atrophied and in combination with the clinical considerations an initial diagnosis of celiac disease is then established. For a number of patients this is correct. There is an increased risk in celiac disease that a malignant lymphoma or some other tumor will later develop in the digestive tract (see chapter 12). If, however, it appears that the patients do not react favorably to a gluten-free diet, then the serious possibility of a malignant lymphoma must be considered. This is also true if it is found that blood serum, urine, or intestinal juices contain pathological immunoglobulins without the light IgA chains. These immunological disorders are characteristic of malignant lymphoma in young adults between 20 and 40 years of age who come from countries around the Mediterranean Sea. Today in the Netherlands this so-called Mediterranean lymphoma that occurs most frequently in the duodenum and proximal jejunum is encountered in migrant workers from Morocco, Greece, and Tur-

key. In the earliest stage of the disease, the lymphoma causes only edema of the mucosa over a large area. The folds are broadened and the intestinal wall is only slightly if at all thicker (fig. 10.31). This edema cannot be distinguished from the edema resulting from hypoalbuminemia. It is also difficult to differentiate it from a moderately pronounced lymphedema whereby the intestinal wall is not yet thickened and has still retained its pliancy. On the basis of our observation that this edema can be temporary, we believe that it should be considered a nonspecific prodromic phenomenon that presumably is due to a hypoalbuminemia. When the latter is treated, the edema disappears. During the subsequent months, sometimes even years, nodular elevations and thick ridge-like mucosal swellings several centimeters in length can develop. Like the edema, these nodules can also disappear temporarily or become less apparent. This is seen mainly in those parts of the small bowel that contain the

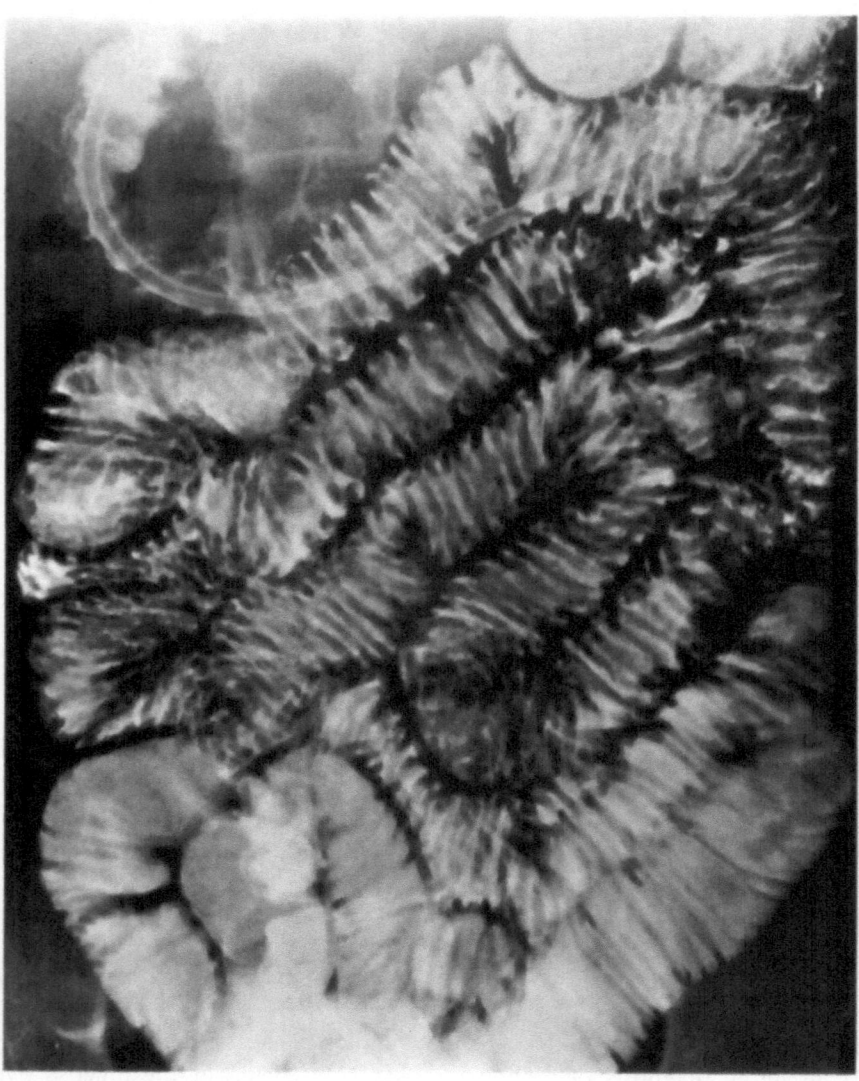

Fig. 10.31. Edematous mucosa and slightly thickened intestinal wall of the jejunum in a 24-year-old man; not recognized at that time as a possible early malignant lymphoma.

most lymphoid tissue, such as the distal ileum, duodenum, and proximal jejunum (fig. 10.32). In this stage, the differential diagnosis certainly should include Crohn's disease localized to the duodenum – especially when cobblestones are also seen (fig. 10.33). In addition to granulomas in the duodenum, abnormalities are seen in the distal ileum in one-half of the cases. By means of biopsies, the presence of Crohn's disease can quickly be excluded.

The problems of differential diagnosis are much greater when a segment of the jejunum or ileum shows coarse, somewhat irregular mucosal folds. This is especially true when the intestinal wall is not at all or barely thickened and has retained a fairly good motility and pliancy (fig. 10.34). The mucosal surface can show multiple small ulcerations, but it can also be completely intact if the spread of the lymphoma is submucosal. It is impossible to differentiate such a case, irrespective of whether there are mucosal ulcerations or not, from the changes that are due to a moderately pronounced ischemia. The completely different set of complaints and the clinical course of these two diseases as well as the age of the patient may be an important indication of the correct diagnosis. The final solution to this dilemma is not produced until a follow-up examination is carried out 4–6 weeks later. In the case of ischemia, obvious changes are always seen: the abnormalities have disappeared or fibrosis is evident. If there are multiple ulcerations, the differential diagnosis may also include an enteritis but here adequate treatment will certainly produce a change for the better in 4–6 weeks. If, on the other hand, a lymphoma is involved, then quite frequently there is little or no

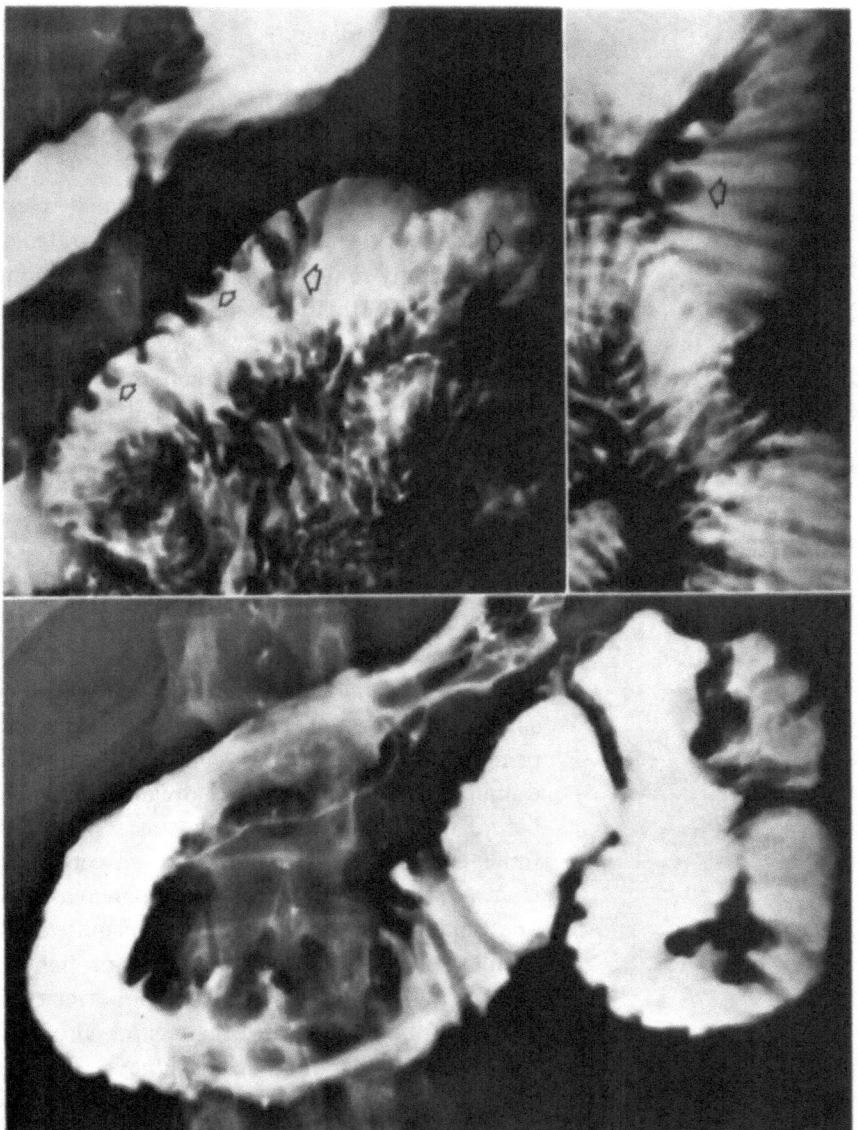

Fig. 10.32. The same patient as seen in fig. 10.31, one year later. In the duodenum and proximal jejunum the mucosal folds have disappeared for the most part and, in the lumen, nodular lumps are seen that may or may not originate from the folds. Crohn's disease was considered at first but the diagnosis of malignant lymphoma was soon apparent. Celiac disease was not considered because of the nodular mucosal swellings.

change, even if the follow-up examination is two or three months later. The complaints can be few and may only be due to the fact that malabsorption has led to several nutritional deficiencies. Adequate treatment of these deficiencies can cause the superficial ulcerative changes to decrease; they may even temporarily disappear for the most part. Mainly because of the clinical well-being of the patient and the fact that the biopsies only show signs of chronic infection and aggregates of plasma cells and lymphocytes in the lamina propria, the diagnosis of lymphoma is often barely considered.

A third manifestation of lymphoma that can cause considerable problems in differential diag-

nosis is when superficial spread over a large intestinal segment causes total obliteration of the mucosa (fig. 10.35). The process can be chronic, lasting for many years. A large area of the intestinal mucosa may be covered with small ulcerations causing a close resemblance to Crohn's disease in an acute stage. The intestinal wall is fairly stiff and slightly thickened, the lumen moderately dilated or narrowed. No contractions can be seen and the loops lie in an orderly fashion in the abdominal cavity with a minimum number of coils, curves, and folds. Because of the superficial character of the ulcerations, there is no fibrotic shriveling and stenoses do not develop, as in Crohn's disease and

312

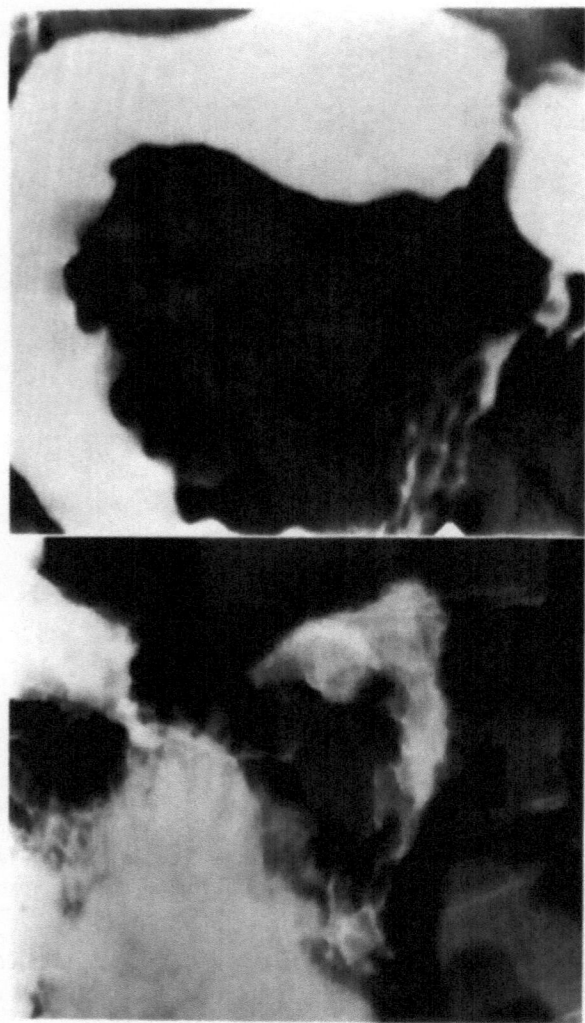

Fig. 10.33. Two patients with cobblestones in the duodenum due to lymphosarcoma.

after ischemia.

If the mucosa in the duodenum or jejunum has atrophied, an alternative possibility could be celiac disease. However, an eventual secondary infection in conjunction with this latter disease reacts quite quickly to the proper treatment augmented with a gluten-free diet. The ulcerations then rapidly disappear while the intestinal wall becomes obviously thinner. In lymphoma the ulcerative changes in the intestinal wall will disappear only with difficulty or not at all, and they also soon recur. A small intestine lymphoma should therefore seriously be considered if there are extensive and often ill-defined changes in the intestinal wall in a patient with relatively few complaints. Sometimes in the event of prolonged uncertainty, a diagnostic lapar-

otomy is unavoidable.

6. Metastasis

Although metastatic tumors in the small intestine or invasion of the mesentery are demonstrated even less frequently radiologically than primary tumors, they are frequently found at autopsy. In our patient material, metastases were demonstrated in less than one-fifth of patients with a benign or malignant tumor in the small bowel. Almost half of these cases of metastatic tumors involved metastasis from melanoma. This high percentage is probably due to the fact that this group of patients is subjected to periodic follow-ups. Whenever occult rectal bleeding occurs, an examination of the small intestine is performed automatically.

On the other hand it is certainly possible that metastases from tumors are demonstrated only sporadically because the complaints are due to the primary tumor or metastases in other organs. These dominate markedly or have already led to death before the small intestine metastases produce definite complaints. In addition to direct invasion from adjacent organs such as the pancreas, colon, or stomach, metastases are also transmitted to the small intestine by the bloodstream or lymphatic system (fig. 10.38A). The primary tumor can therefore be found in these organs and also in the esophagus, lungs, mammae, kidneys, uterus, or ovaries. Metastases from the ovary in particular can be extensive in the intestine, mesentery and peritoneum. In contrast to the malignant primary tumors of the intestine that cause obstruction within a relatively short time, most metastases as a rule do not give rise to such complaints until much later. Metastases spread from the mesentery into the intestinal wall or grow intramurally from the subserous vascular network on the opposite side. Although they not only grow outward from the intestinal surface but also bulge into the lumen, they cause obstruction only at a much later stage (fig. 10.36). Metastases cause ulcerations and central necrosis more often than primary tumors, and fusion with adjacent organs or tissues is also more extensive (fig. 10.37). Metastases localized in the mesentery cause a compression effect on the intestine that is accompanied only by stretching of the

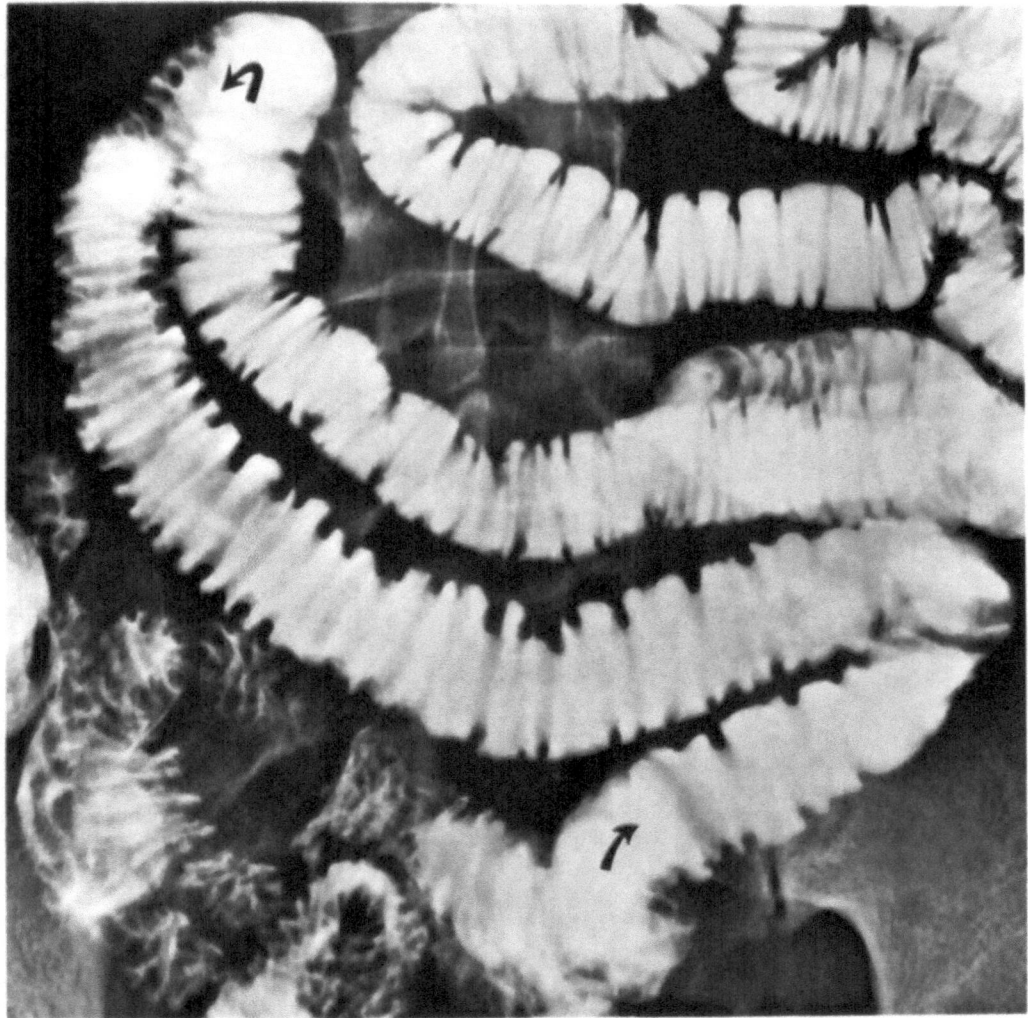

Fig. 10.34. Patient with a probable lymphoma of the ileum growing along the surface. The intestinal wall is thickened and the mucosal folds are irregular and obviously broadened; motility is fairly well preserved. Clinically there was a clear malabsorption and a fairly marked loss of weight. The mucosal biopsy showed an increase in the number of plasma cells in the lamina propria. Only little progress of the abnormalities six months later. Patient has since refused further follow-up examinations.

mucosal folds or flattening of the mucosal contours. This is caused when the growing tumor is fused with the intestinal wall. Diffuse metastasis in the mesentery causes the mesentery to become thicker as well as stiffer and shorter. The intestinal loops attached to the shortened mesentery also become – of necessity – shorter. The mucosal folds along this tract are then very close together. Moreover, these loops lie in a more or less stretched, organized fashion and are visualized without interference from other loops.

Diffuse carcinomatosis in the abdominal cavity is as a rule not a difficult diagnosis (fig. 10.38B). The characteristic radiological abnormalities cannot be confused with those of any other disease, not even a generalized lymphosarcoma. Whenever multiple polypoid masses are seen in the intestinal lumen, the diagnostic conclusion of metastasis is obvious if a primary tumor is known to exist elsewhere. Even if necrosis and ulcerations are observed in these tumors, a lymphoreticular malignancy of the nodular type or a leiomyo(sarco)ma can be considered, but benign polypoid formations need not be included in the differential diagnosis.

If a primary tumor is not known to exist, then multiple nodular abnormalities are probably due to metastasis if they have increased in size and number on a follow-up examination several weeks later. For

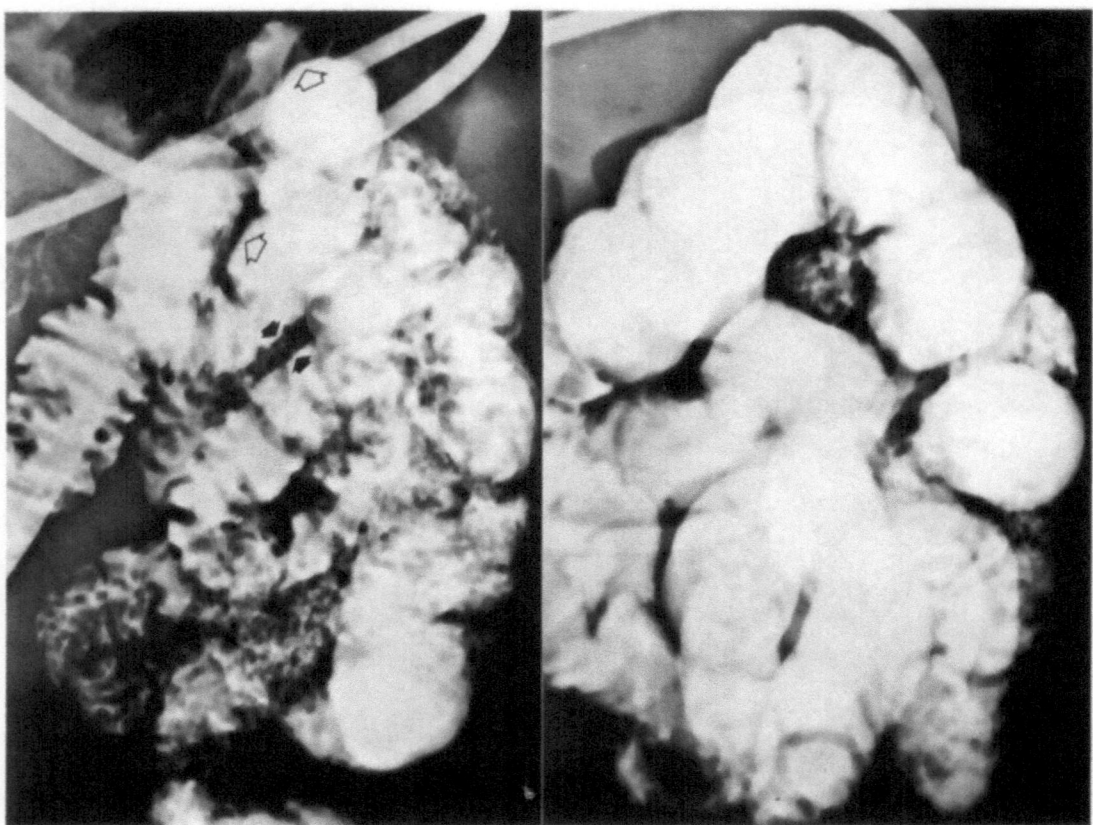

*Fig. 10.35*A. In a relatively proximal part of the jejunum an irregular decrease in the mucosal relief (open arrows) as well as a slight thickening of the intestinal wall (between the solid arrows) is seen in a segment about 10 cm long. The likely diagnoses reported were (1) ischemic changes due to vasculitis or arteriosclerosis, (2) early malignant lymphoma, or (3) possibly celiac disease although this is less likely because the site is not truly proximal. Two years later the jejunum had obviously become even smoother (right) and the diagnosis of malignant lymphoma was confirmed by lymph node biopsy.

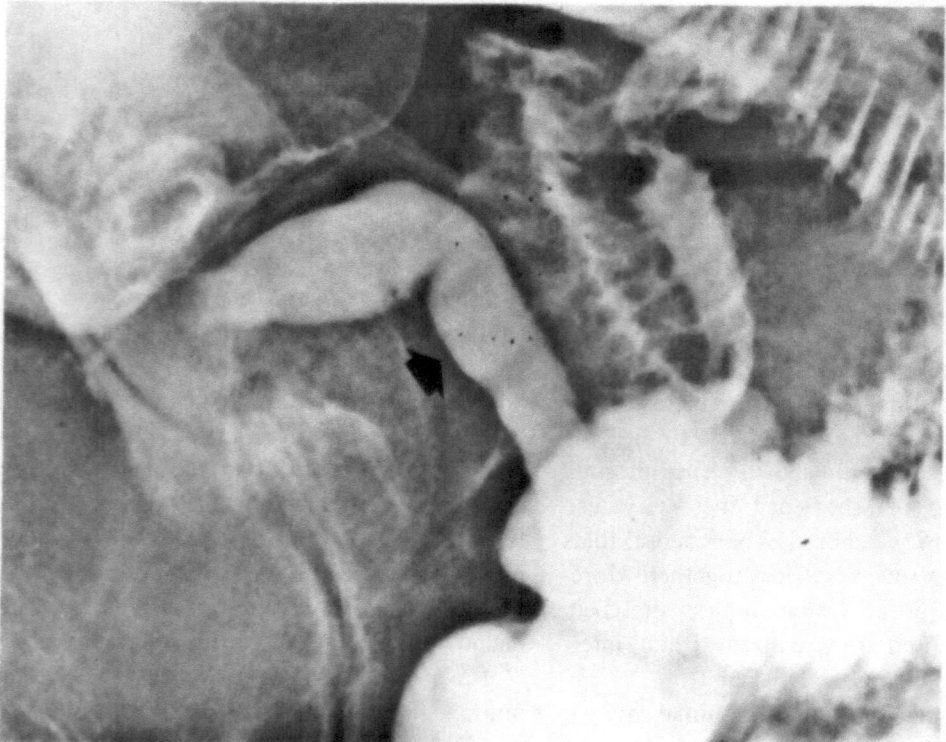

*Fig. 10.35*B. Slight narrowing and stiffening of the wall of the distal ileum without any sign of mucosal relief. Thickened mucosal folds in the proximal loops. Hodgkin's disease.

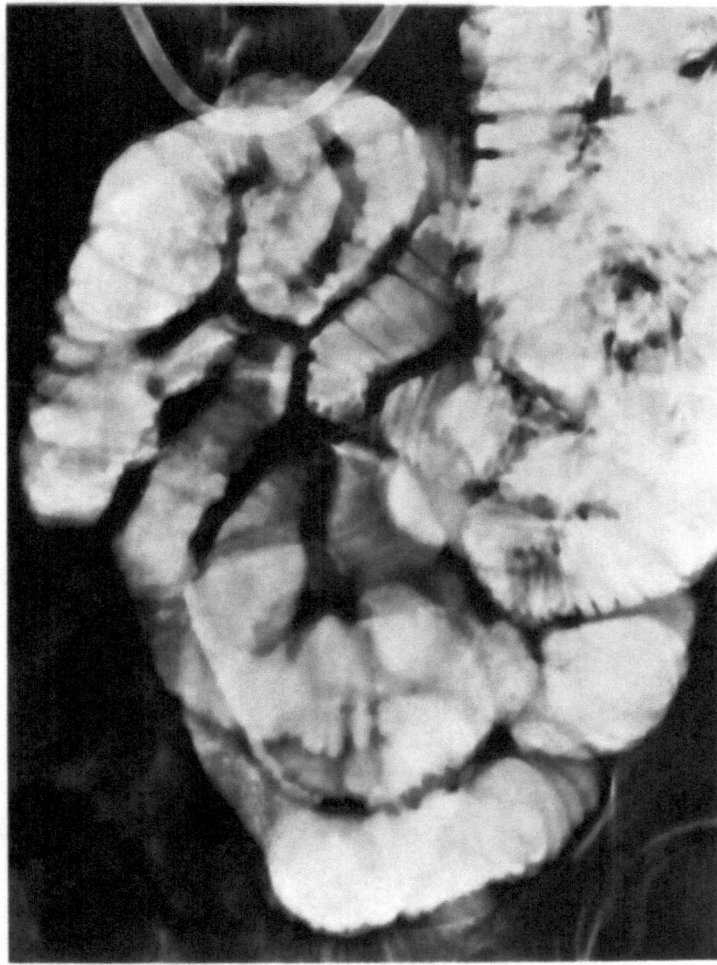

Fig. 10.35c. Malignant lymphoma involving almost the entire ileum with thickened rigid intestinal wall and obliterated mucosal folds. The lumen of the intestine is slightly dilated.

solitary metastases, which are undoubtedly the most difficult to diagnose, a high rate of growth is highly indicative of a malignant disease.

With the exception of general symptoms such as loss of weight, malaise, and anorexia, clinical symptoms of metastasis in the small intestine may be absent. They also may be due solely to hypochromic anemia as a result of occult blood loss.

Of the tumors that metastasize to the gastrointestinal tract, melanoma is the most important. The complaints caused by metastasis in the small intestine can be the first sign of an unrecognized melanoma. Sometimes metastases are encountered in the digestive tract while the primary tumor cannot be demonstrated. In such cases it is assumed that the metastasis originated from a primary site on the skin that disappeared spontaneously. Autopsy of patients who died of melanoma has shown that the frequency of metastasis to the small intestine is 58%, somewhat less than that for the lungs (70%) and the liver (60%). Even without metastasis to the lung or liver, metastasis only to the digestive

tract has been demonstrated. The frequency is highest for the proximal small intestine and decreases distalward.

Roentgenological examination of the small bowel should therefore be carried out whenever it is important to establish the presence of hematogenous metastases. If metastases via the bloodstream have already been proven, then there is no indication for the examination. Metastases to the stomach and colon, as well as other organs, are seen much less frequently (25%). The ratio of the frequencies for stomach, small intestine, and colon is in the same proportion as their respective surfaces, which is typical of melanoma. For other tumors such a distribution does not exist and the small intestine is often spared. The exception of melanoma is attributed to the fact that changes in immunological defence decrease the intrinsic protection of the small intestine against carcinogenic influences.

It is assumed that melanoma does not occur as a primary disease in the digestive tract, since no melanoblasts are found in the entodermal epithe-

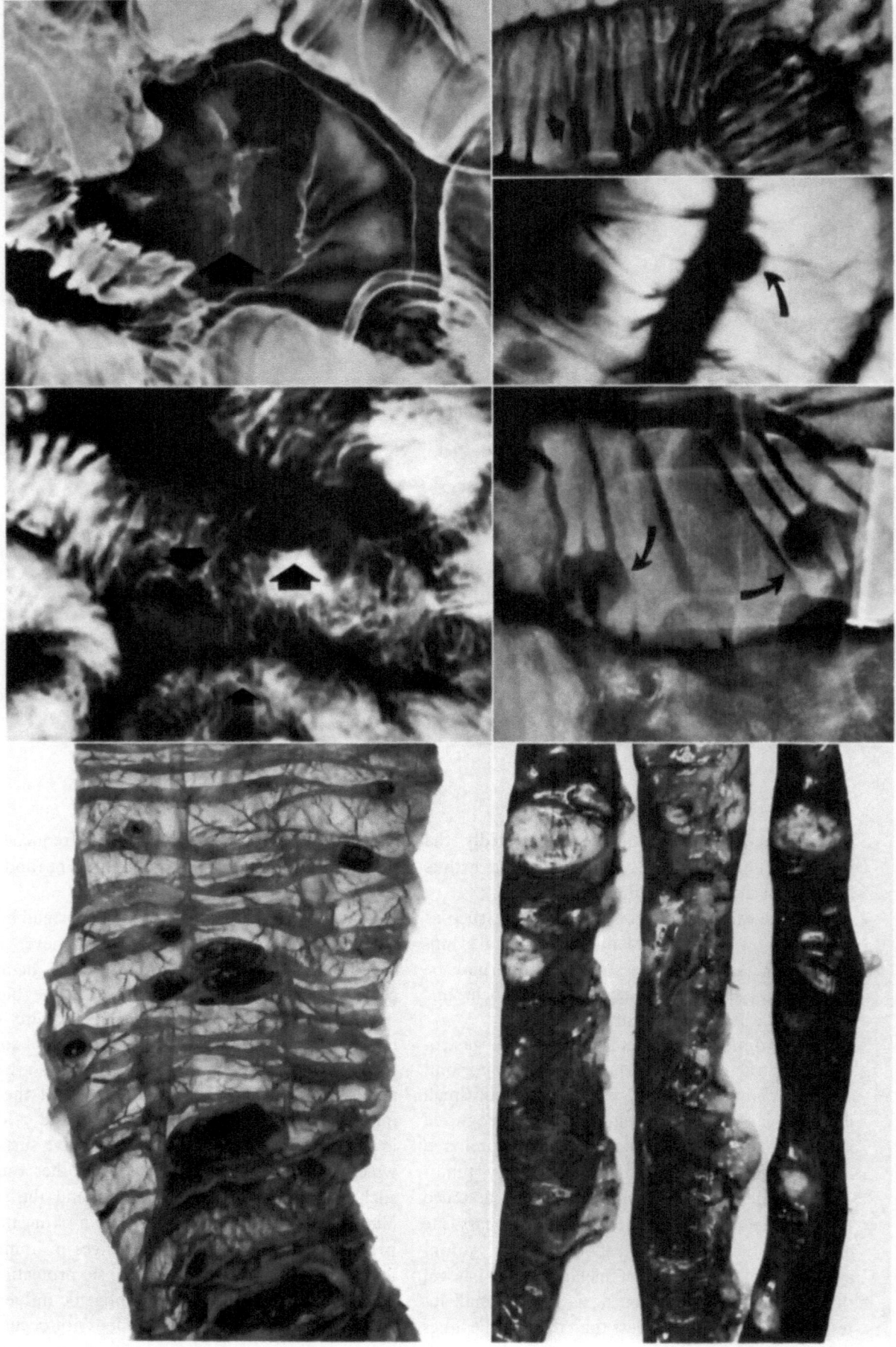

Fig. 10.36. Diverse examples of metastases in the small bowel. The x-rays and the pathology specimen show that they bulge out from the intestinal wall as well as into the lumen.

lium of the digestive tract.

In metastasis transmitted by the bloodstream, the lesions are usually multiple and are generally localized on the antimesenteric side. There can also be a number of metastases of equal size localized within a specific area of the arterial supply in the intestine. The metastatic melanoma spreads from the submucosa into the lumen as a nodular or polypoid, usually amelanotic growth. Thus the roentgenological aspect is that of a nodular or polypoid filling defect. Since there is no adhesion to the surroundings, these nodules can easily cause an intussusception with intermittent obstruction of the intestine.

Central ulceration in a metastasis is seen frequently and can, if it is deep, give the characteristic roentgenological aspect of a 'target lesion' or 'bull's eye' (fig. 10.39). If the ulcerations are superficial, then they are difficult to recognize radiologically. Diagnosis will include leiomyoma and leiomyosarcoma, as well as nodular lymphosarcoma and metastasis from a Kaposi's sarcoma – a fairly rare vascular tumor with a high risk of hemorrhage. If the central ulcerations are missing, then carcinoid lesions must be considered in addition to metastasis

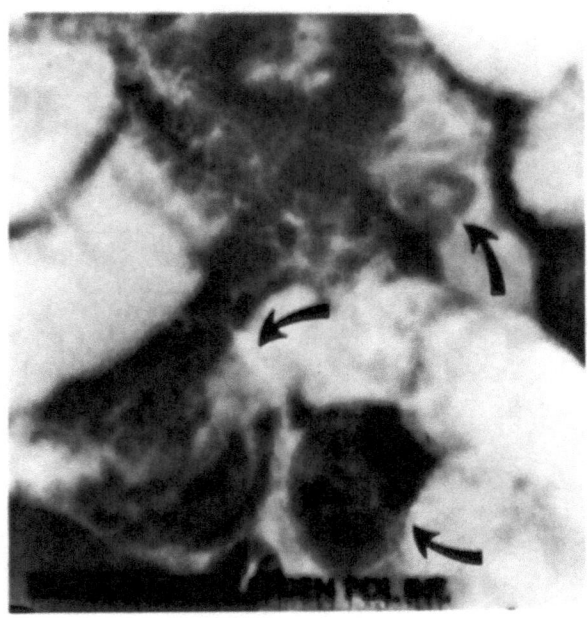

Fig. 10.37. Metastases of a reticulum cell sarcoma, one with central necrosis.

from carcinoma. In contrast to metastasis of melanoma, carcinoids are much more likely to be found in the distal part of the intestine.

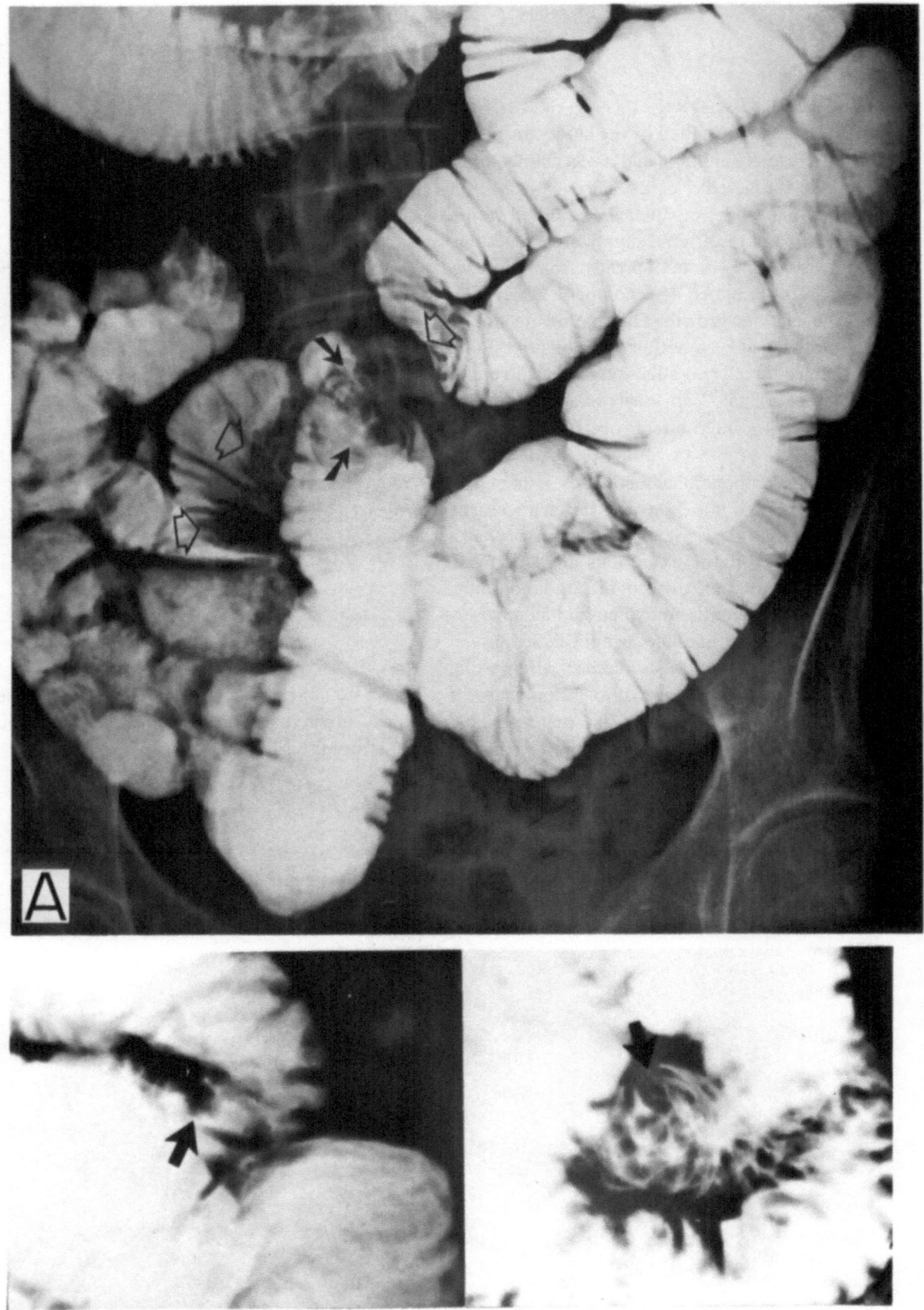

Fig. 10.38A. Stenosis, about 3 cm long, in the jejunum caused by metastasis of a tumor in the cecum (between the solid arrows). At the stenosis the tumor has invaded the mesentery (open arrows) (top). Small metastatic growth in the upper jejunum (arrows) could be visualized only by means of extremely careful compression (bottom).

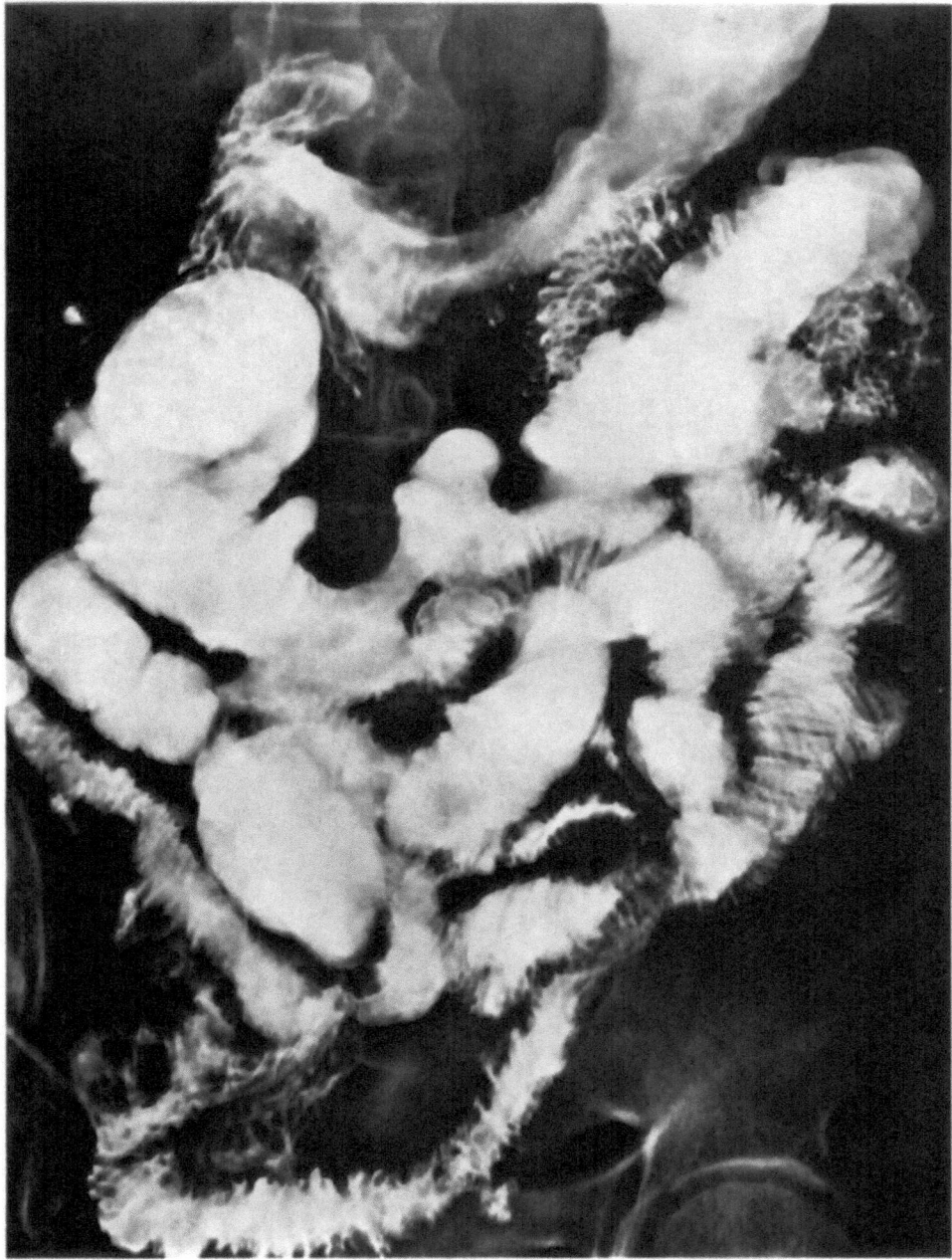

*Fig. 10.38*B. Tumor of the stomach with an extensive peritoneal carcinomatosis.

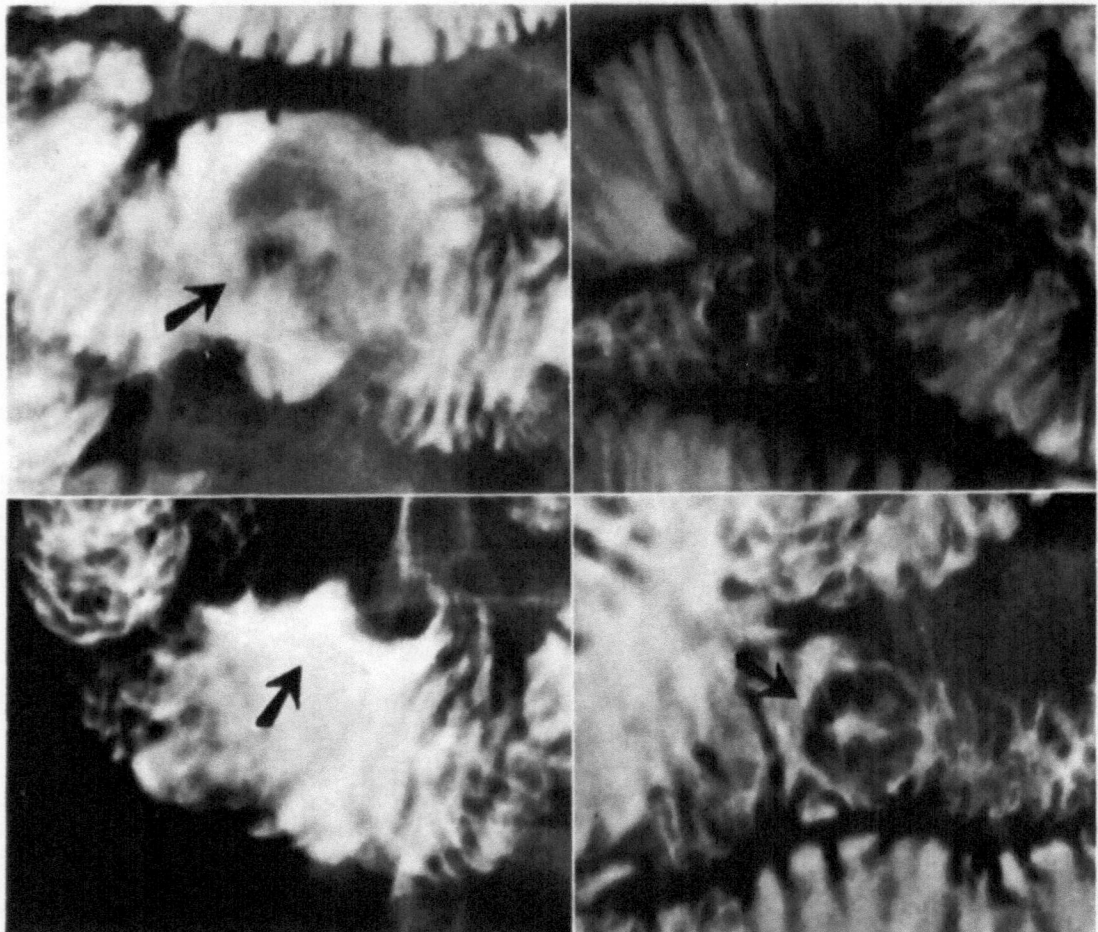

Fig. 10.39. Several examples of melanotic metastases, including one very small one with central necrosis. On the left, a so-called 'bull's eye' is seen en face (top) and in profile (bottom).

Bibliography: chapter 10

Balthazar EJ (1978) Carcinoid tumors of the alimentary tract. Gastrointest Radiol 3: 47–56.

Bancks NH, Goldstein HM, Dodd GD (1975) The röntgenologic spectrum of small intestinal carcinoid tumors. Am J Roentgenol 123: 274–280.

Dodds WJ (1976) Clinical and röntgen features of the intestinal polyposis syndromes. Gastrointest Radiol 1: 127–142.

Hodes PhJ, Stein GN, Finkelstein AK (1973) Tumor atlas of the gastro-intestinal tract. Year Book Medical Publishers.

Marshak RH, Lindner AE, Maklansky D (1979) Lympho-reticular disorders of the gastrointestinal tract: röntgeno-graphic features. Gastrointest Radiol 4: 103–120.

Meyers MA (1975) Metastatic seeding along the small bowel mesentery. Am J Roentgenol 123: 67–73.

Oddson TA, Rice RP, Seigler HF, Thompson WM, Kelvin FM, Clark WM (1977) The spectrum of small bowel melanoma. Gastrointest Radiol 2: 281–291.

Smith SJ, Carlson HC, Gisvold JJ (1977) Secondary neoplasms of the small bowel. Radiology 125: 29–33.

See also the nos. 28, 84, 97, 140 of the bibliography on page 187 and following.

11. VASCULAR DISEASES

Although certainly not rare, abnormalities of the small intestine resulting from an impaired circulation are often not recognized. Fortunately some improvement in this situation can be observed. The failure to establish this diagnosis can be attributed to several reasons. The radiological examination techniques are frequently inadequate and the mucosal changes caused by this type of lesion are not sufficiently well known. Also the clinician often does not consider the possibility of a vascular disorder – not even when it is quite serious. Finally this disorder may sometimes be characterized either by a very mild course or by sudden severe episodes. These are, however, so short that the patient does not consider it necessary to consult a physician. In a number of these cases the abnormalities that persist after such an accident eventually give rise to definite complaints. The roentgenograms then made are 'silent witnesses' of that which occurred several weeks or months before.

Obstructions of the blood flow in the intestinal wall can, depending upon the manner in which they develop, be classified as arterial or venous disorders or hemorrhage. Such a differentiation is not always straightforward since a combination of causes is also possible.

1. Ischemia due to impaired arterial flow

1) The most common cause of a reduction in arterial flow is arteriosclerotic changes in the wall of the superior mesenteric artery (fig. 11.1AB). If the constriction from arteriosclerosis develops gradually, there is sufficient time for formation of collaterals with the celiac trunk, inferior mesenteric artery, and vessels in the abdominal wall. Thus occlusion of the superior mesenteric artery need not lead to serious complaints (fig. 11.1c).

2) Mechanical obstruction of the intestine from adhesions or bands, volvulus, or internal hernia is usually accompanied by obvious impairment of the circulation, arterial as well as venous (fig. 11.2).

3) After surgery involving the major vessels in the abdomen, there may be a temporary decrease in the blood flow through the superior and inferior mesenteric arteries (fig. 11.3A). In addition it is occasionally necessary to sacrifice the latter, which sometimes plays a prominent role in the collateral circulation to the small intestinal vessels. Otherwise a necrosis of the wall of the bowel may be the result (fig. 11.3B).

4) Microemboli, occurring in polycythemia vera or as a result of valvular disease, atrial fibrillation, or a myocardial infarction, can cause sudden occlusion of the relatively small vessels (fig. 11.4).

5) Vasculitis in arteries or small veins, as seen in Buerger's disease, Schönlein-Henoch disease (fig. 11.6), or rheumatoid arthritis, causes thrombosis and multiple occlusions in these vessels (figs. 11.4 and 11.5A). This can also occur in many collagen diseases, accompanied by abnormal skin conditions, such as periarteritis nodosa (fig. 11.7), lupus erythematosus, or dermatomyositis.

6) Vasoconstrictors, for instance ergotamine preparations, can also cause a temporary reduction in the blood supply in the intestinal wall.

2. Graft versus host syndrome

Several months after a bone marrow transplantation, the radiologist may be confronted with abnormalities in the ileum and colon that at least radiologically strongly resemble those seen in ischemia of the peripheral vessels. The mucous membrane as well as the underlying layers of the intestinal wall become markedly edematous and

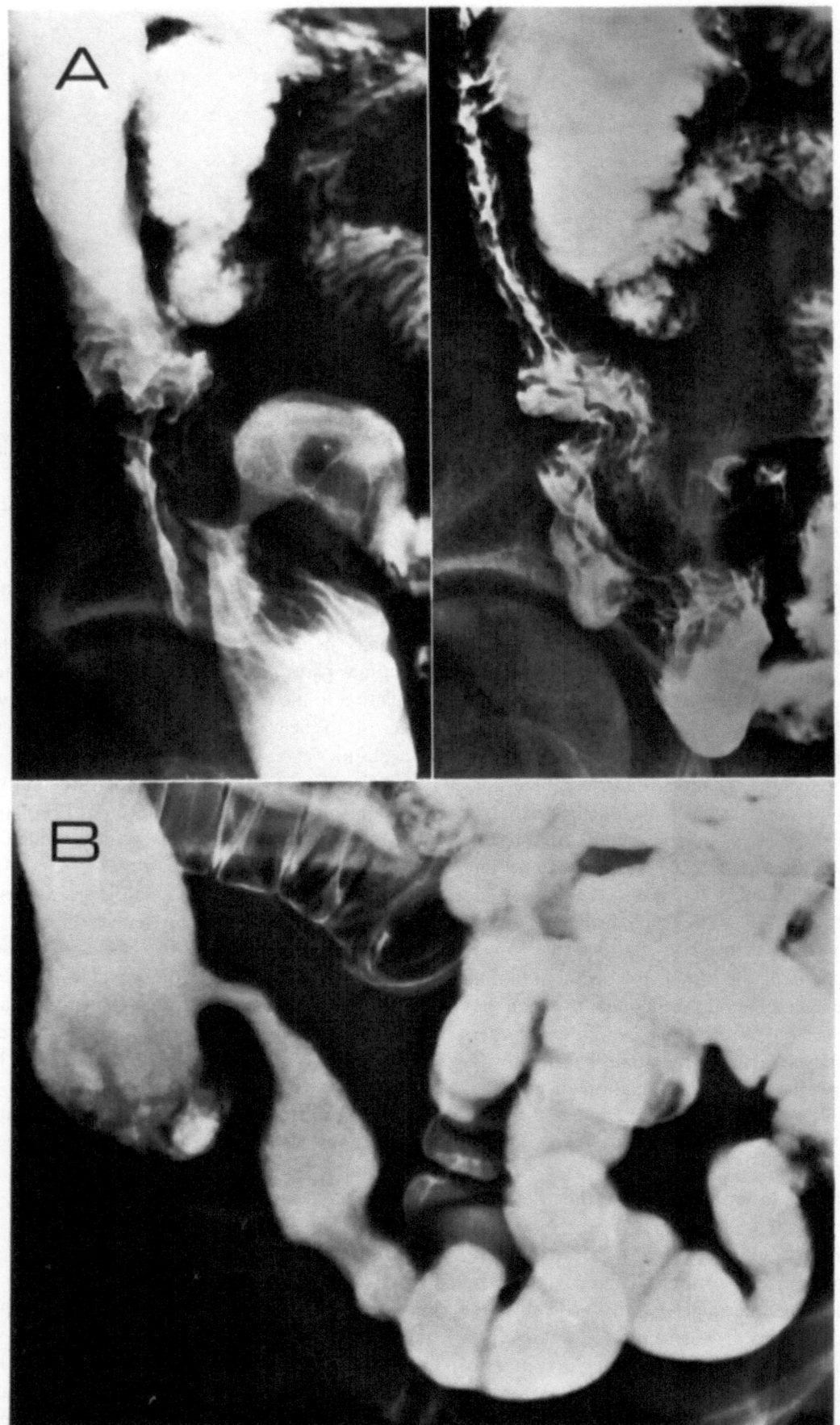

*Fig. 11.1*AB. Two patients after recovery from ischemia. (A) A 50-cm segment of the distal ileum shows pathological fold relief as well as multiple deformations and fusion with adjacent loops. Surgery and subsequent pathological examination revealed a vasculitis and an ulcer 30 cm long. Because of the youth of the patient a vascular disease was not considered. (B) Smooth wall in a 50-cm segment of the cecum and distal ileum. Wide-open Bauhin's valve no longer functions. In this case, differentiation from Crohn's disease on the basis of radiological examination is impossible.

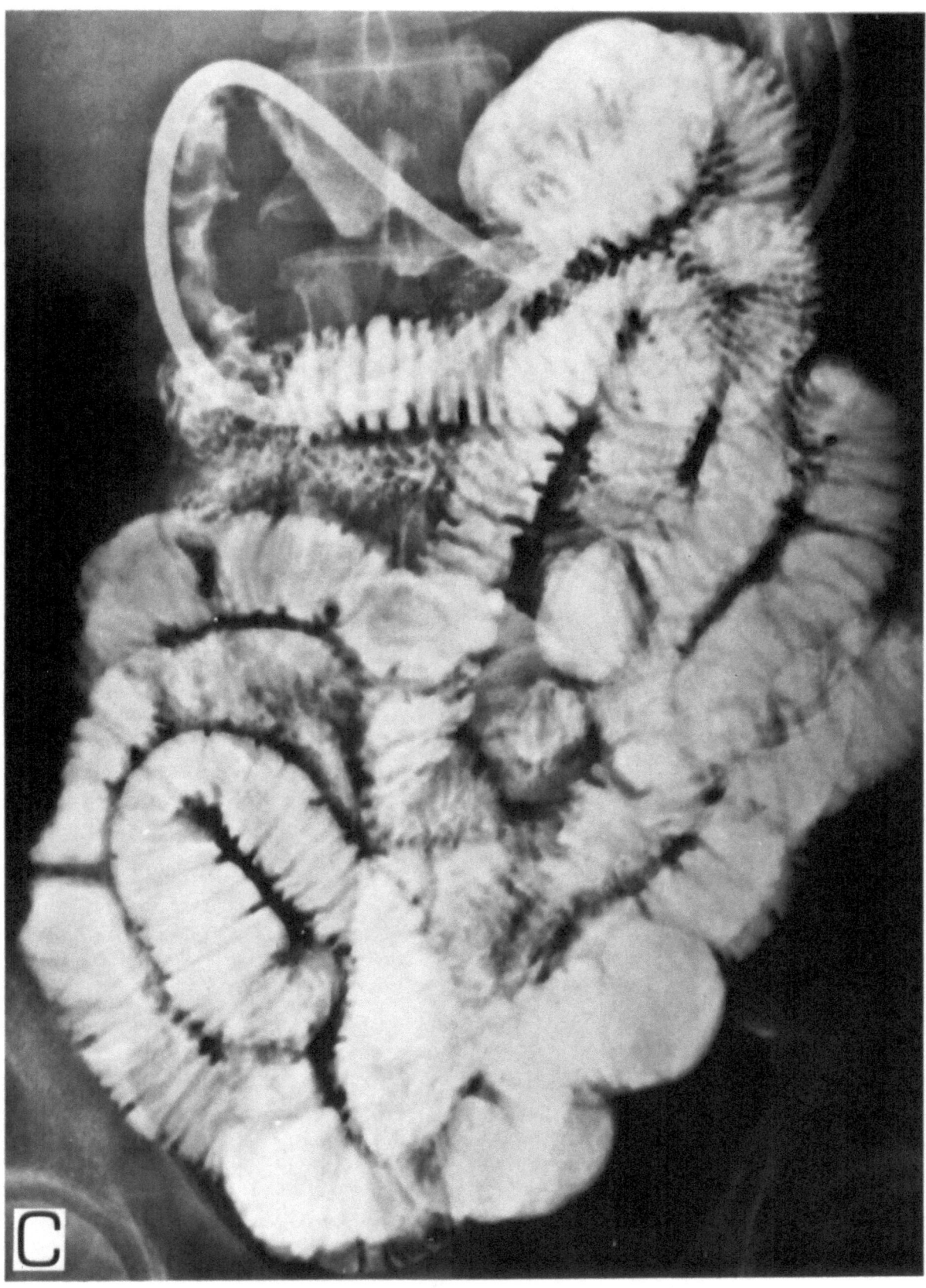

Fig. 11.1c. If a vascular occlusion has developed gradually so that there is time for the formation of collateral circulation, then a total occlusion of the superior and inferior mesenteric arteries need not necessarily cause an abnormal pattern in the small intestine. (See also page 324.)

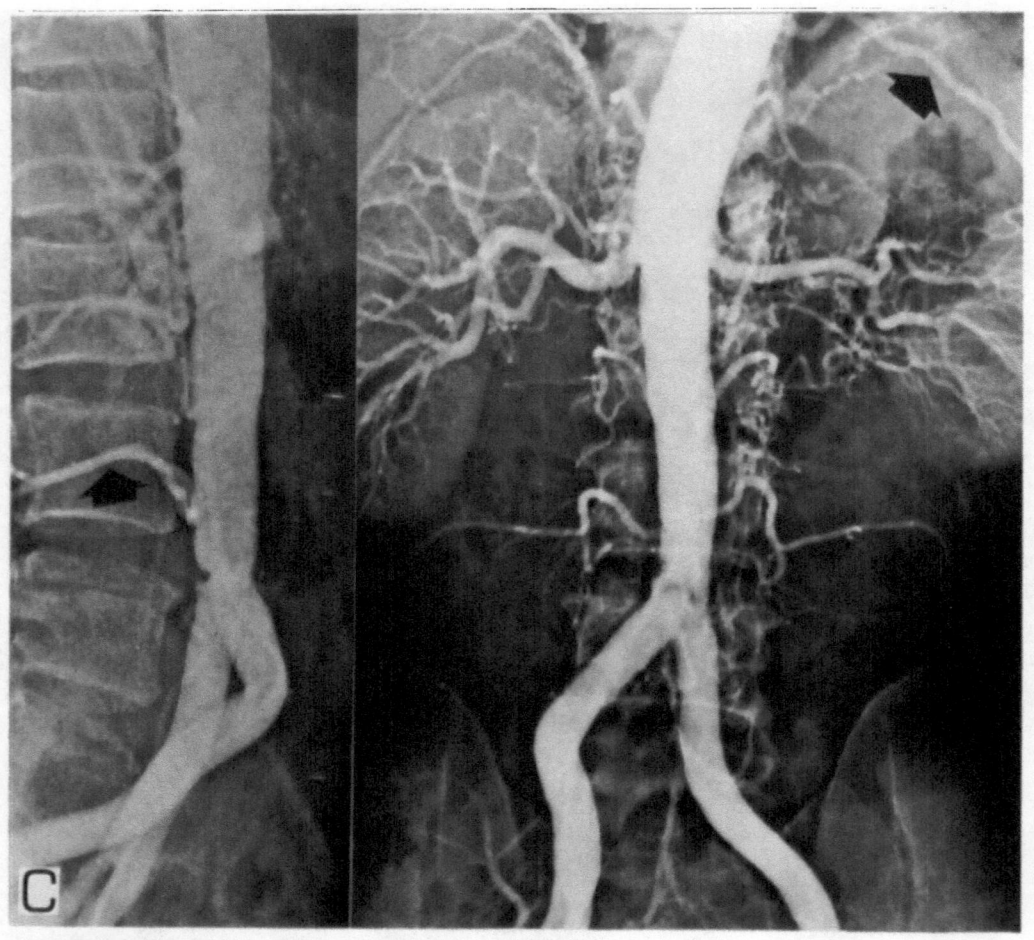

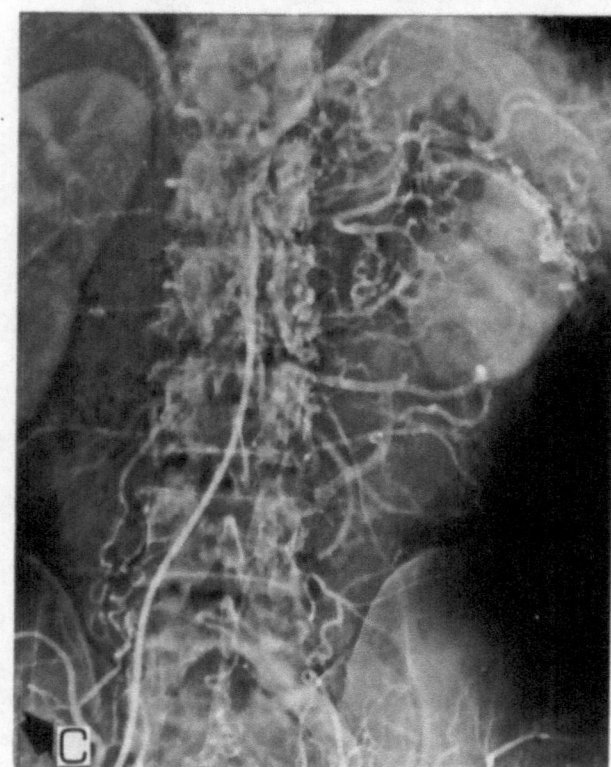

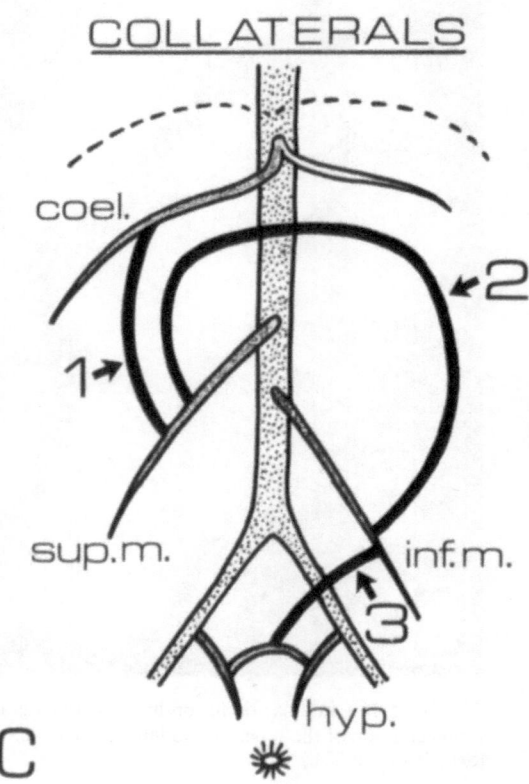

COLLATERALS

coel.

1

2

sup.m.

inf.m.

3

hyp.

C

Fig. 11.1c. See legend on page 323.

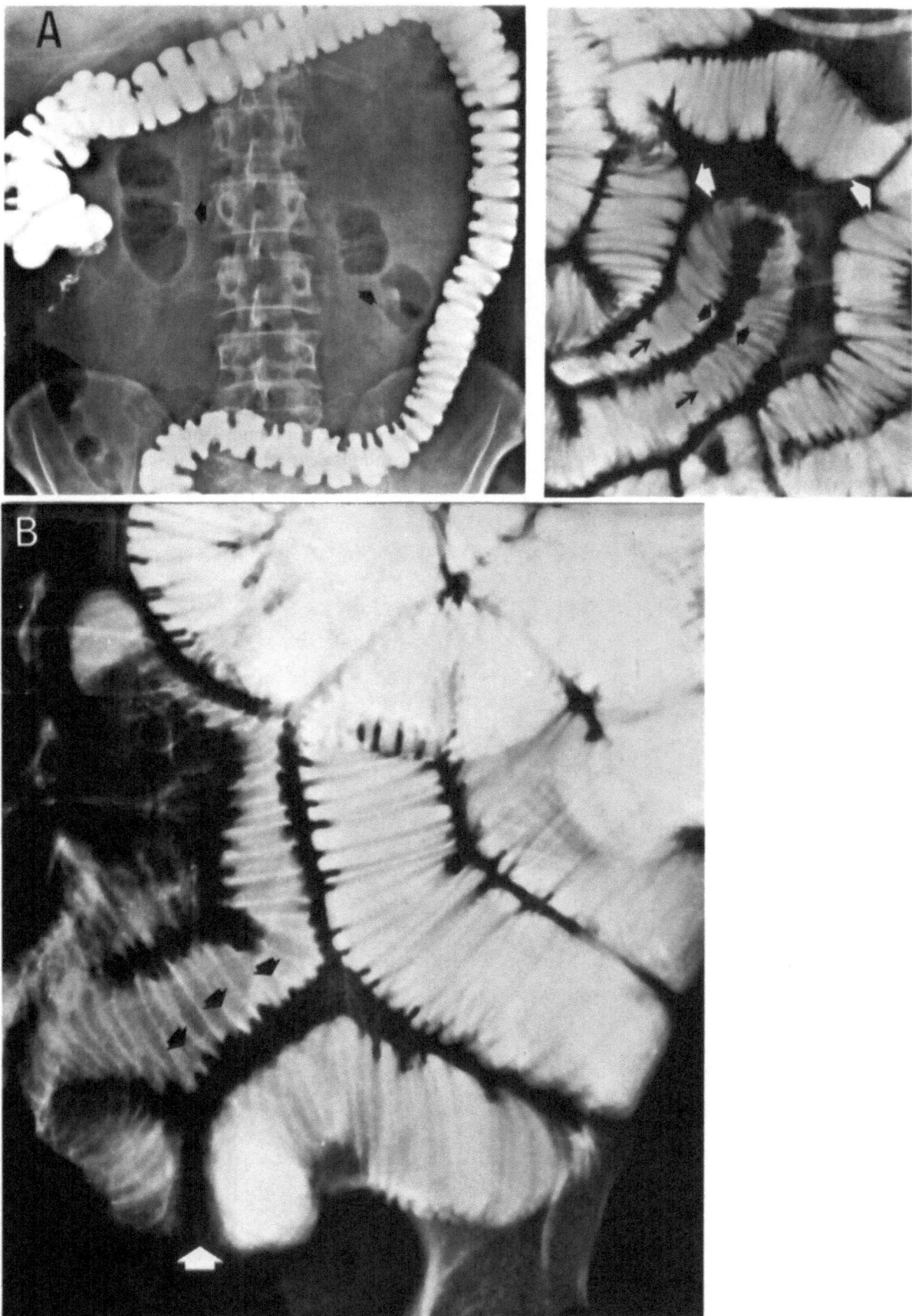

Fig. 11.2. Two cases of vascular abnormalities as a result of constricting bands crossing over the intestine. (A) An examination of the colon was performed because of vague abdominal complaints (left). All films showed two intestinal loops that were filled with gas and slightly dilated. Abnormalities in the small bowel were suspected and an enteroclysis examination was performed (right). This showed a band (thin solid arrows) at the site of the gas accumulation on the left. The intestinal loop here has an obviously thickened wall with subtle signs of 'thumbprinting' (thick sold arrows). On the distal side of the gas accumulation on the right, the wall is thickened over more than 10 cm while the folds are edematous and swollen. (B) Ileus due to bands (solid arrows). In this case the intestinal mucosal folds are only clearly thickened on the distal side of the band (open arrow). It most probably is the venous flow that is disturbed.

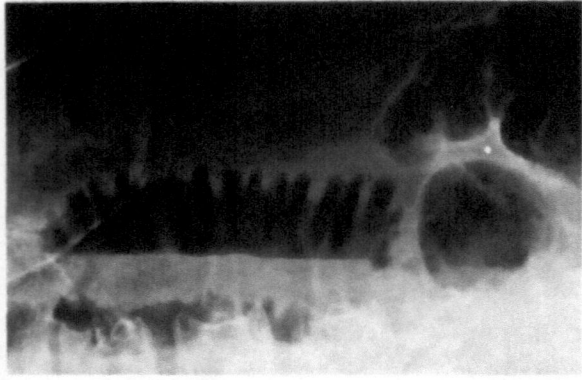

Fig. 11.3A. Ileus after bifurcation of a prothesis. Markedly swollen mucosal folds, possibly due to ischemia of the intestine since recovery was spontaneous.

widespread superficial erosions can develop. The epithelium is necrotic and the villi are shorter or have disappeared altogether. The lamina propria contain inflammatory infiltrates with lymphocytes, plasma cells, and histiocytes. The tiny blood vessels in the intestinal wall are often thrombotic and the fibrin coating the serosa leads to peritonitis and numerous adhesions. Angiographic examination reveals no visible abnormalities in the large vessels. The last stage can be the development of stenoses with prestenotic dilatations from fibrosis at the sites of extensive inflammation. The mucous membrane is almost entirely obliterated so that folds are no longer seen, and the intestinal wall appears com-

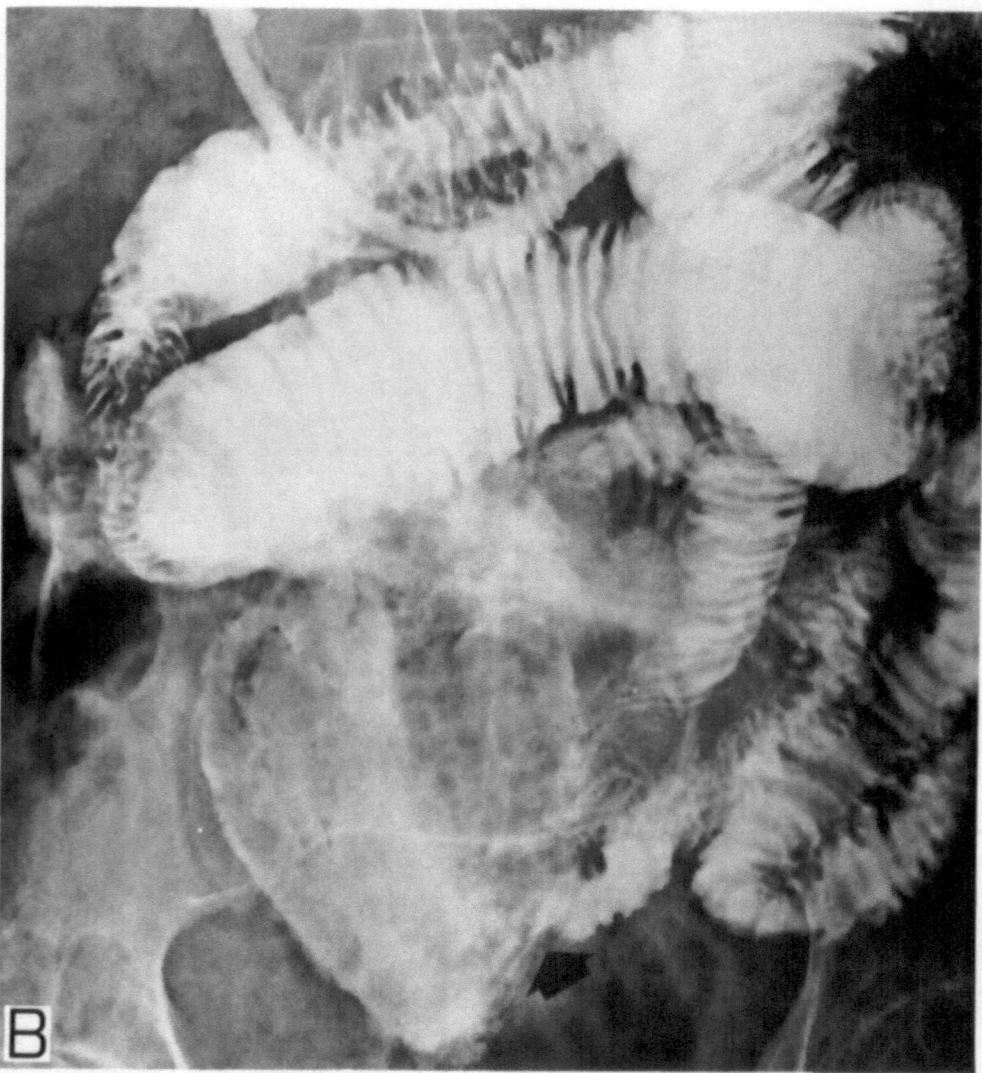

Fig. 11.3B. Perforation of the jejunum due to postoperative ischemia. Both mesenteric arteries were occluded. There is contrast fluid in the abdominal cavity and effacement of mucosal folding proximal to the site of necrosis.

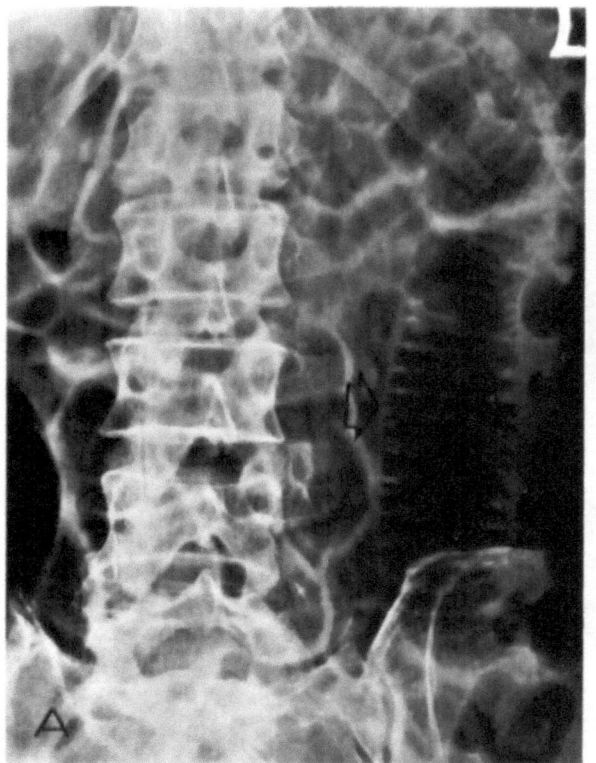

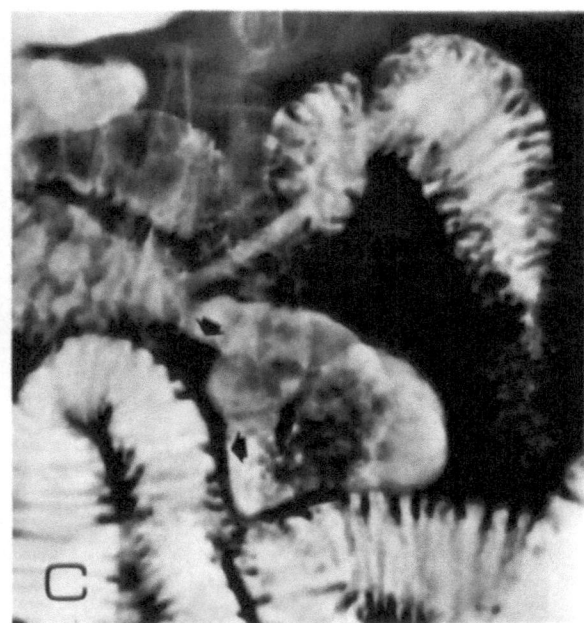

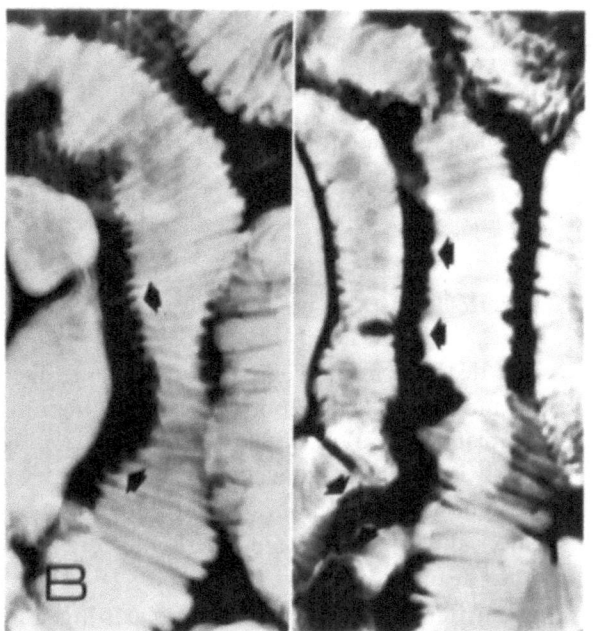

Fig. 11.4. Vascular accident in the small bowel of a patient with atrial fibrillation. (A) There were clear signs of an ileus, both radiologically and clinically. (B) In the distal jejunum, one loop contains highly edematous swollen mucosal folds; this is called 'thumbprinting'. The bowel wall is obviously thicker. No peristaltic movements could be seen in this region. (C) Several weeks later a definite clinical recovery was apparent. The roentgenograms now showed complete obliteration of the mucosal relief in the involved segment. The intestinal lumen is slightly narrower, thickening of the wall is reduced and signs of peristalsis could be seen during fluoroscopy.

pletely smooth. At present it is not known whether this should be considered a true rejection reaction or not (see fig. 11.5B).

3. Impaired venous flow

1) As a result of inflammatory processes in the intestinal wall or the mesentery, venous thrombosis can occur. In this region, however, a venous thrombosis is less common than an arterial thrombosis

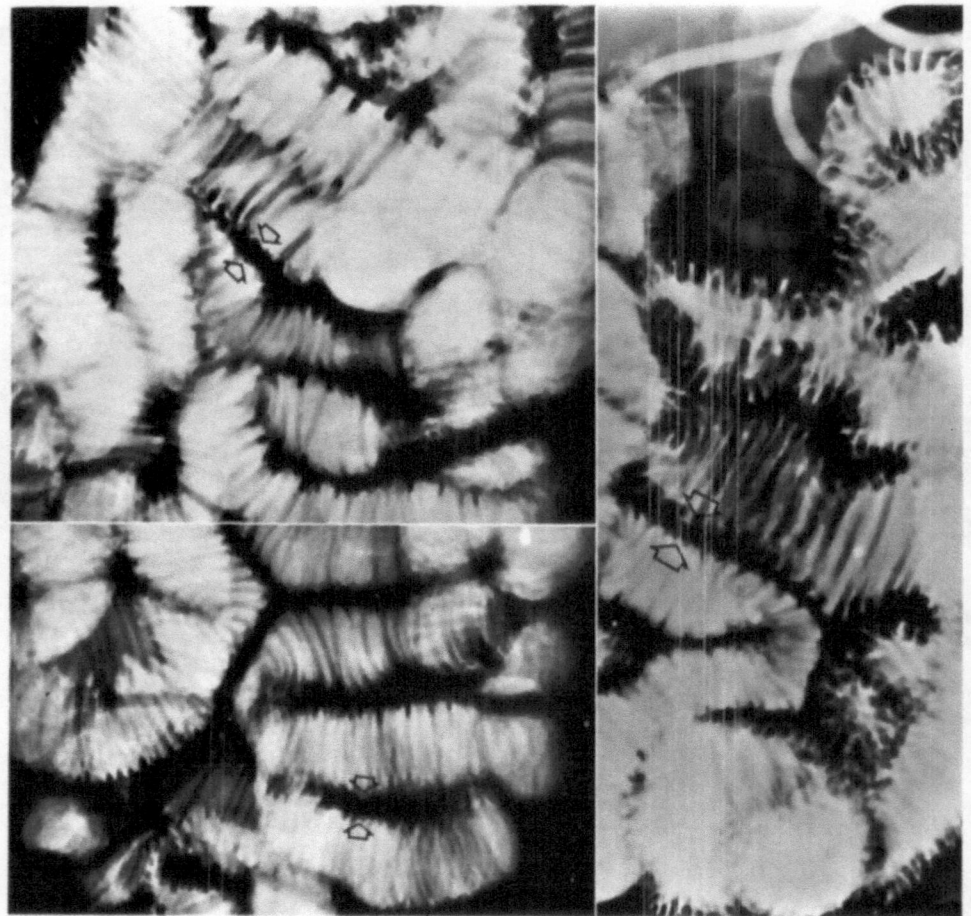

Fig. 11.5A. Mesenteric arteritis of unknown origin, found during surgery, in a 10-year-old boy. The mucosal folds are moderately broadened and the wall is thickened throughout most of the intestine (arrows). For comparison, the thickness of a normal bowel wall in youngsters can be seen at the right. In this child, the mucosal folds lie so close together that they have the so-called 'stacked coin' appearance.

(fig. 11.8).

2) The blood flow can also be impaired when the veins in the mesentery are constricted by compression or invasion of cysts or tumors in the mesentery. Such processes grow slowly and there is therefore sufficient time for an adequate collateral circulation to develop. Swollen mucosal folds therefore are usually caused by lymphedema when tumors or cysts are present.

3) The blood flow in the efferent veins is more likely to be impaired by volvulus, other strangulation already exists from arteriosclerosis or some other disorder.

4) Finally, severe congestive heart failure or portal hypertension from liver cirrhosis can also cause a serious reduction in the venous flow (fig. 11.9). In these cases there will be no chance for adequate collateral circulation to develop.

4. Periodic vascular insufficiency

1) A decrease in the heart minute volume, due for instance to hypertension, can lead to abdominal complaints as a result of an inadequate blood supply in the intestinal wall. This is particulary true if the decrease is temporary and a marginal circulation already exists from arteriosclerosis or some other disorder.

2) After a copious meal, a preexisting critical blood flow in the intestinal wall can suddenly become inadequate, causing severe abdominal cramps. This is called 'intestinal angina'. Such a marginal circulation in the intestinal wall is usually due to the simultaneous occurrence of a stenosis at the junction of the superior mesenteric artery and the celiac trunk. Not only arteriosclerosis but also fibromuscular hyperplasia can cause such stenosis.

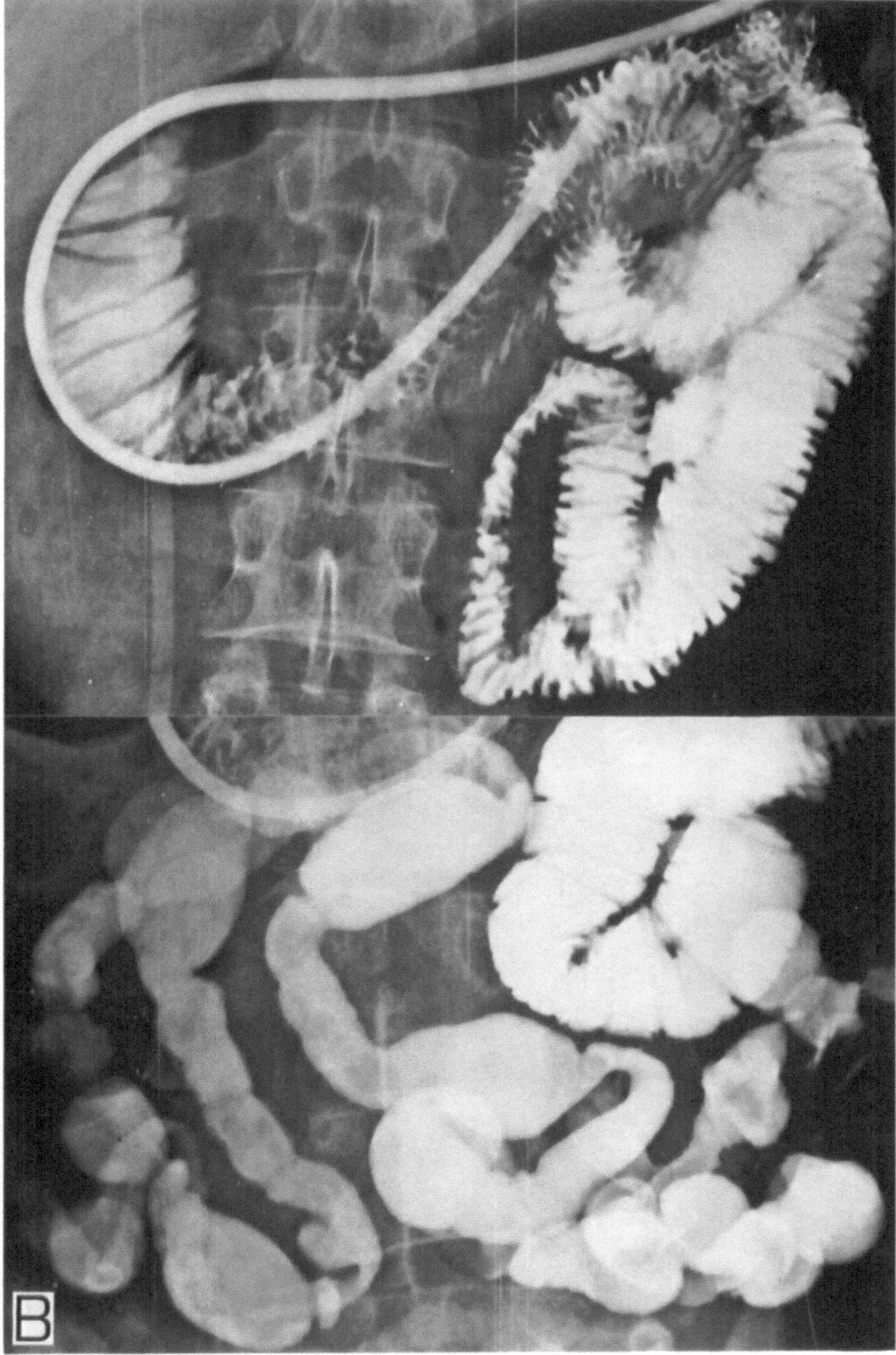

*Fig. 11.5*B. Extensive ischemic abnormalities in the ileum after bone marrow transplantation: the so-called graft versus host disease. There are multiple stenoses and longitudinal ulcers with pseudodiverticula-like shriveling (arrows). The abnormalities do not differ much from those seen in fig. 11.15. However, since angiography revealed no abnormalities, it indicates that the vascular occlusions were predominantly peripheral. (See also pages 330 and 331.)

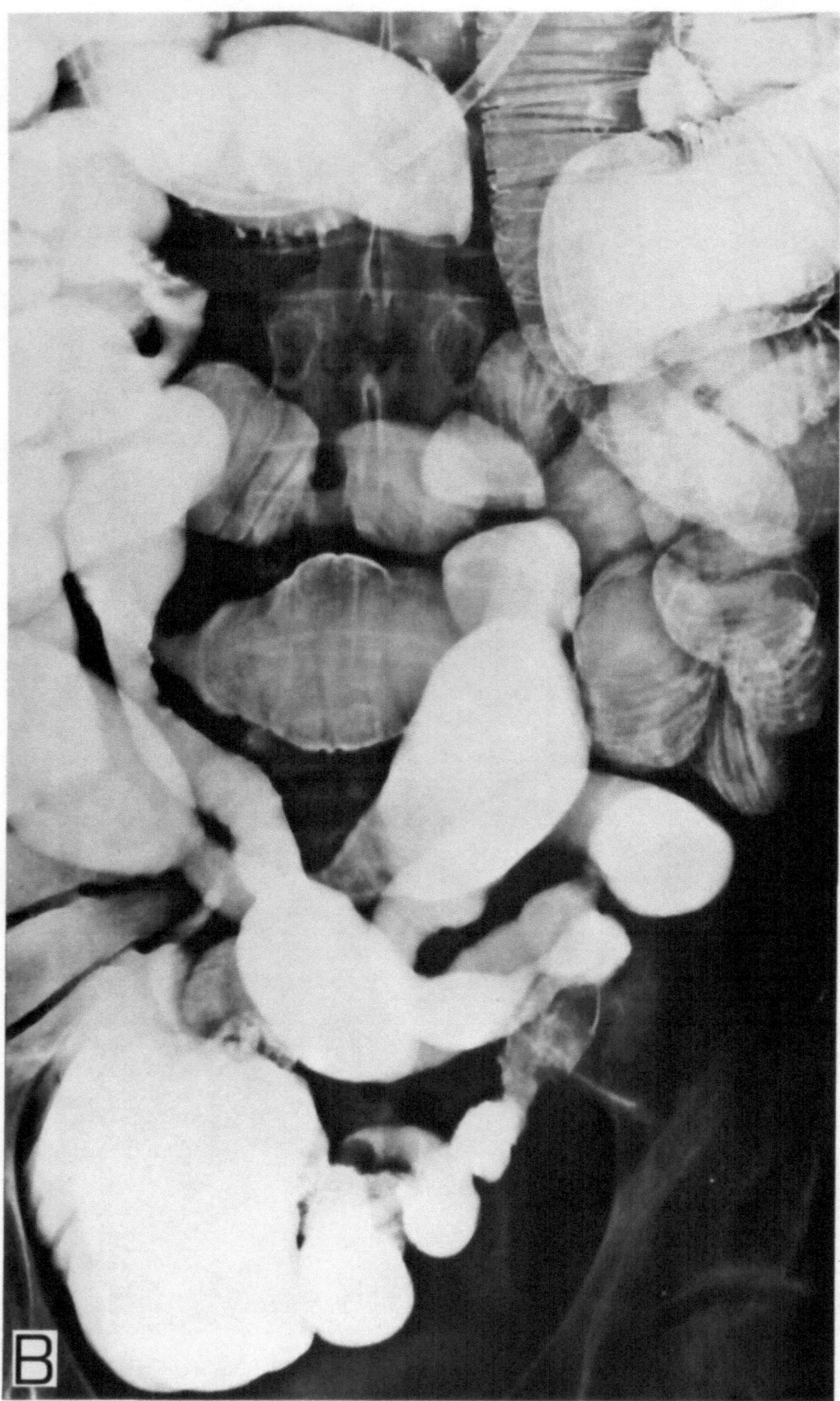

*Fig. 11.5*в. See legend on page 329.

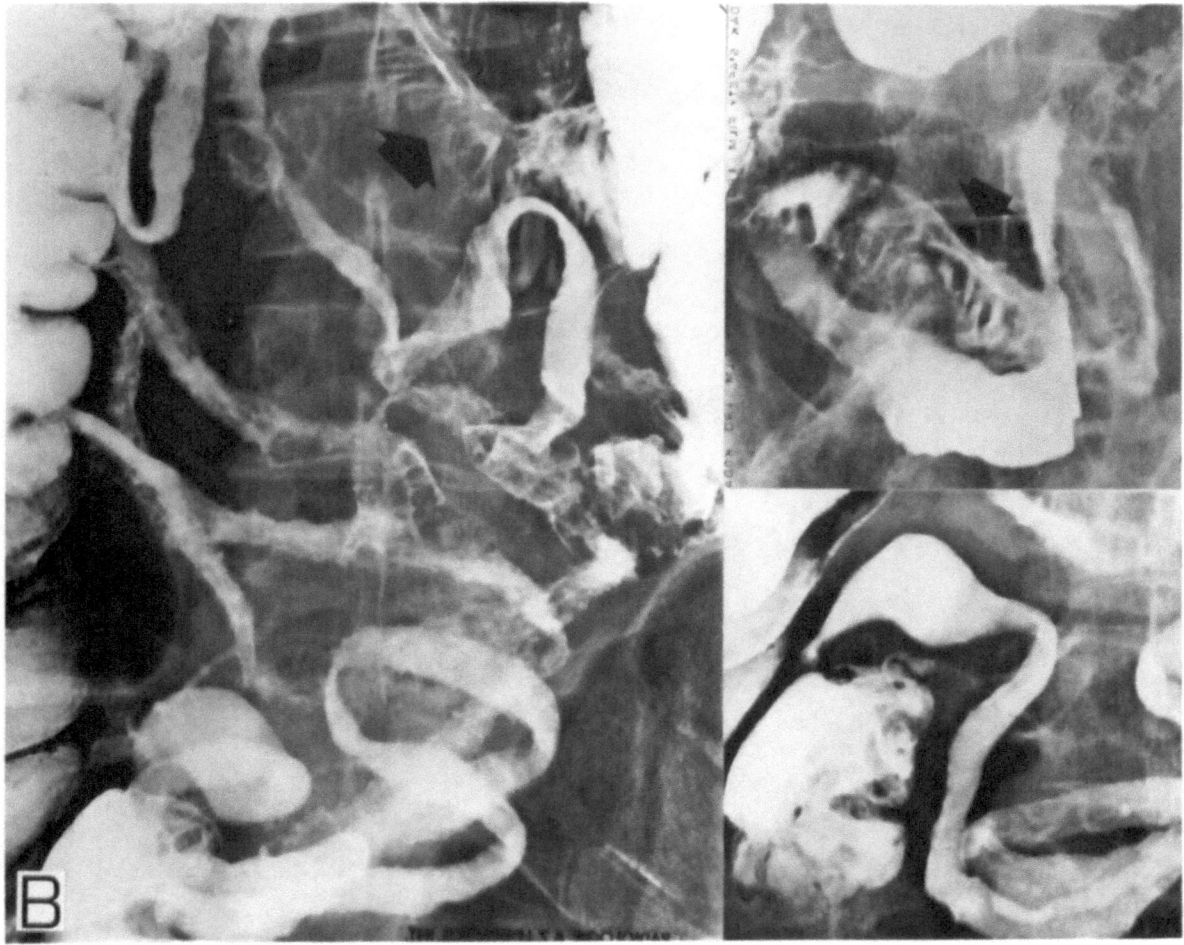

Fig. 11.5B. See legend on page 329.

To establish the diagnosis, abdominal aortography with lateral exposures is necessary. An examination of the small intestine with a contrast fluid reveals no abnormalities in these patients. The complaints that occur 1–2 h after eating are too short and not severe enough to cause visible changes in the mucous membrane.

5. Hemorrhage

A frequently occurring but often completely unrecognized vascular condition in the intestinal wall is the intramural hematoma. The hematoma can be small and heals spontaneously or within several weeks after treatment without persistent abnormalities (fig. 11.10). However, if the diagnosis is not recognized, the hematoma can become very large and cause total obstruction of the intestinal lumen.

The intestinal wall may then become necrotic and perforate, usually causing the death of the patient. The most common cause of hematomas in the intestinal wall is a disturbance of the coagulation mechanism from treatment with anticoagulants or the use of drugs containing aspirin (fig. 11.11A). Much less common is bleeding due to a hemorrhagic diathesis such as hemophilia or a vitamin K deficiency (fig. 11.11B). Blunt trauma to the abdomen in itself is a frequent cause of hematomas in the intestinal wall. It is also often a concurrent cause in patients with a preexisting enhanced bleeding tendency. Because it is fixed against the spinal column, the second half of the duodenum is the most vulnerable part of the small bowel. Hematomas are indeed encountered in this segment more often than in any other. Polypoid mucosal swelling from a hematoma can, especially in the proximal part of the small intestine, enhance per-

332

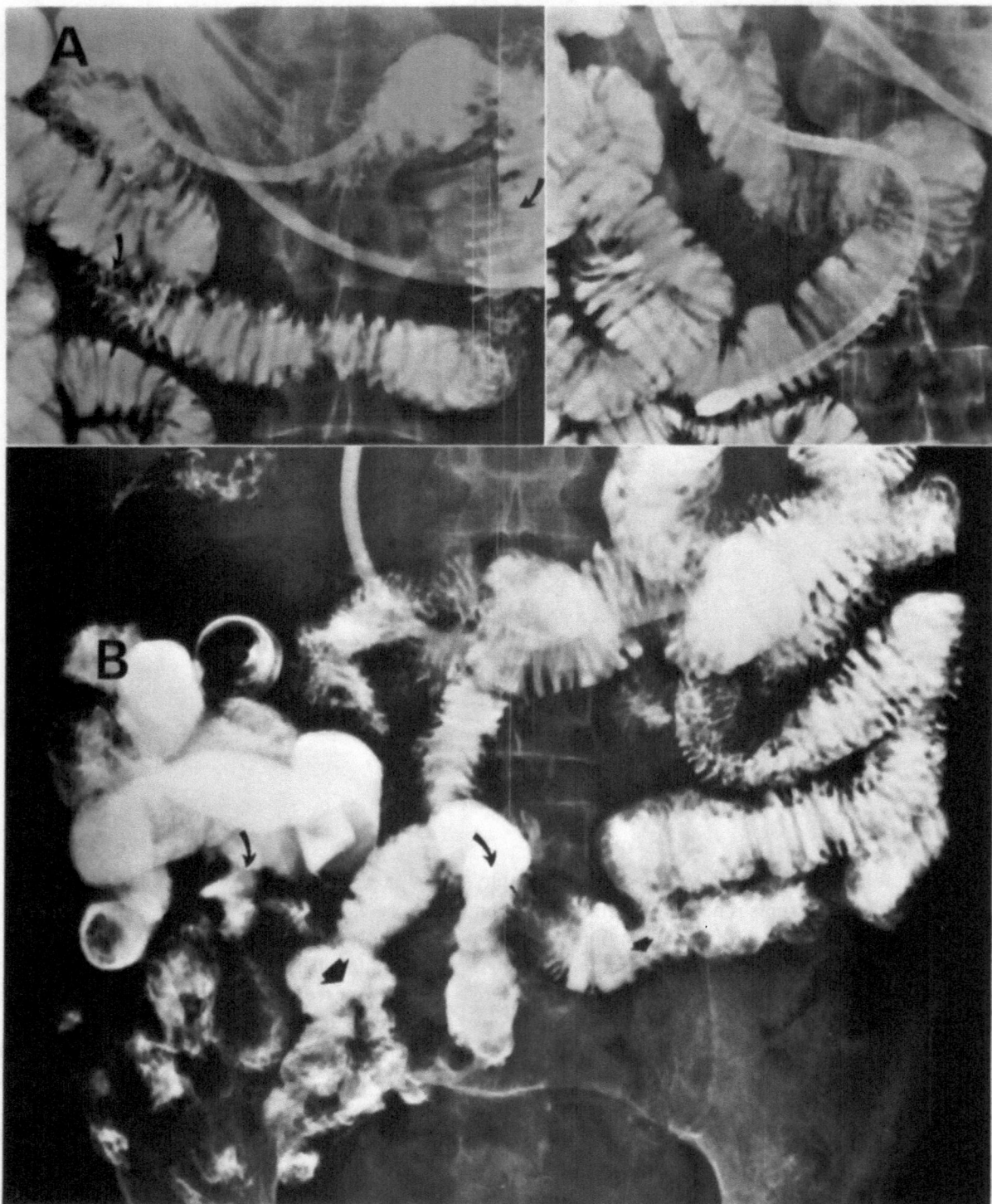

Fig. 11.6. Two patients with rectal bleeding due to Schönlein-Henoch disease. (A) Several decimeters of highly edematous swollen mucosal folds in the proximal jejunum (left), probably due to diffuse submucosal bleedings only. As so often in these patients, recovery was spontaneous and the mucosa appeared normal two weeks later (right). (B) The abnormalities can, however, also be more widespread as well as more pronounced so that complete recovery does not follow. Then the mucosal relief in several areas will be pathologically changed or completely absent. There will be an obvious hypermotility in the proximal ileum in the lower right quadrant. Similar abnormalities can be encountered in other diseases that are accompanied by arteritis – for instance dermatomyositis (see fig. 12.24).

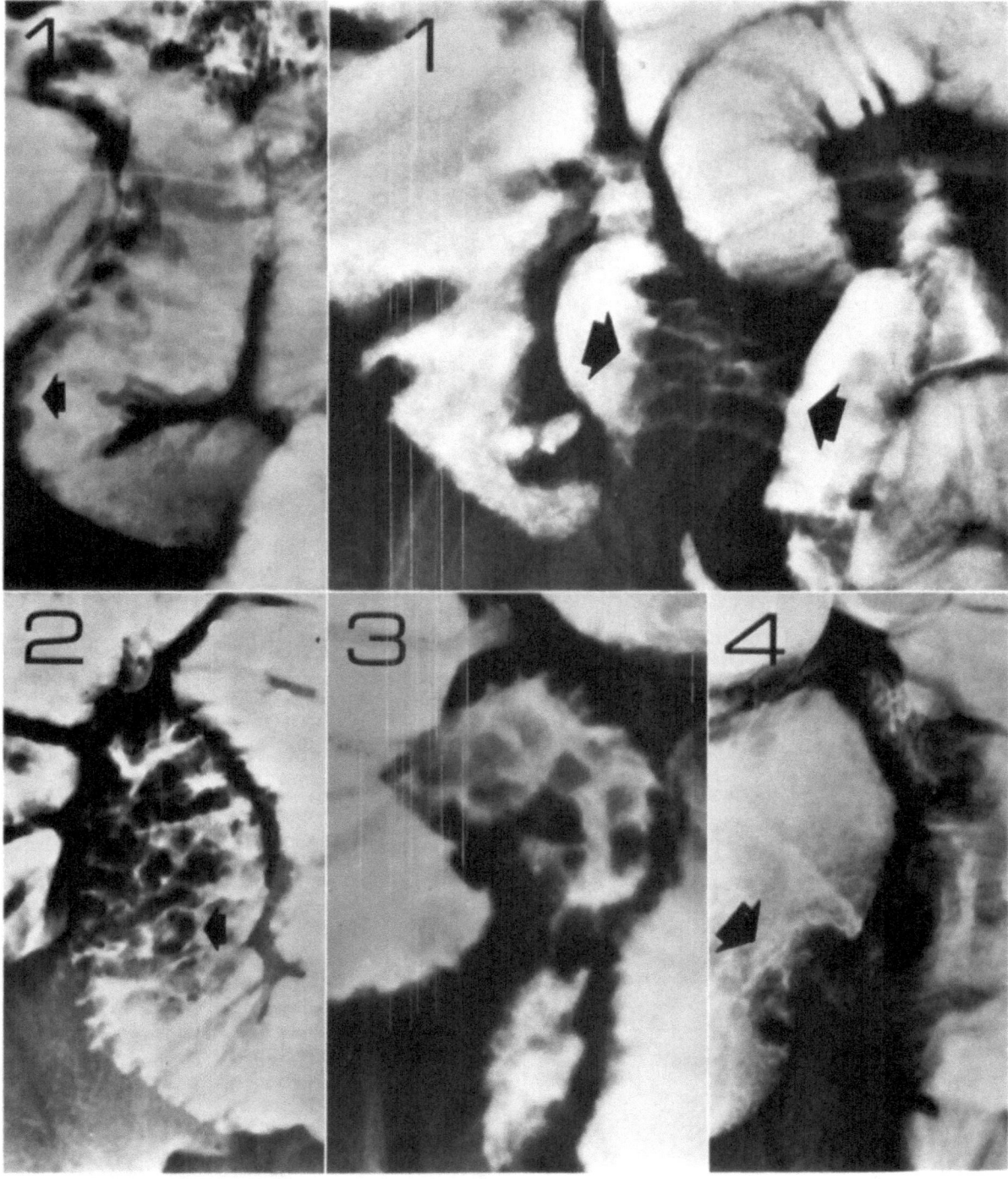

333

Fig. 11.7. Four cases of periarteritis nodosa with coarse mucosal folds and granuloma-like abnormalities. Some probably have a central ulcer crater. Several months later, one of the patients (no. 1) showed a cobblestone pattern that could not be distinguished from Crohn's disease.

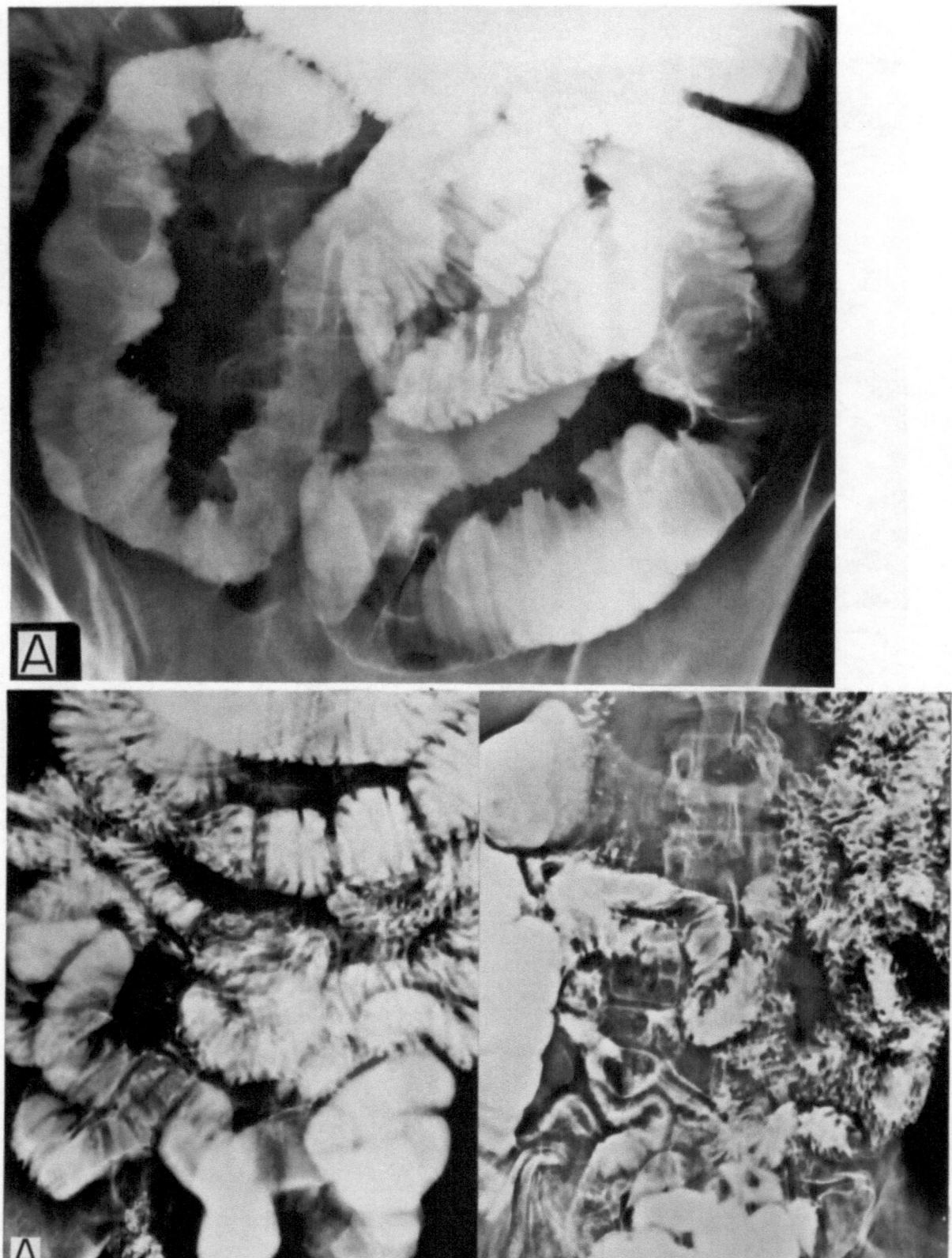

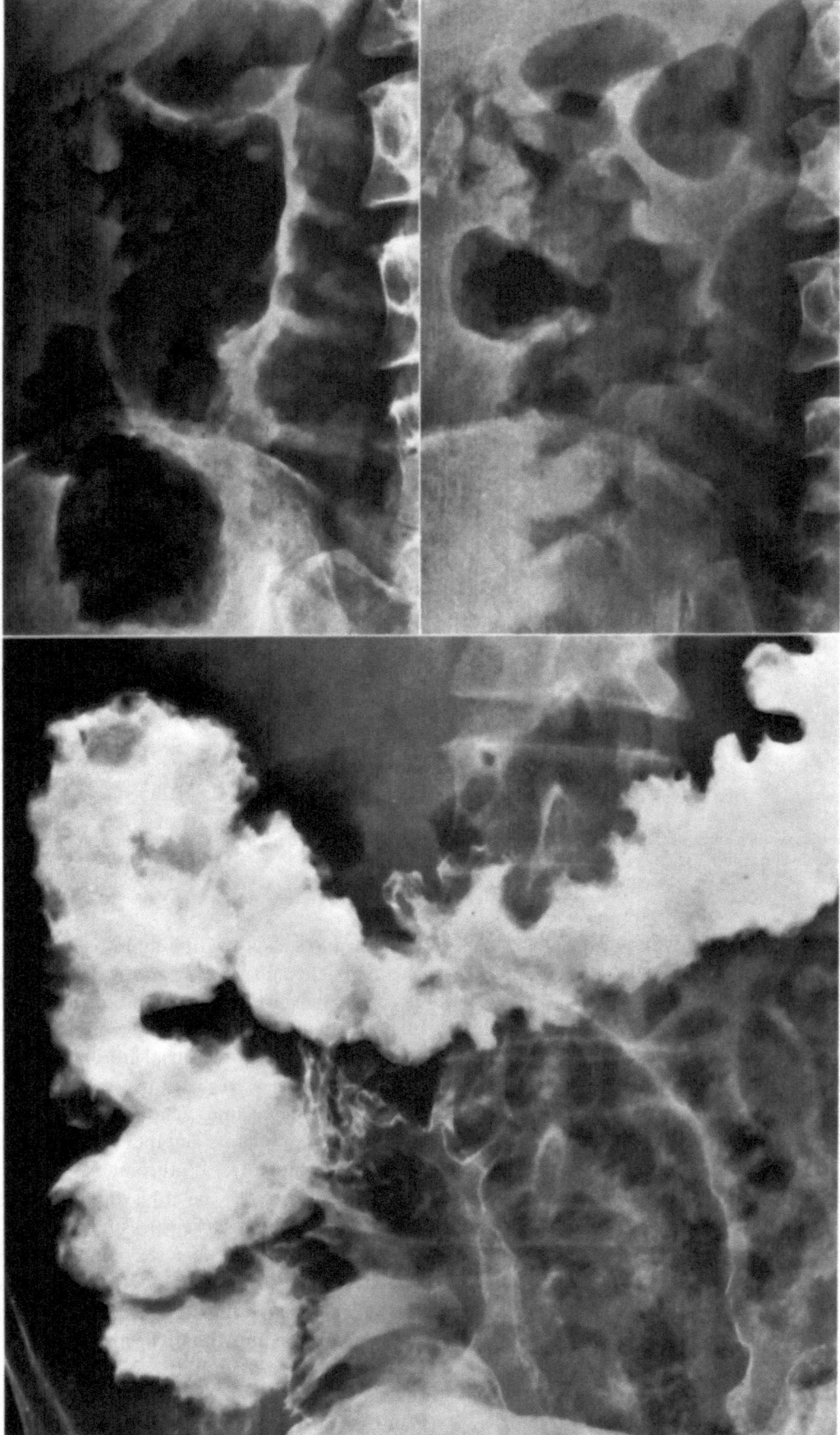

*Fig. 11.8*ʙ. Thrombosis of the superior mesenteric artery. Acute abdomen for two days. Bloody diarrhea and fever. The abdominal survey film showed gaseous distention, especially in the colon. Multiple nodular defects in the ascending colon; 24 h later the abnormalities had obviously increased (top right). The distance between the loops of the small bowel that now were also filled with gas had definitely increased (not shown). The colon examination performed the next day showed multiple defects arising from the wall that must be hematomas in the mucosa. The hematomas were not palpable during surgery; we have found that this is not uncommon.

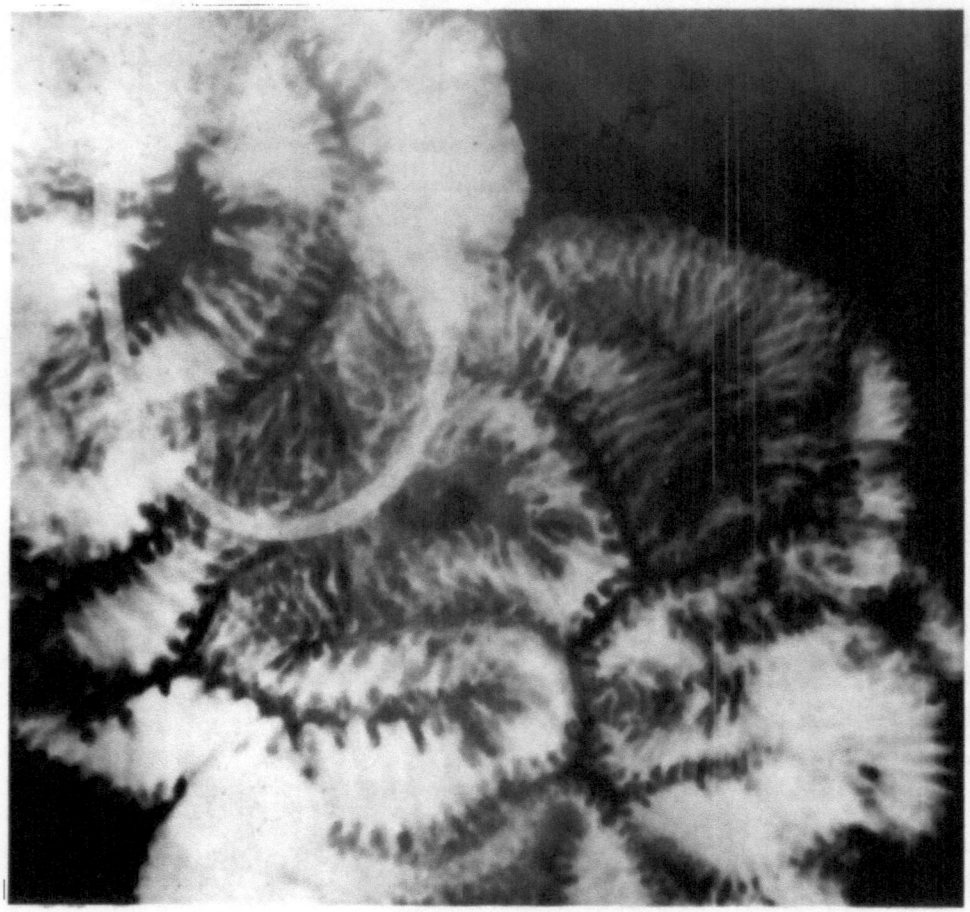

Fig. 11.9. Edematous swollen omega-shaped mucosal folds throughout the small bowel from a pronounced impairment of the venous flow as a result of liver cirrhosis. The liver is small; the spleen is greatly enlarged.

istalsis markedly. It may thereby cause an intussusception of the intestinal segment, containing the hematoma into the distal loop.

Hemorrhage occurs not only in the intestinal wall but also in the mesentery, where it causes a local but marked increase in the space between adjacent intestinal loops. The resulting roentgenogram resembles that of a mesenteric cyst. In practice, however, differentiation between these two disorders should never be difficult because the subsequent clinical findings and histories differ completely.

5.1. Clinical symptomology
The phenomena due to a vascular accident can vary considerably according to the length of the involved intestinal segment and the rate at which the occlusion develops. Here, too, an important factor is whether or not the collateral circulation can and will develop rapidly. Arterial occlusion occurs more frequently than venous occlusion, develops fairly suddenly, causes shock with a more or less serious ileus or subileus and severe pain in the abdomen. Quite often the history or a subsequent physical examination will clearly indicate the possibility of a vascular accident, such as atrial fibrillation or an advanced arteriosclerosis. The pulse rate sometimes can be of immediate value. Venous thromboses can cause the same complaints, but they usually develop much more gradually. If thrombosis develops slowly, then there may be no symptoms at all. In general the patient suffers least from the frequently multiple but always very small ischemic occlusions caused by vasculitis. Although obstipation may occur, abdominal pain and diarrhea are the most frequent complaints. The history as well as a brief physical examination usually provides several indications of a disease accompanied by vasculitis. Thus, an examination of the skin and inquiry about joint complaints can be most useful.

Vascular occlusions occur in the colon somewhat more frequently than in the small bowel. In con-

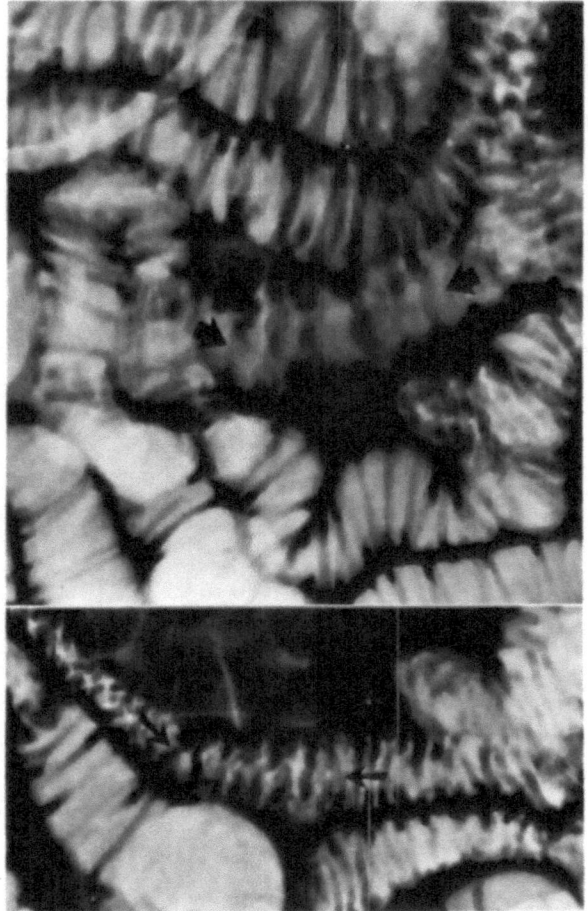

Fig. 11.10. Swollen mucosal folds in a jejunal loop that crossed the spinal column after a blunt trauma of the stomach. Complete recovery within three weeks.

trast, mucosal bleeding is seen in the small intestine more often than in the colon. Complaints due to hemorrhage can differ even more than those caused by vascular occlusion. In mild cases there is only slight discomfort in the abdomen. In a severe case there will be obstruction with vomiting and rectal bleeding. With a hematoma, these complaints are fairly subacute – thus they develop more gradually than those of an arterial occlusion and more acutely than in most cases of venous occlusion.

5.2. Roentgenological findings

Venous thrombosis causes a hemorrhagic infarct in the intestinal wall that becomes thicker and stiffer. The films reveal an increase in the space between the infarcted intestine and the adjacent intestinal loops. The mucosal folds become swollen due to the increased venous pressure and the subsequent development of edema. The spaces between the numerous folds in the jejunum become so thin that they resemble the thorns on a rose bush – sharply pointed at the tips and concave on either side (fig. 11.12BC). In the involved intestinal loop these thorny protrusions that enclose the swollen folds are found on both sides of the lumen at approximately equal distances from one another. The

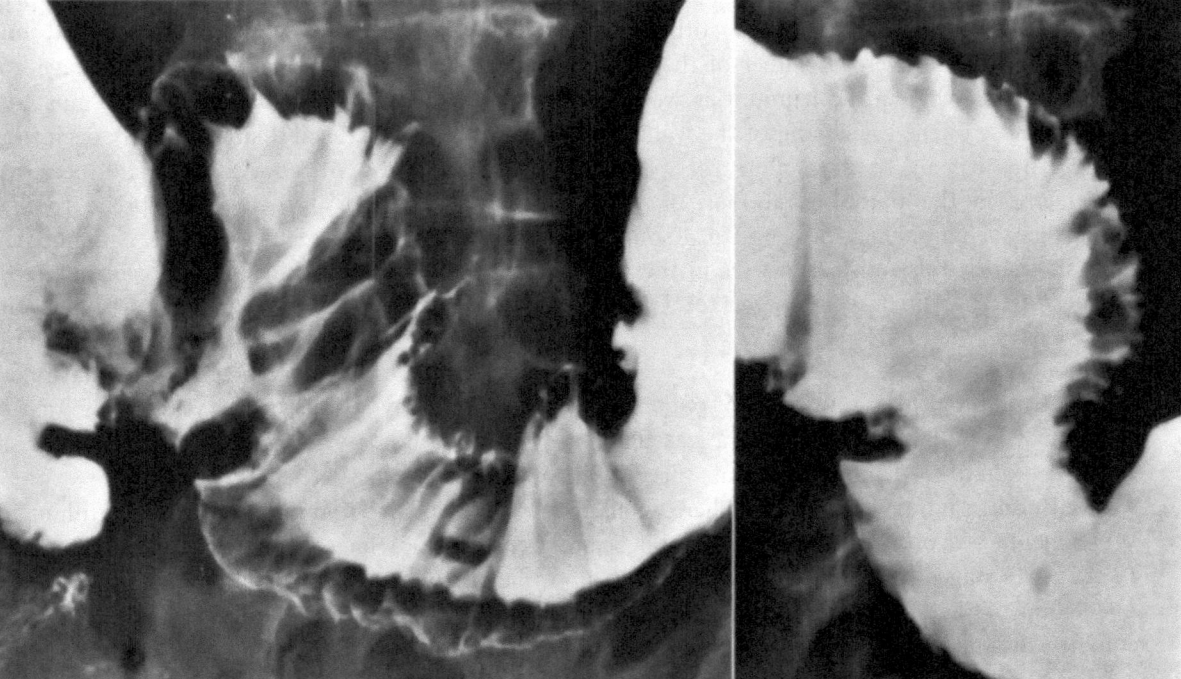

Fig. 11.11A. Submucosal hematomas in the transverse colon in a patient with an enhanced bleeding tendency as a result of incorrect anticoagulant therapy. Complete recovery two weeks later.

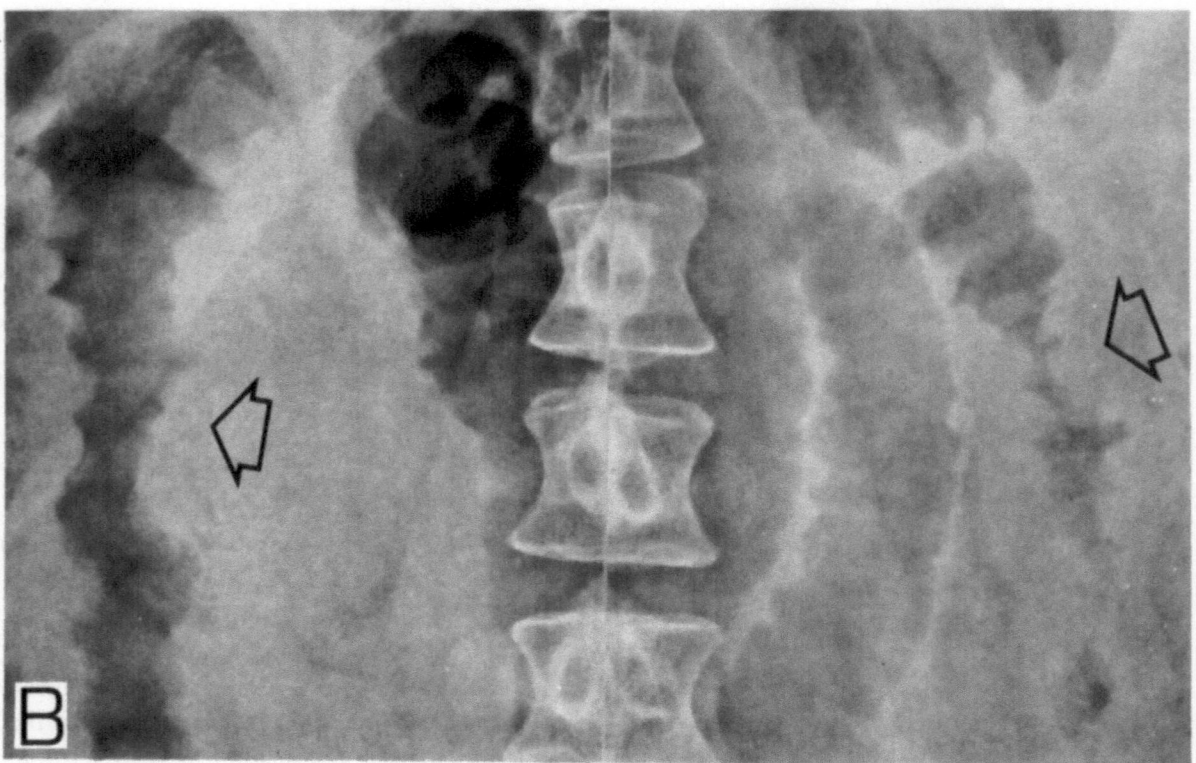

*Fig. 11.11*ʙ. Persistent gas in several dilated intestinal loops. The irregular aspect, the so-called 'thumbprinting' sign, is from hemorrhage in the intestinal wall. Patient has hemophilia.

impressions of these broadened mucosal folds on the contrast column are also called 'thumbprinting'.

In the ileum the folds are so scarce and so much shorter that the pattern is that of a stiff tube with smooth walls. The average caliber of the intestine decreases somewhat in the jejunum as well as the ileum because of the thickening of the wall. Under fluoroscopy it can be seen that the peristaltic movements in the pathological loop are clearly diminished or completely missing. In a somewhat later stage, peristalsis also decreases in the rest of the intestine, sometimes resulting in a total paralytic ileus.

The first radiological examination of patients with abdominal complaints resembling a vascular accident is often a plain abdominal survey film without contrast fluid. Sometimes there is also a supplementary exposure using a horizontal beam. In the early stages these films show a solitary air-filled loop of the small bowel that obviously can contain the abnormal mucosal folds described above. Another characteristic, because of the local absence of peristalsis, is that this gas-filled loop remains unchanged on repeat films taken several hours later.

The increased vulnerability of the intestinal wall,

a result of the vascular insufficiency, can lead to secondary infections and mucosal ulcerations. The ulcers develop quickly and are at first so superficial that they usually cannot be visualized on the roentgenograms. As a result of damage to the muscle bundles, after the mucosa the most vulnerable to anoxia, local dilatations may occur that do not result from a stenosis. Later still, necrosis and the inflammatory process will spread to the less sensitive connective tissue of the submucosa and subserosa. The pliability of the wall of the bowel although changed by edema, is only slightly diminished. The mucosal folds can disappear completely or become more irregular. This irregularity can be enhanced by lesions in the vessel walls that cause intramural hemorrhage; they develop as a result of the necrotizing enteritis.

We can also find multiple polypoid filling defects from hemorrhages in a still intact mucosa. These hemorrhages can be massive and cause pseudo-tumors that bulge far out into the intestinal lumen (fig. 11.13ʙ). As a result of gas-producing intestinal bacteria or open communication with the intestinal lumen, accumulations of gas may become visible within the intestinal wall (fig. 11.13ᴀ). They can be differentiated from the gas seen in pneumatosis intestinalis because the latter develops in an in-

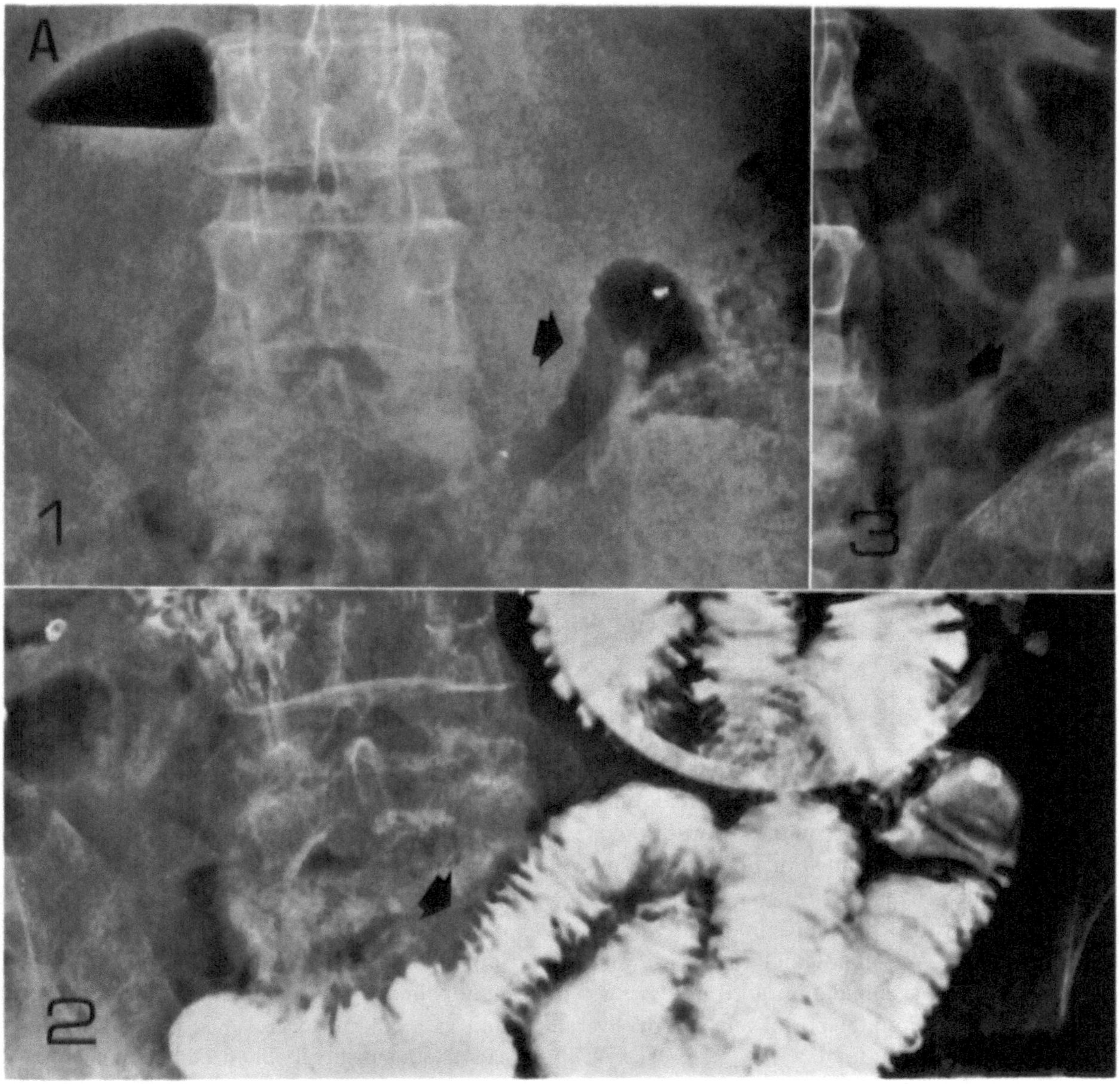

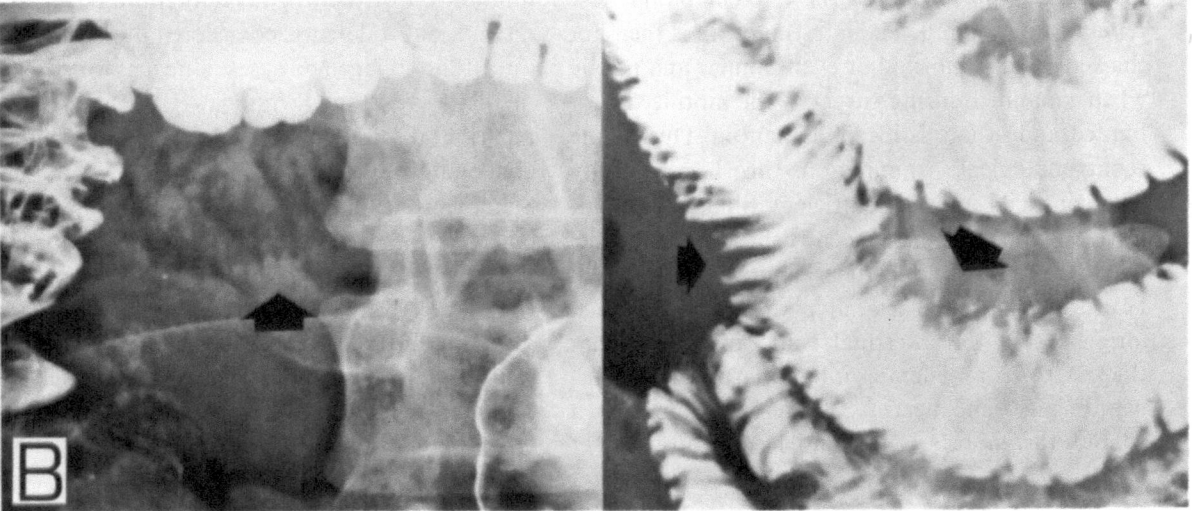

*Fig. 11.12*A. (1) Intestinal loop filled with gas in a patient with acute abdominal pain. The mucosal folds are flattened and obviously broadened. The enteroclysis examination performed the following day shows the same abnormalities in the same loop. The swelling of the mucosal folds has possibly even increased. (2) Several days later an abdominal survey film revealed an intramural film of gas in the intestinal wall at the same site, apparently as a result of local necrosis with limited perforation. (3) Fortunately, because of the contained nature of the lesion, recovery was complete.

*Fig. 11.12*B. Slight bleeding in the wall of the jejunum; pattern similar to that seen in fig. 11.12A.

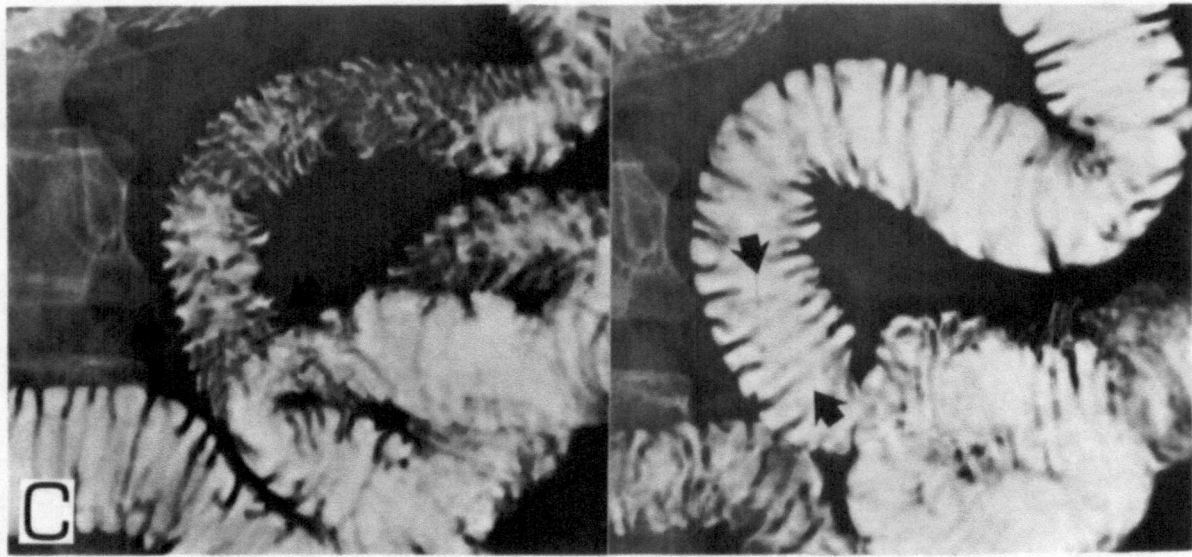

Fig. 11.12c. Unexplained thickening of the folds along a segment of the jejunum about 5 cm long, visible only in the contraction phase. No abnormalities visible in the well-filled state. Misleading pattern of mild edema?

testinal wall of normal thickness and with a normal mucosal pattern. If there are only small quantities of gas, then they appear on the x-ray as thin lines or crevices; a large accumulation of gas can assume the most bizarre shapes.

Total necrosis of the intestinal wall with perforation to the free abdominal cavity as well as a continued gas accumulation until it passes via the intestinal veins into the portal vein and the liver are conditions that are fatal.

The radiological characteristics of an arterial obstruction can only be differentiated from those of a venous thrombosis in the early stages. Arterial occlusion causes a termination of or a decrease in the blood supply whereas the efferent blood flow remains unimpaired. The intestinal wall is then not thickened but is normal or even thinner and is pale when examined during surgery. The motility is not limited and in fact is locally enhanced. During the roentgenological examination this hypermotility and spasticity prevent sufficient filling of an intestinal loop that has recently become ischemic. Dilatation of this loop then cannot be visualized. However, this pure arterial pattern does not last long because the intestinal wall rapidly becomes thickened from edema, inflammatory reactions, hemorrhage, and necrosis. Differentiation from a venous thrombosis is then no longer possible, at

least radiologically.

In Schönlein-Henoch disease, there is an acute arteritis accompanied by pain in the abdomen and the joints, and purpura and nephritis. There is also a submucosal edema with moderately swollen mucosal folds. The larger arteries in these intestinal loops, that appear red during surgery, remain unimpaired so that circulation is barely disturbed and as a rule no necrosis or ulcerations develop. Here, too, motility is enhanced but it encompasses a larger segment than in the early stages of an ischemic infarct. The caliber of the intestine is normal or only slightly decreased.

The etiology of Schönlein-Henoch disease is unknown. For years it was thought to be an allergic disease, but today it is considered more likely to be one of the collagen diseases. Unusual for this group of diseases is that Schönlein-Henoch disease is a recurrent disease. In addition, the relationship with concomitant Streptococci infection is unknown. Schönlein-Henoch disease also differs from other collagen diseases in that it is self-limiting and usually disappears without persistent abnormalities (fig. 11.6A). Recently, however, it has become evident that this differentiation is not clear-cut, and that residual abnormalities can be seen (fig. 11.6B).

There are good arguments for including the collagen diseases in this chapter on vascular dis-

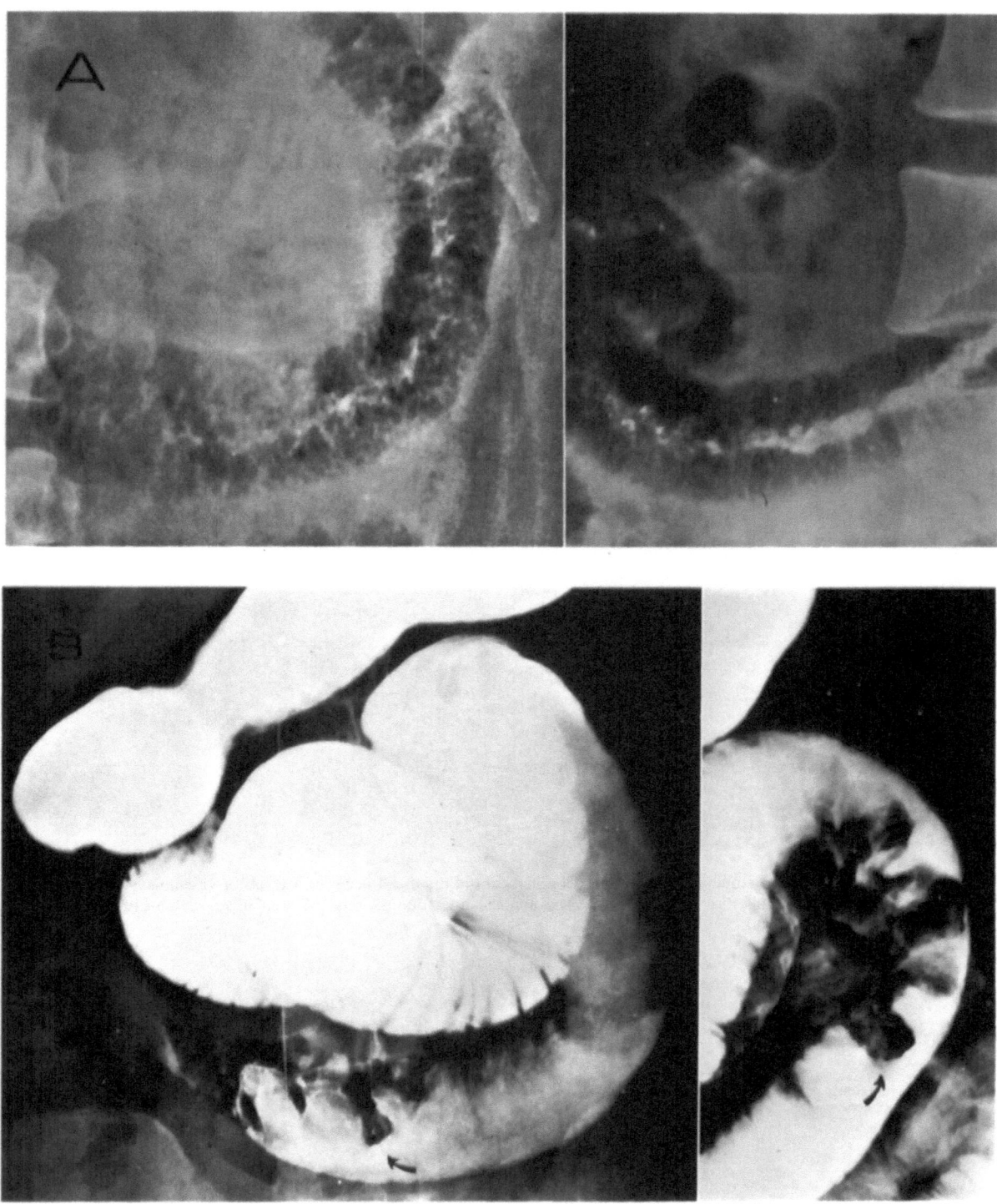

Fig. 11.13. Erratic intramural gas accumulations (A) and large pseudotumors bulging out into the intestinal lumen (B) as a result of submucosal hematomas in a patient with mesenteric thrombosis.

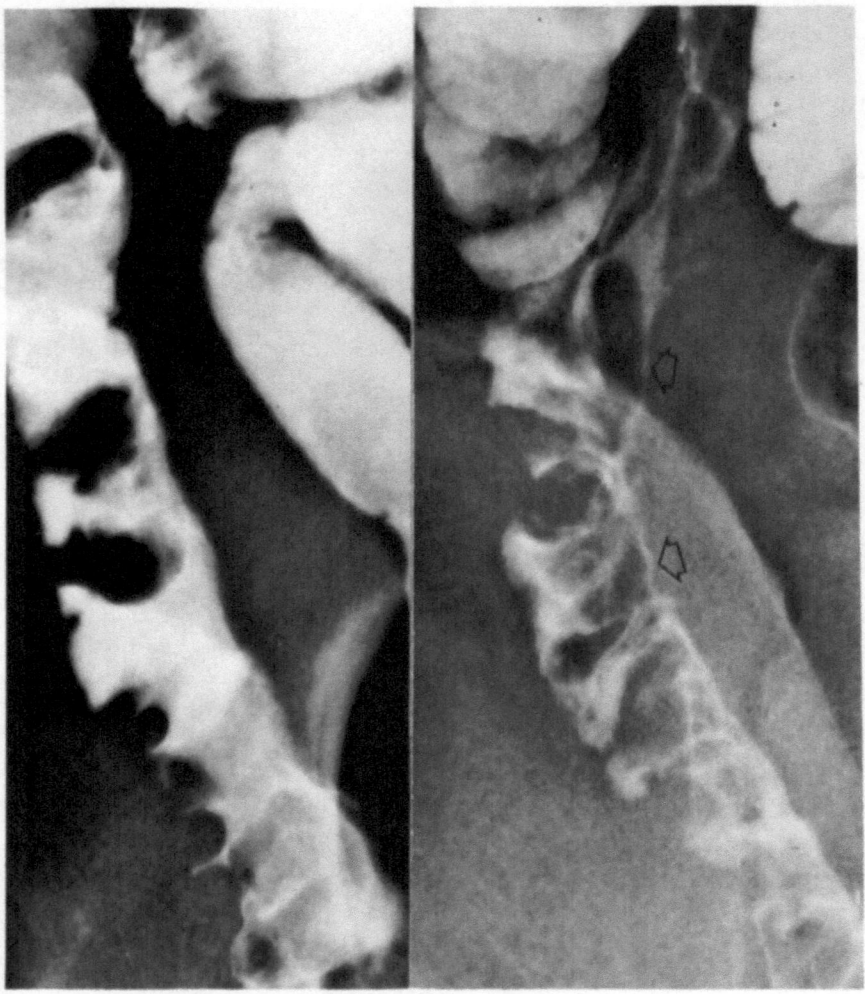

*Fig. 11.14*A. Very long longitudinal ulcer and pseudodiverticula in the distal ileum as a result of vasculitis. Abnormalities similar to those caused by Crohn's disease in fig. 9.12. The abnormalities due to ischemia seen in the colon also appear to suggest Crohn's disease (fig. 11.14B).

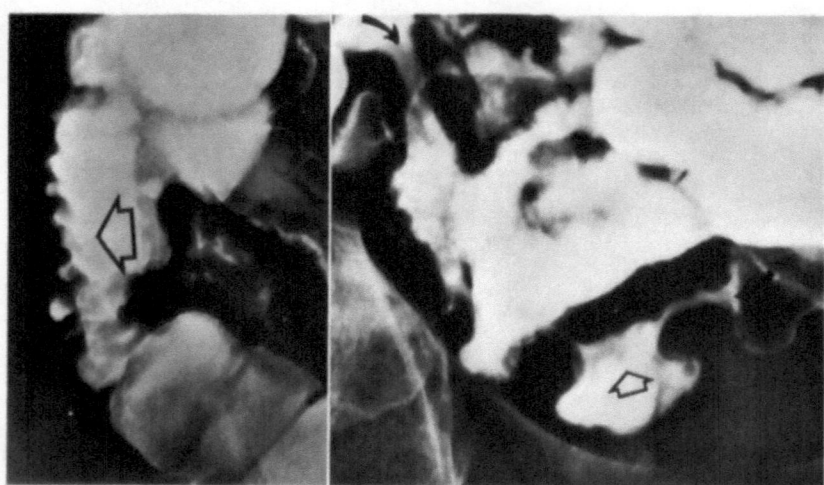

*Fig. 11.14*B. Fibrous remnants after a vascular accident with pseudodiverticula (left), long smooth stenoses and asymmetrically shriveled ulcers (right). Differentiation from Crohn's disease by means of radiological examination is usually not possible.

eases. However, it was decided that, since motility disorders are so common in this disease, they should be included in the chapter on disturbed motility. An exception has been made for Schönlein-Henoch disease for historical reasons.

Hematomas in the intestinal wall due to hemorrhagic diathesis heal in one or two weeks and, in contrast to hematomas of a vascular accident, with restitutio integrum. Radiologically, however, a simple hematoma is not always easy to differentiate from hemorrhage due to a vascular accident. A common hematoma is indicated by the presence of a mesenteric mass due to the hemorrhage in the mesentery. In addition, the caliber of the intestine does not change and peristalsis remains normal.

5.3. Prognosis

The results of ischemia, immediately as well as later, depend upon the location, the extent, the rate of development, and the total duration.

Anatomically, circulation in the distal intestinal wall differs from that in the proximal part. In the ileum the afferent vessels lie in the subserosa, thus on the outer side of the intestinal surface. From here numerous perpendicular branches extend straight through all layers of the intestinal wall in the direction of the lumen. In an intestinal segment with this type of circulation the afferent terminal vessels are not constricted as quickly by the swelling and compression from edema and hematomas as those in the jejunum. There, both the large and the small afferent vessels form a network deep in the submucosa and tunica muscularis. An ischemic attack lasting about 3 h causes necrosis of the mucosa, but the muscularis usually remains intact. The mucous membrane becomes totally atrophied as a result of the necrosis and the mucosal relief disappears. Months later, however, there can be a recovery of the mucosa. Then, adhesions or fusion with adjacent intestinal loops is often seen since a fibrinous

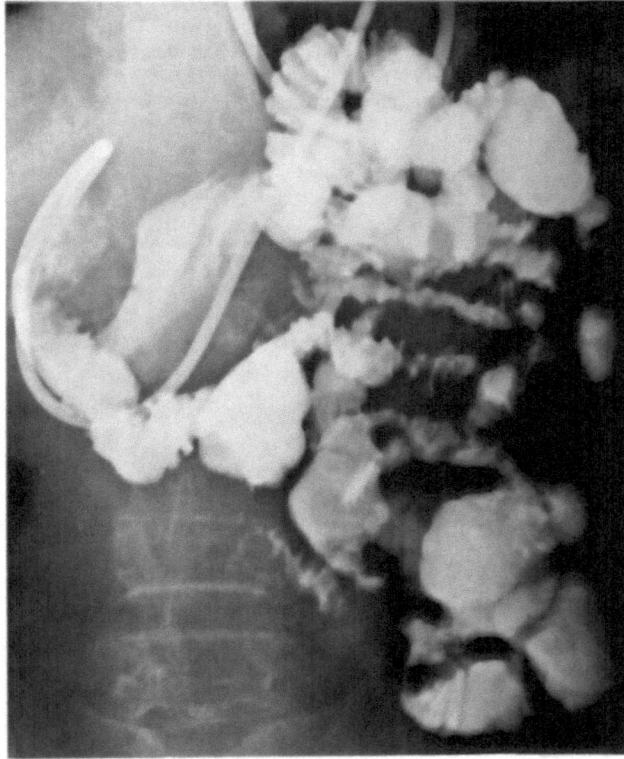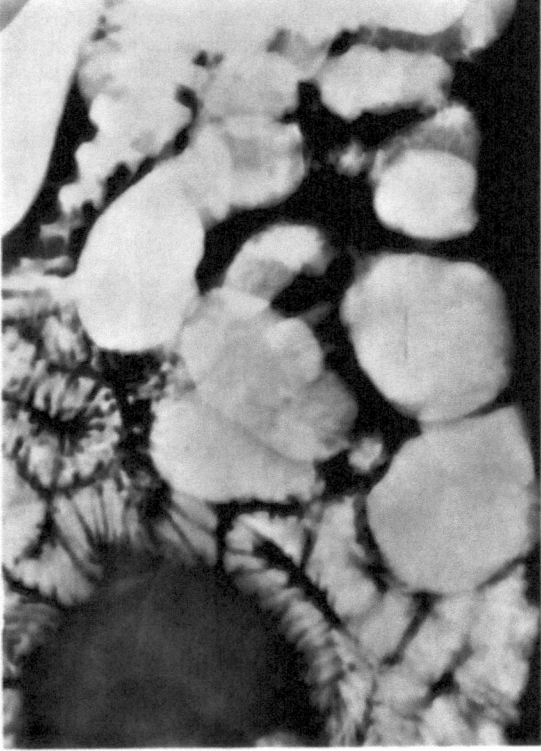

Fig. 11.15. Elderly male with multiple ischemic stenoses several centimeters in length in the jejunum. The mucosal pattern has disappeared in the intestinal segments between the stenoses. An angiographic examination revealed a vascular insufficiency in this part of the small bowel and the appearance of the vessels indicated that the mesentery was shriveled. It is not possible to distinguish here between a state after remission of an inflammatory process, for instance Crohn's disease, and a primary vascular disease. Because of the stenoses, a biopsy instrument could not be introduced so that celiac disease with atrophy of the mucosa and ulcerations also could not be excluded – at least not in this manner.

344

layer coats the intestine as a result of the ischemia.

Anoxia lasting 5–6 h also causes damage to the muscle bundles. Both the inner and the outer intestinal wall now show necrotic changes and ulcerations. The latter heal with the formation of connective tissue and lead, 1–3 months later, to shriveling and stenoses. Ischemic stenoses are usually about 2–5 cm long, have smooth walls, and increase in caliber gradually at the transition to the healthy intestine on each end (fig. 11.15). In the case of tumor, the stenosis is often shorter, has more irregular margins, and the transition to the normal intestine is much more abrupt.

After ischemia, just as after ulcerations in Crohn's disease that heal with fibrotic shriveling, pseudodiverticula and sacculations can develop on the intestines' antimesenteric side with a straight smooth-walled shriveling on the opposite side (fig. 11.14A). In the colon a persistent abnormality of this type is, however, more common than in the small bowel. Ischemic episodes lasting 8–9 h or longer cause total necrosis of the intestinal wall with perforation into the free abdominal cavity. The nerve cells are the least sensitive to anoxia so that intestinal motility as a rule remains unchanged after an infarct.

Bibliography: chapter 11

Balthazar EJ, Einhorn R (1976) Intramural gastrointestinal hemorrhage. Gastrointest Radiol 1: 229–239.

Boley SJ, Schwartz SS, Donaldson RM (1971) Vascular disorders of the intestine. London: Butterworths.

Joffe N, Goldman H, Antonioli DA (1977) Barium studies in small-bowel infarction. Radiological-pathological correlation. Radiology 123: 303.

Gharemani GG, Meyers MA, Farman J, Port RB (1977) Ischemic disease of the small bowel and colon associated with oral contraceptives. Gastrointest Radiol 2: 221–228.

Meyers MA, Kaplowitz N, Bloom AA (1973) Malabsorption secondary to mesenteric ischemia. Am J Roentgenol 119: 352–358.

Pearson KD, Buchignani JS, Shimkin PM, Frank MM (1972) Hereditary angioneurotic edema of the gastrointestinal tract. Am J Roentgenol 116: 256–277.

Reuter SR, Redman HC (1972) Gastrointestinal angiography. Monographs in clinical radiology. Philadelphia: Saunders.

Vascular diseases in the alimentary tract (1972) Clinics in gastroenterology. Philadelphia: Saunders.

Voegeli E (1974) Die Angiographie bei Dünndarm- und Dickdarmerkrankungen. Stuttgart: Thieme.

12. DISTURBED MOTILITY

Many highly divergent diseases can be accompanied by changes in the motility in the small bowel. However, understanding and knowledge of the mechanism responsible for these motility disorders can be considered no more than rudimentary. The infusion technique has shown that motility is disturbed much more frequently than is generally assumed. On the contrary, when the contrast medium is administered orally, hypermotility is sometimes incorrectly diagnosed on the basis of an accelerated transit time. This is seen for instance in achylia gastrica or it may be due to hyperperistalsis of the stomach. In both cases there is an accelerated gastric emptying and therefore a shorter transit time. The elimination of gastric emptying time in the enteroclysis examination has increased the possibilities of comparing transit time through the small intestine.

The greatest contribution toward establishing the diagnosis of disturbed motility is that during this examination the contrast column is followed under intermittent fluoroscopy. Therefore short local changes in motility are as a rule no longer overlooked (figs. 12.1 and 12.2).

Some diseases are accompanied by the strange phenomenon of either an enhanced or a decreased motility, such as occurs in the collagen diseases and diabetes mellitus. Thus not only a hypomotility is seen but also a hypermotility; the latter is due to a mild anoxia of the intestinal wall. In the collagen diseases, this anoxia is due to a vasculitis. In diabetes it is the result of an insufficiency of the peripheral circulation from arteriosclerotic changes in the walls of the arteriolae. If there is a diabetogenic diarrhea, then as a rule there will also be a retinopathy, and the kidney and pancreas functions will be disturbed. The impaired functioning of the pancreas can be such that resorption of diverse food substances is disturbed, resulting in a pancreato-genic steatorrhea.

If motility is not sufficient to propel the contrast fluid distalward quickly, it will be seen that few intestinal loops are in a state of contraction. The barium suspension then will flocculate almost immediately (fig. 12.3).

On the basis of the number of patients and also the number of causative factors, a decreased motility occurs in the intestine more frequently than a hypermotility. As far as the latter is concerned, an enhanced motility throughout the entire small bowel is seen more often than a local hyperperistalsis. Although seemingly paradoxical, most states of hypomotility alternate with periods of hypermotility. These attacks of hyperperistalsis cause most of the patient's subjective complaints and lead him to consult a physician. The causative factors of a disturbed motility of the small intestine can be grouped in several major categories:

A. Neurogenic or humoral
B. Mechanical obstruction; ileus
C. Diseases affecting the intestinal wall
D. Inflammatory processes
E. Allergic reactions
F. Anoxia
G. Disturbed resorption.

A. Neurogenic or humoral factors

Carcinoid lesions and states of fear or emotion cause a pronounced increase in peristaltic movements; this is because of increased adrenalin production. The mechanism of the diarrhea that tends to accompany a hyperparathyroidism is unknown. It is possible that reduced production of gastric acid and the accelerated gastric emptying that is in part the result of the former play a role.

Many of the diseases in this group, however, lead to a decrease in peristaltic movements. The most

346

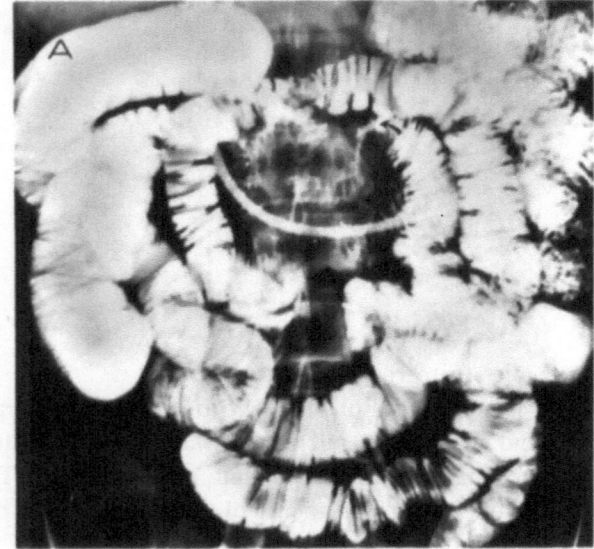

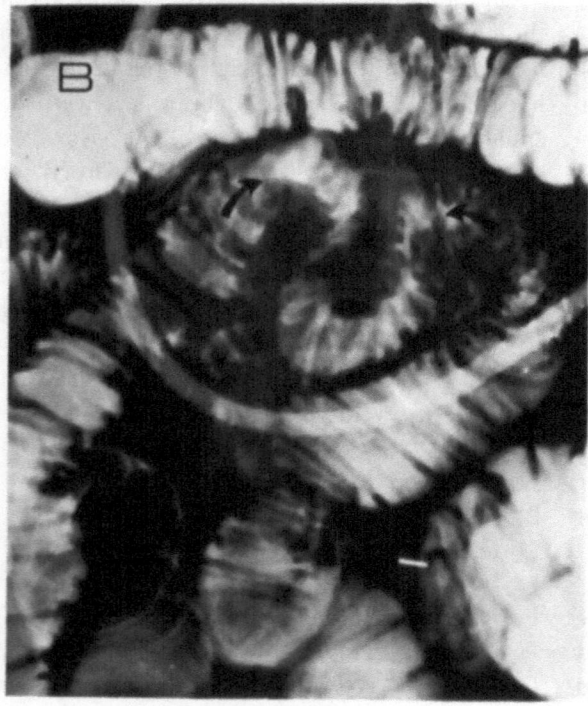

Fig. 12.1. X-rays of a patient with very local enhanced motility of the small bowel without visual abnormalities of the mucosal folds. (A) Radiation enteritis, shortly after irradiation for Hodgkin's disease. After a laparotomy staging procedure, the involved intestinal loops fused with the surroundings and as a result were more susceptible to x-ray damage. (B) A follow-up examination two years later showed that the position of the involved intestinal loop had not changed. Now, however, mucosal changes can be seen. The fold relief has become irregular, the intestinal wall is thickened and rigid, and total dilatation is no longer possible.

common cause is prolonged medication with tranquilizers, sedatives or antispasmodics (see page 352). Other factors are diabetic neuropathy, amyotrophic lateral sclerosis, multiple sclerosis, chronic alcoholism, myoedema, pregnancy, severe abdominal pain, and peritonitis.

Dilatation, sometimes quite pronounced, and reduced peristalsis, particularly in the proximal part of the small intestine, are also encountered in Naish's syndrome (fig. 12.4). This disease, described by Naish and his associates in 1960 (*Gut* 1: 62), is due to degenerative changes in the myenteric plexus. The course is chronic, gradually increases in severity and is characterized by periods of temporary exacerbation or abatement of the complaints. Inadequate mixing of the digestive juices with food substances in the proximal jejunum impairs digestion. In this section of the bowel, rapid flocculation of the barium suspension is also often seen (fig. 12.5). Periods of severe abdominal pain can occur as a result of segmented nonpropulsive small intestine contractions. Histological examination shows that these contractions are due to a marked hypertrophy of the innermost layer of smooth circular muscle in the intestinal wall. The thickened wall is obvious even macroscopically.

Differentiation between this disease and drug-induced atony of the intestine, some cases of amyloidosis, or scleroderma is not always possible by radiological examination alone. To establish the diagnosis in such cases it is particularly important that the history be complete and accurate and that mucosal biopsies be examined histologically.

B. *Mechanical obstruction*
Mechanical obstructions from stenotic processes, bands, or multiple adhesions cause a dilatation of the intestine that increases as the distance from the obstruction decreases. These obstructions cause a prestenotic hyperperistalsis; the peristaltic movements then decrease in a later stage. Even when this latter phenomenon is observed, peristalsis has not changed in the most proximal part of the bowel where the caliber of the loops is also entirely normal (fig. 12.6). This finding is extremely important for differentiation from drug-induced atony. In the latter case, peristalsis in the proximal intestine is also clearly reduced. When a subileus gradually deteriorates, becoming a manifest ileus, dilatation

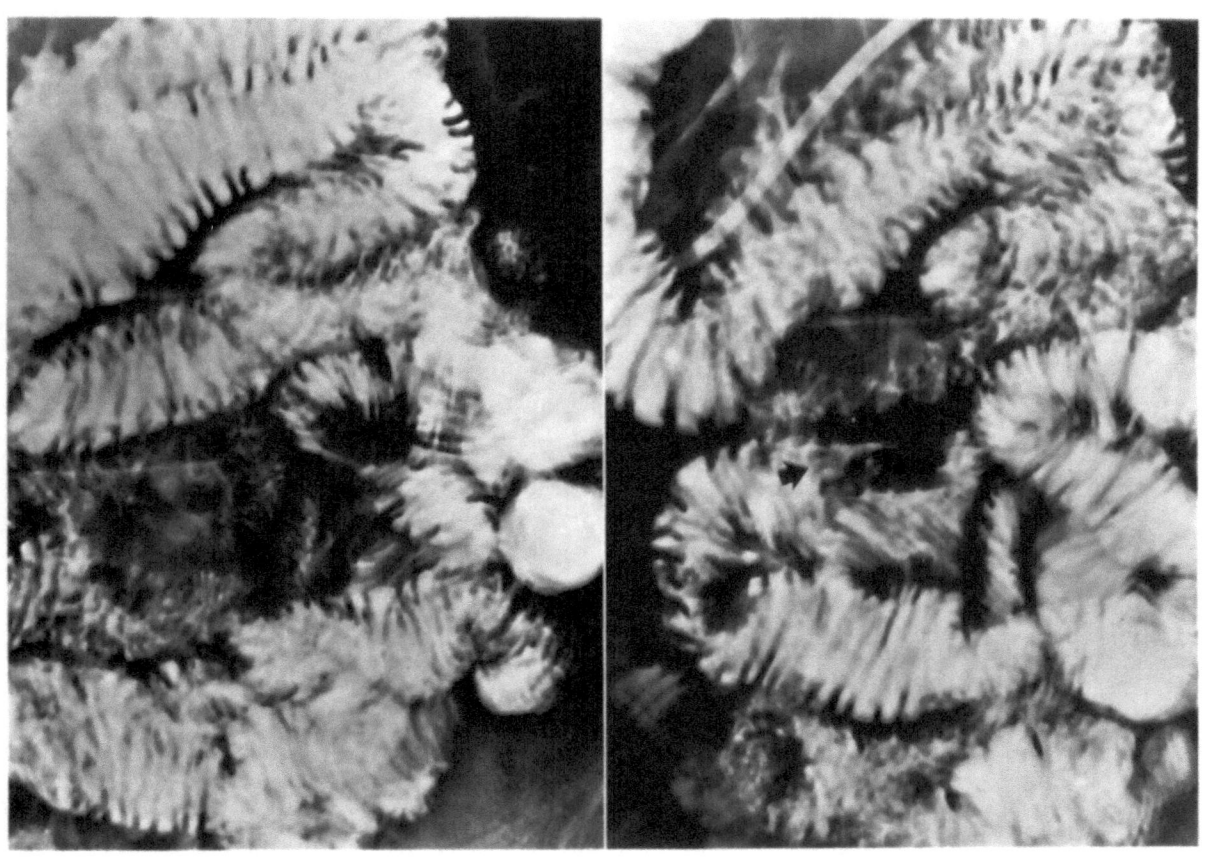
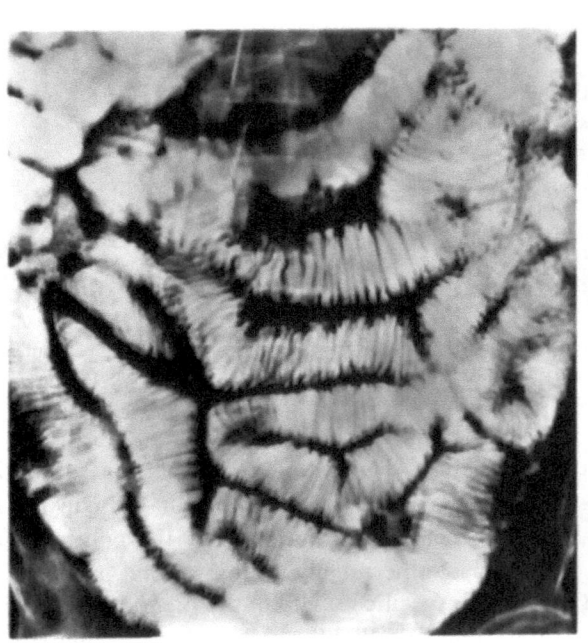
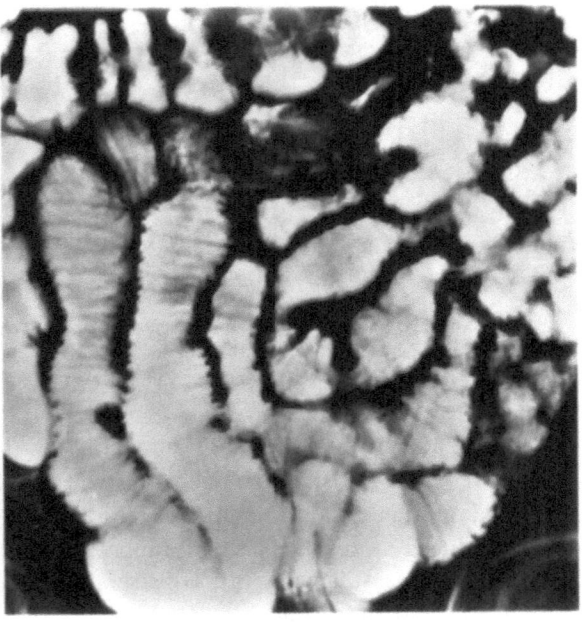

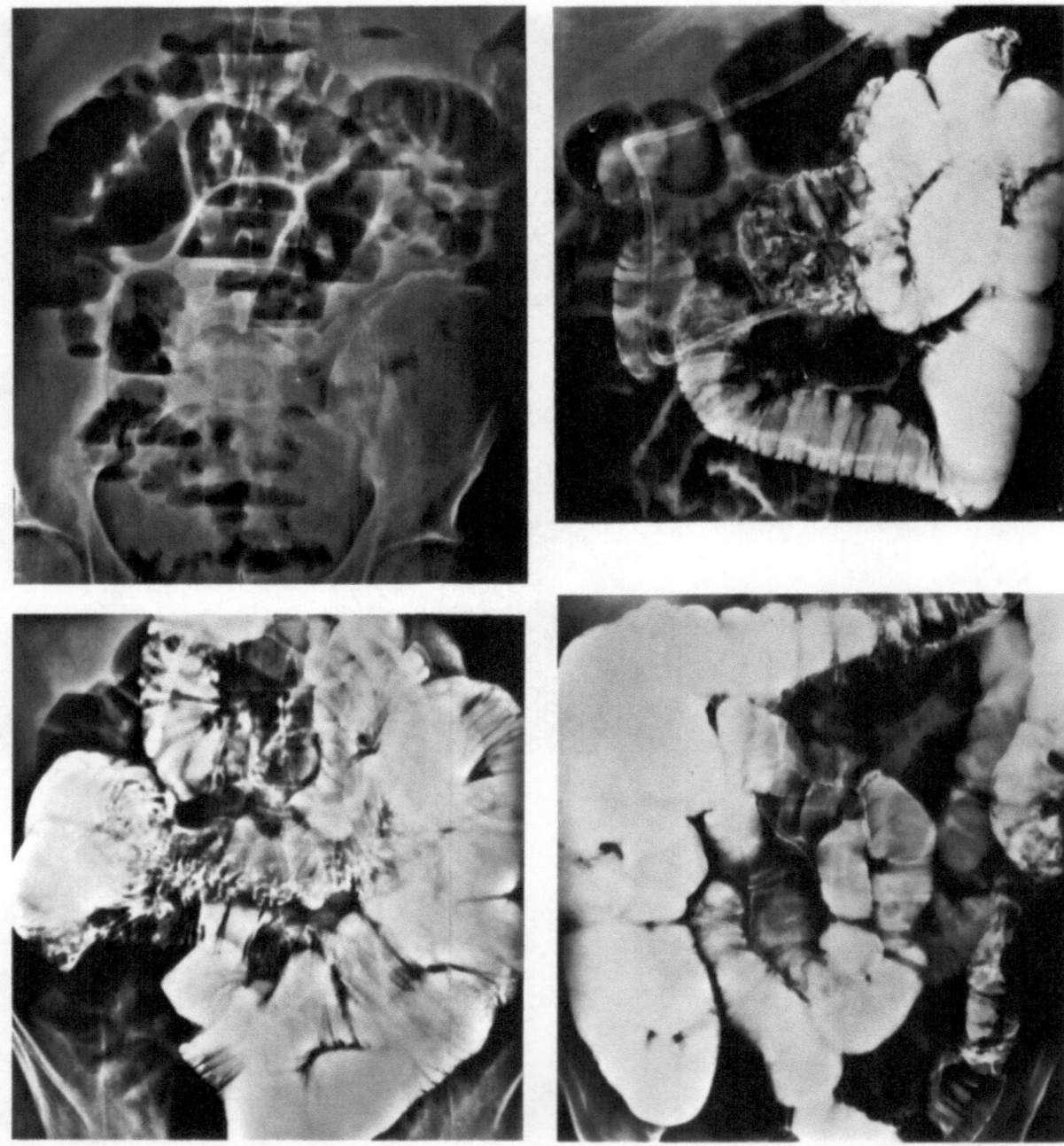

*Fig. 12.4*AB. Two patients with degeneration of the nerve cells in the wall of the bowel (Naish's syndrome). Although the intestinal loops are markedly dilated in both patients, contracted segments can still be seen. During fluoroscopy, vigorous retroperistaltic movements can be observed. Numerous fluid levels in the erect position.

also spreads in the proximal direction so that ultimately the peristaltic movements will be decreased in this area too. Differentiation from a drug-induced atony then becomes more difficult.

If peristalsis still exists, the obstruction is not total. It is then certainly worthwhile to try to demonstrate, by means of the enteroclysis examination, the reason for and the location of the obstruction. Thickening of the barium suspension in the small intestine, feared for so many years, never occurs. On the contrary the contrast fluid becomes rather highly diluted so that in case of an ileus the specific gravity of the first dose of contrast fluid must be slightly higher than normal. In addition it is recommended that the rate of flow be somewhat lower than normal. The administration

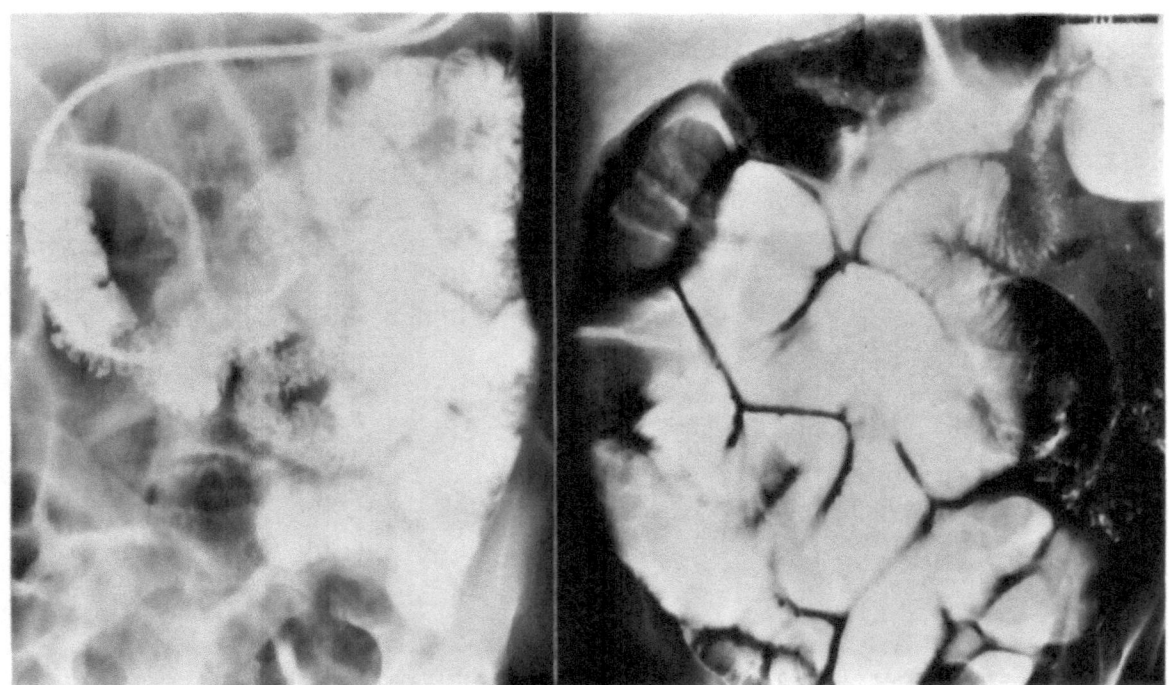

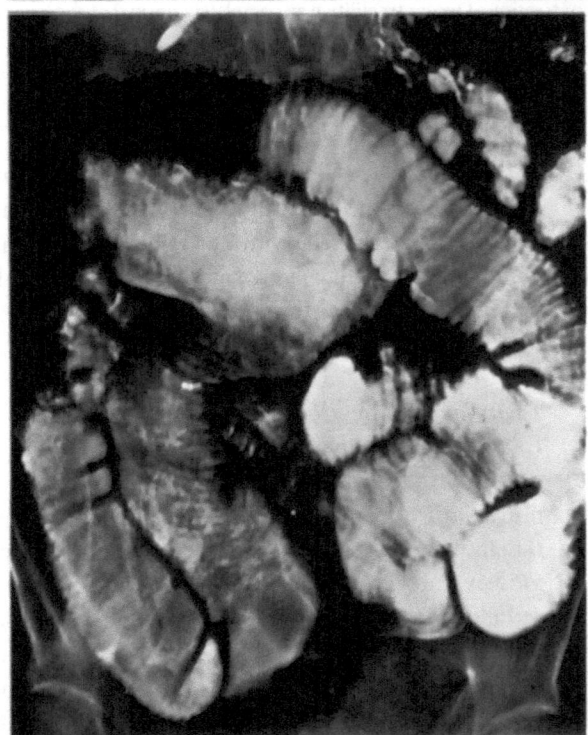

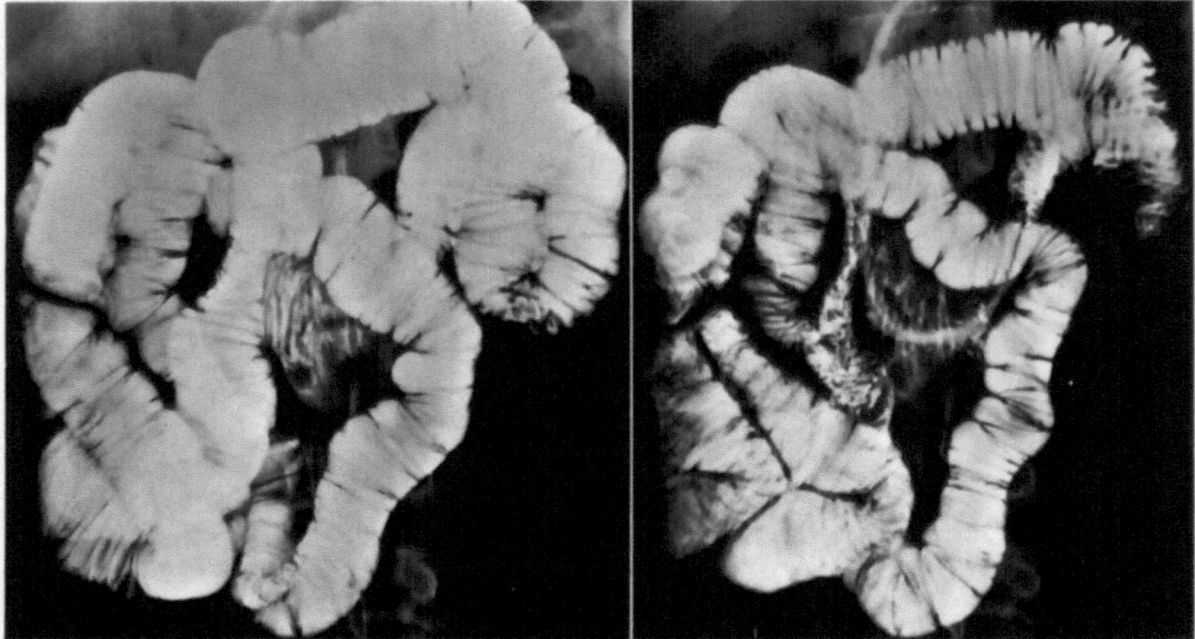

Fig. 12.6. Dilated intestinal loops due to a mechanical obstruction in the distal ileum. In this stage of the enteroclysis examination intestinal segments can no longer be seen that are in a state of contraction. The contractility was completely normal at the beginning of the examination (right).

mentioned elsewhere (page 360), the collagen diseases are frequently accompanied by vasculitis that can eventually result in a local anoxia of the intestinal wall with hyperperistalsis. In amyloidosis, too, motility can be enhanced. In this case, however, it is due to stimulation of the peristaltic movements by abnormal stretching of the intestinal wall. This is a result of the meteorism that can

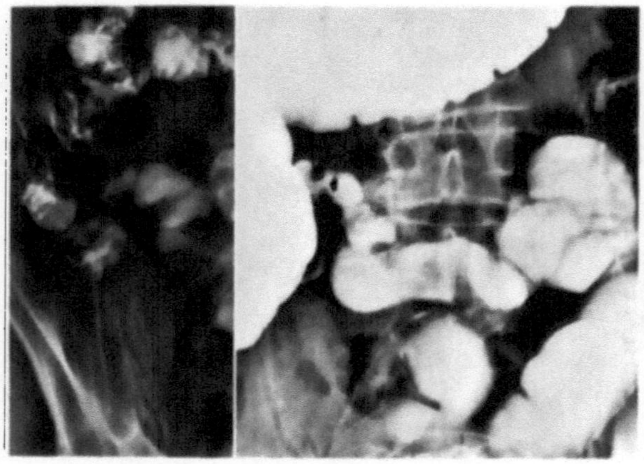

Fig. 12.7. Obstruction in the ileum several centimeters proximal to Bauhin's valve, due to chronic nonspecific inflammation. It was not possible to reach the site of the obstruction in spite of the administration of 2½ liters of contrast fluid. This was, however, achieved quickly during a colon examination with rectal filling and reflux into the terminal ileum.

develop in this disease.

A pronounced decrease in motility without a dilatation of the intestinal loops is also seen in acquired generalized lymphedema. The intestinal wall is then so thick and rigid that peristalsis has become impossible, even if the musculature is intact.

D. Inflammatory processes

Extensive inflammatory processes in the wall of the small bowel can impair the normal function of the musculature mechanically. They can also damage the muscle layers themselves. As mentioned previously, motility in the distal ileum can also be reduced if there is right-sided ulcerative colitis with an inadequate Bauhin's valve. In none of these cases is there a marked dilatation of the lumen. Inflammatory processes on the other hand can also cause a local hyperperistalsis or spasms usually in nearby sections of the small bowel or colon. The origin and the action of these reflex mechanisms are not precisely known.

Chemical enteritis usually causes a decrease in motility; this is seen for example in lead poisoning and uremic enteritis. A disturbed kidney function, whether due to diabetes or not, can lead to an

351

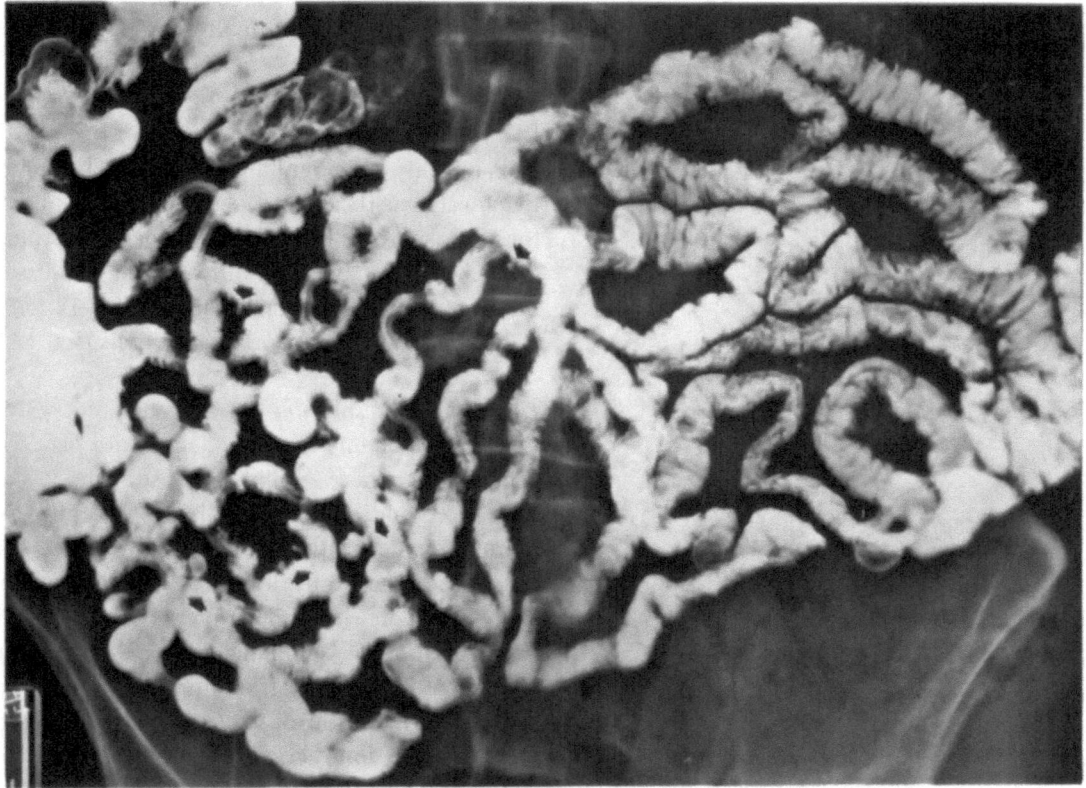

Fig. 12.8A. Hypertonicity of the small intestine with a decreased diameter of the lumen in a very obese patient. This hypertonicity, which is usually caused by a diminished arterial blood flow, is also the cause of the numerous diverticles of different size that can be seen in the ileum.

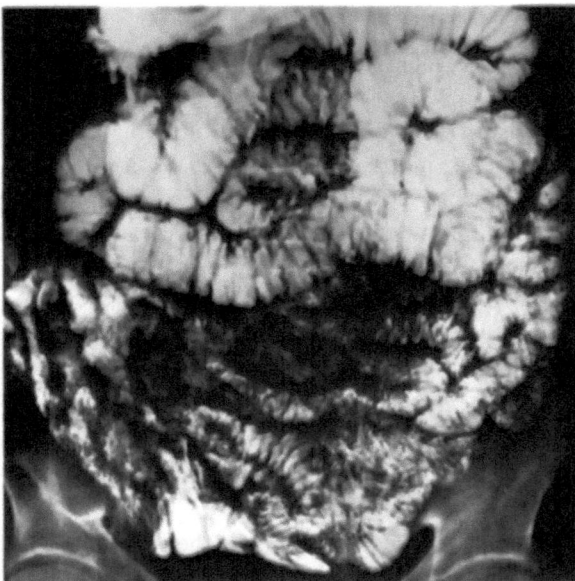

Fig. 12.8B. Pronounced hypermotility of the entire ileum with some stagnation of the contrast fluid in the jejunum as a result of numerous fusions and adhesions in the distal half of the small bowel. Compression showed that all ileal loops were totally fused. The patient complained of considerable rumbling in the stomach and attacks of pain, especially when he assumed certain positions. Occasionally a subileus developed with numerous fluid levels.

increased urea concentration in the blood. The urea can then diffuse into the lumen of the intestine where urea enzyme causes the formation of ammonia leading to a chemical enteritis. This is sometimes accompanied by ulcerations. Ulcerations in the intestinal wall of kidney transplant patients, however, are not due to a chemical enteritis but are the result of changes in the vessels caused by immunosuppressive therapy. The chemical enteritis caused by gastric acid in Zollinger-Ellison disease (page 262) also results in hypermotility. This is probably because the content of the intestine is considerably enlarged as a result of hypersecretion and severe malabsorption.

E. Allergic reactions

Infestations by worms (ascaris) and parasites (*Giardia lamblia*) as well as allergic reactions to food such as milk can cause violent, sometimes local, peristaltic movements with pronounced intestinal narrowing (fig. 12.9A). A local hypermotility can also be encountered in Schönlein-Henoch disease, a possibly allergic vasculitis that as a rule disappears

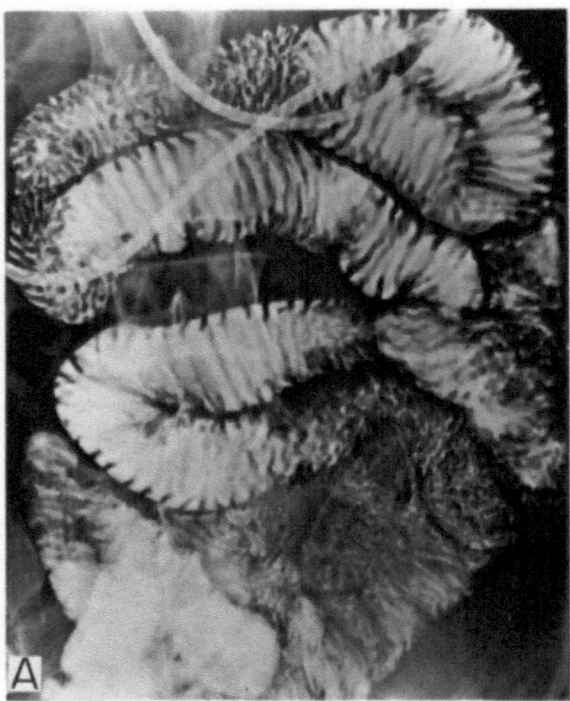

Fig. 12.9A. Dilatation of the jejunum and hypermotility caused by lambliasis. There was no dilatation of the ileum and therefore no reason to consider a celiac disease. Differential diagnosis should include Whipple's disease. Dilatation is rather usual in lambliasis.

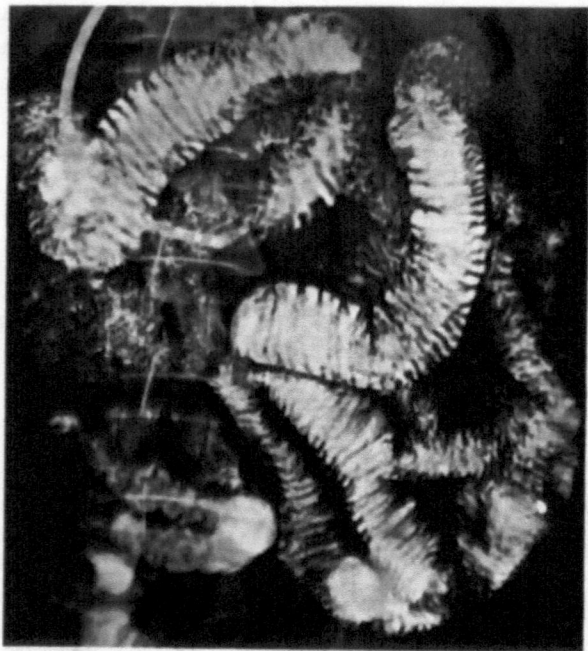

Fig. 12.9B. Active motility of the intestine in a patient with pancreatogenic steatorrhea. The loops in the rest phase have an exceptionally large caliber.

without persistent abnormalities.

F. Anoxia

In all cases involving a mild anoxia of the intestinal wall, motility can be enhanced locally. The lumen of the intestine is then always significantly smaller and the mucosal folds lie very close together. Examples of such diseases are vasculitis in collagen diseases, radiation enteritis, intestinal angina (fig. 12.8A) and vascular insufficiency due to adhesions (fig. 12.8B).

G. Disturbed resorption

Diseases belonging to this category are pancreatogenic steatorrhea, Zollinger-Ellison disease (see page 262), and adult celiac disease (see page 364).

Impaired resorption of food substances, sometimes accompanied by dilution of the contrast fluid, causes an increase in the contents of the intestine. As a result there is enhancement of the peristaltic movements. This 'intestinal hurry' is often accompanied by dilatation of those intestinal loops that are not in a contraction phase. It is then easily distinguished from the 'intestinal hurry' accompanied by a decreased lumen as seen in anoxia or allergic reactions (fig. 12.9B).

1. Drug-induced atony of the small bowel

Disturbed motility in the colon may develop in patients in psychiatric clinics as a result of the prescribed medication. Serious obstipation may then follow that sometimes even leads to complete ileus. In general the radiological examination reveals a long dilated colon that empties only partially or not at all. It is seldom possible to determine whether the long dilated colon was formerly completely normal or whether a preexisting dolichocolon was perhaps a predisposing factor. To prevent frequent recurrence, surgical shortening of the sigmoid is often necessary.

Although it is known that the small intestine will react in a similar manner to the administration of such drugs, few publications on this subject are seen in the radiological literature. Only brief reports have appeared in surgical journals. This can probably be explained because such abnormalities cannot be demonstrated adequately in the small intestine by means of conventional examination tech-

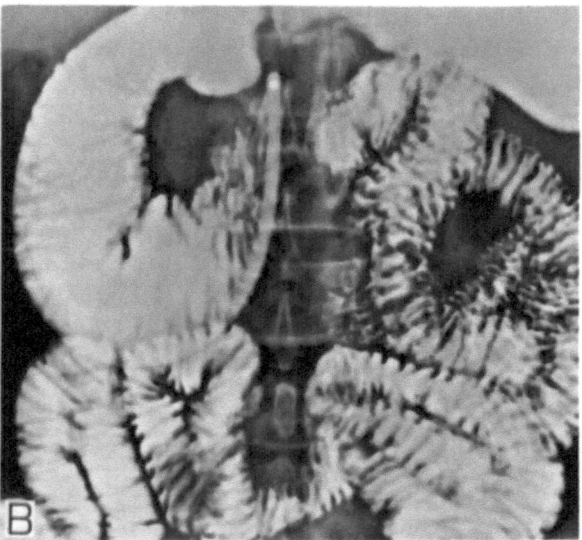

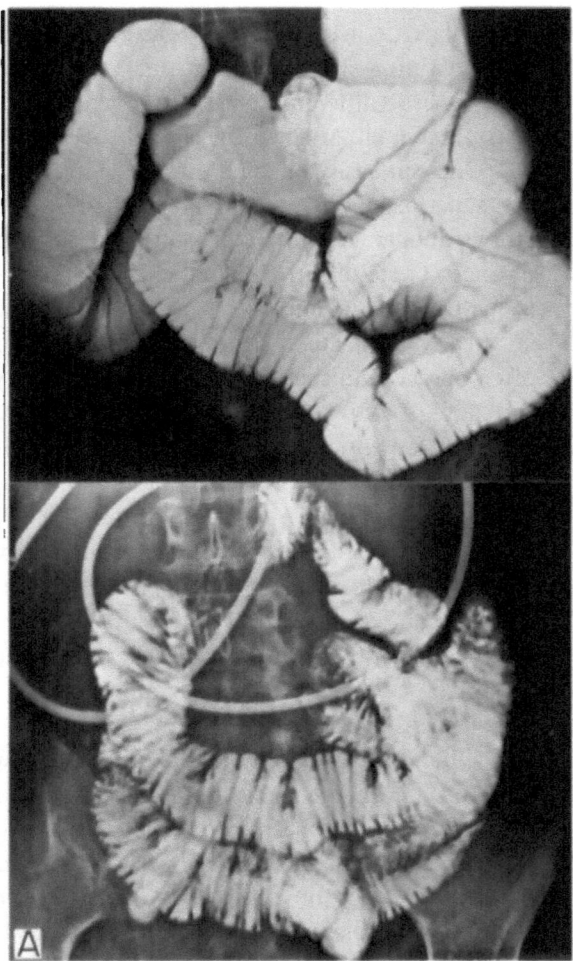

Fig. 12.10B. In this very thin patient, even the moderate use of antispasmodics caused passage to be so retarded in the duodenum at the point where it crosses the aorta that frequent vomiting developed. The motility in the rest of the small intestine was still fairly active.

Fig. 12.10A. Hypomotility and pronounced dilatation of the entire small intestine from prolonged use of antispasmodics and pain relievers. The abnormality is noted during the first few minutes of the examination. The impression of the aorta on the duodenum is often clearly visible in these patients. Retroperistaltic movements in the duodenum are common and there is usually marked reflux of the contrast fluid into the stomach. One year after the above-mentioned drugs had been discontinued almost completely, the motility in the jejunum was normal once again. Some slight dilatation was still visible.

niques. The reason for this is that the dose and the flow rates of the contrast medium in a small bowel examination differ completely from those used in the colon examination.

Since in enteroclysis the flow rate is the same in all patients, we have noted in a number of patients that a strikingly large dose of contrast fluid is required before the cecum is reached. In some patients even with our maximum dose of 1200 ml barium suspension followed by 1200 ml water, the cecum is only reached after 30–45 min. Since this technique is executed under intermittent fluoroscopy, we have also seen in these patients that the

intestinal loops not only are dilated but also show a pronounced decrease in peristalsis. Moreover, in spite of a correct positioning of the tube, reflux of contrast fluid into the stomach occurred fairly regularly. Upon inquiry, there had been prolonged medication with tranquilizers, antispasmodics, or sedatives in all cases. There was no clear difference when these drugs were discontinued for only several weeks before the examination.

Because of the anatomical location, and especially the patient's complaints, dilatations of the small bowel of iatrogenic origin can best be divided into those of the duodenum and those of the entire small intestine. The roentgenograms then show the following:

A) The duodenum shows rather pronounced dilatation, sometimes mainly in the distal segment (fig. 12.10). This is immediately observed during fluoroscopy in the first few minutes of the examination. At the same time it is noted that this widening is accompanied by retroperistaltic pendulum movements. It may have been discovered beforehand that the tube cannot be inserted into the duodenojejunal junction – or only with considerable difficulty. In these patients the tube often becomes lodged at the level of the superior mesen-

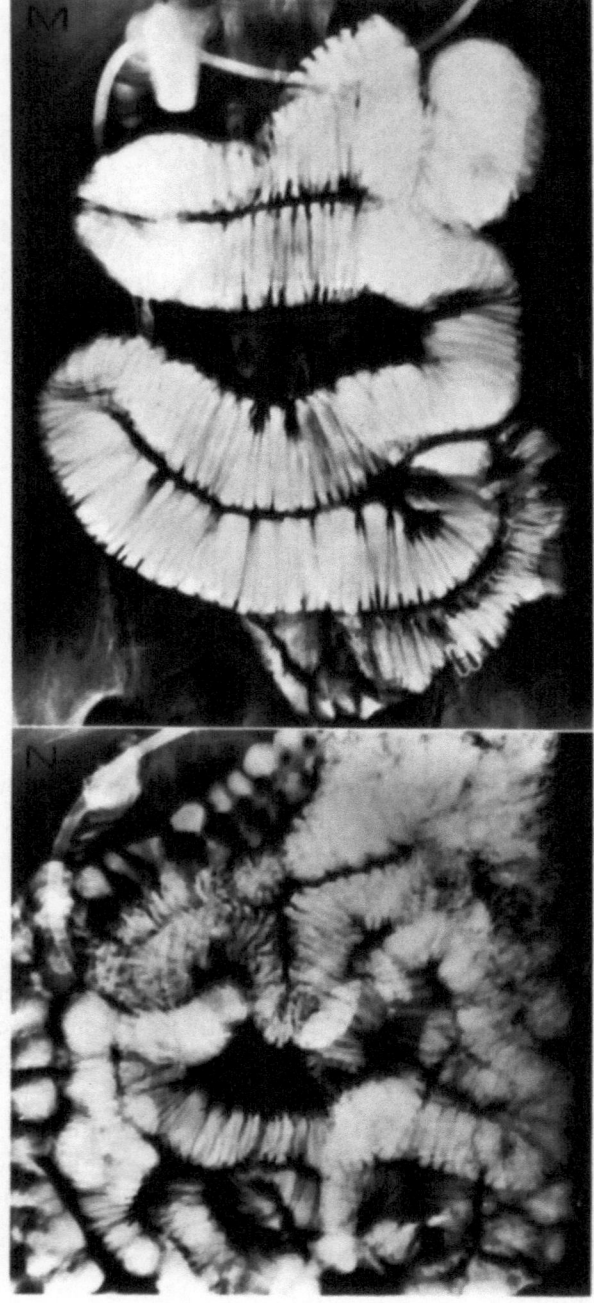

especially true in patients who have become emaciated within a short period of time. In such cases it makes little difference whether the patient lies on his stomach, either side, or his back.

One can easily imagine that the impression of the superior mesenteric artery on a dilated and atonic duodenum would be sufficient to impede passage. Certainly in thin patients the angle between the superior mesenteric artery and the aorta is already so acute. The retroperistaltic motion, often observed in such dilated duodenums, may be the cause of reflux of the bilious duodenal contents into the prepyloric area of the stomach. The pyloric ring is also influenced by drugs that induce atony so that it does not close sufficiently to prevent reflux. Just as esophagitis may develop from reflux of gastric acid into the esophagus, an antral gastritis can be caused by reflux of basic gall into the stomach. The superficial erosions then encountered cannot be easily demonstrated radiologically, but are visible during gastroscopy.

The complaints of these patients are not always easy to differentiate from those caused by a duodenal ulcer. It has been noted that vomiting is a frequent symptom and that hunger pains so classic of ulcer are not obvious or are missing. Some patients have discovered that a certain position, usually the right or left side, will cause them the least discomfort. A light (bread) meal is in general tolerated more easily than a warm meal and small portions better than large. Although obviously indicated, it is clear that antispasmodics and psychopharmaca will have an adverse effect on the complaints – they will increase rather than decrease. Primperan (metoclopramide) is indicated in these cases. This drug causes an increase in the tone of the musculature of the intestinal walls, enhances gastric emptying, and decreases retroperistaltic motion (fig. 12.11). Duration and dose are of course dependent upon the severity of the complaints. In general, recovery takes many weeks and sometimes even months. It is recommended then to gradually decrease the dose (fig. 12.12).

Another way in which the treatment clearly differs from that of an ulcer is diet. If the angle between the aorta and the superior mesenteric artery is acute, it is particularly important to improve the patient's nutritional state and thereby increase this angle.

Fig. 12.11. (M) Dilated jejunal loops and practically no peristaltic movements. (N) After administration of metoclopramide through the tube or by injection, the tone of the intestine usually increases, dilatation decreases and motility improves.

teric artery. When it is pushed further, it curls back in the direction of the pylorus.

This apparent obstruction, caused by an acute angle between the aorta and the superior mesenteric artery, is encountered only in thin patients. This is

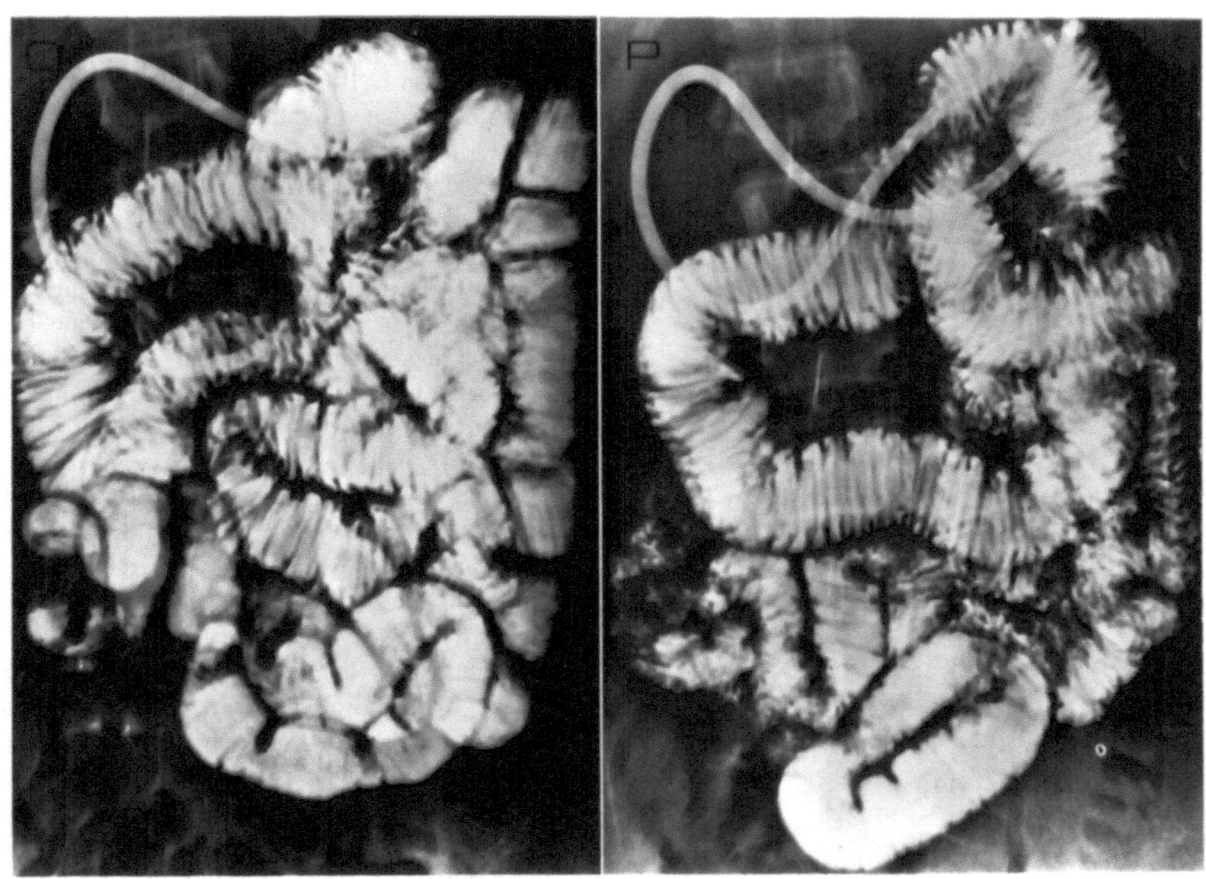

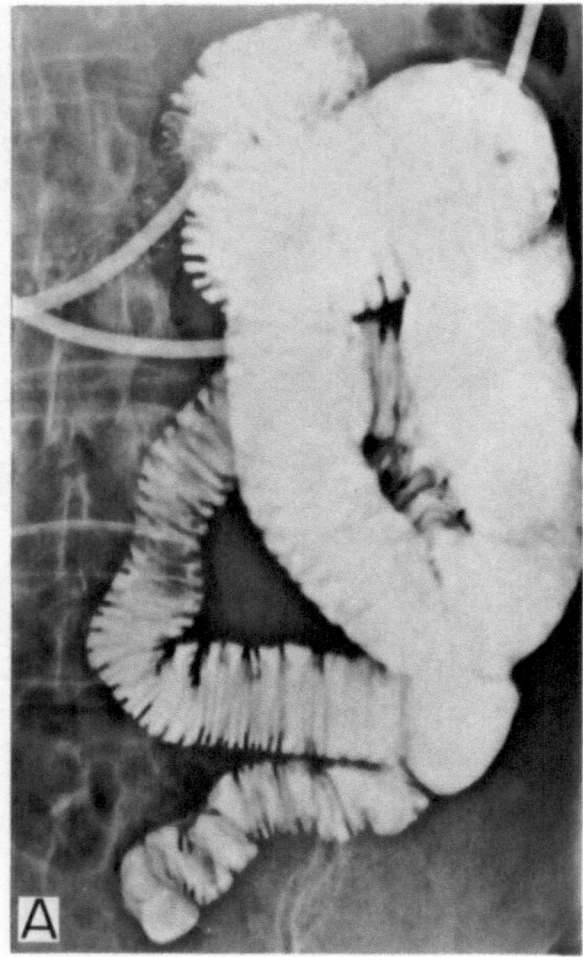

*Fig. 12.13*A. A 57-year-old woman with invalidating stomach cramps as a result of a severe drug-induced atony of the small bowel. There is pronounced dilatation with a total lack of peristalsis in the jejunum. The ileum appears practically normal (page 357). Dilatation of the ileum is only seen in even more severe cases that are called 'paralytic ileus'.

the obstruction caused by a space-occupying process can in general easily be differentiated from a pseudo-obstruction from the administration of drugs. In the former case the average caliber of the proximal intestinal loops can be completely normal and peristalsis may be undisturbed or sometimes even increased. If the obstruction is pronounced, the caliber of the intestine will increase distalward, and just before the site of the obstruction there may be a clear prestenotic dilatation (fig. 12.18). Moderate dilatation and a decrease in the peristaltic movements in the ileum are sometimes also accompanied by atrophy of the mucosa in the region of the ileocecal junction. With normal motility in the

jejunum, this can also be due to the chronic use of laxatives (fig. 12.19). In case of drug-induced atony, on the other hand, dilatation of the loops and lack of peristalsis appear as dominating symptoms in the proximal part of the intestine.

Unfortunately the reason for the stagnation in the flow of contrast medium that may develop at the ileojejunal junction, or in the proximal ileum, is still a matter of conjecture. At present, it appears to be a temporary mechanical twisting, or a torsion of the intestine.

In the small bowel there may appear to be different obstructions, apparently physiological in origin, that impede an accelerated flow of contrast medium. It is obvious that this is also true of adhesions and bands that develop after surgery. The latter, however, are easily demonstrated on spot films. The function of the radiological examination by means of enteroclysis may perhaps best be compared with that of a water-loaded urography for the urinary tract. In pyknics the small intestine is as a rule shorter than in asthenics; the mesentery is shorter and also contains more fat. As a result, the loops of the small bowel lie in a very orderly fashion with respect to one another. The physiological potential sites of obstruction may then be absent. Specifically, we have never seen a stagnation of the flow at the level of the superior mesenteric artery nor at Treitz's ligament in pyknics.

The significance of these radiological findings (dilatation and decreased motility) should now be obvious in many cases. In other cases – those patients with few or vague complaints – this question is not yet answered. It is possible that the 'unphysiological' rapid flow of the contrast medium causes the temporary stagnation.

However, this stagnation often correlates so closely with the complaints of the patient that it probably does not occur only during enteroclysis. It probably is a true representation of an actual phenomenon. Our experience with two patients in our series supports this assumption. Both underwent a conventional gastrointestinal examination one week before enteroclysis. The enteroclysis examination lasted 40–45 min – which is exceptionally long, in spite of the administration of 1800

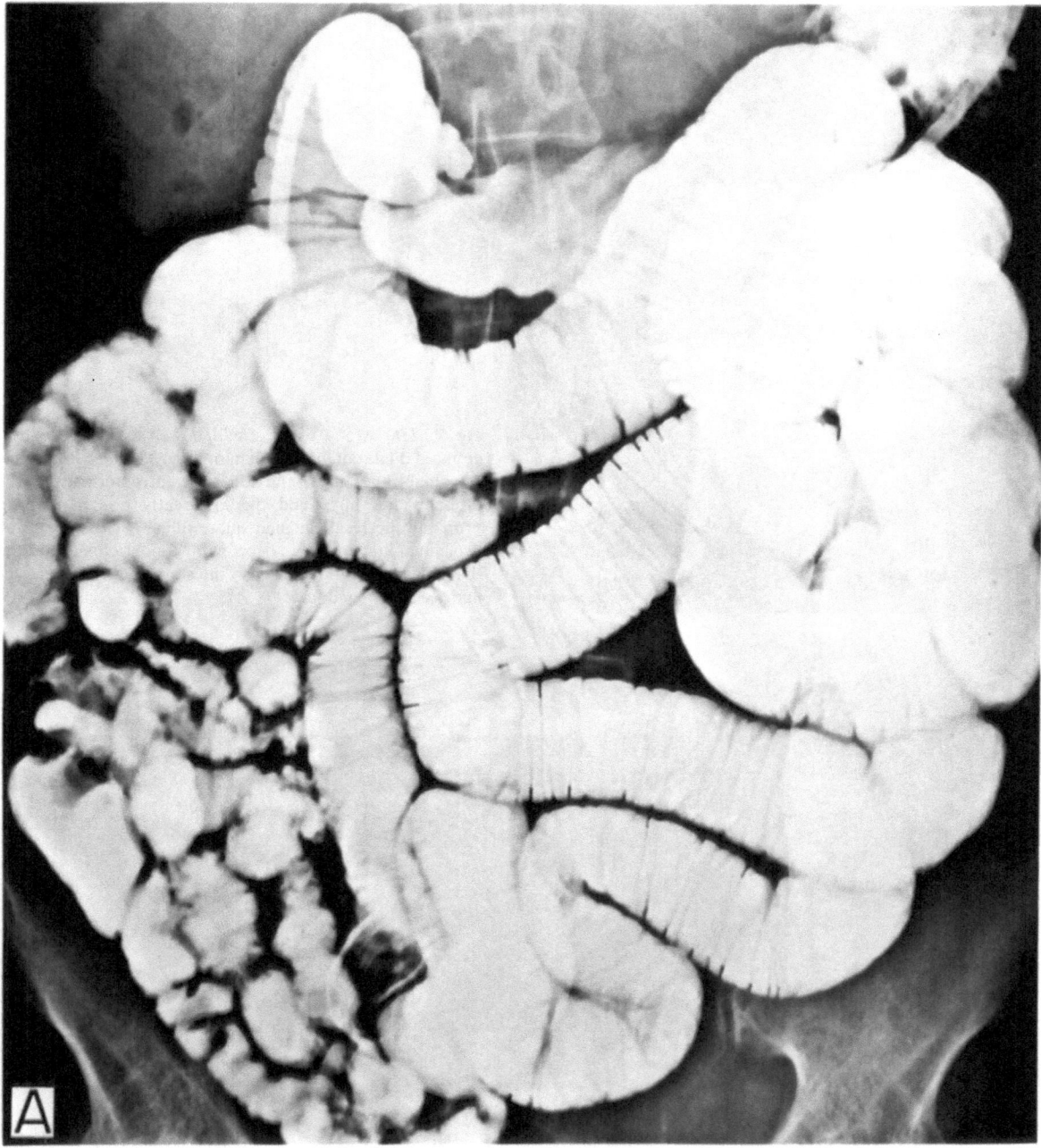

*Fig. 12.13*A. See legend on page 356.

ml contrast fluid. During the oral gastrointestinal examination of these patients, the rate of flow was more 'physiological'. We noted that in spite of the administration of passage accelerating drugs, it was 8 h (instead of the normal 1–2 h) before the cecum was reached. Under comparable physiological conditions, such as after the consumption of a normal meal, it can apparently take quite some time before the small intestine is empty. Our observation that

transit in patients with a dilated intestine and decreased persistalsis is impeded by food remnants from the previous day can now also be explained.

It is known that tranquilizers, sedatives, and antispasmodics tend to decrease the tone and peristalsis in the intestine quite effectively. Excessive and prolonged use of these medications can even lead to a total ileus. Of course the transition from a

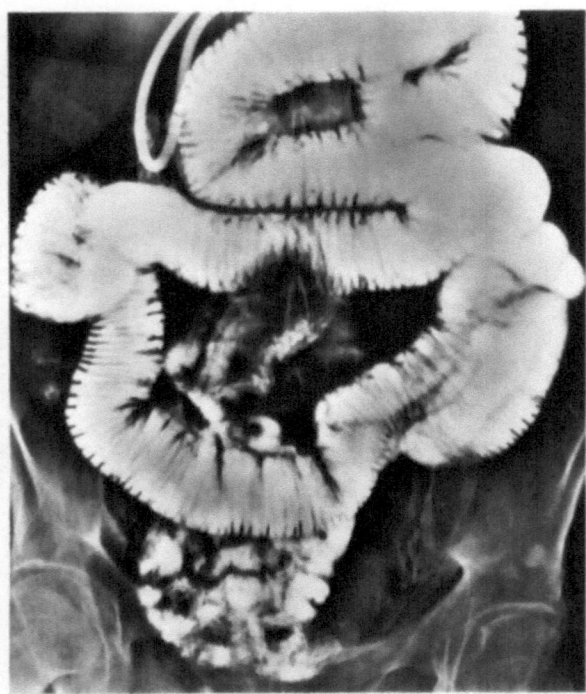

*Fig. 12.13*B. Atony of the small bowel accompanied by pronounced dilatation of the jejunum only. The tone in the ileum is presumably not high, and the apparently normal diameter is probably not high, and the apparently normal diameter is probably the result of inadequate filling. In the region of the ileojejunal junction there is probably a physiological bottleneck that either is not found in every intestine or only impedes transit under certain conditions.

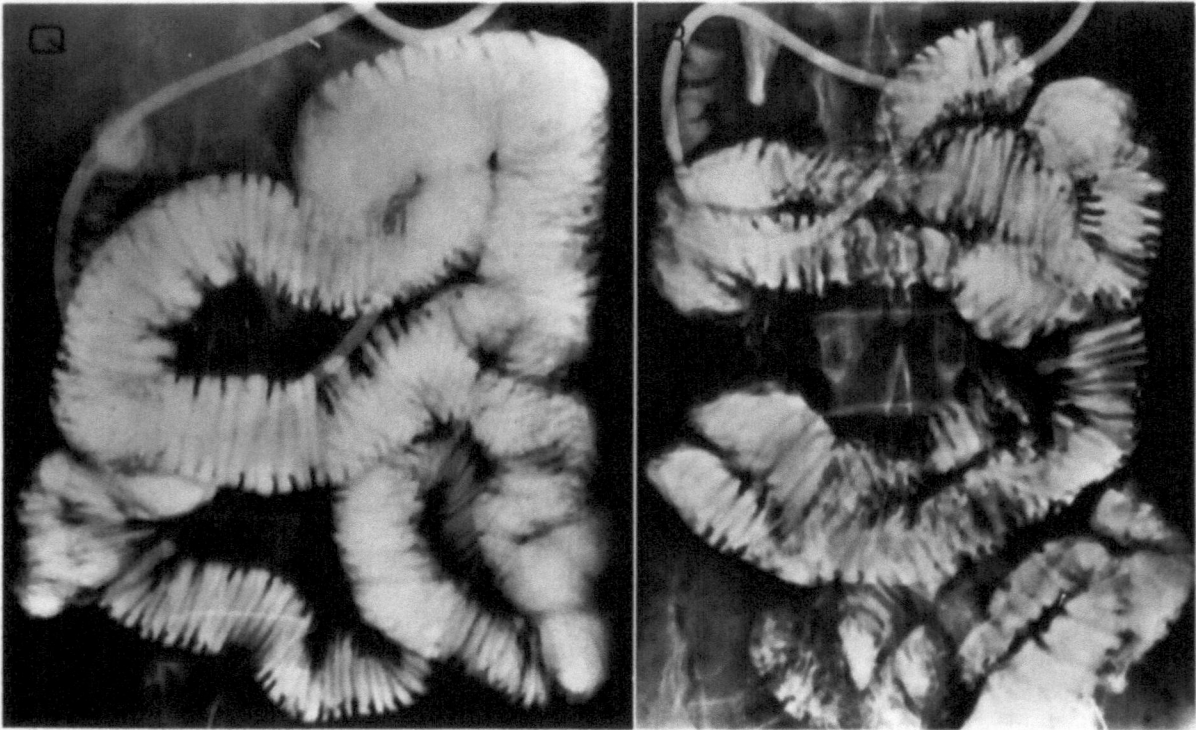

Fig. 12.14. (Q) Dilated jejunal loops and stagnation of the passage to the ileum of unknown origin. (R) Several minutes later the stagnation suddenly disappeared. Although there are fewer intestinal loops in the contraction phase than normal, an atony is not at all certam.

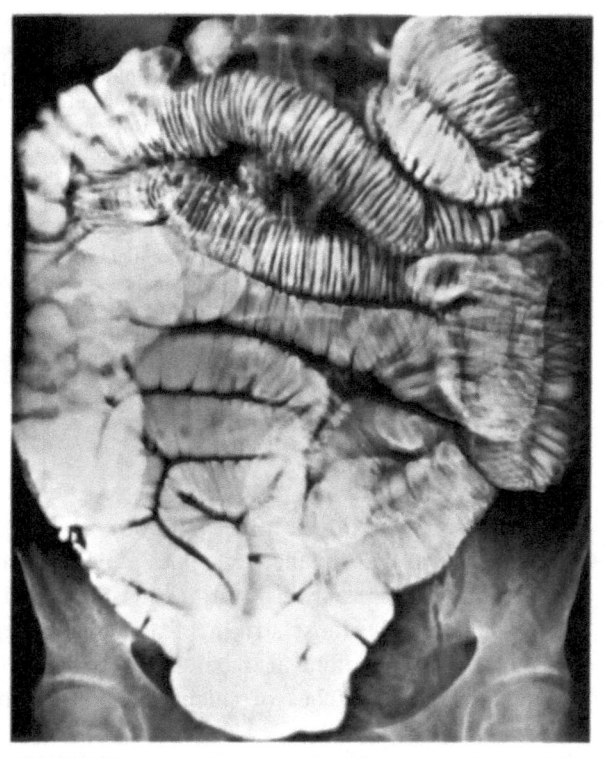

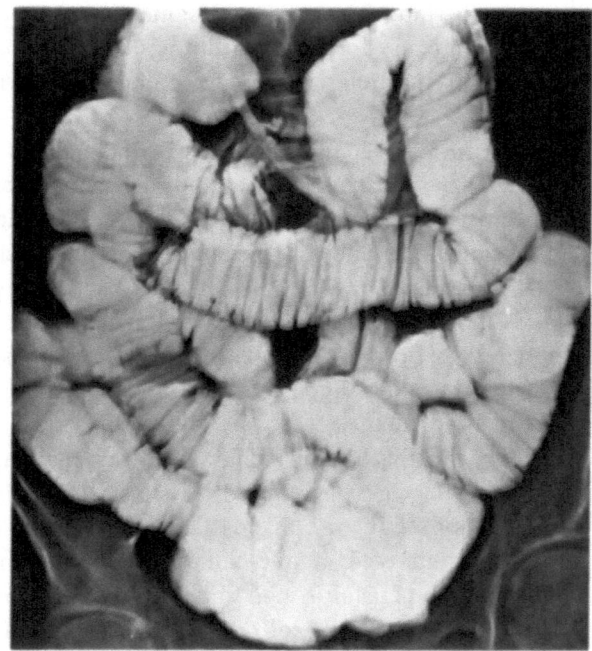

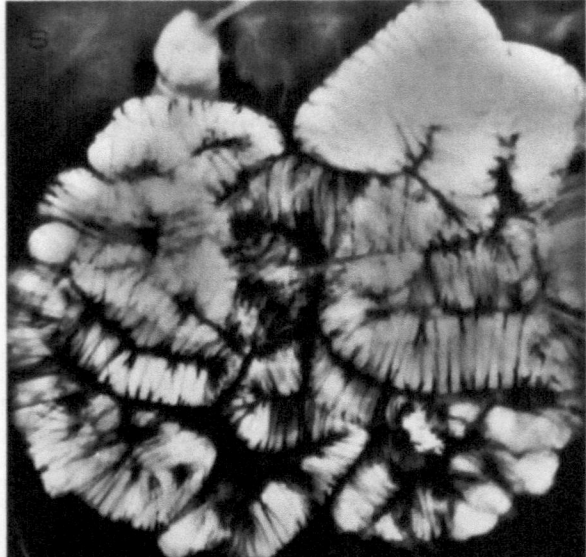

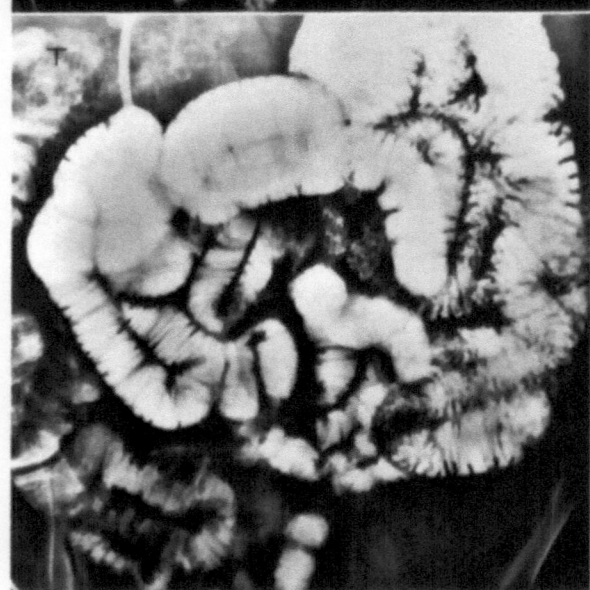

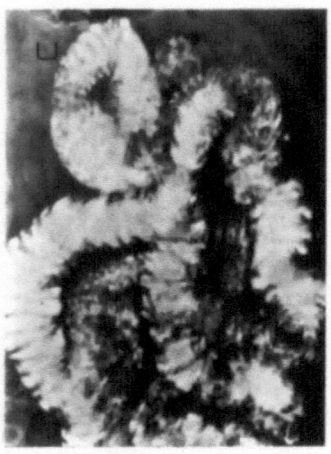

Fig. 12.16. (S) Moderately pronounced atony of the small intestine from prolonged medication with tranquilizers. Because the patient complained of recurrent attacks of abdominal pain, antispasmodics were prescribed and the complaints increased. (T) All drug therapy was discontinued for three months; at the end of this period some improvement in the motility could be observed. Subjectively, however, the complaints had diminished considerably. For the previous examination, 1300 ml contrast fluid were required to reach the cecum; this time only 900 ml were used. (U) 1½ years later, a follow-up examination showed that peristalsis and the caliber of the intestine had become completely normal. We have found that an improvement in motility always precedes normalization of the tone of the intestine. The patient's complaints almost always disappear sooner than the radiological abnormalities.

fibrosis, the skin becomes smooth and tightly stretched so that the face resembles a mask. A sharp prominent nose and a mouth that is smaller than normal are the most striking features. Hyperpigmentation can often also be seen and hard thick subcutaneous patches of calcium deposits can be felt.

In the internal organs, the same sclerosing process can cause for example fibrosis of the myocardium or the lungs with the accompanying symptoms.

Fibrin deposits in the intima of the walls of the small arteries cause stenoses and therefore ischemic necrosis for example in the fingertips (Raynaud's phenomenon) and diverse internal organs, including the small bowel. In the digestive tract the layers of smooth muscle become atrophied and are replaced by fibrous tissue. This leads to a decrease in peristalsis, then hypotonic dilatations and finally sometimes stenoses.

The most well-known characteristic, occurring in 80% of the cases, is reduced peristalsis and a slight dilatation of the esophagus. Less well known but still encountered in one-half of the patients is a decreased peristalsis and dilatation in the small intestine. The degree of dilatation can vary and is sometimes so local that sacculations are observed (fig. 12.20). In this stage the patients complain of a 'full stomach' and bothersome flatulence. Obstipation can be so marked that obstruction sometimes develops. The duodenum and jejunum are affected the most so that in a later stage malabsorption may also occur. Obstipation may be replaced then by steatorrhea. Less common, and often not recognized if the other classic symptoms of the

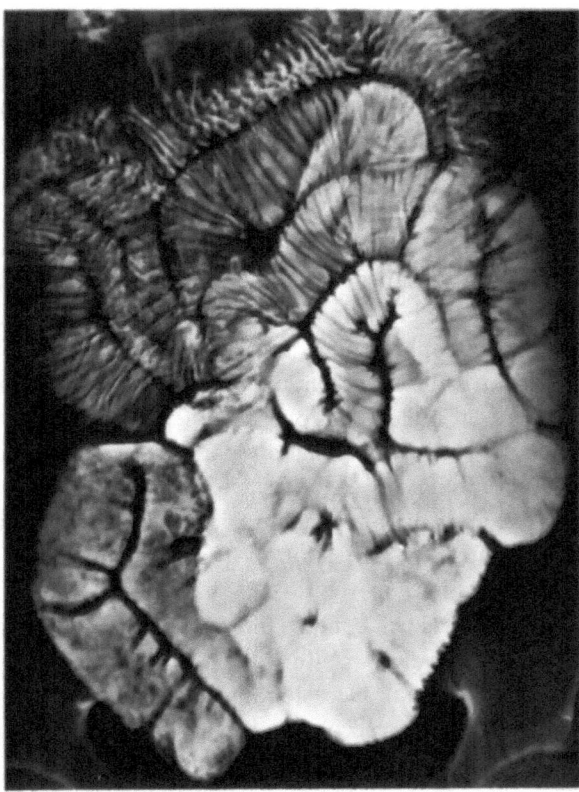

Fig. 12.17. Drug-induced atony of the intestine. In the distal ileum there are food remnants from the previous day that act as an additional mechanical obstruction and impede passage.

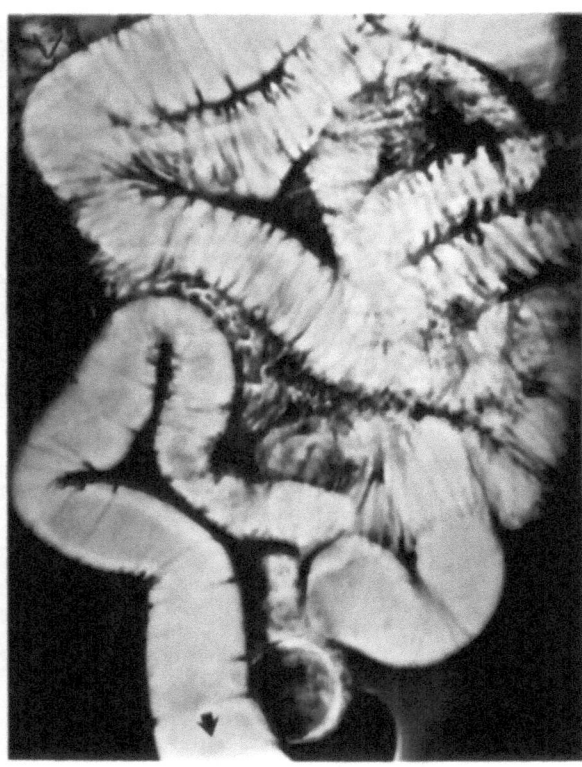

Fig. 12.18. (v) Strikingly pronounced increase in dilatation of the distal ileum that appeared to be due to stagnation of the flow of contrast fluid due to a tumor in the cecum. Motility in the jejunum was completely normal.

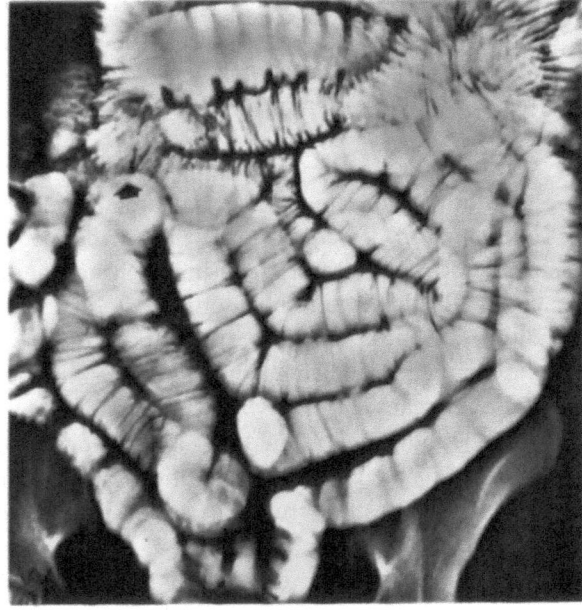

Fig. 12.18. (w) Patient with subileus from mechanical obstruction of the transit through the small intestine from bands in the lower abdomen (thin arrows). Although more difficult to recognize than in patient v, it can be seen that dilatation is more pronounced in the ileum than in the jejunum. Also the jejunum still shows states of contraction, especially in the upper right quadrant (thick arrow).

disease are missing, are the abnormalities of the stomach. In most cases, a definite atony is seen with dilatation of the stomach and a decrease in peristaltic movements, just as in the esophagus. On the other hand, a change in the wall of the stomach due to scleroderma can resemble a linitis plastica or even a local stenosis in the pars antralis or the pylorus. An uneven dilatation of the jejunum together with sacculations need not be due to scleroderma. We have seen this combination once in a chronic alcoholic with Wernicke's syndrome (fig. 12.21).

2.2. Periarteritis nodosa

This disease, in contrast to the other collagen diseases, occurs predominantly in males. The skin conditions consist of red spots and subcutaneous nodules mainly on the dorsal side of the hands and feet, the tensor side of the extremities, and on the face.

362

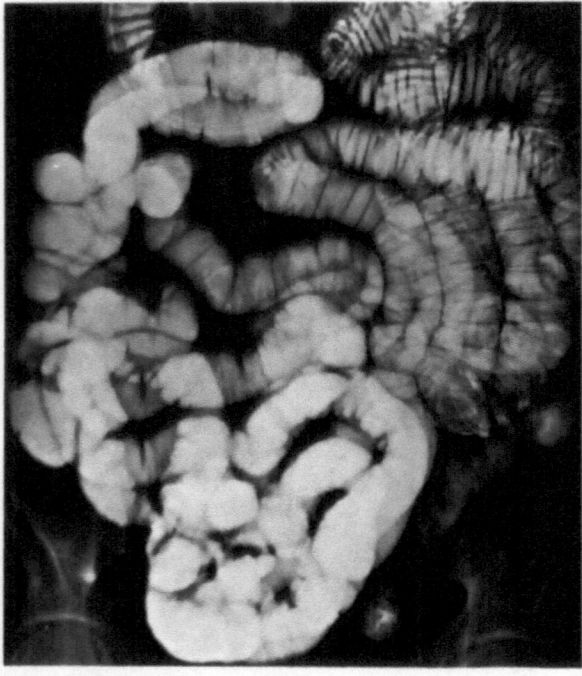

Fig. 12.19. In rare cases a diminished peristalsis in the ileum can be from the chronic use of laxatives. In the classic case, atrophy of the fold relief is seen that extends to the cecum. Moreover, dilatation is not as pronounced as in patients who use spasmodics. In the beginning of the examination, contractions in the jejunum are completely normal; this was also the case in this patient. As soon as large quantities of contrast fluid are required to reach the cecum (here 1000 ml barium suspension followed by 1000 ml water), the loops in the jejunum also became dilated and peristalsis decreased (enteroenteral reflex mechanism).

Pathologically the disease is characterized by an inflammatory process in the walls of the medium-sized and small arteries, causing occlusion and necrosis. Erythrocyte sedimentation rate and temperature are increased. There is leukocytosis with a shift to the left and sometimes also an eosinophilia. Various organs can be involved. Often abnormalities of the kidneys, heart, and lungs are found. In about one-half of the cases, manifestations also occur in the small intestine. In contrast to scleroderma, however, the abnormalities are localized in the distal jejunum and the ileum. The radiological characteristics are similar to those of vascular occlusion. They consist of edema, ulcerations, hemorrhage, and sometimes also perforation (fig. 12.22). Partly because of the localization, differentiation from Crohn's disease is sometimes impossible. This confusion can persist for some time since these two diseases can have highly similar courses. As in Crohn's disease the appendix may also be involved; this occurs fairly frequently in periarteritis nodosa (see fig. 11.7).

2.3. (Systemic) Lupus erythematosus (SLE)

The skin abnormalities in this disease include a butterfly-shaped exanthem around the eyes and across the bridge of the nose. The skin there is scaly and atrophied and during exacerbation of the disease, the exanthem may become slightly elevated or even bullous. In one-half of patients, there is a polyserositis, lymphadenopathy, or abnormalities of the internal organs such as the kidneys, heart, spleen, liver, or intestine because of a constricting arteritis. In three out of four patients there are complaints of the joints. Certain multinucleate leukocytes will contain the LE bodies characteristic of this disease. Quite often there is also a hyperglobulinemia. Occasionally Raynaud-like abnormalities are seen on the fingers similar to the skin conditions on the face. Abdominal complaints can be due to a peritonitis as well as an arteritis.

If the vascular abnormalities are only slight, then one will observe only hypermotility as a result of anoxia (fig. 12.23). If the abnormalities are more serious then in the distal ileum they can only be distinguished with difficulty from Crohn's disease or not at all.

As in scleroderma and drug-induced atony of the bowel, the duodenum can be markedly dilated leading to the development of a superior mesenteric syndrome.

The prognosis of the disease is poor; many of the patients die as a result of severe damage to the liver or kidneys.

2.4. Dermatomyositis

In addition to erythematous and edematous changes in the skin, characterized in particular by periorbital edema, inflammations of the transverse striated muscles lead to necrosis. These are the major features of this frequently fatal disease. The muscles affected most frequently are those of the pelvis, shoulder, and neck. Rapid fatigue of the eye muscles sometimes causes double vision. If the diaphragm and the intercostal muscles are involved, a pronounced dyspnea will develop. One-half of the patients also have deglutitory complaints. If accom-

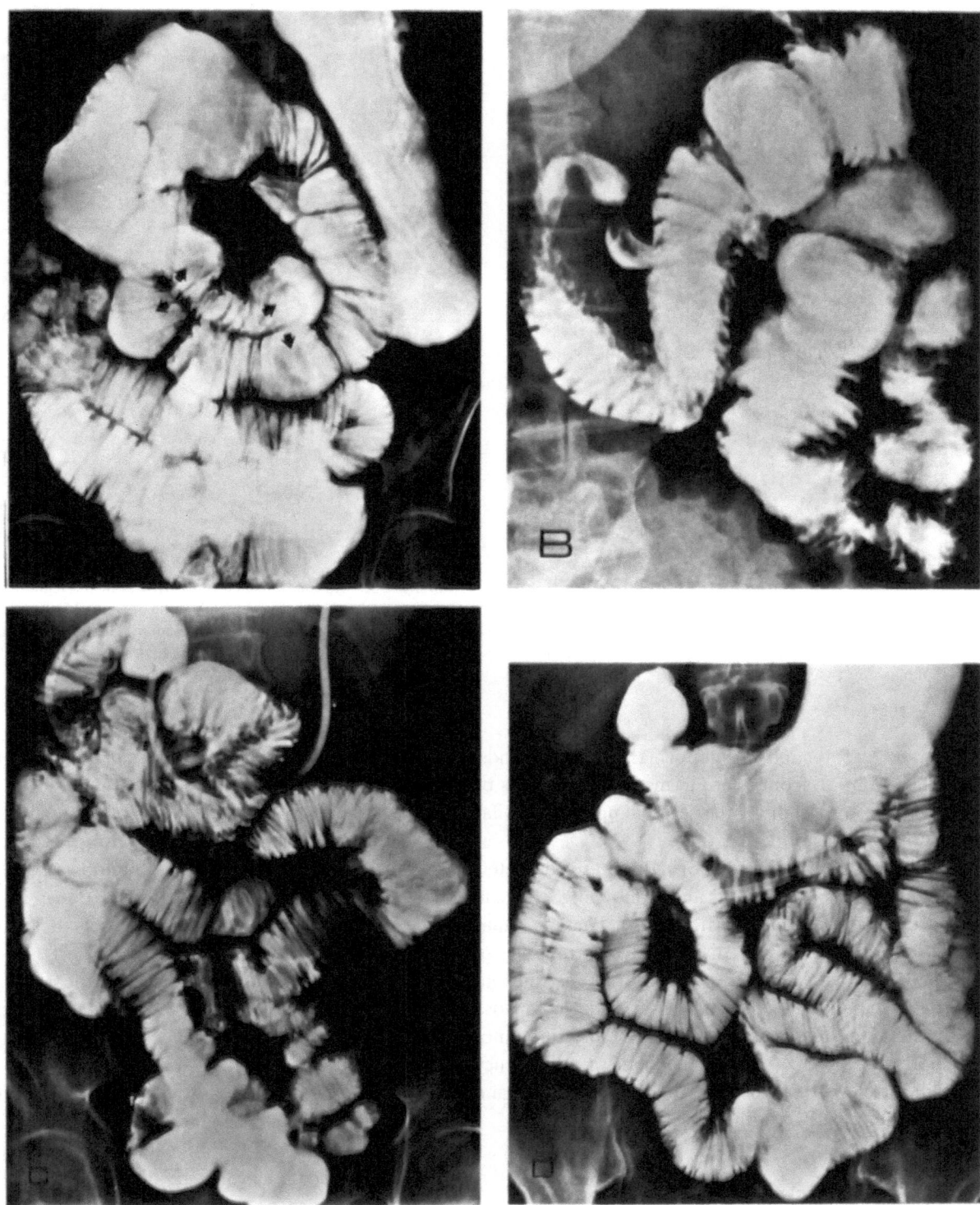

*Fig. 12.20*A–F. Six patients with scleroderma and the resulting abnormalities encountered in the small intestine. (A) Very large stomach with pronounced dilatation of the descending limb of the duodenum. The jejunum that is also dilated shows several local sacculations (arrows) but there are also contractions in the right upper quadrant. This patient also had abnormalities of the skin and esophagus. (B) Sacculations in the jejunum. (C) Unequal dilatations in the jejunum but also many contracted loops (in contrast to a drug-induced atony, where this is not seen). In this patient there were also abnormalities of the hands and esophagus. (D) Abundant reflux into a normal-sized stomach. Dilatation of the duodenum and jejunum without sacculations or contracted intestinal segments. This patient also had abnormalities of the esophagus. Differentiation from a drug-induced atony of the small bowel is not possible. (See E and F on page 364.)

364

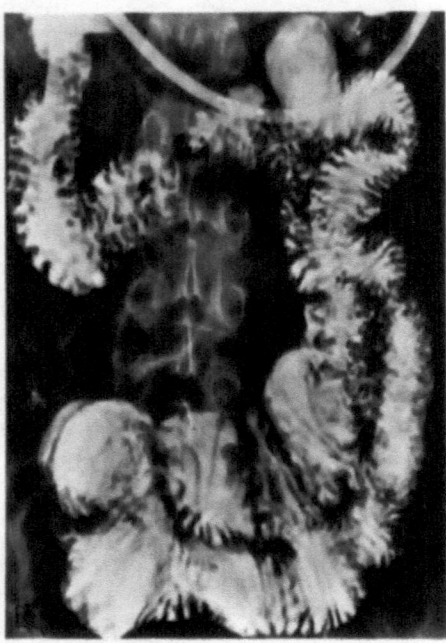

Fig. 12.20ᴇ. Sacculations in the jejunum. Motility was fairly normal at first but became clearly disturbed within several minutes. In this patient, abnormalities of the skin, hands, and esophagus were also seen.

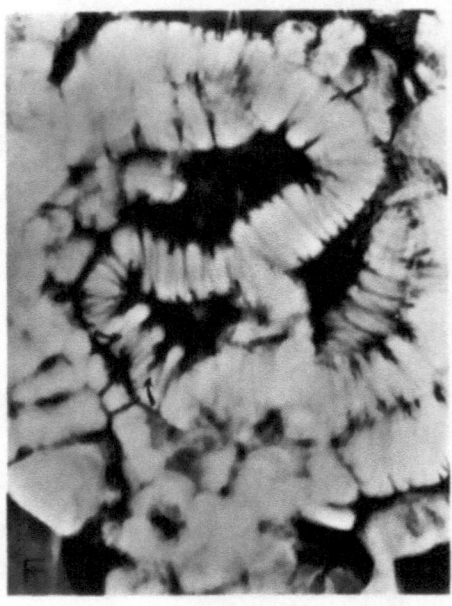

Fig. 12.20ꜰ. Minimal sacculations (arrows) in the jejunum in a patient with scleroderma. It is of course not possible to establish whether this configuration is incidental, and thus should be considered normal, or shows subtle abnormalities due to scleroderma.

panied by Raynaud-like abnormalities in the hands, differentiation from scleroderma can sometimes be difficult – especially if the skin changes are similar to those of scleroderma.

The gastrointestinal abnormalities are characterized by diffuse ulcerations and hemorrhage that can spread over a large area (fig. 12.24). These vascular lesions are caused by a disseminated thrombosis of the small vessels. Microscopically there is thickening of the intima of the small arteries in the mucosa or submucosa. A specific part of the intestine is not preferred. In 10%–15% of the cases, a malignancy will develop somewhere in the digestive tract and quite frequently in other organs.

3. Adult celiac disease (W.F.H. Müller)

Celiac disease is encountered in small children as well as adults. The classic case is characterized by fatigue, loss of weight, and diarrhea. The stools are usually pulpy, voluminous, and pale, and will float in water. Watery diarrhea can also develop. The steatorrhea can be latent; there are also cases with obstipation. These patients frequently present com-

pletely different symptoms such as pain in the joints and neurological abnormalities.

As a result of a marked decrease in the Ca resorption, osteomalacia can develop and tetanic cramps can occur. A defective vitamin K resorption can cause purpura, a vitamin B_{12} deficiency, a megaloblastic anemia, and a decreased Fe absorption and iron deficiency anemia.

Abdominal pain, often resembling the dyspeptic symptoms of a duodenal ulcer, is a frequent complaint. These highly variable atypical symptoms make it difficult to establish a diagnosis.

The symptoms can be acute, for instance after traveler's diarrhea, pregnancy, or a stress situation. The course of the disease can also be stealthy. Sometimes the patient himself does not realize that he is sick, since he has learned to live with his complaints. The nature of this illness was not recognized in the past. This has led to a multitude of terms, including celiac disease, adult celiac disease, idiopathic steatorrhea, primary malabsorption, sprue, celiac sprue, free-gluten disease, and gluten-induced enteropathy.

In 1953, Dicke showed that children with 'celiac disease' improved when wheat was omitted from

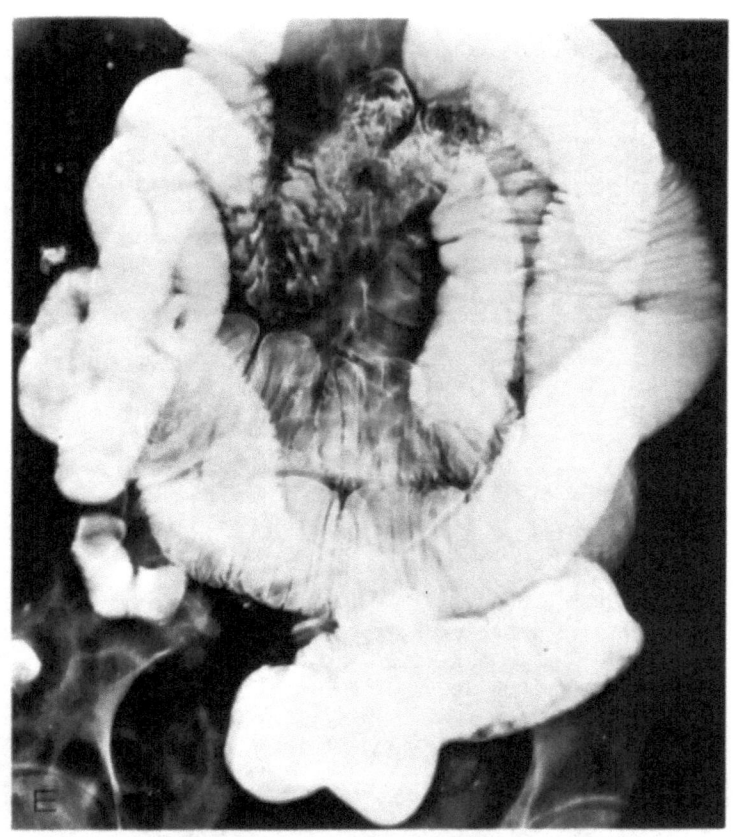

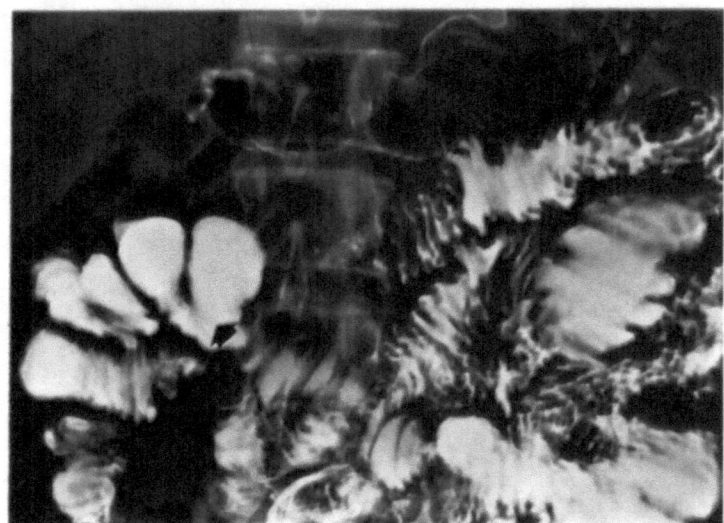

366

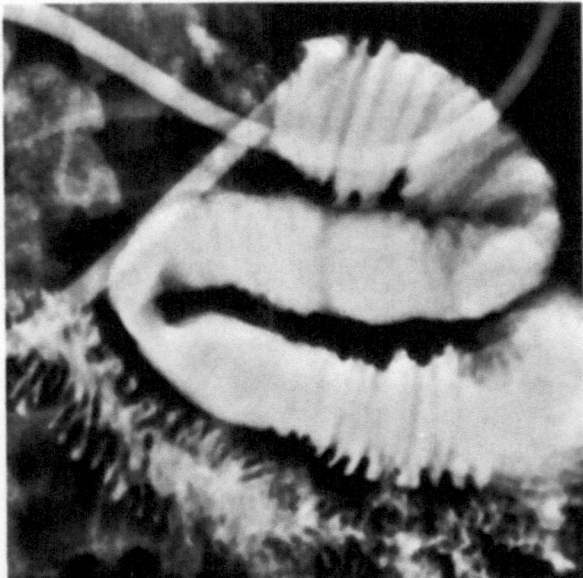

Fig. 12.22. Periarteritis nodosa in a 16-year-old girl. Mucosal folds have disappeared and the wall of the proximal jejunum is thickened over a length of about 20 cm. The differentiation between ischemic abnormalities and infiltration of the mucous membrane by a lymphoreticular malignancy is almost impossible. The rather abrupt edges of the lesion, the lack of nodular swellings, and the completely normal mucosa in the rest of the small intestine are more likely to indicate a vascular origin of the abnormalities. The fact that thickening of the intestinal wall is only local and that the mucosa in the duodenum is normal (not visible here) exclude celiac disease. Because of the lack of cobblestones in the jejunum – otherwise so numerous – and the absence of an edematous swollen mucosa at the edges of the lesion, Crohn's disease also need not be considered.

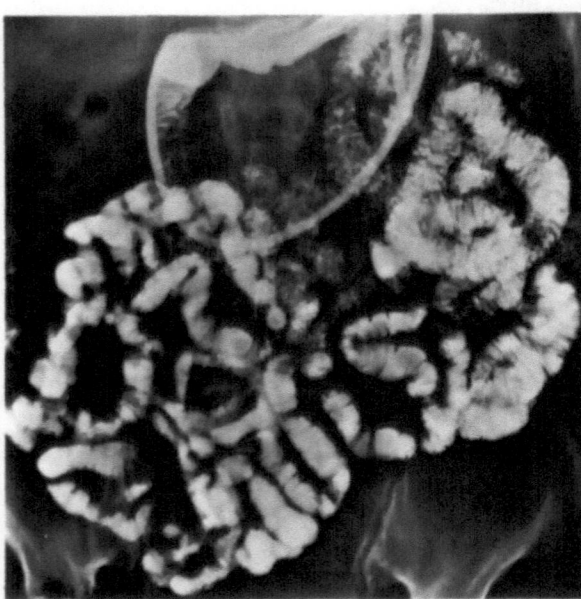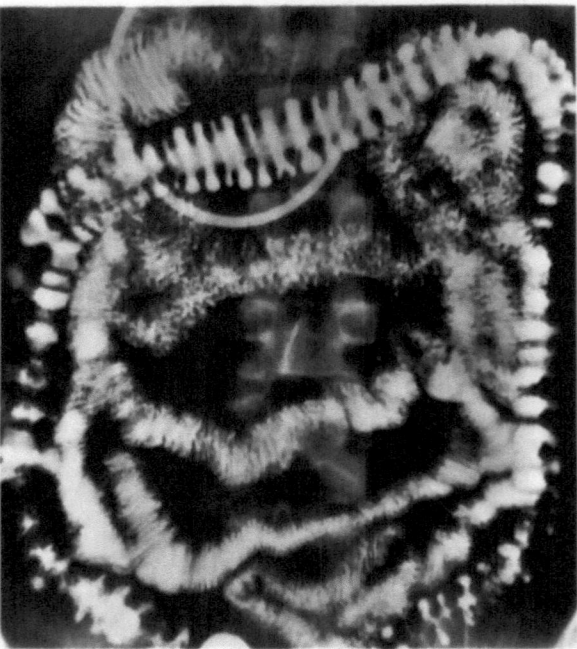

Fig. 12.23. Two patients with chronic abdominal cramps as a result of SLE. The loops of the small bowel show a pronounced hypermotility, but no ischemic mucosal lesions can be found. Many of the loops are in the contraction phase and the lumen of the intestine is obviously smaller than normal. Since the colon can also be quite spastic, it is sometimes possible in these cases to fill both the large and the small intestine with only 400 ml barium suspension.

established in 10%–18% of the first-degree relations of each patient. According to Rubin, this disease is therefore definitely not simply acquired through exogenous factors alone – specifically gluten. It is also genetically determined. The pattern of transmission is as yet unknown. There exists an important indication of the genetic origin of this pathological reaction to gluten. This is the frequent occurrence of the histocompatibility antigens HL A1 and HL A8 in patients with celiac disease. But, since these antigens can also be found in normals, other factors must also be involved.

The frequency of celiac disease in England is 1:2000; in West Ireland it is 1:300 (1973). No exact figures are available for the Netherlands, but at the Celiac Symposium held in 1974, it was estimated at

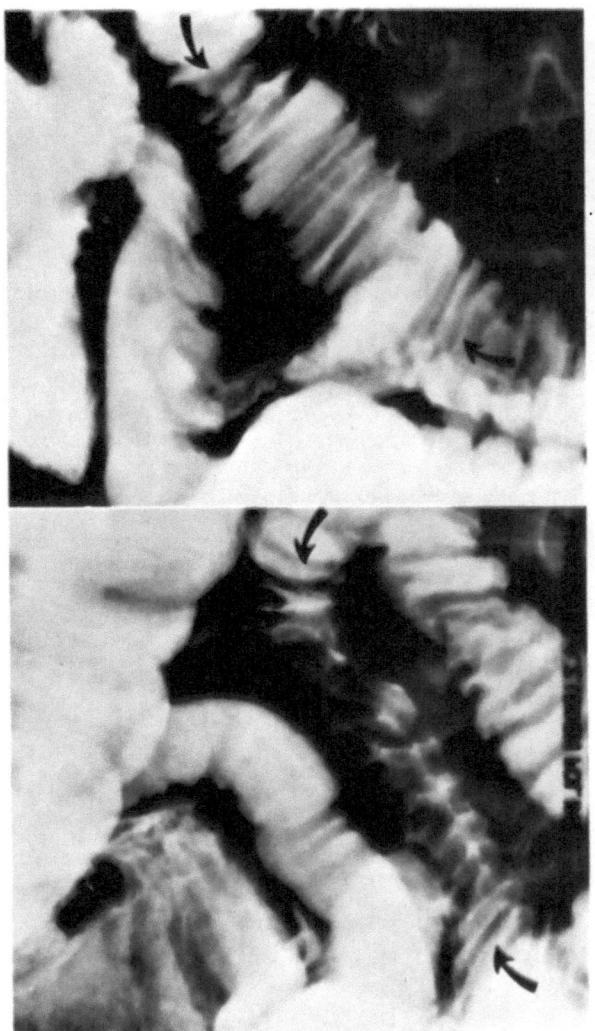

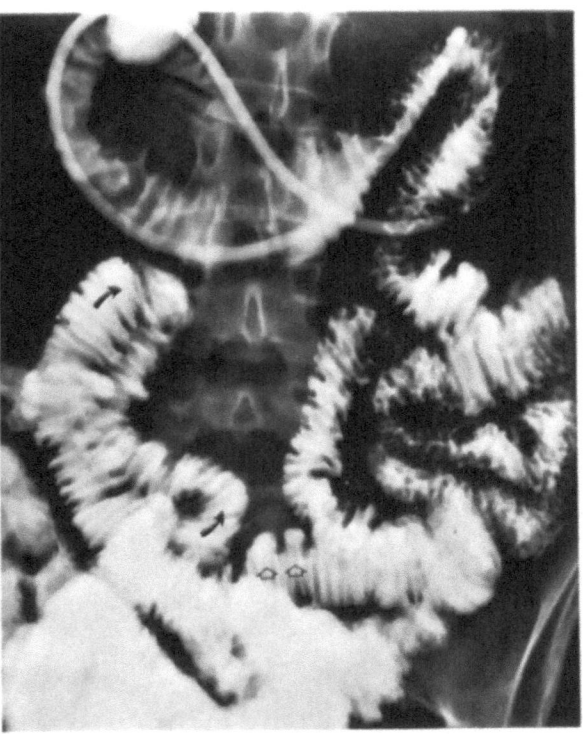

Fig. 12.24. Diffuse vascular abnormalities in the small intestine of a patient with dermatomyositis. Coarse and also irregular mucosal relief in the region of the ileojejunal junction (solid arrows). In the duodenum, too, the folds appear fairly coarse; the degree of filling here is, however, moderate. As in the patient with scleroderma in fig. 12.20F, a number of small sacculations can also be seen (open arrows).

about 1:1000. This means that there are approximately 13,000 patients with celiac disease in the Netherlands.

3.1. Radiological appearance

In 1953, Mackie was the first to describe a radiological abnormality of the small bowel in nontropical sprue. He observed an abnormal nonpropulsive peristalsis. In 1934, Snell and Camp described smooth contours in the jejunum and duodenum. In subsequent years, diverse publications appeared describing flocculation and segmentation of the barium suspension. Golden called this phenomenon the 'deficiency pattern'. However, flocculation and segmentation are not at all specific for celiac disease. This is also encountered in numerous other diseases even when a so-called

'high stable' barium suspension is used.

By administering larger quantities of the barium suspension, Schwishuk et al. and Marshak were able to visualize the mucosal patterns as well as the dilatation more clearly. Ishell et al., however, found that in spite of using a 'nonflocculating' suspension for patients with celiac disease, flocculation and segmentation were still observed more frequently than dilatation of the small intestine. With the enteroclysis method, a large dose of contrast medium is administered rapidly. The disturbing disintegration of the barium suspension can then be avoided under all conditions – even if the preparation is not particularly stable. However, the transit rate of the contrast fluid in patients with celiac disease can be so accelerated that it is impossible to obtain adequate filling of the intestinal loops even

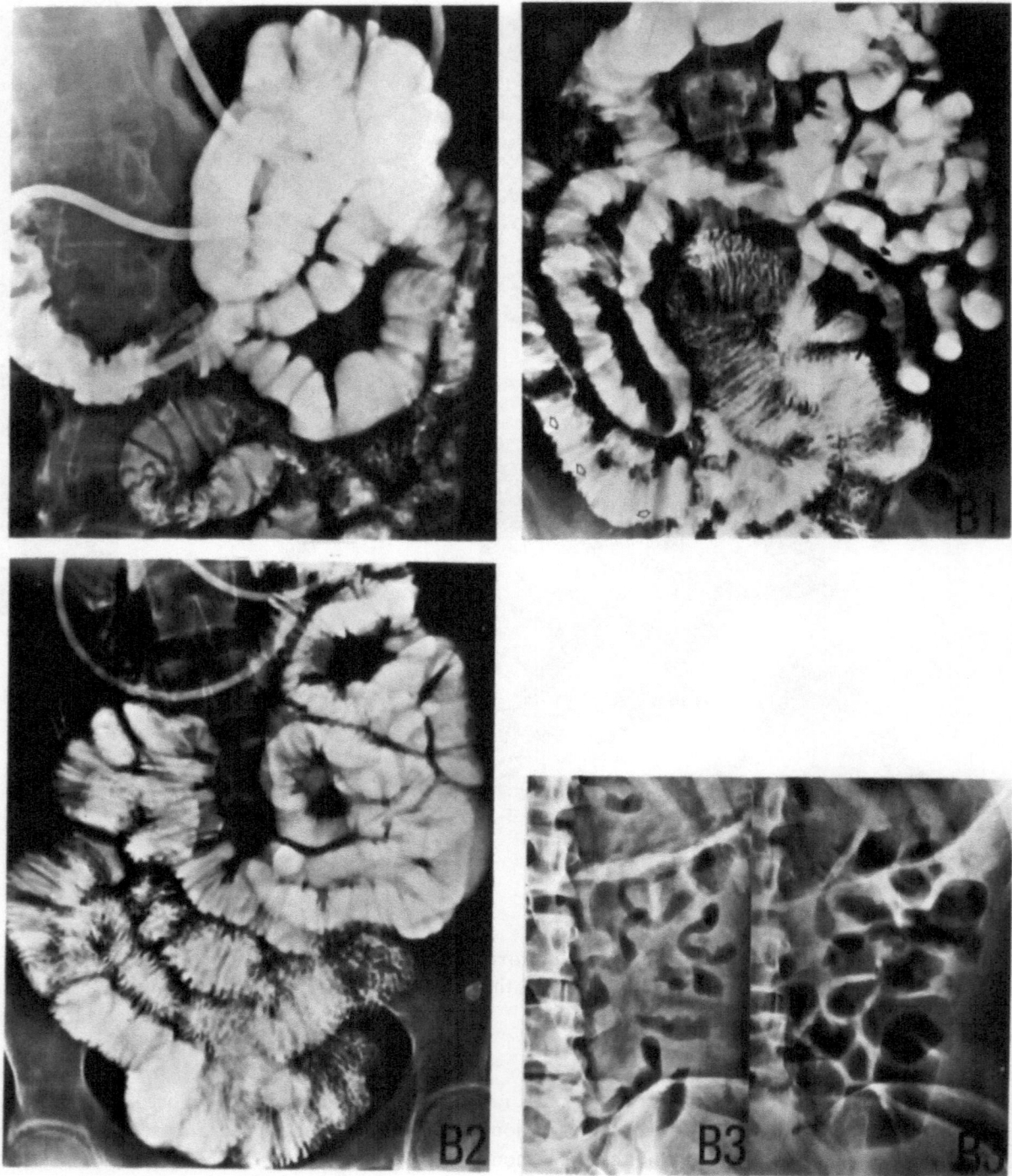

369

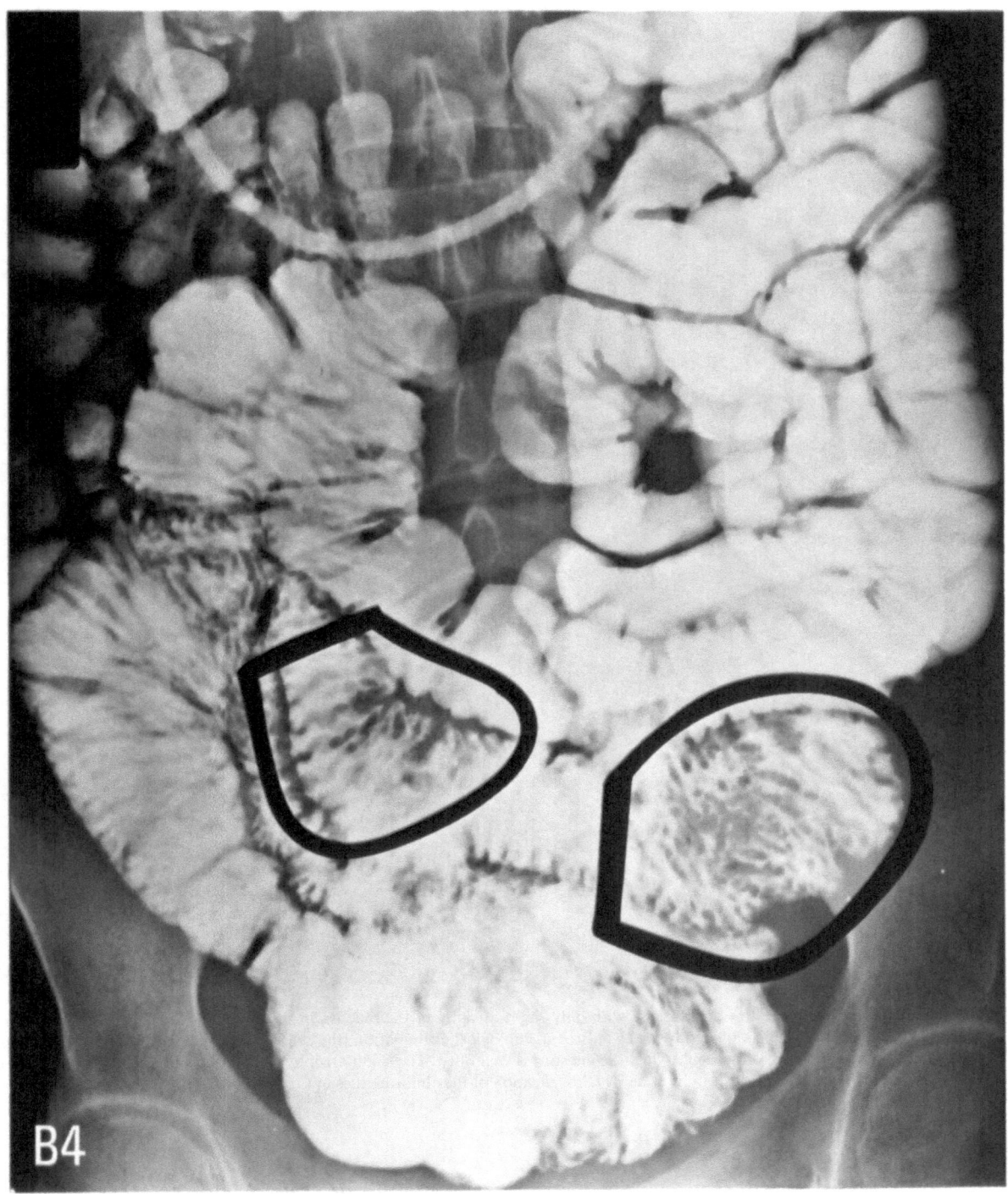

Fig. 12.25. See legend on page 368.

370

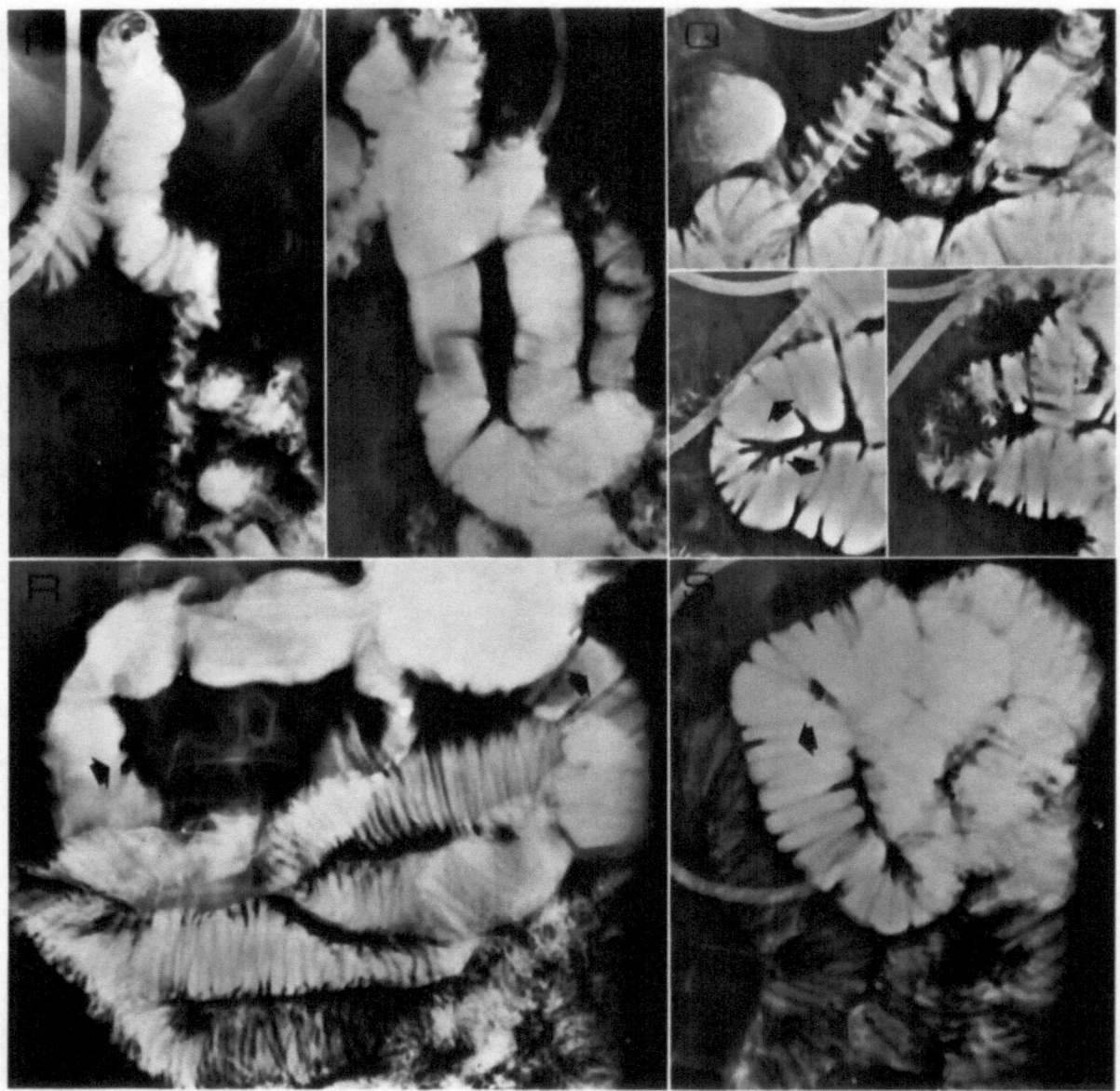

*Fig. 12.26*A. Four patients with celiac disease with only slight atrophy of the mucosa in the jejunum. For all of these patients the presence of this disease was discovered by means of roentgenological examination (the celiac disease provocative test). In patients P and Q, the abnormalities are only visible when the intestine is well filled. The slight atrophy of the folds in patient S is similar to that seen in the patient with amyloidosis in fig. 12.35(1). Localization of the abnormalities in the most proximal part of the jejunum led us to consider celiac disease first.

with enteroclysis. Therefore when celiac disease is suspected, it is essential that the flow rate of the contrast fluid is even greater than the normal 75 ml/min. The barium suspension must be diluted with water to reduce viscosity so that it will flow through the infusion system more quickly. The specific gravity of the barium suspension can be reduced by dilution from s.g. 1.25 for normal patients to s.g. 1.20 without objection. The decrease

in contrast intensity that results from the decrease in specific gravity can be compensated for by lowering the exposure voltage 10 or 20 kV. A characteristic of celiac disease is smooth margins in the jejunum. It is always easiest to discover these smooth contours in a well-filled segment of the bowel.

The importance of a rapid contrast medium flow is demonstrated in fig. 12.26. Rapid flow is nec-

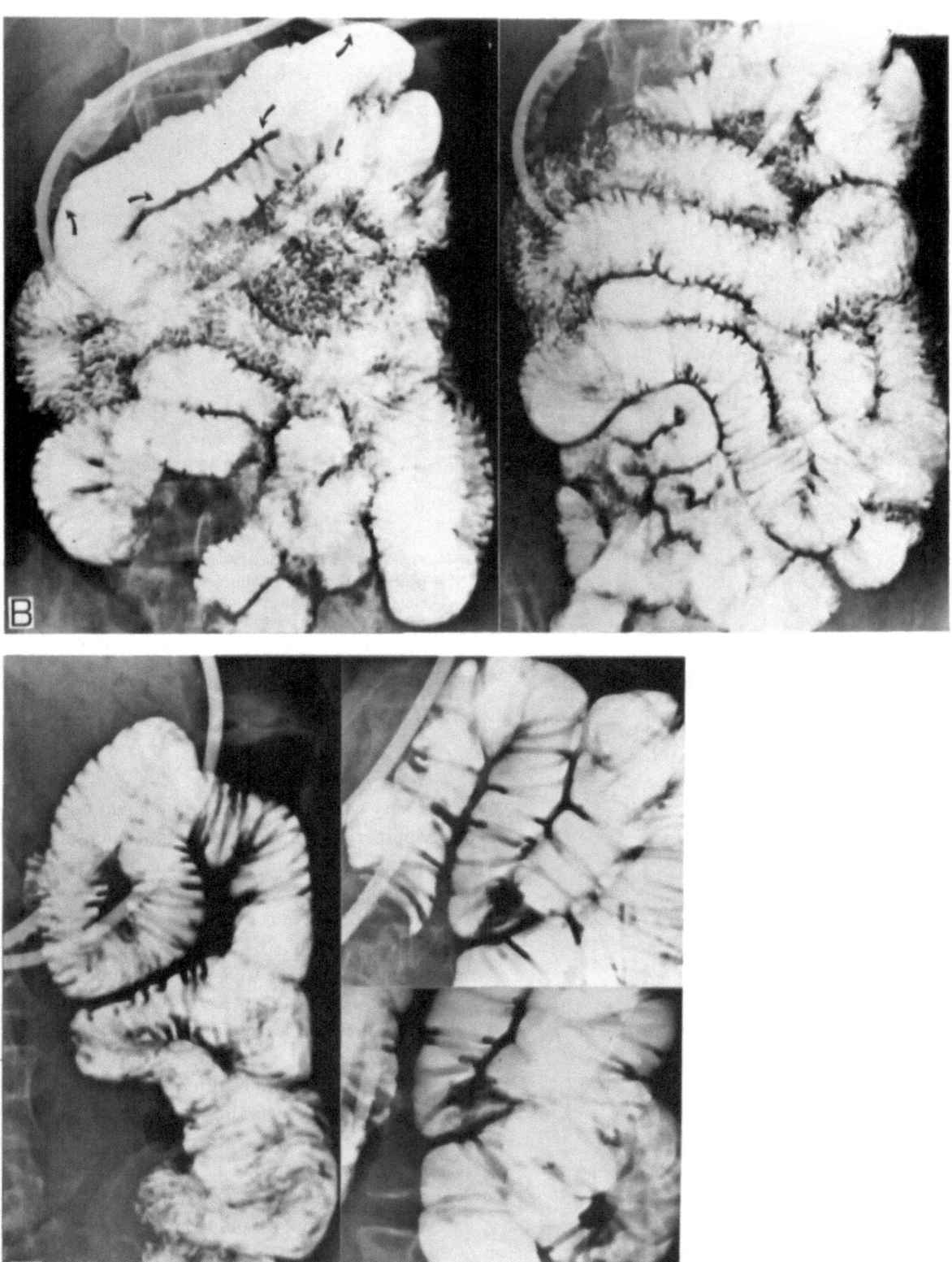

*Fig. 12.26*B. Two cases of subtle mucosal atrophy in the proximal jejunum in celiac disease that is visualized only in the well-filled state. The folds are shorter than normal and the distance between the folds has increased. In these cases, too, the diagnosis was established from the roentgenograms.

372

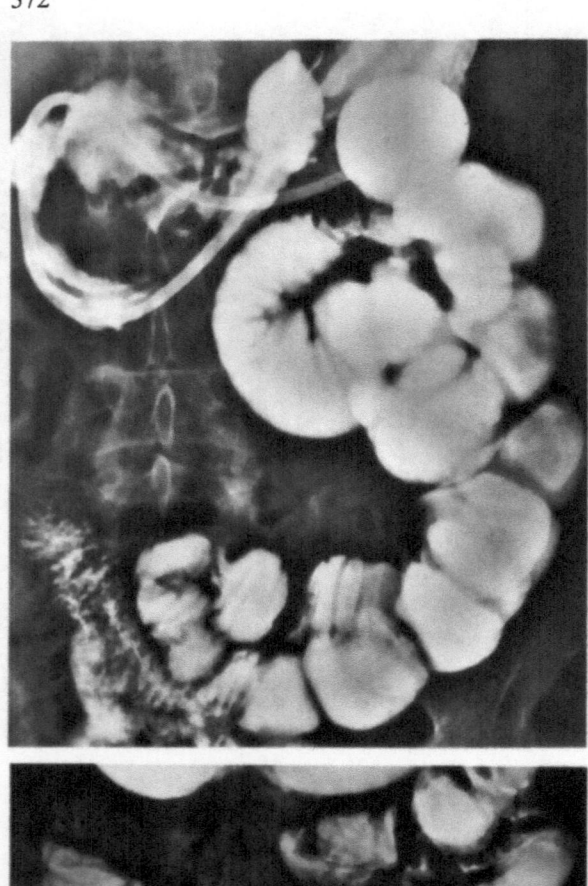

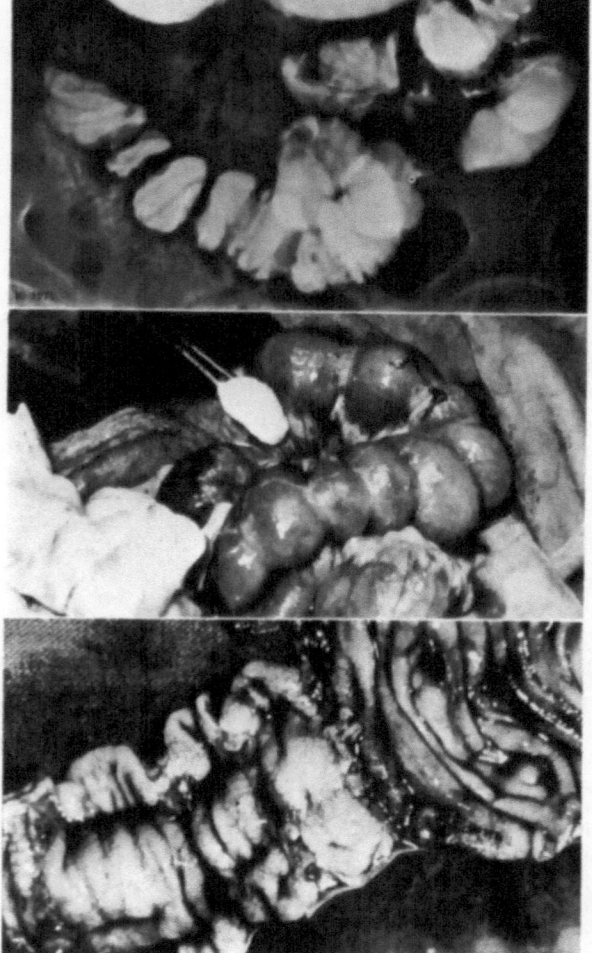

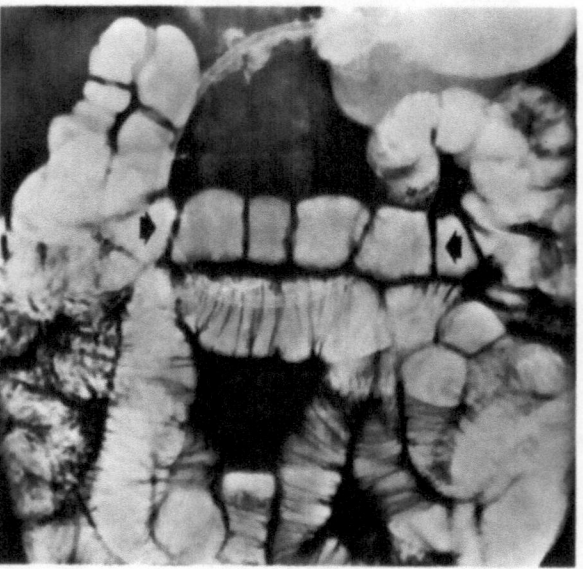

Fig. 12.27. Two patients with a colon-like haustration in the jejunum. The abnormalities seen in the patient on the right closely resemble the ischemic abnormalities in fig. 11.15. During surgery they appeared to be caused by spasms and cicatrization at the site of circular ulcerations. These stenotic ulcerations in this patient possibly resulted from atrophy of the vascular system. On the surgical photographs, the colonization pattern is clearly visible and also, in the open intestine, the atrophied mucosal relief in the jejunum.

essary when trying to detect a slight decrease in the number and flattening of the mucosal folds that suggest celiac disease. The radiologist's tentative diagnosis would have been missed with a slower flow rate inherent in the oral administration of the contrast medium.

In some cases a well-filled jejunum may show the haustral-like pattern seen in the colon; these structures are caused by spasms (fig. 12.27). In celiac disease, a gastric examination shows that the folds in the duodenum are often coarse and asymmetrically thickened. This is in itself hardly specific and is therefore not sufficient to establish this diagnosis – especially if there are no mucosal abnormalities in the jejunum. An enteroclysis examination of this same duodenum would, however, reveal the flattened folds and thus the probable diagnosis, when combined with a good case history.

A disadvantage, albeit of little importance, of the infusion method is that the duodenum often cannot be visualized in a well-filled state since the tip of the tube should be located at Treitz's ligament in order to avoid reflux into the stomach. At the end of the

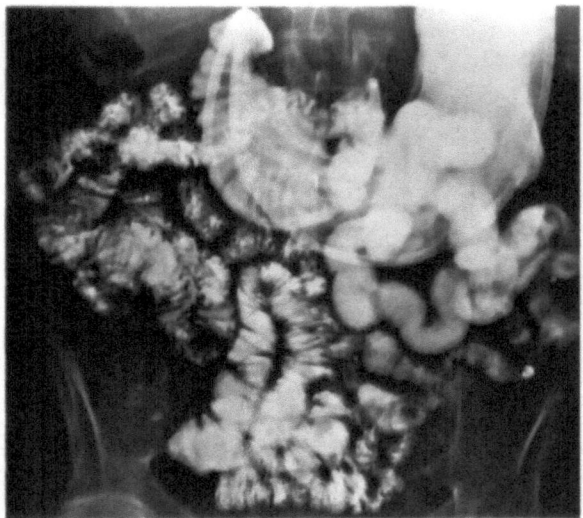

Fig. 12.28. Misleading pattern suggesting celiac disease. This is because of the abnormal position in the upper left quadrant of the ileum that at this moment shows few mucosal impressions (disintegration of the head of the contrast column!).

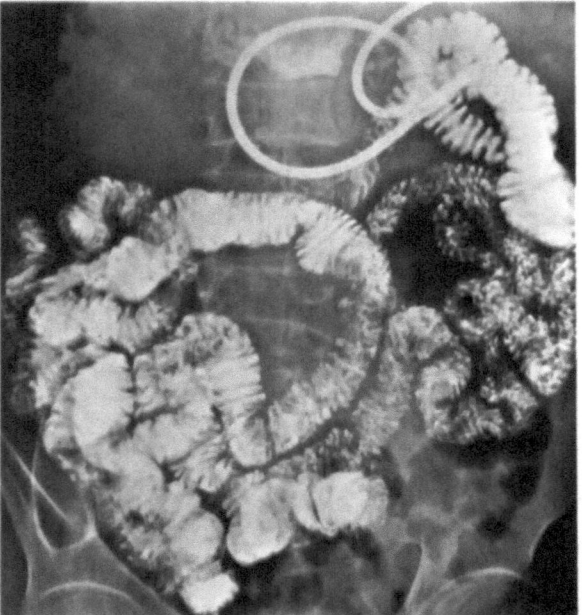

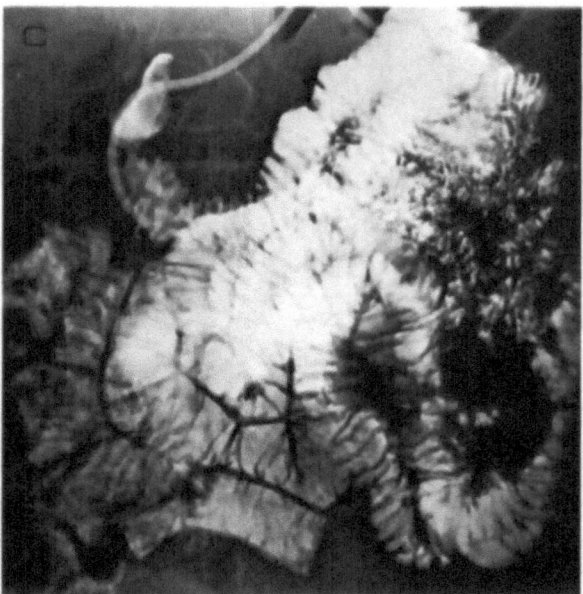

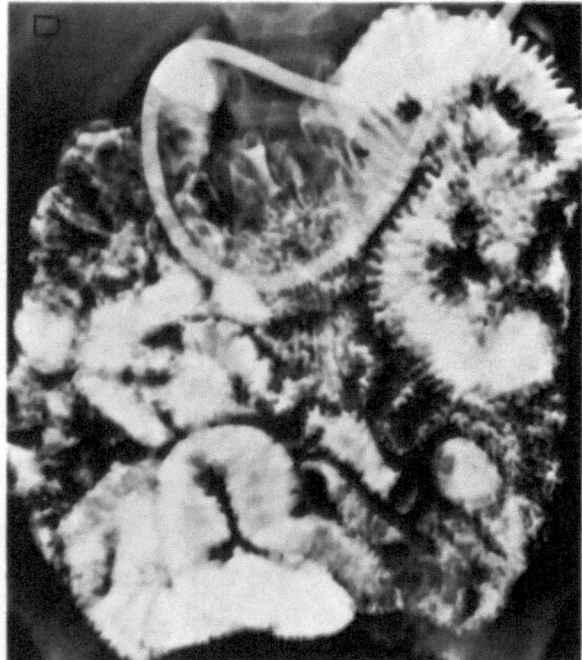

Fig. 12.29C–D. For legend see following page.

examination, the tube can be slightly pulled back into the descending duodenum and this area adequately filled.

The mucosal folds in the jejunum in patients with celiac disease can show interesting variations. We have observed the following groups of abnormalities.

3.1.1. Group 1. In about one-half of the patients with celiac disease, the mucosa in the duodenum and the jejunum is smooth. This could be due to a flattening of the circular folds that have become shorter, and an increase in the distance between the folds. This is the so-called 'moulage' sign, a true representation of atrophied mucosa (fig. 12.25). In contrast, 'pseudomoulage' (see fig. 4.7AB) also shows a smooth

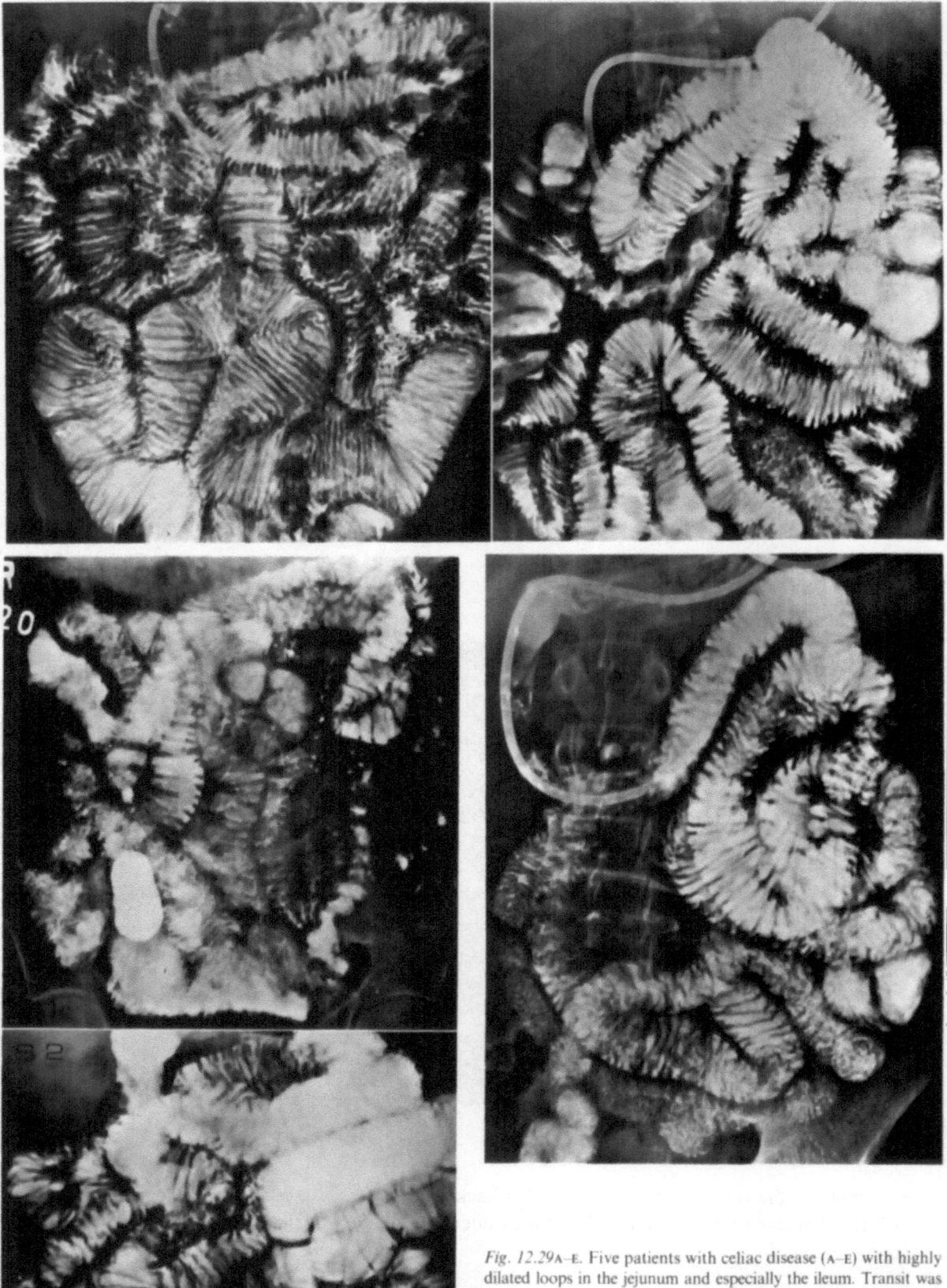

*Fig. 12.29*A–E. Five patients with celiac disease (A–E) with highly dilated loops in the jejunum and especially the ileum. Transit was so rapid that it was not possible to fill the intestine adequately. Patients A–C also showed considerable radiological improvement after treatment (right column). There was no follow-up examination of patient D, a 10-year-old child. Patient B, one of our first cases after the introduction of the (at that time not yet perfected) enteroclysis method (B2). He had been examined shortly beforehand by the conventional passage technique (B1) that produced a pronounced flocculation and dilution of the contrast fluid.

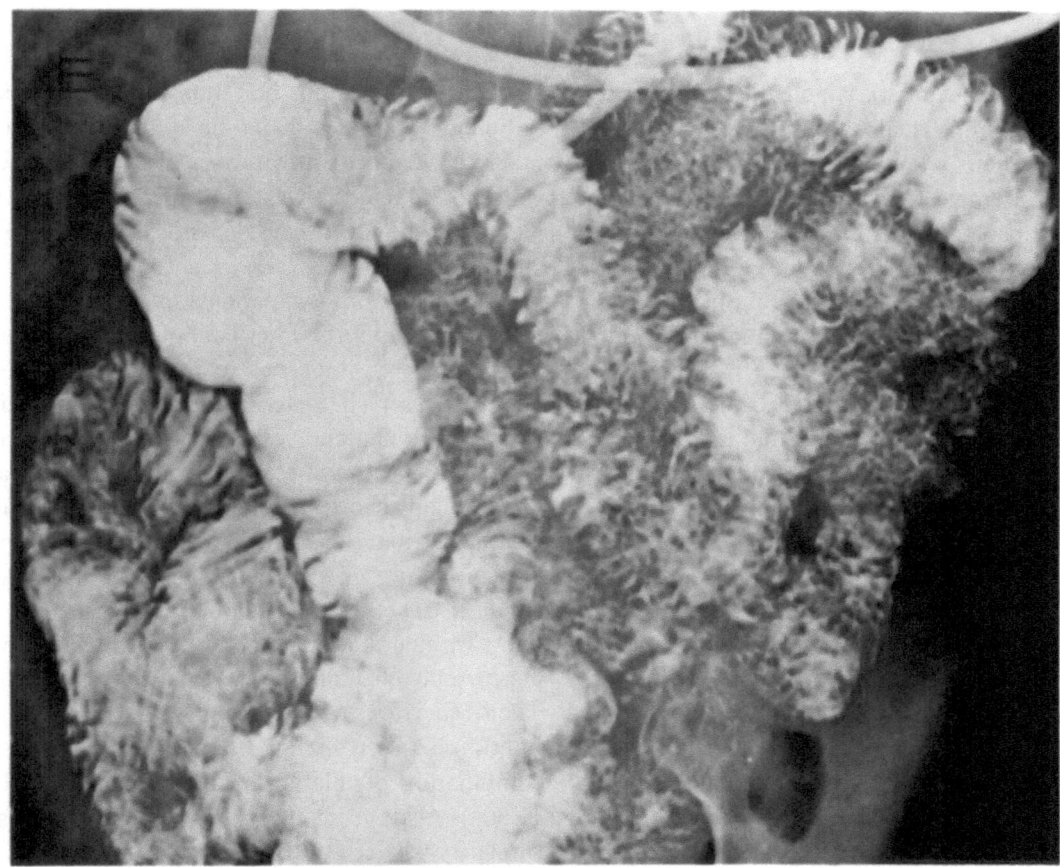

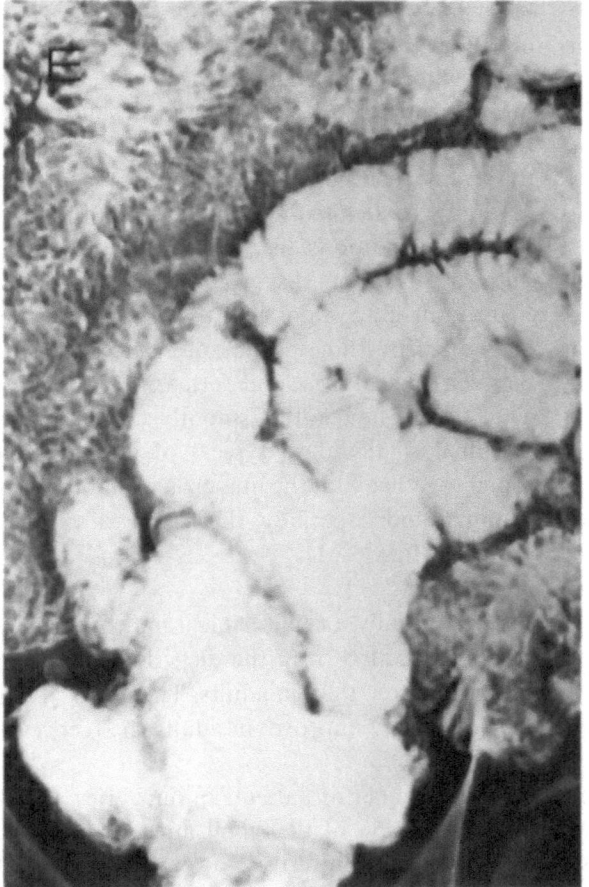

*Fig. 12.29*E. Transplantation patient who had complained of diarrhea for two weeks. The roentgen examination showed a clear dilatation of the jejunum and ileum together with a hypermotility and a pronounced tendency toward flocculation of the contrast medium. On the basis of these findings the diagnosis of celiac disease was established; this was subsequently confirmed by means of a biopsy.

mucosal surface from stasis and thickening of the contrast medium. Visualization of the mucosa that still exists is then no longer possible. As a result of a positional anomaly (malrotation) of the small intestine (see page 373), ileal loops may be found in the upper left quadrant. Pronounced filling of these loops produces fairly smooth contours and this misleading pattern must be differentiated from that described above for celiac disease (fig. 12.28).

In celiac disease, peristalsis in the smooth atrophied jejunal loops is abnormal and nonpropulsive. The ileal loops are frequently dilated with numerous mucosal folds. This might be considered an attempt to compensate for the decrease in the mucosal surface in the jejunum ('jejunization', fig. 2.3).

3.1.2. Group II. In about one-quarter of the patients with celiac disease, we have seen a striking dilatation of both the ileal and the jejunal loops (fig. 12.29). The diameter of the jejunum as well as the ileum may even be 40–55 mm (in enteroclysis the normal value is a maximum of ± 35 mm). Peristalsis is active and the intestine is highly contractile so that the transit time is exceedingly short (the cecum can be reached within 5 min). In spite of a high flow rate of the contrast medium, it is difficult to obtain adequate filling of the intestinal loops. A pronounced dilution of the barium suspension occurs as a result of excess intestinal juice in the intestinal lumen. It is possible that this large quantity of fluid is not due to hypersecretion but to a disturbed water resorption. Patients in this group, like those of group I, usually have the most severe clinical symptoms. There is a definitely disturbed resorption of diverse food substances such as fats, Fe, Ca, and vitamin B_{12} as well as a marked protein loss in the digestive tract. This so-called protein-losing enteropathy is accompanied by a generalized edema of the mucosal folds in the small bowel. These swollen folds are clearly visible on the x-rays; in addition it is seen that the thickness of the intestinal wall has also increased.

3.1.3. Group III. In the remaining 25% of the patients with celiac disease, rapid transit and dilatation of the intestinal loops can also be found. They are not as pronounced as in group II and therefore are not specific for celiac disease. The diagnosis in these cases generally cannot be established by means of radiology. These patients have only mild complaints. There are known cases of celiac disease in which the diagnosis was confirmed by biopsy but the roentgenograms revealed no abnormalities at all.

For this group of patients in particular, the radiological abnormalities cannot be differentiated from those seen in dermatitis herpetiformis. In the latter disease, characterized by bilateral itching, there are papular and vesicular lesions on the tensor side of the extremities. The transit time is also exceptionally short. In some cases almost the entire small intestine is in a state of contraction, a phenomenon that can also be encountered in carcinoid (fig. 12.30A). Strangely enough, the risk that patients with dermatitis herpetiformis will also have a concurrent celiac disease is statistically fairly high. Then, contrary to the decreased caliber of the intestine as seen in fig. 12.30A, we may find the combination of dilatation and hypermotility (fig. 12.30B). Aside from this there are many points of similarity between these two diseases. For example, we can find the full range of flat villi — from normal to even a complete 'snowflake' atrophy. As in celiac disease, we will also see various degrees of malabsorption, steatorrhea, and thickened mucosal folds from the loss of protein. It is peculiar that these abnormalities of the digestive tract also react favorably to a gluten-free diet. We have found that the skin conditions likewise improve although a number of authors disagree.

It is not always possible to differentiate clearly between these three groups of celiac patients, nor between celiac disease and dermatitis herpetiformis. Thus for instance the smooth contours in the proximal small bowel typical of group I can be found together with the numerous dilatations in the jejunum and especially the ileum described for group II (fig. 12.31).

There is usually a rapid clinical improvement after gluten is omitted from the diet; this is more often true in children than in adults. The mucosal lesions may obviously improve; in adults the recovery can be incomplete.

For a number of patients in our series, a follow-up examination of the small intestine was carried out from two months to two years after the gluten-

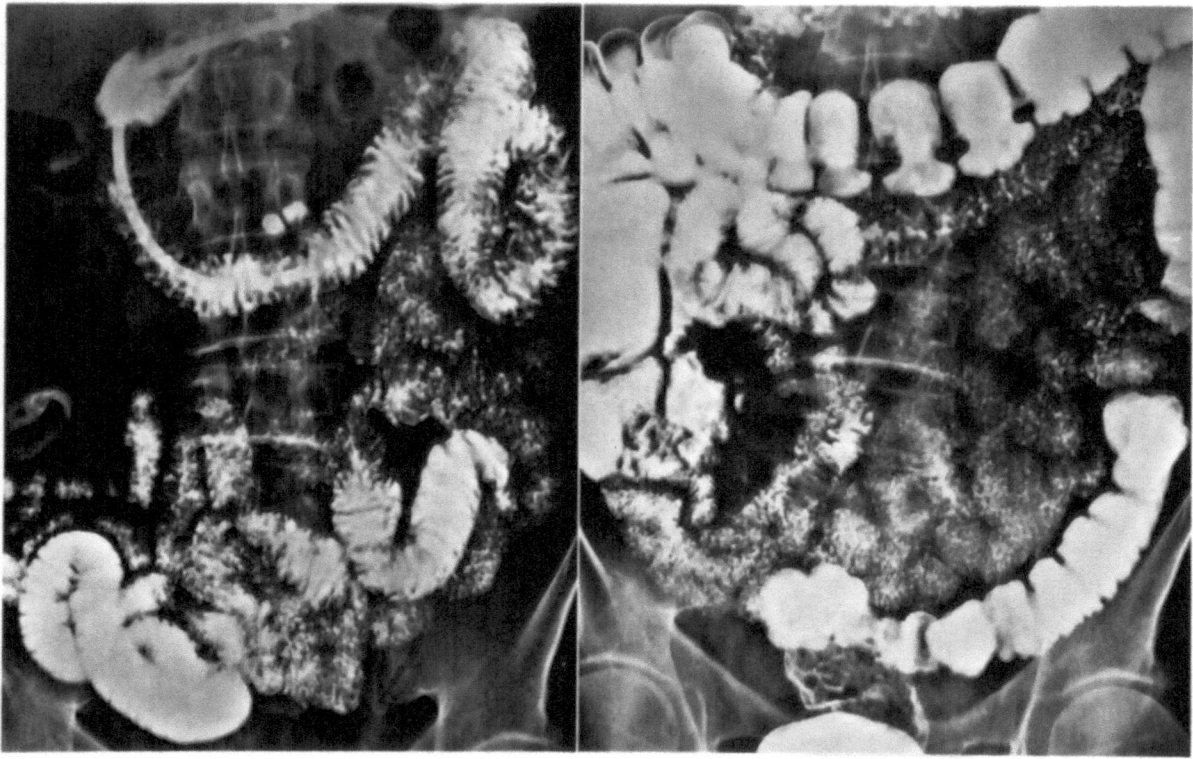

Fig. 12.30A. Two stages of the examination of a patient with dermatitis herpetiformis. Transit was exceptionally fast, almost the entire small bowel is in a state of contraction. The loops are not dilated and there is no atrophy of the mucosa in the jejunum.

free diet was instituted (fig. 12.29). In all our cases, dilatation, hypersecretion, and mucosal edema when present had disappeared or diminished (mainly patients from group II). An essential recovery of the smooth mucosal surface (mainly patients from group I) was never seen. Apparently therefore the mucosal folds never reappear once an intestinal loop has become atrophied.

3.2. Complications

3.2.1. Malignancies. Since the publications by Golden in 1936 and Mackey and Fairley in 1937, it has been known that there is some connection between steatorrhea and the development of malignant lymphoma. At first steatorrhea was thought to be secondary to the infiltration of malignant cells into the small intestinal wall and occlusion of the lymphatic channels. In 1962, Golden and his associates suggested that intestinal lymphoma could develop as a complication of adult celiac disease. This was confirmed by Harris, who examined 250 patients with celiac disease and found 40 cases of malignancy. Of these 40 patients, 16 had carcinoma of

the digestive tract. The esophagus was the most common localization, relatively speaking (fig. 12.33). Although the greatest turnover of cells occurs in the proximal part of the small intestine, carcinoma seldom develops in the duodenum and jejunum (fig. 12.34). Four patients had malignancies elsewhere in the body. There were 20 patients with lymphoma, one-third of which did not originate in the intestinal wall. The malignancies occur more frequently in males than females. It also appeared that within one family the number of patients with adult celiac disease in conjunction with a malignancy was larger. If a gluten-free diet is followed for at least 12 months, the risk of carcinoma will decrease, but not that of lymphoma. A tumor must always be included in the differential diagnosis when patients do not improve on a gluten-free diet or have new complaints after a temporary remission. This is also the case when there is obstruction of perforation in addition to symptoms such as loss of weight, diarrhea, and skin problems. In celiac disease, both humoral and cellular immunological disorders are known. It can be seen that these factors, whether genetically

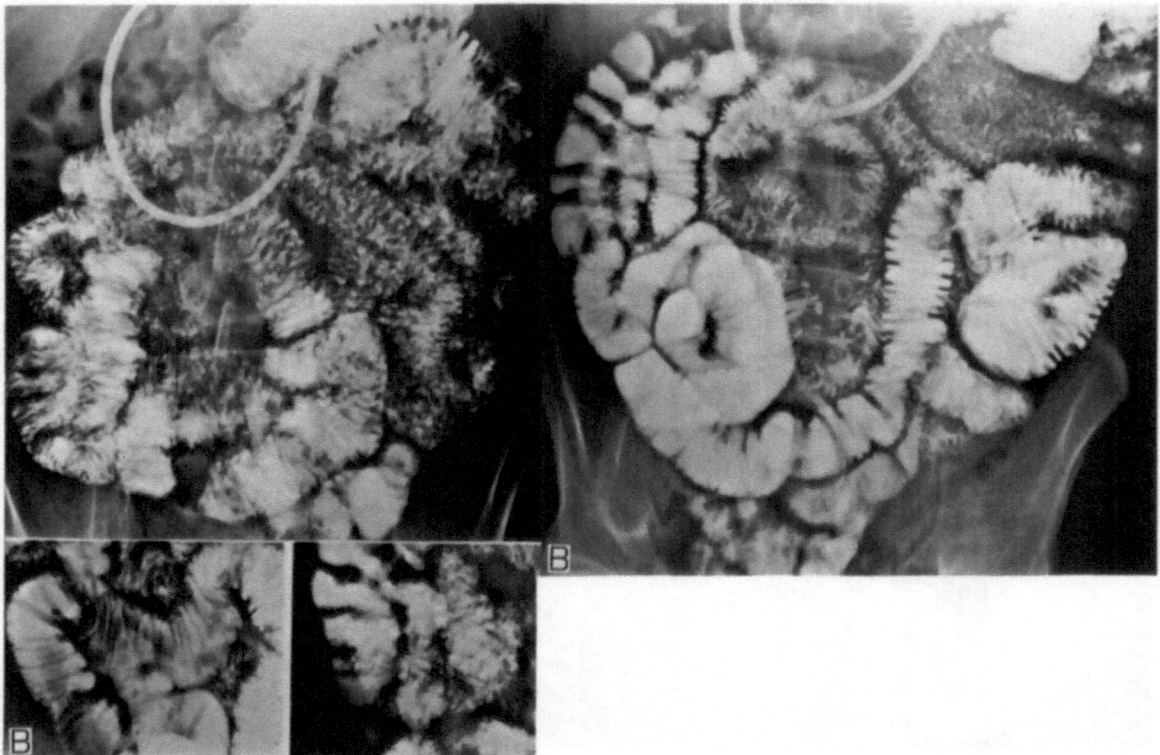

*Fig. 12.30*B. Combination pattern of celiac disease and dermatitis herpetiformis with dilatation of the jejunal and ileal loops together with hypermotility. There is a strong tendency toward flocculation of the barium suspension (left). After treatment of the celiac disease, the tendency toward disintegration has disappeared and the caliber of the jejunum has normalized (right).

determined or not, could play a role in the development of a malignancy.

Biochemical parameters indicating incipient lymphoma are a low albumin concentration, a high alkaline phosphatase content, and an increased serum IgA level.

There are reasons to assume that an immature or abnormal immune system is a predisposing factor for the development of malignancies because of failure of the so-called 'immunological surveillance'. Potential neoplastic cells that develop from errors in cell division are not recognized as such and are therefore not removed.

To discover mucosal abnormalities caused by malignancies in celiac disease at an early stage, it is essential that the examination is not thwarted by flocculation or segmentation of the contrast medium. More so than for any other disease of the small intestine, the use of enteroclysis is therefore an absolute necessity.

3.2.2. Ulcerations. If patients with celiac disease no longer react favorably to a gluten-free diet, then not only malignancy but also ulcerations must be included in the differential diagnosis. In addition to the symptoms of the malabsorption, these patients may also complain of vomiting and severe pain in the upper abdomen. The ulcerations may be solitary or multiple and, as a result of spasms or fibrotic shriveling, they can cause a haustral-like pattern in the jejunum. The most dangerous complications are hemorrhage and perforation; eventually transit may also be impaired. The disease is usually fatal in such cases unless the ulcerous and stenotic jejunal section is removed in time and the patient follows a gluten-free diet.

3.2.3. Intussusceptions. According to the literature, nonobstructing intussusceptions may develop — possibly causing the colic-like pain in the abdomen. This hypothesis in itself seems highly unlikely. The roentgenograms illustrating these reports show that probably all of these cases were incorrectly interpreted because of inadequate filling and misleading patterns. In any event we have never been able to demonstrate this phenomenon in our patients

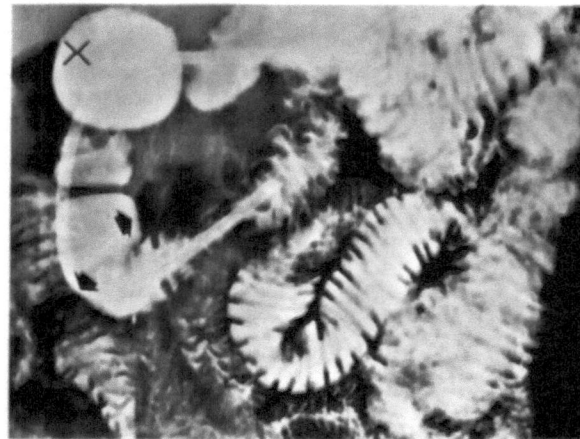

Fig. 12.31. It is not always possible to classify the abnormalities found in patients with celiac disease in one particular group. Transitional forms are also encountered. The differentiation between a dermatitis herpetiformis and celiac disease is likewise difficult. Furthermore these two diseases often develop together, as in these two patients. Here the radiological aspect of group II (pronounced dilatations in the proximal jejunum) is found together with an atrophy of the folds of Kerkring in the proximal duodenum that is characteristic of group I.

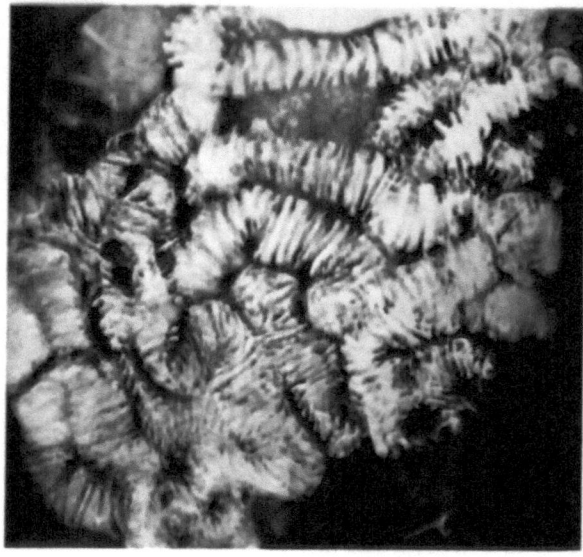

with the enteroclysis method.

3.2.4. Results of malabsorption. The disturbed resorption of a number of food substances causes deficiencies that can lead to the following complications:

1) Severe hemorrhage in the intestinal wall or the retroperitoneal cavity disturbed coagulation mechanism from vitamin K deficiency.
2) A reduced Ca resorption may give rise to tetanic cramps and osteomalacia.
3) Several cases can be found in the literature of volvulus as a result of a marked increase in the size of the colon (fig. 12.32). Enlargement of the colon in patients with celiac disease can be from:
   a) an increase in the bulk of the feces as a result of malabsorption;
   b) a decrease in the muscular tone due to a K deficiency.

4. Amyloidosis

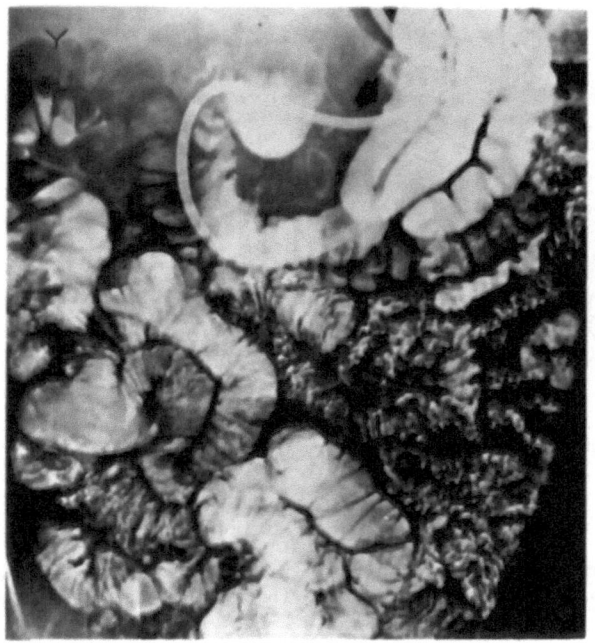

Amyloid is a protein substance that can be deposited in tissue by an unknown mechanism without demonstrable cause. It is assumed that an immunologically determined disturbance of plasma cell function is involved. In addition to this so-called primary amyloidosis, there is also a secondary amyloidosis. These amyloid deposits occur in conjunction with various diseases such as chronic infections, multiple myeloma, and lymphoreticular malignancies. Amyloid deposits can be local but may also be spread diffusely throughout all layers of the wall anywhere in the digestive tract. Furthermore the deposits can be small or quite large. In the latter case they can form nodular masses and bulge into the contrast column such that differentiation from lymphoreticular malignancy can be difficult

380

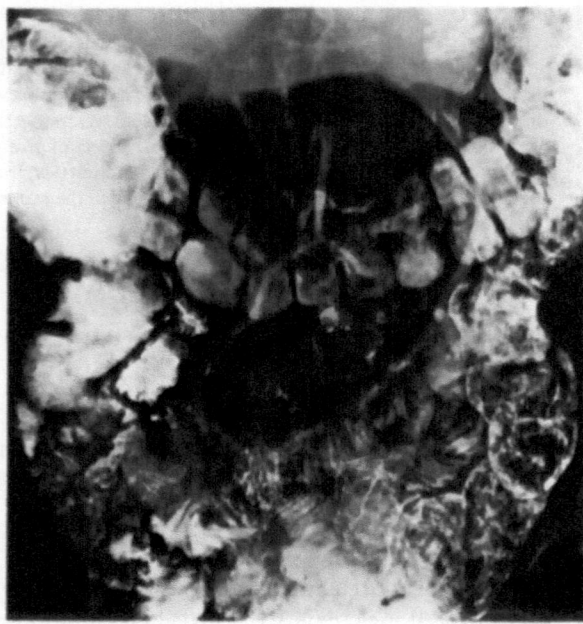

Fig. 12.32. A dolichocolon, a long and voluminous sigmoid that is filled with gas in this x-ray, has caused volvulus. The development of volvulus is a common complication in celiac disease. It is not known exactly whether the increase in the volume of the sigmoid is from an increase in feces or from changes in musculature tone of the large and the small intestine as a result of disturbed mineral resorption.

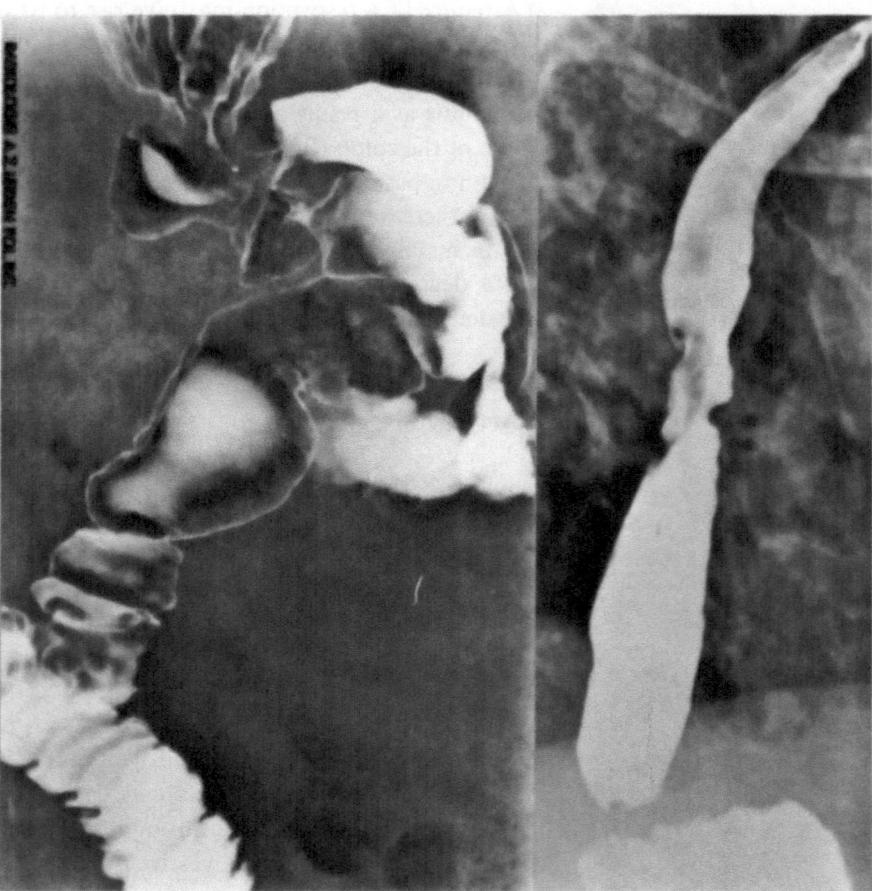

Fig. 12.33. Routine control examination after gastric resection; there is clearly visible atrophy of the mucosa in the jejunal loops just beyond the anastomosis. This is from celiac disease that had not yet been recognized elsewhere. There was also a carcinoma of the esophagus.

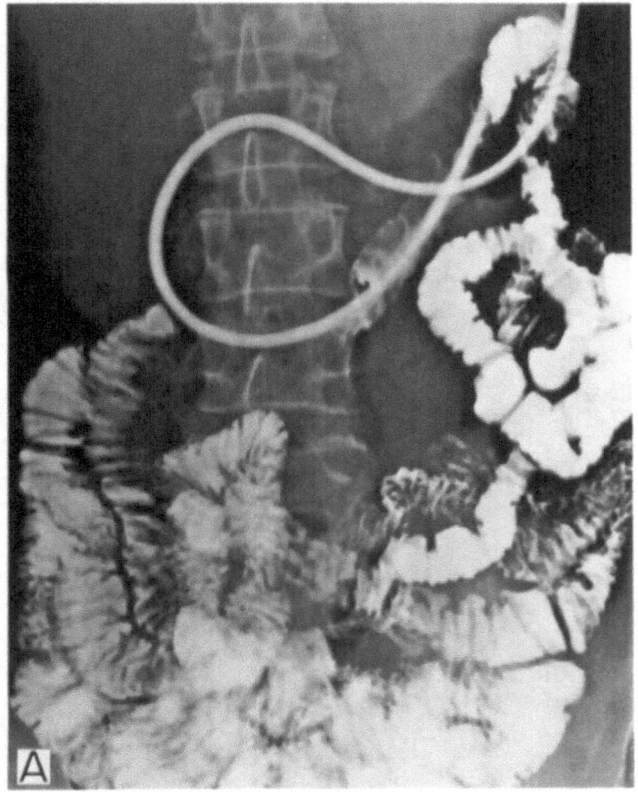

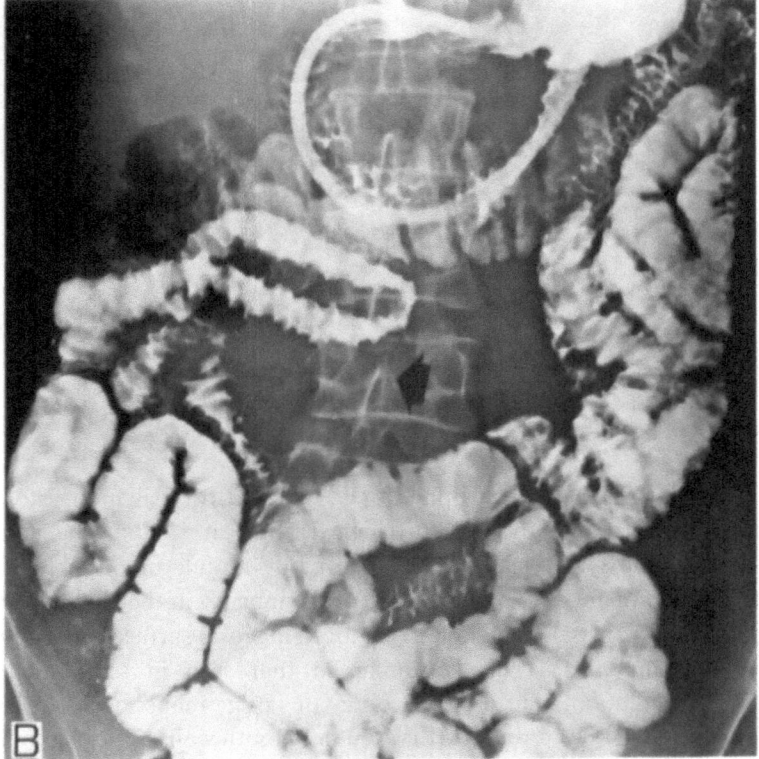

*Fig. 12.34*A–C. Patient with celiac disease: there is obvious atrophy of the mucosa in the jejunum with thick folds and coarse nodular defects distalward from a lymphoreticular malignancy (B and C). An examination cartied out elsewhere (A), where the rate of flow was too low, did not reveal the malignant changes. (See also page 382.)

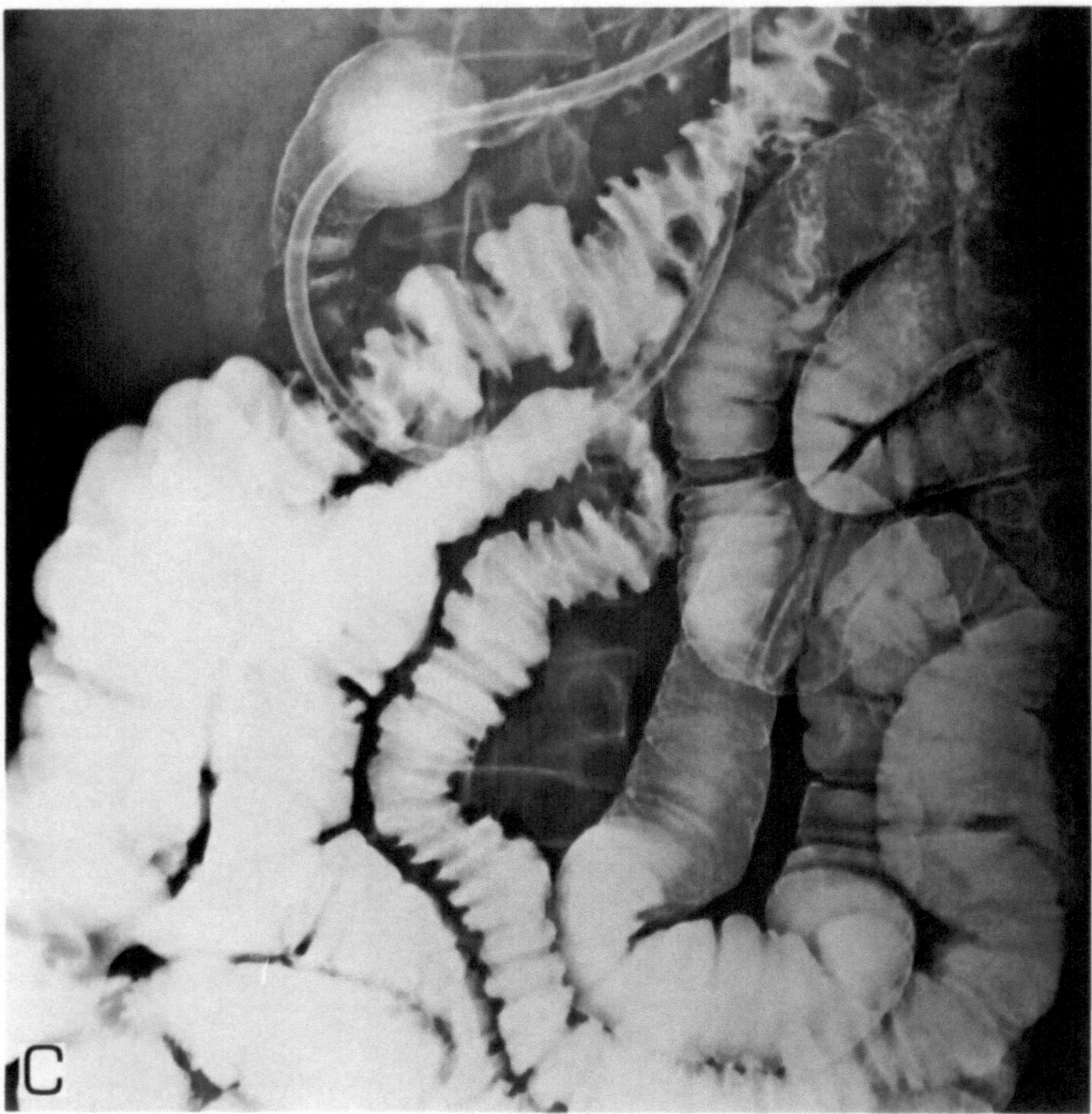

*Fig. 12.34*C. See legend on page 381.

(fig. 12.37). Depending upon localization of the deposits, resorption and motility can become seriously disturbed, leading to a malabsorption syndrome and fairly severe meteorism. The complaints from localization in the small intestine consist mainly of painful cramps. This is accompanied either by diarrhea as a result of gas accumulation, or by a pseudo-obstruction because of the severely disturbed motility (fig. 12.38). The lumen of the small intestine can be obviously dilated, the intestinal wall thickened, and the mucosa atrophied.

If atrophy of the mucosal folds is moderate, they become broadened and flat so that the mucosal surface appears, lightly undulatory (fig. 12.35). A severe atrophy of the mucosa in the ileum produces a completely smooth mucosal surface without folds. This is similar to that seen in reflux ileitis in ulcerative colitis or after remission of Crohn's disease (fig. 12.36). Smooth walls in the jejunum are usually from celiac disease: then there is definitely no dilatation of the lumen since the muscular layers are intact.

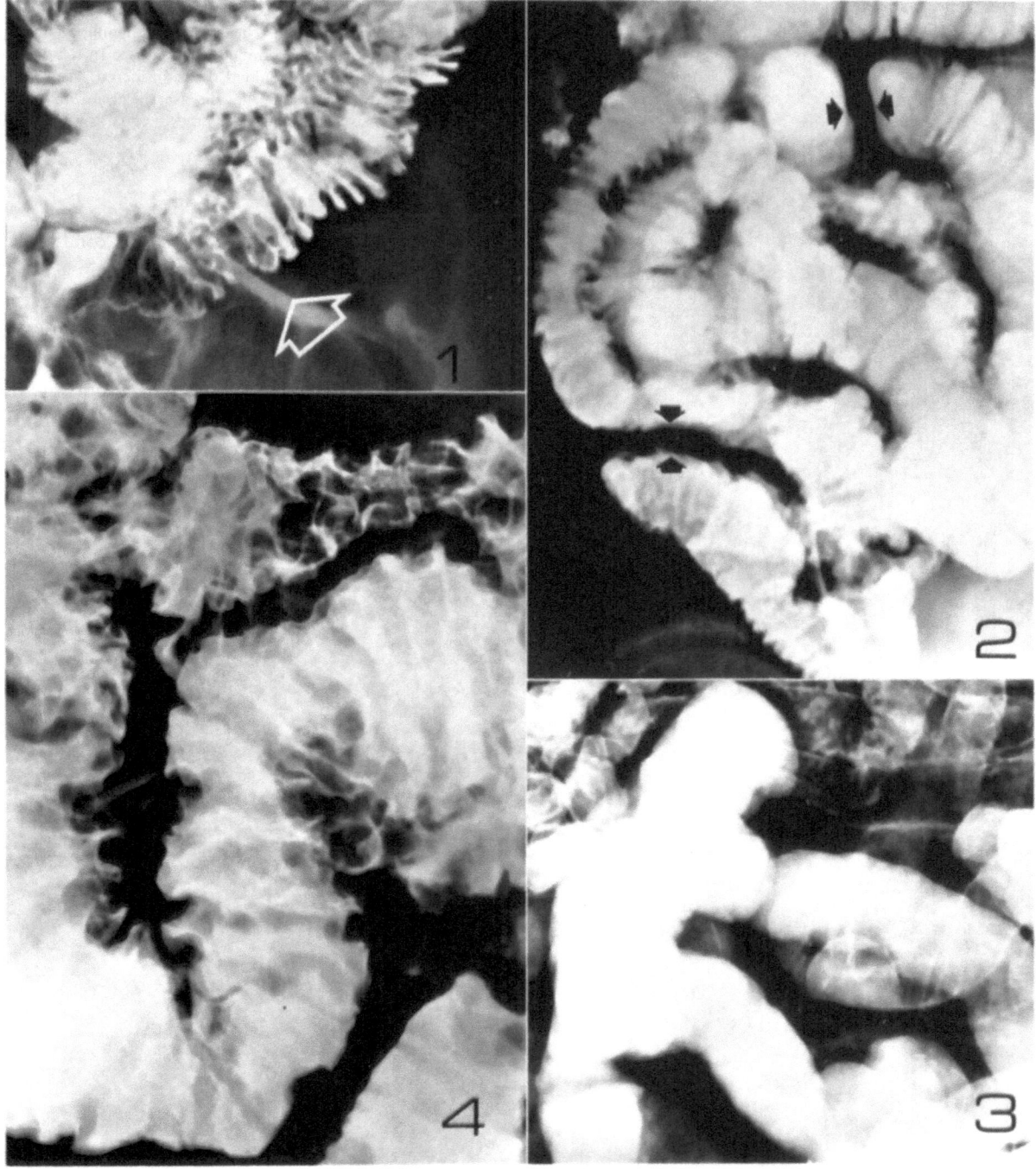

Fig. 12.35. Abnormalities, increasing in severity, in four patients with primary amyloidosis of the small intestine. (1) Decreased motility in the small bowel and mucosal folds with a slightly undulant course in some regions (arrow). (2) No clear-cut abnormalities in the jejunum (not shown). In the ileum the mucosal relief is flattened and the intestinal wall is thickened. Differentiation from a lymphoma (compare fig. 10.35) is not really possible. After remission of Crohn's disease the intestinal wall is neither as thick nor as rigid (stiff). (3) Flat mucosal relief throughout almost the entire small bowel (detail of the patient shown in fig. 12.36). (4) Greatly thickened intestinal wall and broad irregular mucosal folds that in places can no longer be recognized. There are multiple nodular amyloid deposits and unequal dilatation of the intestinal lumen (detail of the patient shown in fig. 12.37).

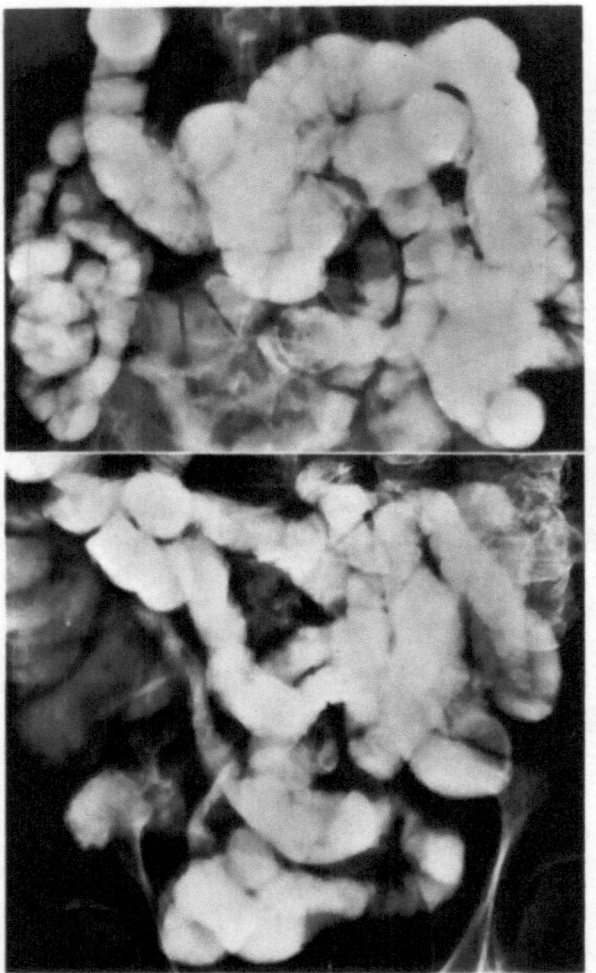

Fig. 12.36. Flat mucosal relief in the duodenum, jejunum, and ileum of a patient with primary amyloidosis. In the differential diagnosis, lymphoma should also be considered. After remission of Crohn's disease and in celiac disease, the abnormalities would be less extensive and the rigidity and unequal thickening of the wall seen here would be missing.

In amyloidosis the lumen may be dilated. If it is not, then differentiation from celiac disease may be difficult and must be based on the findings in the ileum (fig. 12.36). In the colon, atrophy of the mucosa cannot be distinguished roentgenologically from the destruction caused by the chronic use of laxatives. Amyloidosis can only be differentiated radiologically from ulcerative colitis because there are (almost) no ulcerations in the former.

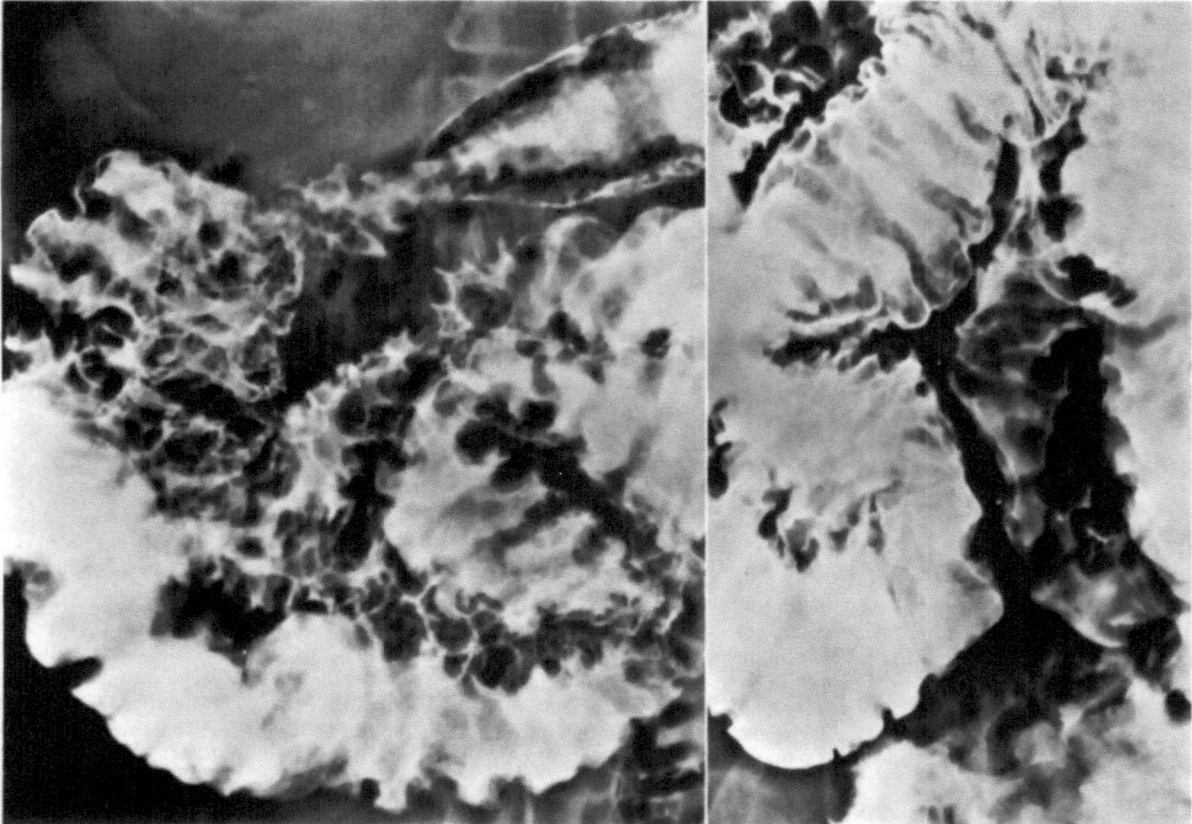

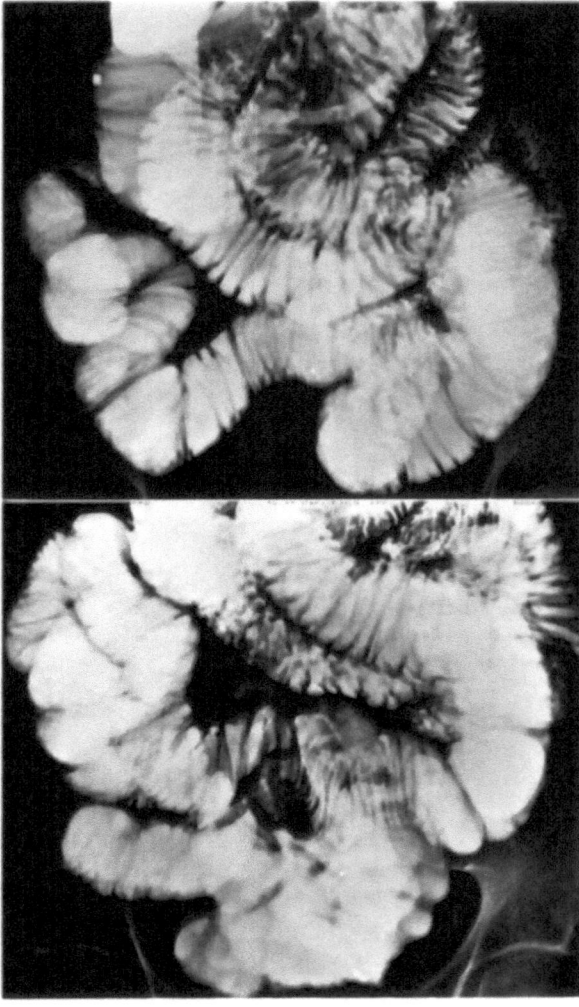

Fig. 12.38. Pseudo-obstruction of the small intestine from disturbed motility in a patient with amyloidosis. There are diverse contractions, especially in the jejunum. Although differentiation from scleroderma or drug-induced atony is most difficult, the presence of sacculations would suggest scleroderma. This degree of dilatation of the ileum and a more pronounced decrease in peristalsis in the jejunum would indicate a drug-induced atony.

Bibliography: chapter 12

Cummings JH (1974) Laxative abuse. Gut 15: 758–766.

Dyer NH, Dawson AM, Smith BF, Todd IP (1969) Obstruction of bowel due to lesion in myenteric plexus. Br Med J 1: 686.

Hyson EA, Burrell M, Toffler R (1977) Drug-induced gastrointestinal disease. Gastrointest Radiol 2: 183–212.

Maldonado JE, Gregg JA. Pagreen AL, Brown NJ (1970) Chronic idiopathic intestinal pseudo-obstruction. Am J Med 49: 203.

Moss A, Goldberg Hl, Brotman M (1972) Idiopathic intestinal pseudo-obstruction. Am J Roentgenol 115: 312.

Naish JM, Capper WM, Brown NJ (1960) Intestinal pseudo-obstruction with steatorrhoea. Gut 1: 62.

Nicolette CC, Tully TE (1971) The duodenum in celiac sprue. Am J Roentgenol 113: 248–254.

Seaman WB (1972) Motor dysfunction of the gastrointestinal tract. Am J Roentgenol 116: 235.

Literature about celiac disease can be found in: Müller WFH (1976) Radiological examination of the small intestine in celiac disease. Leiden.

See also the nos. 3, 8, 11, 14, 29, 35, 43, 52, 59, 66, 76, 97, 184, 194, 196, 206, 231 and 240 of the bibliography on pages 187 and following.

Fig. 12.37. Primary amyloidosis of the small intestine. Both the obviously thickened intestinal wall and the markedly broadened mucosal folds, which can still be recognized here and there, contain numerous pea and marble-sized lumps. The lumen of the intestine shows multiple unequal dilatations without stenoses. In a lymphoreticular malignancy, either there are no pronounced dilatations at all or they are due to a stenosis; in addition, in patients with this disease larger spaces between the intestinal loops are to be expected.

13. CONGENITAL ANOMALIES

1. Abnormal positioning of the entire small bowel: disturbed rotation or fixation

In 90% of the adults, the jejunum is located in the left upper quadrant and the ileum in the right lower quadrant of the abdomen (fig. 13.1). According to Zimmer, a small convolution usually lies in the middle, forming the transition between these two segments of the intestine. The lack of this 'intermediate convolution' may be the most common anomaly. The small intestine usually leaves the retroperitoneal space and enters the abdominal cavity to the left of the spinal column. However, in rare cases Treitz's ligament can also lie in the middle, in front of the spinal column, or even to the right of the latter (fig. 13.2).

Variations in the normal position of the mass of intestinal loops are frequently encountered. They are probably dependent upon the size of the liver at the time of the reduction of the physiological herniation (fig. 13.3). During this reduction, the jejunum may not pass behind the superior mesenteric artery into the left half of the abdomen but instead remains on the right side. We then are confronted with an inversion of the small intestine. In these cases the ileum lies in the middle or to the left in the abdominal cavity (fig. 13.4). If the ileum is found on the left side, the distal segment can lie in the lower, middle or upper abdomen. It is therefore possible that the last ileal loop coming from the left will cross the abdomen diagonally to end up at the cecum in the lower right quadrant (fig. 13.5).

If the entire colon is found in the left half of the abdomen, then the second stage of the rotation phase did not occur at all. The radix mesenterii then will extend more or less vertically from top to bottom. Usually the entire mass of jejunal loops is also located in the right half of the abdomen and the duodenojejunal junction is approximately in the

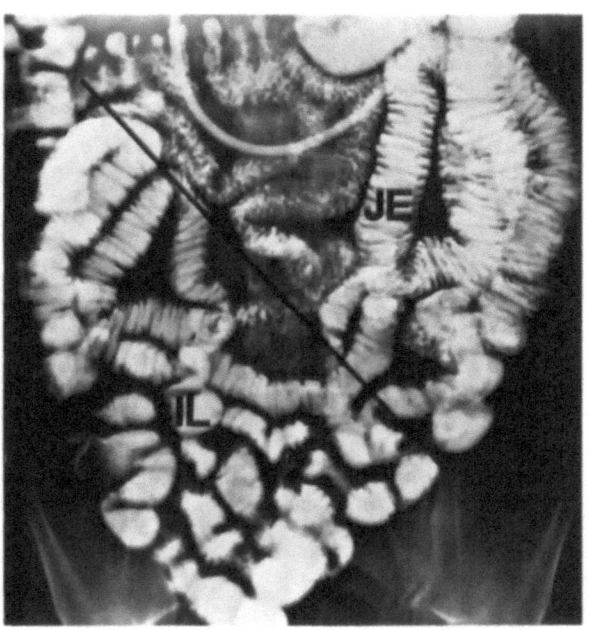

Fig. 13.1. Most common position of the small bowel. Jejunum in left upper quadrant; ileum in right lower quadrant. The line separating these two convolutions is diagonal, running more or less perpendicular to the radix mesenterii which extends from the upper left to the lower right.

center (fig. 13.6). An even more unusual situation occurs when only part of the jejunum passes behind the superior mesenteric artery into the left upper quadrant. Treitz's ligament then is also in the normal position to the right of the spinal column (fig. 13.7).

If the omphalomesenteric duct is far removed from Bauhin's valve, most of the ileal loops may end up in the right half of the abdomen during the second stage of rotation (fig. 13.8). If the ascending colon does not drop, the cecum may also be found in the upper right quadrant. The relationship between the failure of the ascending colon to drop and a distal ileum that is high in the right upper quadrant is not clear. It is striking that this com-

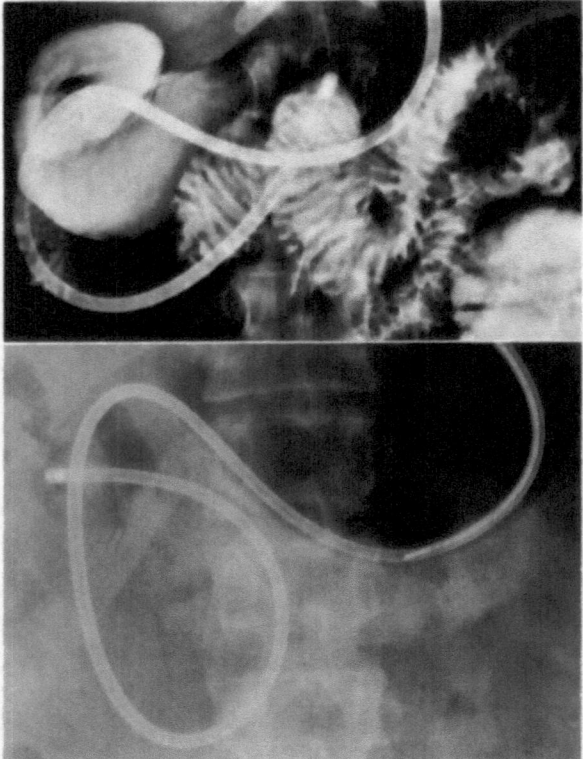

Fig. 13.2. Treitz's ligament may also be found in the center in front of the spinal column (top) or next to it on the right (bottom).

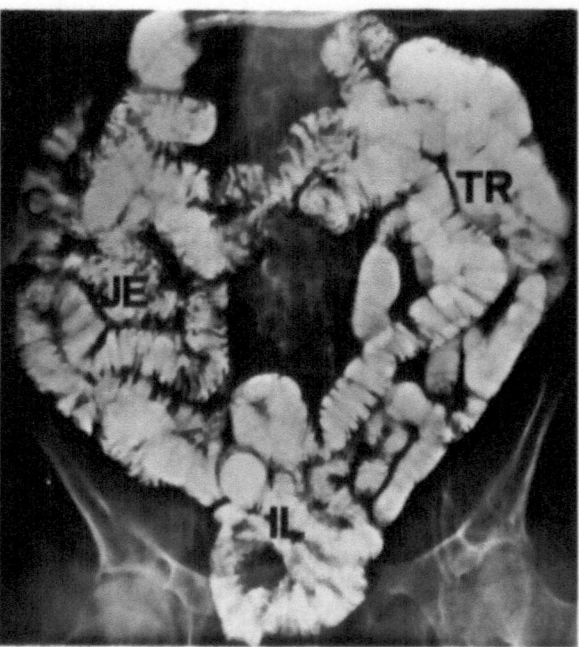

Fig. 13.4. If after reduction of the physiological herniation the jejunal loops do not pass behind the superior mesenteric artery to the upper left quadrant but remain on the right, then the ileal loops are forced to lie more or less in the left half of the abdomen. In this case the transition (TR) between the jejunum and the ileum is in the upper left quadrant. In contrast to a total inversion, the duodenum and the cecum are in the normal position here. Furthermore in this patient, the ascending colon barely descended so that the cecum (C) is in the right upper quadrant.

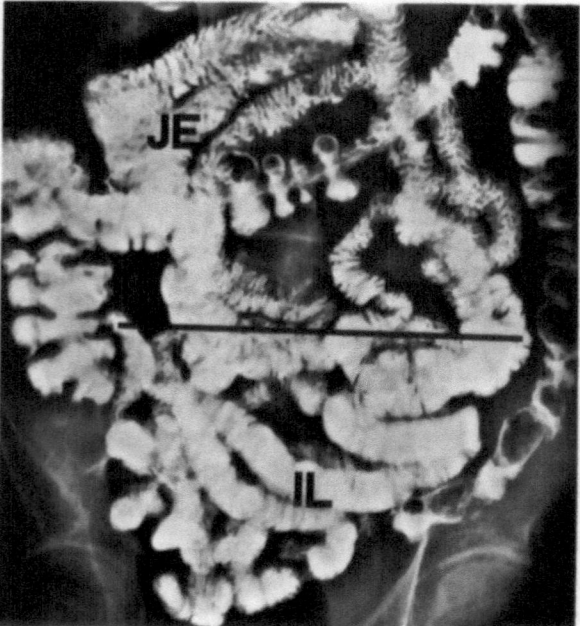

Fig. 13.3. A fairly frequently encountered variation in the position of the mass of loops of the small intestine is when the jejunum lies more or less in the middle of the upper abdomen with the ileum directly underneath.

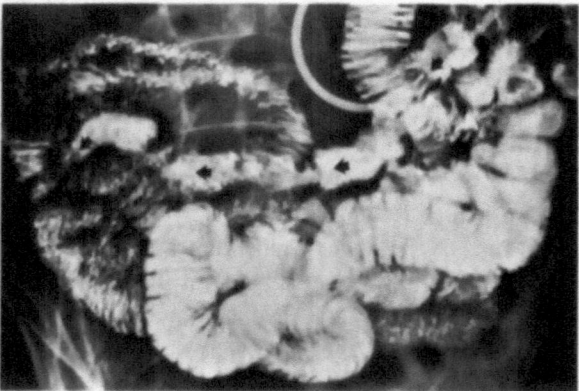

Fig. 13.5. The jejunum is in the right half of the abdomen and the ileum in the left. The distal ileum crosses the abdomen diagonally from left to right (arrows).

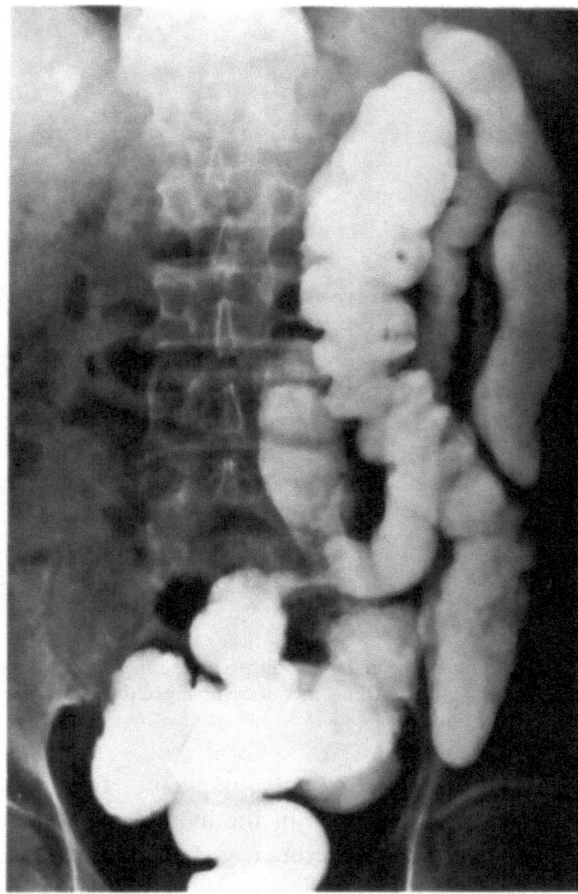

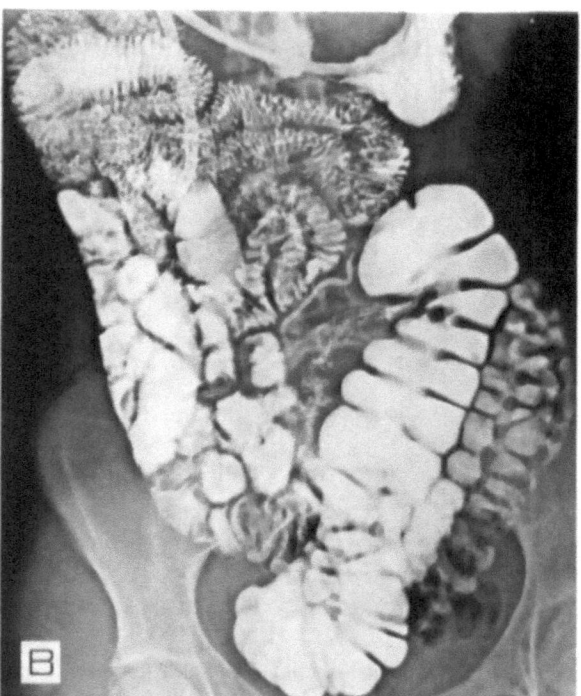

Fig. 13.6B. Patient with vague abdominal complaints and periodic cramps. There is a rotational anomaly of the large and the small intestine. The appendix is located near the navel. There was pronounced hypermotility so that the small intestine and the entire colon could be filled with 600 ml contrast fluid within 6 min. Hypermotility is not unusual in patients with a rotational anomaly. Presumably hypermotility can be attributed to anoxia of the small intestine resulting from a (temporary) disturbance of the blood flow. The rapid passage and decreased oxygenation of the intestinal wall often cause malabsorption with quick flocculation of the contrast fluid, as seen in this patient.

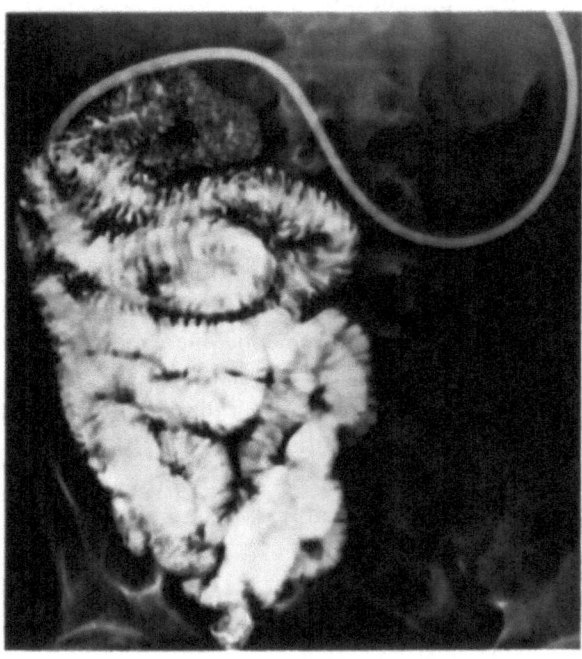

Fig. 13.6A. Lack of rotation of the mesentery and the intestine. The colon lies on the far left in the abdomen and the small bowel on the right. Treitz's ligament is in the middle.

bination is encountered regularly (fig. 13.9).

Lack of fixation of the cecum after descent can lead to excessive mobility and eventually to a lateral Bauhin's valve (fig. 13.10). When fixation of the cecum is retarded, it may show pronounced growth in length. A low cecum may develop if in the final stage descent of the ascending colon continues too long. In all of these cases the cecum can end up deep in the minor pelvis and may in addition become very voluminous (fig. 13.11). If the cecum and the sigmoid then become filled with feces, they can block the minor pelvis so completely that the ileum is severely compressed (fig. 13.12).

Quite rare are the cases of total stomach–intestine inversion. In this anomaly the jejunum lies in the middle of the upper abdomen, the ileum in the middle of the lower abdomen and the stomach and the cecum to the left.

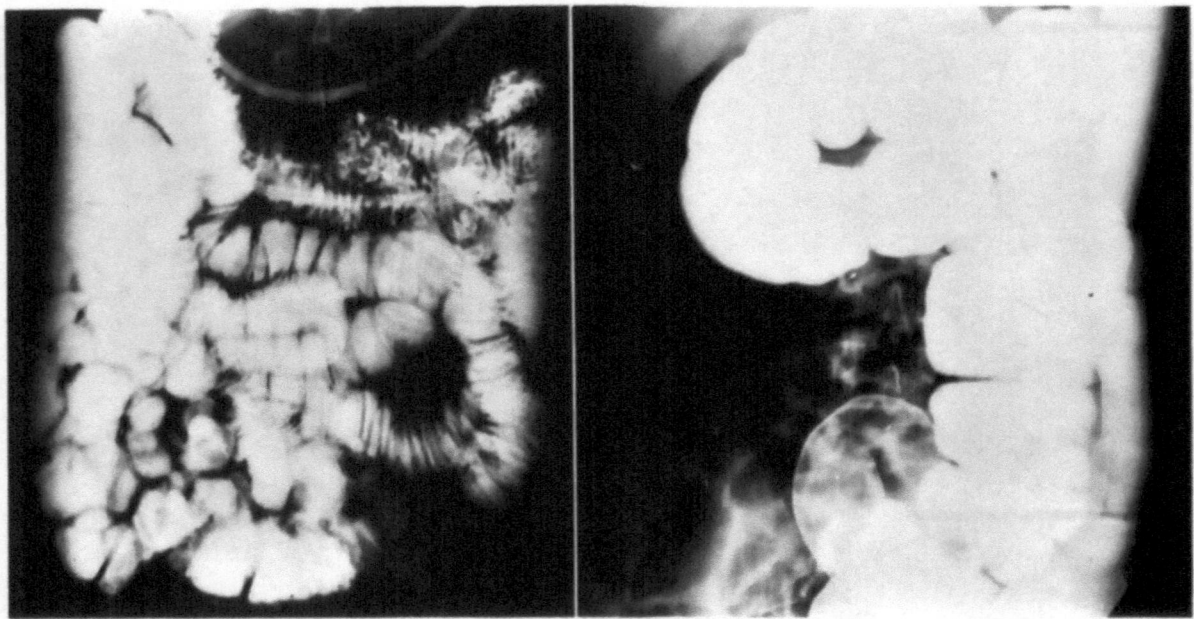

Fig. 13.7. Although the intestine failed to rotate as in fig. 13.6, the proximal jejunum was displaced during reduction of the physiological herniation to the upper left quadrant. Possibly a liver of unusual size or a difference in the timing of the reduction of the physiological herniation played a role in the abnormal course of events in figs. 13.6 and 13.7.

Although it is a striking abnormality, malrotation during embryonal development is often overlooked, or is at least not included in reports. Fortunately this negligence seldom has consequences since most developmental anomalies do not give rise to complaints. This is not always true since some inversions can be reduced rather easily and can cause intermittent complaints. In particular temporary inversion of the most proximal jejunal loops sometimes occurs (fig. 13.13). Probably as a result of some torsion of the involved intestinal segment, slight vascular disorders may develop. The ease with which temporary inversions can occur increases as the length of the intestinal mesentery increases and that of the radix mesenterii therefore decreases.

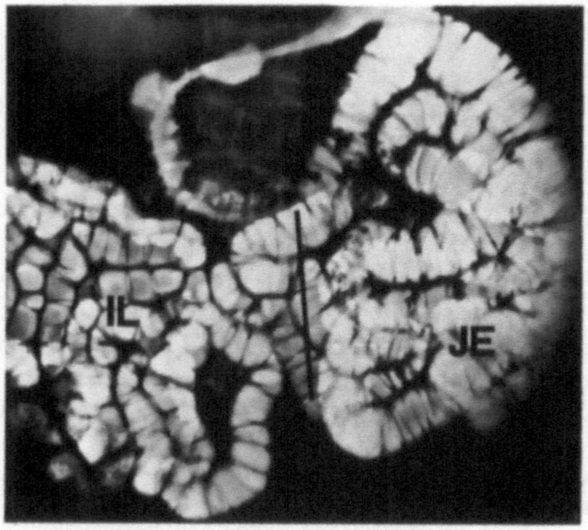

Further questioning may reveal that some patients have colic-like attacks of abdominal pain whenever they assume an abnormal position. Examples are bending over, climbing (or descending) the stairs quickly, etc. – especially when making sharp thrusting movements. There must be personal contact between the physician and the patient in these cases before a correct diagnosis can be established. The diagnosis will certainly be missed if survey films taken by a laboratory assistant are considered sufficient.

2. Abnormal or fixed positioning of several intestinal loops: internal hernia

In about the eleventh fetal week, rotation of the digestive tract is completed and the small intestine

Fig. 13.8. If the omphalomesenteric duct is far from the cecum, there is an increased risk that during reduction of the physiological herniation a large section of the ileum will end up in the right half of the abdominal cavity.

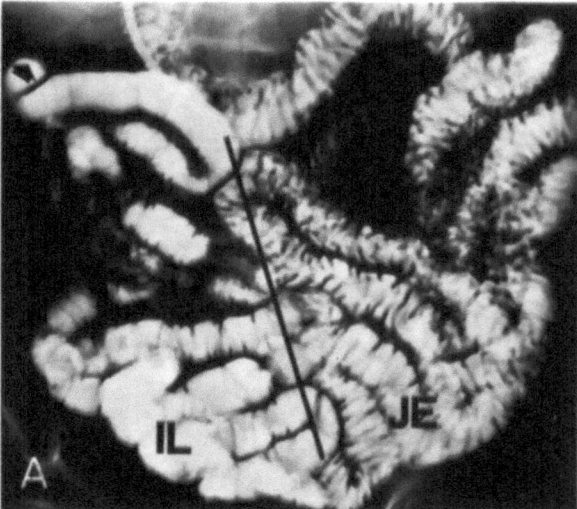

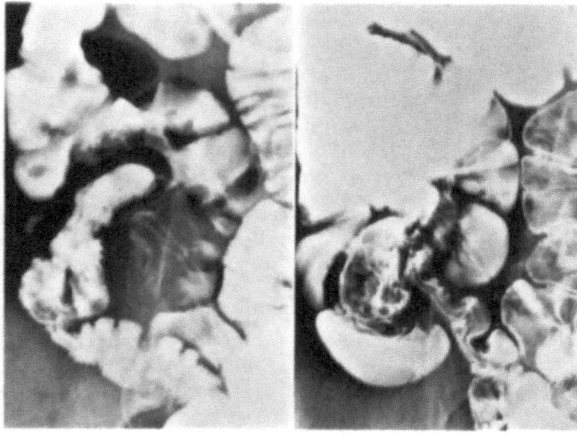

Fig. 13.10. Excessive mobility of the cecum; Bauhin's valve will then sometimes assume a lateral position.

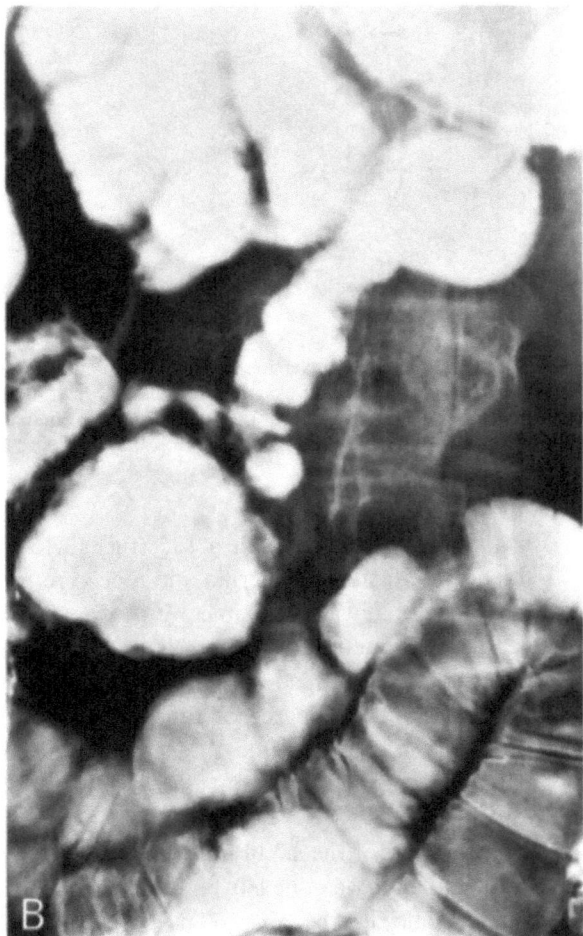

Fig. 13.9. (A) The jejunum is to the left in the abdomen, the ileum to the right. Since the ascending colon failed to drop, the cecum (not yet filled here) and Bauhin's valve are situated under the liver in the upper abdomen. (B) Ileum in the right upper quadrant and incomplete descent of the cecum. The jejunum was in the left half of the abdomen and the transition between the two parts of the intestine was found in the middle of the lower abdomen.

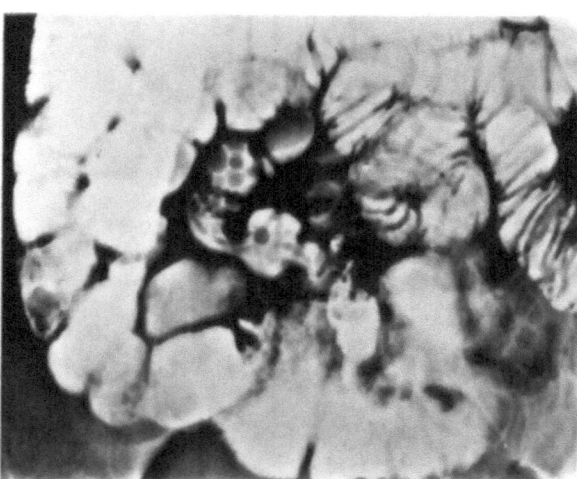

Fig. 13.11. Excessive lengthwise growth of the cecum because descent of the ascending colon lasted too long; this may sometimes be accompanied by abnormal fixation. See also fig. 7.30.

and the colon assume their final positions in the abdomen. After this phase a number of bands or adhesions form between several intestinal loops and the surrounding tissue that serve to fix these loops in position. If these bands or adhesions develop before the intestine has assumed its final position, then the abnormalities described above can occur. If they are inadequate or completely missing then, as we have seen, pathological mobility can develop locally. An incomplete or partial fixation can, however, also be such that the intestinal loops can herniate through the resulting opening. Such hernias are found in the region of the ileocecal valve,

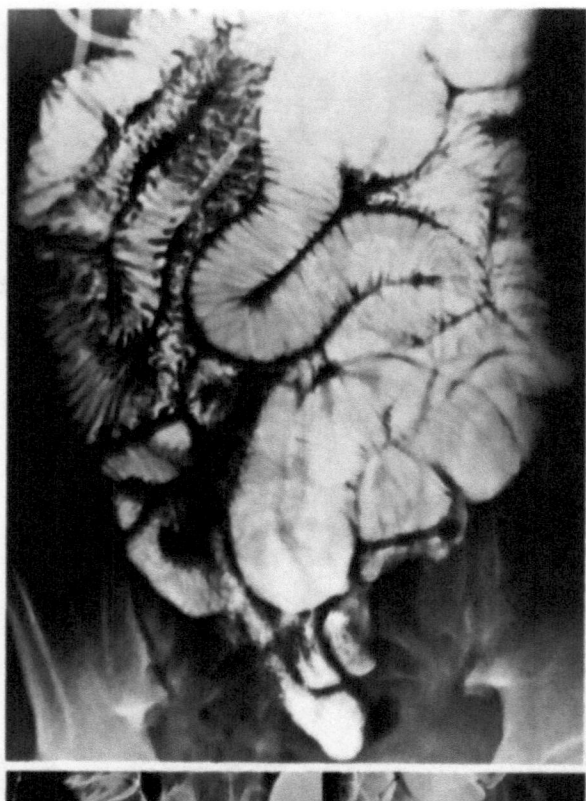

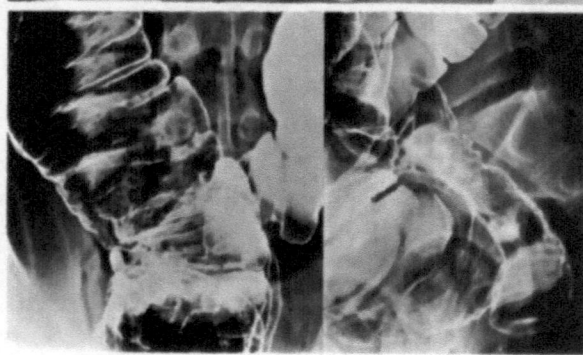

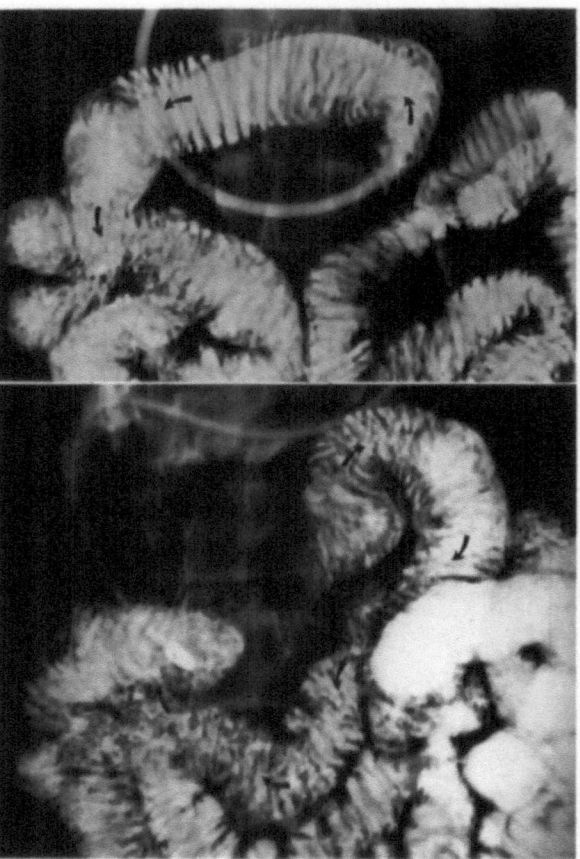

Fig. 13.13. Temporary inversion of the most proximal part of the jejunum. During the first examination this loop was located in the right upper quadrant (top); in a subsequent examination it was approximately in the middle (bottom).

Fig. 13.12. If the sigmoid and a deep-seated voluminous cecum both contain large quantities of feces, they can block the entrance to the minor pelvis. The distal ileum will become somewhat constricted and temporary obstruction can develop; this is recognized by the ileal loops' dilatation that increases in the distal direction.

the so-called retrocecal hernia, and in the duo-denojejunal flexure, where left and right paraduo-denal hernias develop (fig. 13.14). The latter type in particular accounts for half of all internal hernias. It can become quite large and cause alarming clinical signs that resemble the clinical findings of obstruction in the proximal intestine.

In the region of the ileocecal valve, a fairly deep sac can develop, especially if the mesentery of the distal ileum is long. A mass of ileal loops can easily

become fixed within such a sac (fig. 13.15). Dif-ferentiation between a hernia and a deep retrocecal fossa is not always possible by means of roent-genology. Sometimes the fossa is so small that the intestinal loop trapped within it can be forced free by increasing the degree of filling (fig. 13.16). In general it is not possible to use compression or palpation to force loops out of a hernia or a deep fossa.

Herniation of the small intestine through defects in the mesentery can be left-handed as well as right-handed. They can become so large that they include practically all the loops of the small intestine.

Congenital or traumatic defects in the mesentery, the mesocolon, or the mesosigmoid can cause compression of a large or small segment of the small intestine (fig. 13.17A). Such abnormalities can also result from an inflammatory process or surgery (fig.

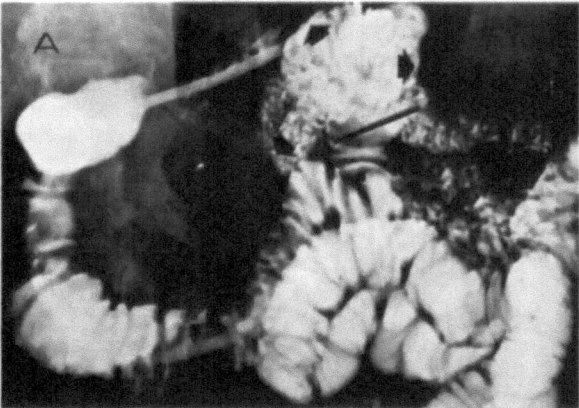

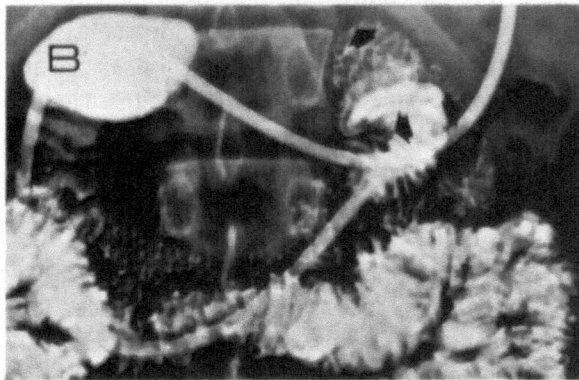

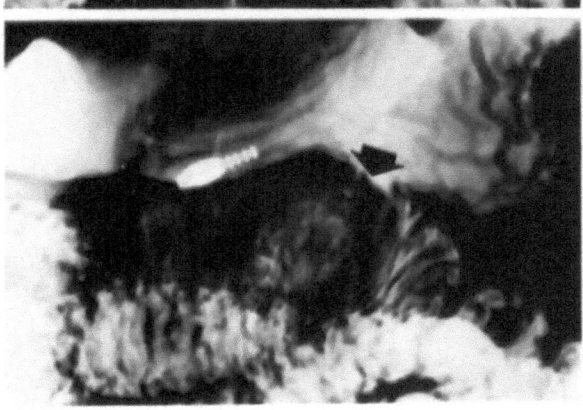

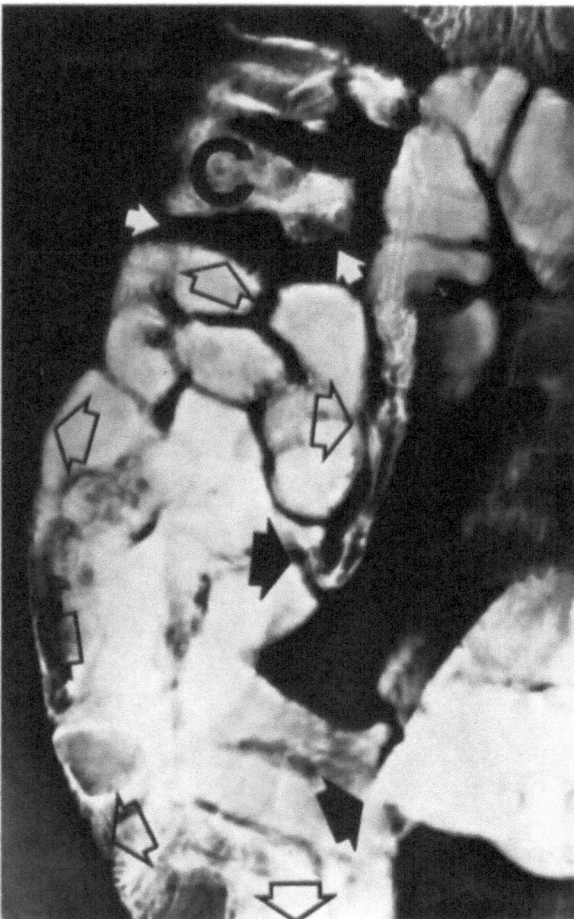

*Fig. 13.15*A. Large sac (open black arrow) containing fixed ileal loops filled with air. The afferent and efferent ileal loop indicated black arrows. C, secum.

Fig. 13.14. Two cases of paraduodenal herniation. (A) There were only slight intermittent complaints so that surgery was not necessary. (B) The hernia is small but the complaints were quite severe (top). During complaint-free periods, the herniation was not visible (bottom).

13.17B). Another common type of herniation is through the transverse mesocolon. The intestinal loops, part of the omentum, or both end up behind the stomach, causing a clear impression on the pars antralis (fig. 13.18).

Finally an inguinal or abdominal herniation may also be encountered. In addition the foramen of Winslow can be too large so that the intestinal loops pass easily into the lesser peritoneal sac. In order to determine the diagnosis, lateral exposures are often essential, especially in the event of an abdominal hernia at the site of an old surgical scar. Sometimes in this type of hernia, anterioposterior exposures will reveal nothing since the orifice can be missed rather easily in this direction. It is also important that the contrast column be followed under fluoroscopy since intestinal motility in and in front of the hernia is often locally but clearly disturbed. There may be an obstruction or locally reduced motility. Usually there is a pronounced hypermotility and the patients complain of recurring colic-like attacks of abdominal pain localized exactly at the site of the hernia. Another characteristic is that the afferent and efferent loops of the compressed intestine taper slightly at the hernial orifice that is in itself invisible.

394

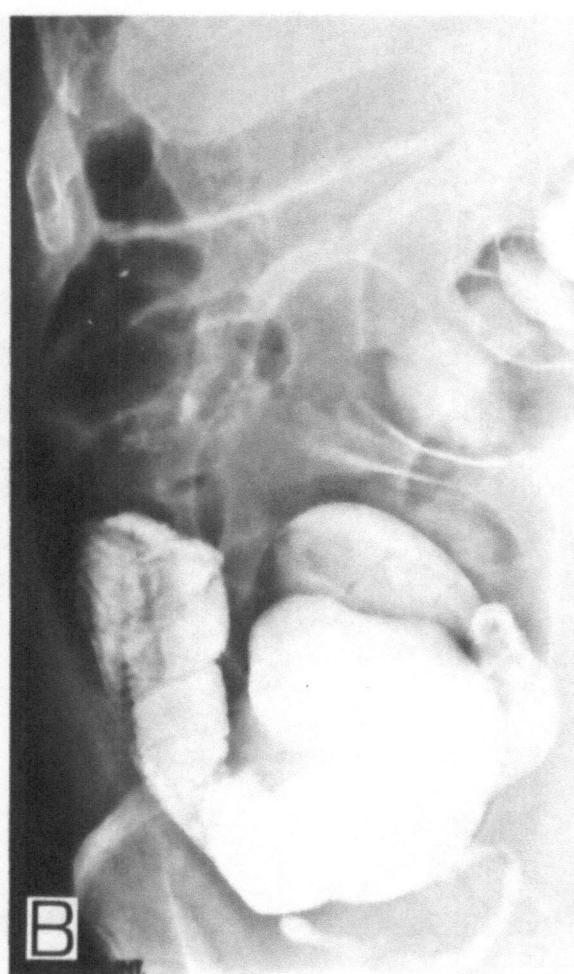

*Fig. 13.15.*B. The last meter of the ileum is located on the lateral side of the ascending colon under the liver in the right upper quadrant. Usually, as here, this is not the result of herniation whereby the ileum passes behind the colon. It is the result of a long mesentery that passes in front of the colon. This condition is quite different from the one in fig. 13.15A!

They also lie close together and are absolutely fixed so that they cannot be moved by palpation. If survey photographs of the abdomen are made before the contrast medium examination, it will be noted that several intestinal loops consistently lie close together and are filled with air. Moreover, when the patient is filmed upright, these loops show fluid levels.

According to numerous reports in the literature, a preoperative radiological examination almost never yields a diagnosis of 'internal hernia'. We have found, however, that this disorder with its fairly classic history is easily recognized. The possible diagnosis must be at least considered, and the roentgen examination must be carried out by using the enteroclysis technique with intermittent fluoroscopy.

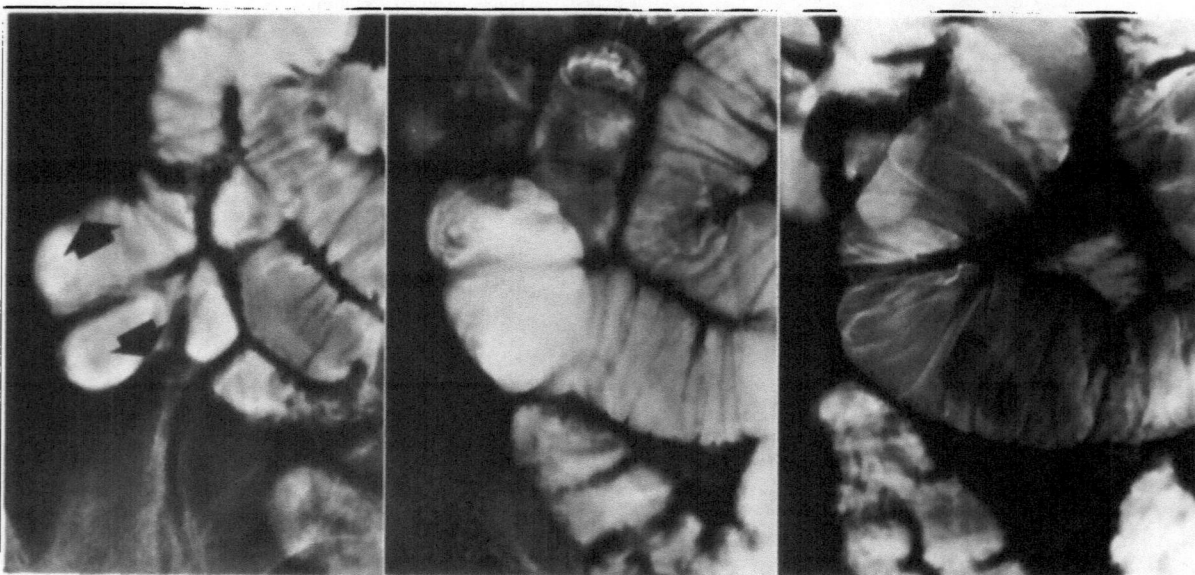

Fig. 13.16. Segment of ileal loop in shallow retrocecal fossa (arrows) that was freed (from left to right) by means of maximum filling (water infusion).

395

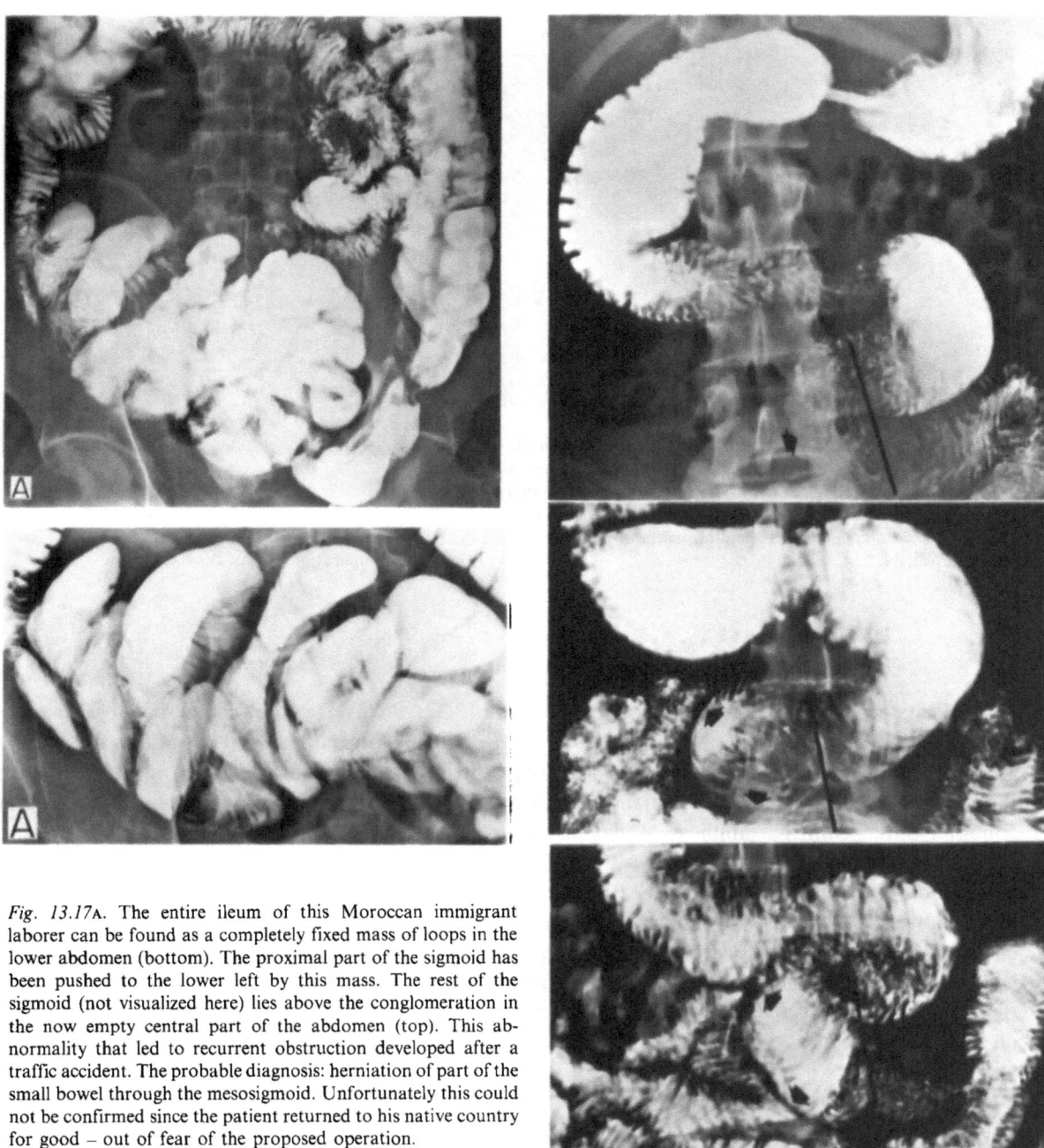

*Fig. 13.17*A. The entire ileum of this Moroccan immigrant laborer can be found as a completely fixed mass of loops in the lower abdomen (bottom). The proximal part of the sigmoid has been pushed to the lower left by this mass. The rest of the sigmoid (not visualized here) lies above the conglomeration in the now empty central part of the abdomen (top). This abnormality that led to recurrent obstruction developed after a traffic accident. The probable diagnosis: herniation of part of the small bowel through the mesosigmoid. Unfortunately this could not be confirmed since the patient returned to his native country for good – out of fear of the proposed operation.

*Fig. 13.17*B. Herniation of a segment of the proximal jejunal loop through a small defect in the mesentery (straight black line) that developed after surgical removal of a mesenteric cyst. Proximal to the herniation is a prestenotic dilatation. On the distal side is local, pronounced hyperperistalsis that caused the colic-like attacks of abdominal pain.

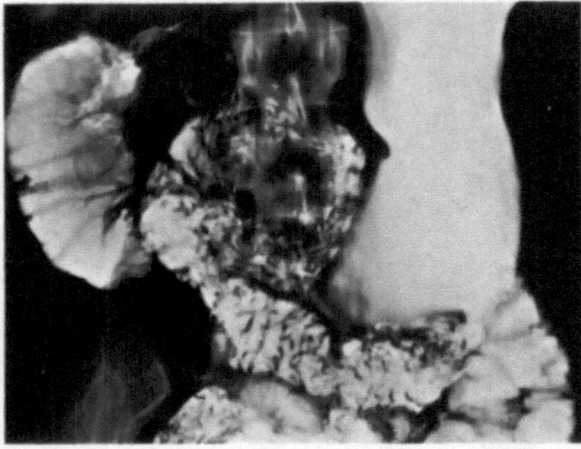

Fig. 13.18. Compression effect of proximal jejunal loop on the posterior pars antralis of the stomach. This is encountered in cases of herniation through the transverse mesocolon (or through a dilated foramen of Winslow into the lesser sac). In this case there were no complaints and therefore surgical confirmation was not available.

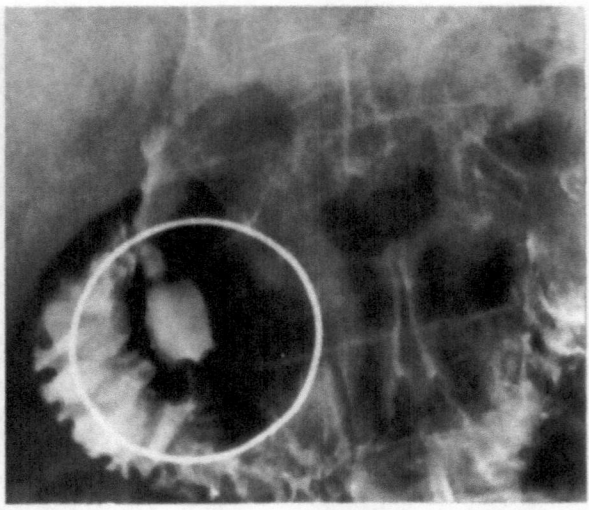

Fig. 13.19. Duplication cyst in the duodenum.

3. Duplications

Although duplications can occur anywhere along the entire length of the small intestine, they are most common in the ileum. The duplication may become filled with contrast fluid if there is an open communication with the intestinal lumen (fig. 13.19). Often, however, this is not the case and the space is enclosed. An accumulation of secretion in this space will cause the so-called duplication cyst. Sometimes the only indication of these cysts is an impression on adjacent loops.

4. Diverticulosis

Small groups of two to three diverticula are frequently found in the small intestine, almost always in the duodenum. Larger groups of four to six, localized in the proximal jejunum, are a somewhat less frequent finding. In our departments we have encountered this in one out of every 200 examinations of the small intestine (fig. 13.20); 20–30 diverticula spread throughout the entire jejunum are found in one of every 800 patients (fig. 13.21). In diverticulosis, the number and size of the diverticula decrease gradually in the distal direction (fig.

13.22). A diverticulosis in the ileum is therefore a rare phenomenon. In our series this was seen only twice in 4000 examinations (fig. 13.23). Diverticulosis seldom causes complaints. Occasionally, however, a volvulus may develop as well as a diverticulitis or dyspeptic complaints from a disturbance in the bacterial flora as a result of stasis. Mechanical complications can develop especially if the diverticula are extremely large. If the mesentery is extra long, then as a result of changes in posture, pronounced changes in the position of the loops can occur. Torsion of a diverticulum may easily develop leading to necrosis and perforation (fig. 13.24). Perforation can occur during duodenal intubation if the location of the diverticulum is unfavorable (fig. 13.20c). In our experience we have had the tube in diverticula but not yet seen perforation in 10,000 cases.

Acquired diverticula are usually located on the mesenteric side of the intestine where the wall is the weakest due to the presence of vascular openings. The wall of such a diverticulum is thin and, like false diverticula in Crohn's disease, does not contain the muscular layer.

False diverticula in Crohn's disease are easily differentiated from other diverticula because they form in an obviously diseased intestinal wall (fig.

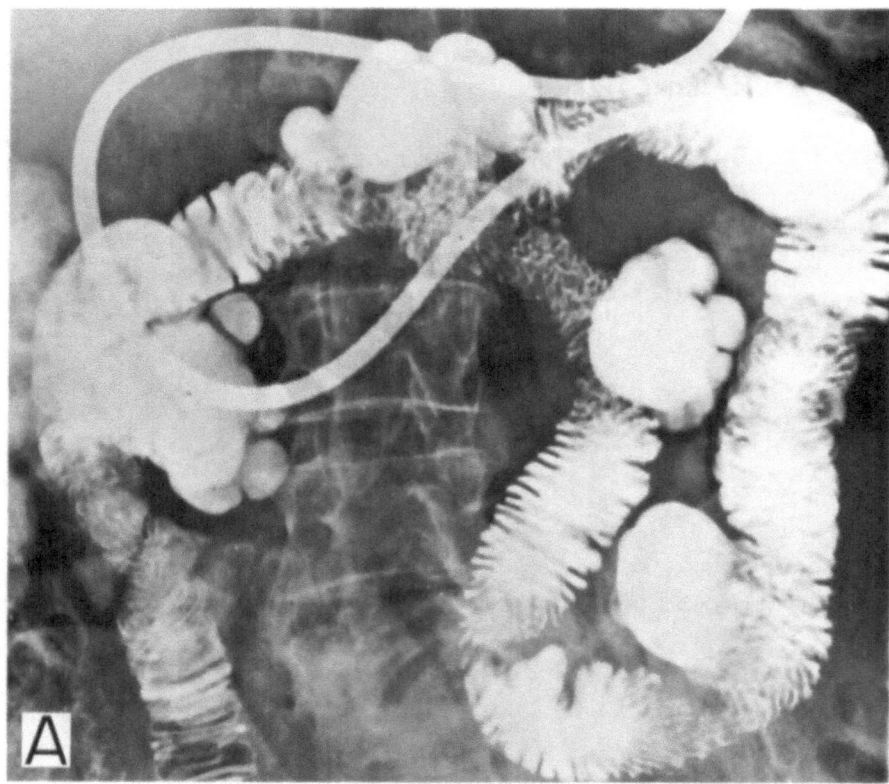

*Fig. 13.20*A. Multiple large jejunal diverticula, some of which also contain a number of diverticula on their surface.

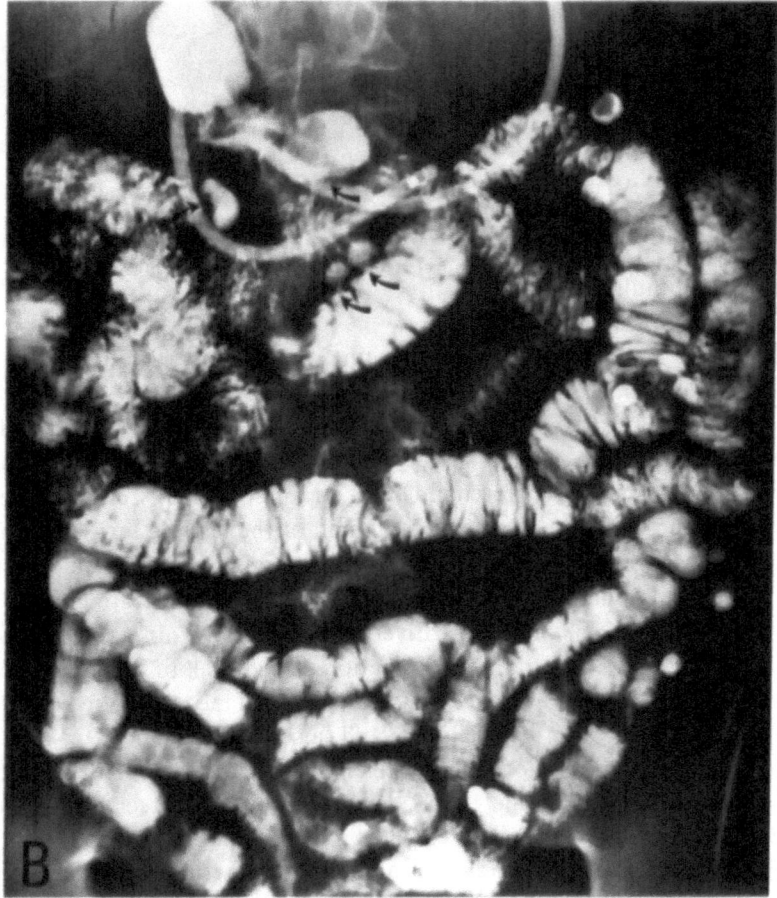

*Fig. 13.20*B. Four diverticula in the duodenum and proximal jejunum. The more intensive white small round shadows in the left half of the abdomen are from residual contrast fluid in colonic diverticula after an enema one week prior to the enteroclysis examination.

398

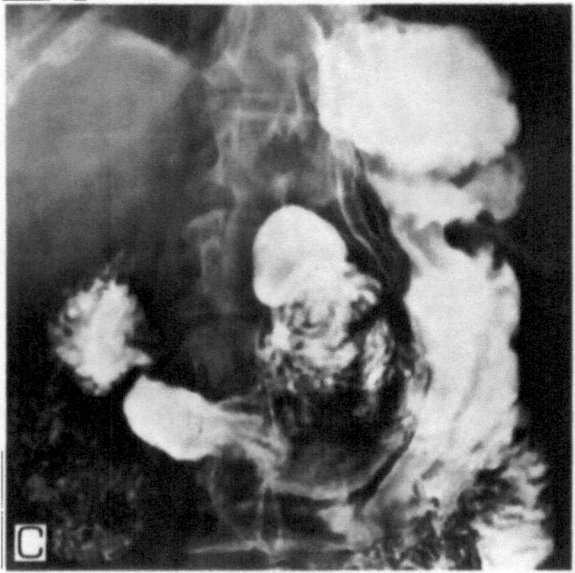

Fig. 13.20c. Large diverticulum in duodeno-jejunal flexure. Danger of perforation by duodenal intubation.

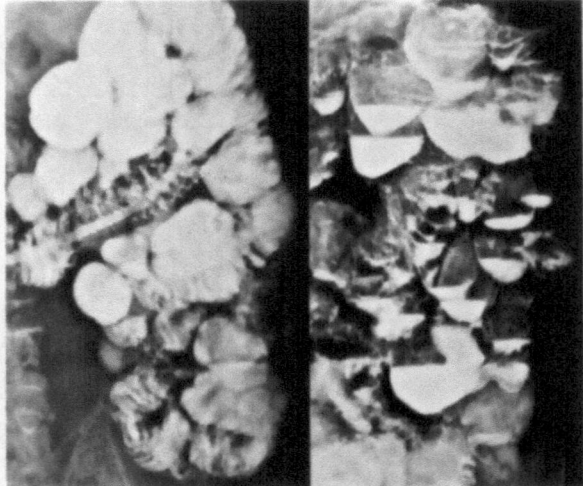

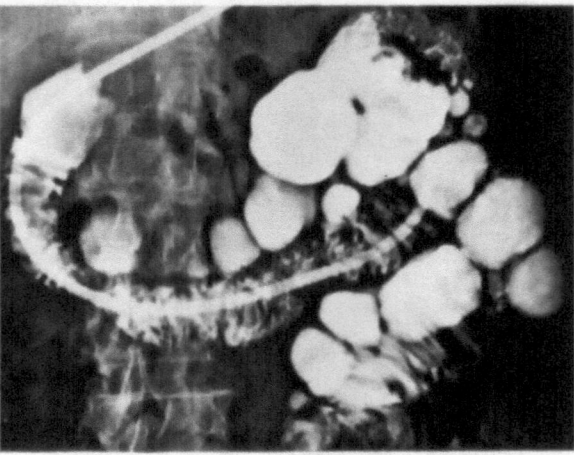

Fig. 13.21. Numerous large diverticula in the duodenum and jejunum. They are visualized most easily when the intestine is in the contraction phase and is therefore relatively empty. When the patient is erect, there are numerous fluid levels.

13.25).

Congenital diverticula are on the antimesenteric side of the intestine. They involve the tunica muscularis and are therefore contractile.

The mucosal folds in the intestinal wall can be followed through the neck of the diverticulum. However, in practice this cannot always be determined with certainty so that differentiation between a congenital anomaly and an acquired diverticulosis is usually not possible (fig. 13.26).

One must be careful not to consider all multiple sac-like bulges in the intestine diverticula. One such case for example, is illustrated in fig. 13.27. Four or five diverticula-like formations are seen to originate from one point and appear to vary in size from 2 to 20 cm. It was found that they developed from multiple autoamputations after a hernia during adolescence was treated surgically. It was no longer possible to determine whether erroneous ligation played a role in the development of this peculiar anatomical phenomenon.

5. Meckel's diverticulum

Every serious radiologist is greatly disappointed if his findings are not confirmed by specialists from other disciplines. In the case of an examination of

the small intestine, this means the findings of the surgeon and the pathologist.

One abnormality that usually is not identified until surgery or autopsy, and seldom diagnosed beforehand by the radiologist, is Meckel's diverticulum. Although all of the leading textbooks mention Meckel's diverticulum and list the complications, radiological illustrations are sparse. A Meckel's diverticulum is only observed during a transit examination of the small bowel in those rare instances when the contrast medium ended up in the diverticulum and also was retained in the sac noticeably longer than in the rest of the intestine (fig. 13.28). A diverticulum is occasionally also recognized when it is particularly large. This failure of radiological diagnosis must be attributed mainly

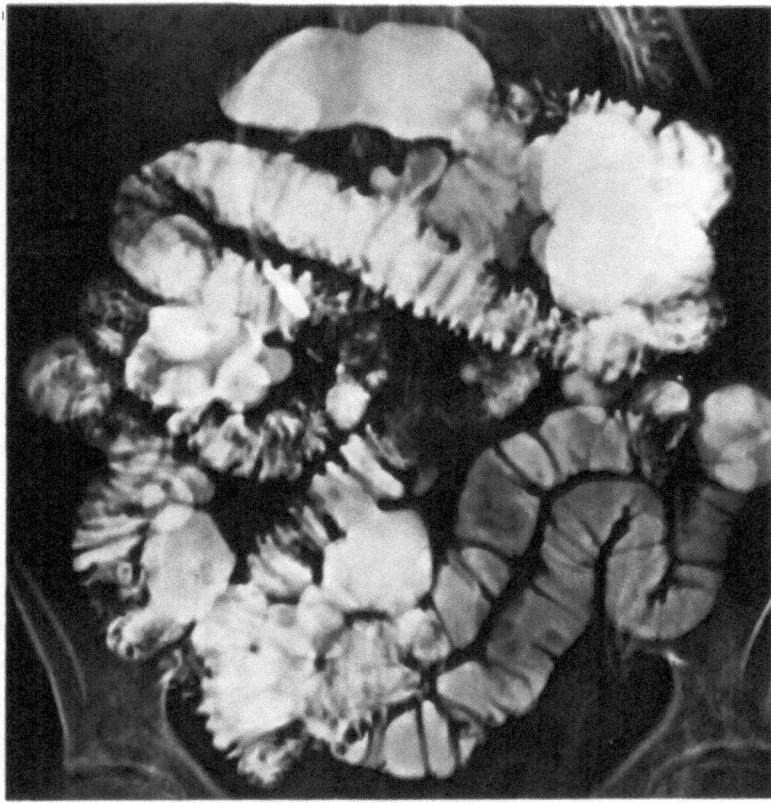

Fig. 13.22. Jejunal diverticulosis. The size and number of the diverticula decrease in the distal direction.

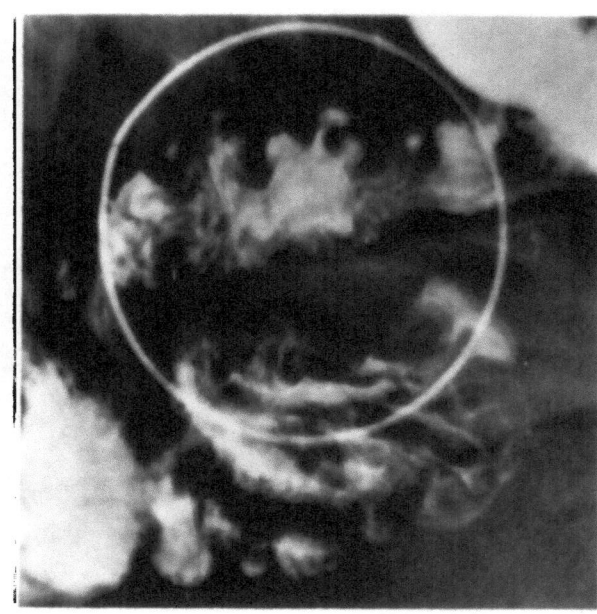

Fig. 13.23. Six small diverticula in the distal ileum. Ileal diverticulosis is a rare phenomenon.

to an inadequate examination technique. The low diagnostic score in part is also because the clinical course can sometimes be so acute that the patient must undergo immediate surgery. Therefore there is no time for a radiological examination of the small intestine. This is especially true since it had usually proven to be of little value. Since the small bowel examination can now be carried out quickly by means of enteroclysis, the disappointing results regarding the diagnosis of a Meckel's diverticulum have certainly improved. Now by means of enteroclysis, a Meckel's diverticulum is found in one out of every 150 patients. We believe, however, that a Meckel's diverticulum is still overlooked in an approximately equal number of cases. In one of our patients this happened because during the examination we concentrated too heavily on a concomitant jejunal tumor. In two other cases we were diverted by Crohn's disease (fig. 13.29A). This is understandable, especially in one of these cases where a local

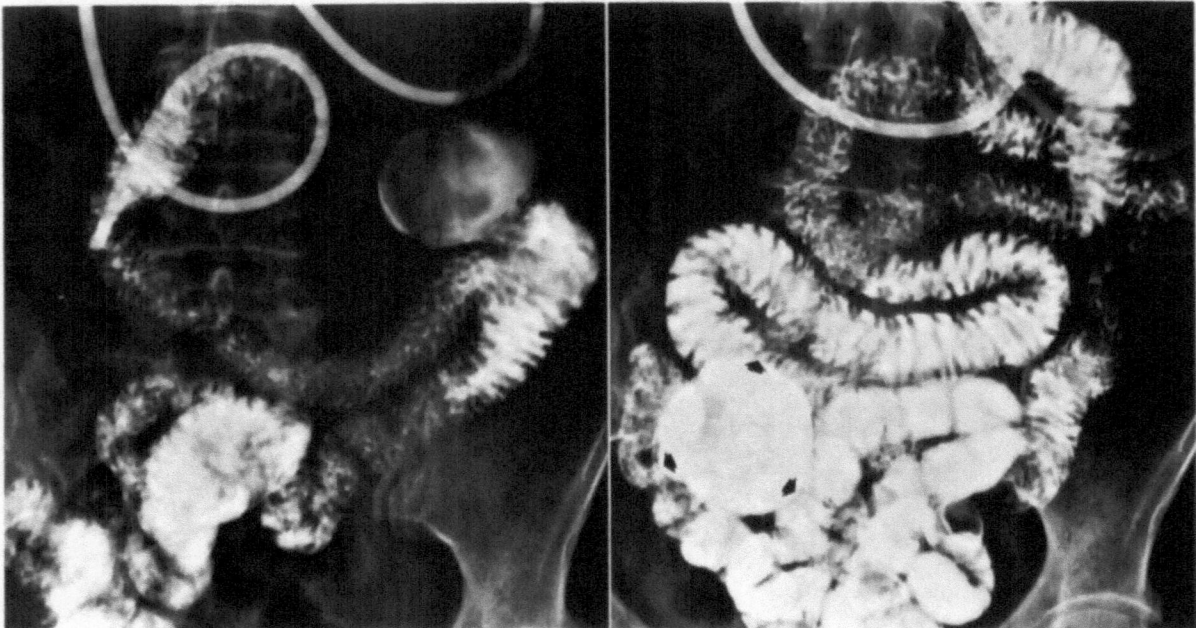

Fig. 13.24. Large highly mobile diverticulum in the proximal jejunum. With changes in the patient's posture, the neck of such a diverticulum can easily twist, producing the symptoms of an acute abdomen. The danger of necrosis and perforation is a real possibility.

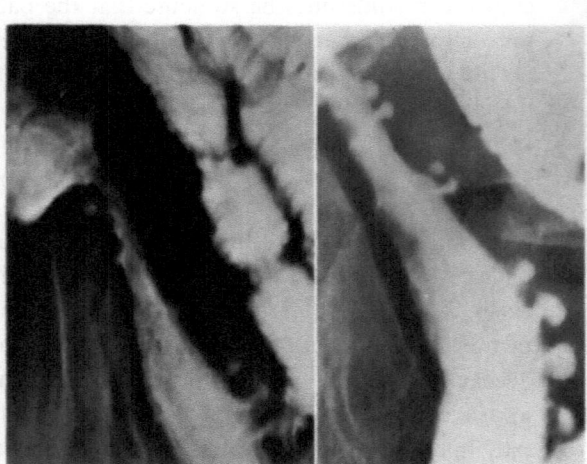

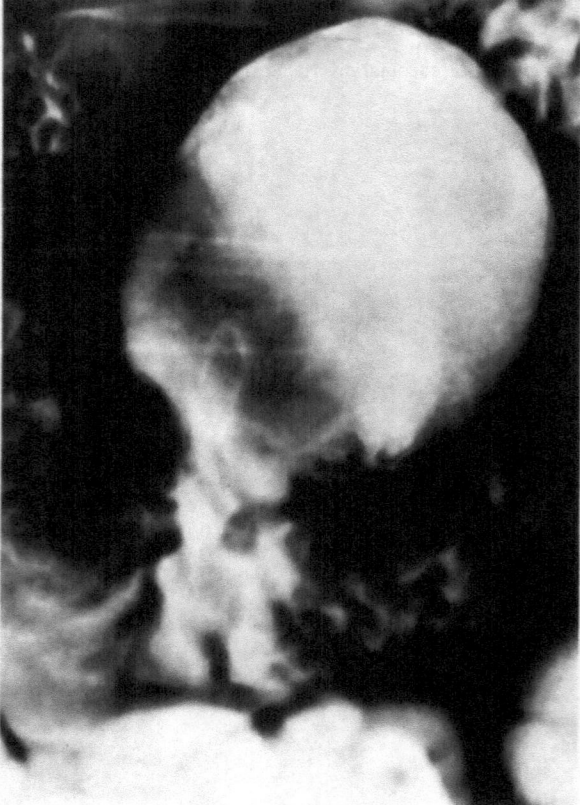

Fig. 13.25. False diverticula in Crohn's disease are easily distinguished from true diverticula. They develop in a clearly diseased intestinal wall, as in this case where mucosal folds can no longer be seen.

Fig. 13.26. Large solitary diverticulum in the small intestine probably congenital in origin since the mucosal folds of the intestinal wall can be followed easily through the neck of the diverticulum.

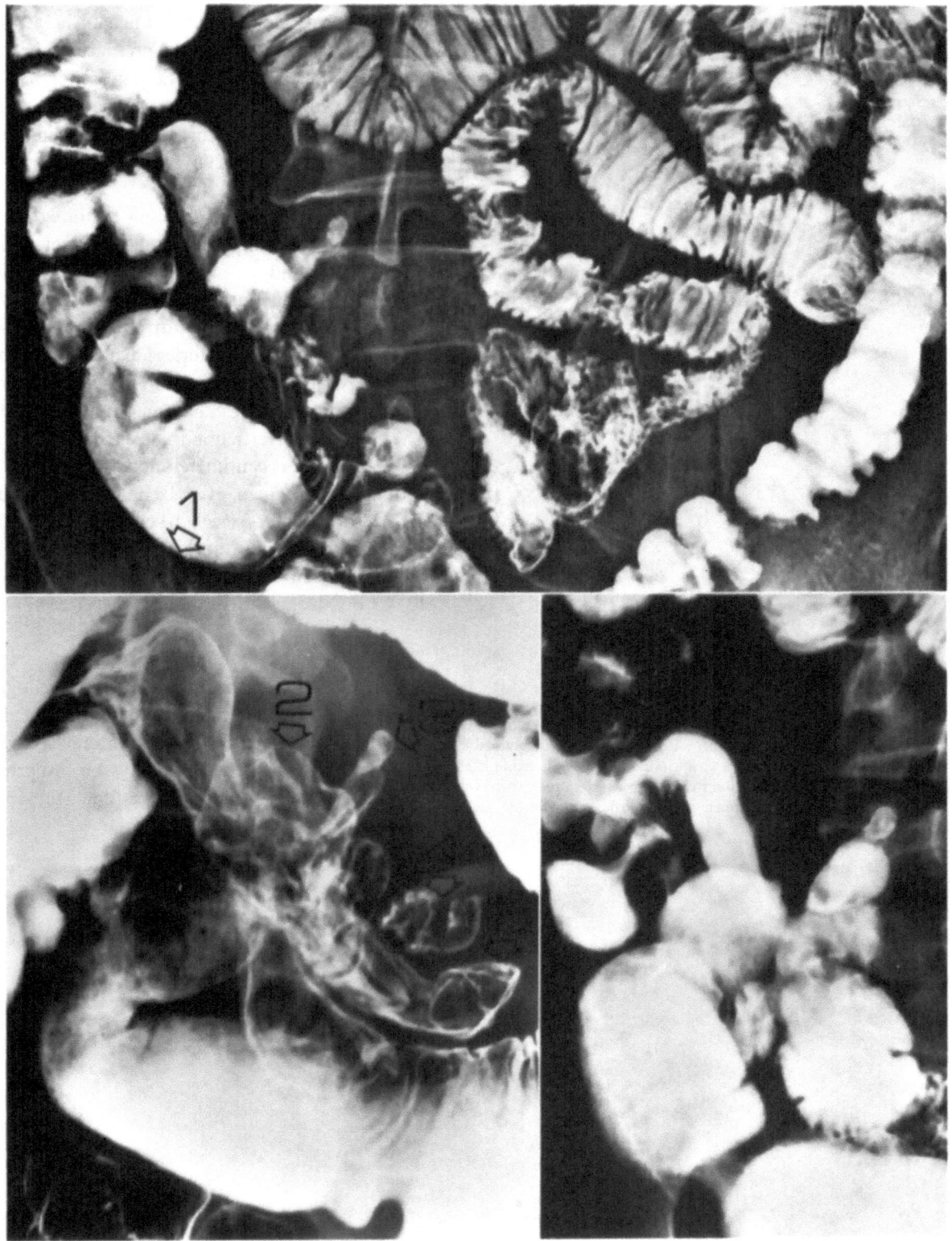

Fig. 13.27. Five sac-like bulges, extending from one point in the ileum. These developed due to constrictions and autoamputation of the intestinal lumen after an incarcerated inguinal hernia was treated surgically. It is no longer possible to determine whether artificial ligation is involved here.

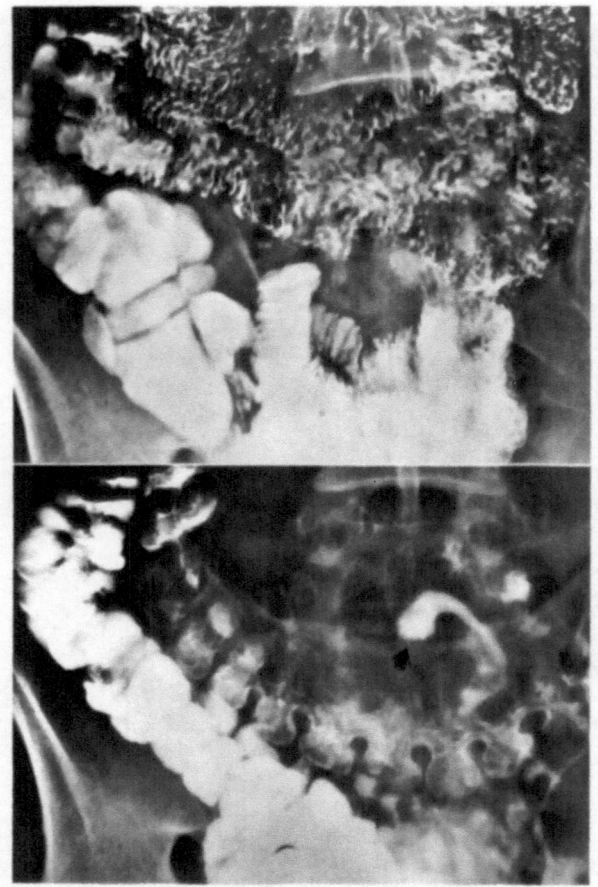

Fig. 13.28. A Meckel's diverticulum can be discovered easily, even if no effort is made to do so, if contrast fluid is retained in the diverticulum after the transit examination is completed (bottom). On the survey film (which was at that time carried out in the conventional manner), the diverticulum was not seen (top).

dilatation was incorrectly assumed to be a prestenotic dilatation because of the presence of the string sign. If the Meckel's diverticulum itself has also been affected by Crohn's disease, then there is little danger of overlooking this unique combination of abnormalities (fig. 13.29B).

A Meckel's diverticulum develops because the proximal end of the omphalomesenteric duct remains open. It is found at autopsy in 1%–2% of adults. Normally this duct atrophies during an early stage of fetal development. The diverticulum is always located on the antimesenteric side of the intestine. It is usually about 80 cm from the ileocecal valve although this distance can range from 20 to 100 cm. The Meckel's diverticulum can be very small (fig. 13.30) or several centimeters long (fig. 13.31A). In extreme cases it can even be 30 cm long, but in general it does not exceed 10 cm. Depending upon the degree of obliteration and/or persistence of the omphalomesenteric duct, there are three types (fig. 13.32) of Meckel's diverticulum (Arey 1947).

Type A. The most common type is a blind sac that is not connected with the navel. The roentgenograms can be surprising and misleading because the diverticulum is free to move in the abdominal cavity. The diverticulum will therefore always be projected in different positions on successive films (fig. 13.33).

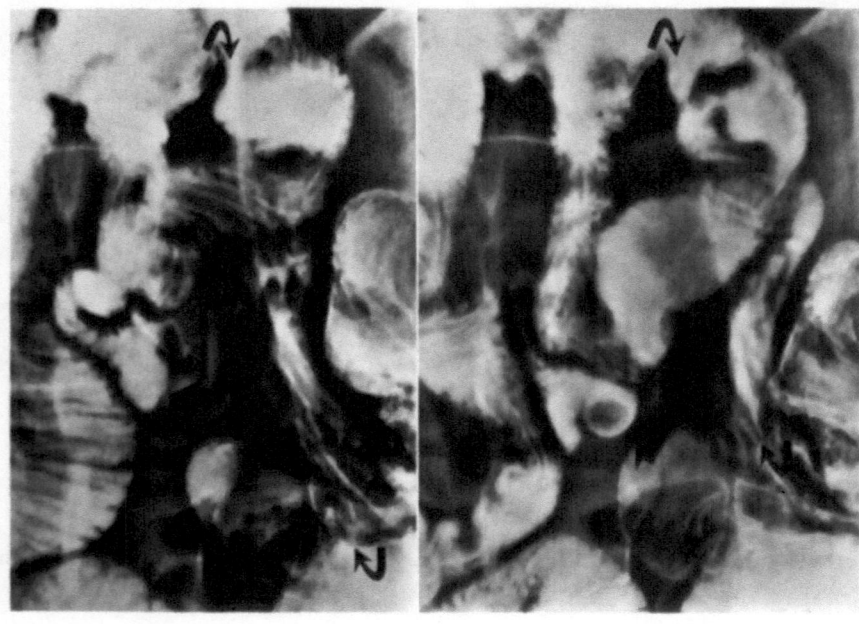

*Fig. 13.29*A. Small Meckel's diverticulum (thick solid arrow) that was overlooked because attention was distracted by scar formation (thin solid arrows) from Crohn's disease.

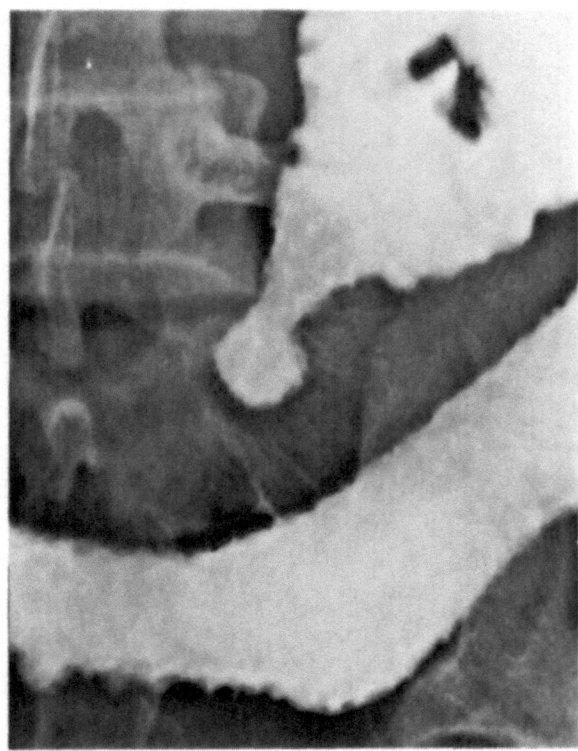

*Fig. 13.29*B. Extensive active Crohn's disease in the distal ileum. The disease has also spread to the fairly small Meckel's diverticulum that was also present.

Type B. This type of Meckel's diverticulum, encountered less frequently, is a blind sac that is attached to the navel by a fibrous residual band of the omphalomesenteric duct. In contrast to type A, this diverticulum is always localized in approximately the same position because of its fixation. Often the tip of the diverticulum will point in the direction of the navel in all projections.

Type C. A rare type of Meckel's diverticulum develops when there is an open channel leading outside the body. Externally a polyp-like bulge is seen that contains the fistula opening. Roentgenological diagnosis of this type is not difficult since it is easily demonstrated by injecting contrast medium into the fistulous tract.

In general the wall of the diverticulum is the same as that of the small bowel (70%). However, the diverticulum can also be partially or completely lined with heterotopic tissue. In 15%–20% of the cases

this tissue is gastric mucosa, but duodenal or colonic mucosa is also encountered and sometimes even pancreatic tissue (4%). A peptic ulcer in a Meckel's diverticulum is not an unusual finding. Pathologists have known this for more than a century. Tumors in and calcification of the diverticulum are rare findings. Autopsy studies have shown that the Meckel's diverticulum is encountered in men more frequently than in women in a ratio of 3:1. It often occurs also in combination with other congenital anomalies.

5.1. Clinical symptoms

All of our patients with a surgically confirmed Meckel's diverticulum were clearly anemic; in most cases there was even visible rectal bleeding. In addition it was striking that almost all of these patients had had complaints for years. They had for this reason been examined radiologically several times although a satisfactory explanation had yet to be established. Some patients complain of abdominal pain or recurrent high temperatures, others only of fatigue. Physical examination often reveals a site that is sensitive to pressure; sometimes resistance is also encountered during palpation. A Meckel's diverticulum can be present without ever causing complaints. On the other hand a sudden Meckel's perforation with peritonitis can cause a life-threatening situation.

5.2. Radiological examination

Many suggestions have been made concerning small bowel examination technique aimed at improving diagnosis and thus increasing the chance of visualizing a Meckel's diverticulum. A large group of radiologists hoped to solve this problem by fractional oral administration of the barium suspension (Prevot 1936; Mendelsohn 1952; Bischoff and Stampeli 1955; Berne 1959). They believed that the diverticulum was almost never visualized because it was hidden by other intestinal loops. Others (Grossman et al. 1950; Wagner et al. 1955; Arcomano et al. 1962; Grollman and Sachs 1965; Miller with his retrograde small bowel examination 1965) preferred a colonic examination. By means of retrograde filling of the distal ileal loops, the diverticulum would be filled (fig. 13.34). Obviously the diverticulum can be visualized more easily in this manner since other intestinal loops are no longer projected over the

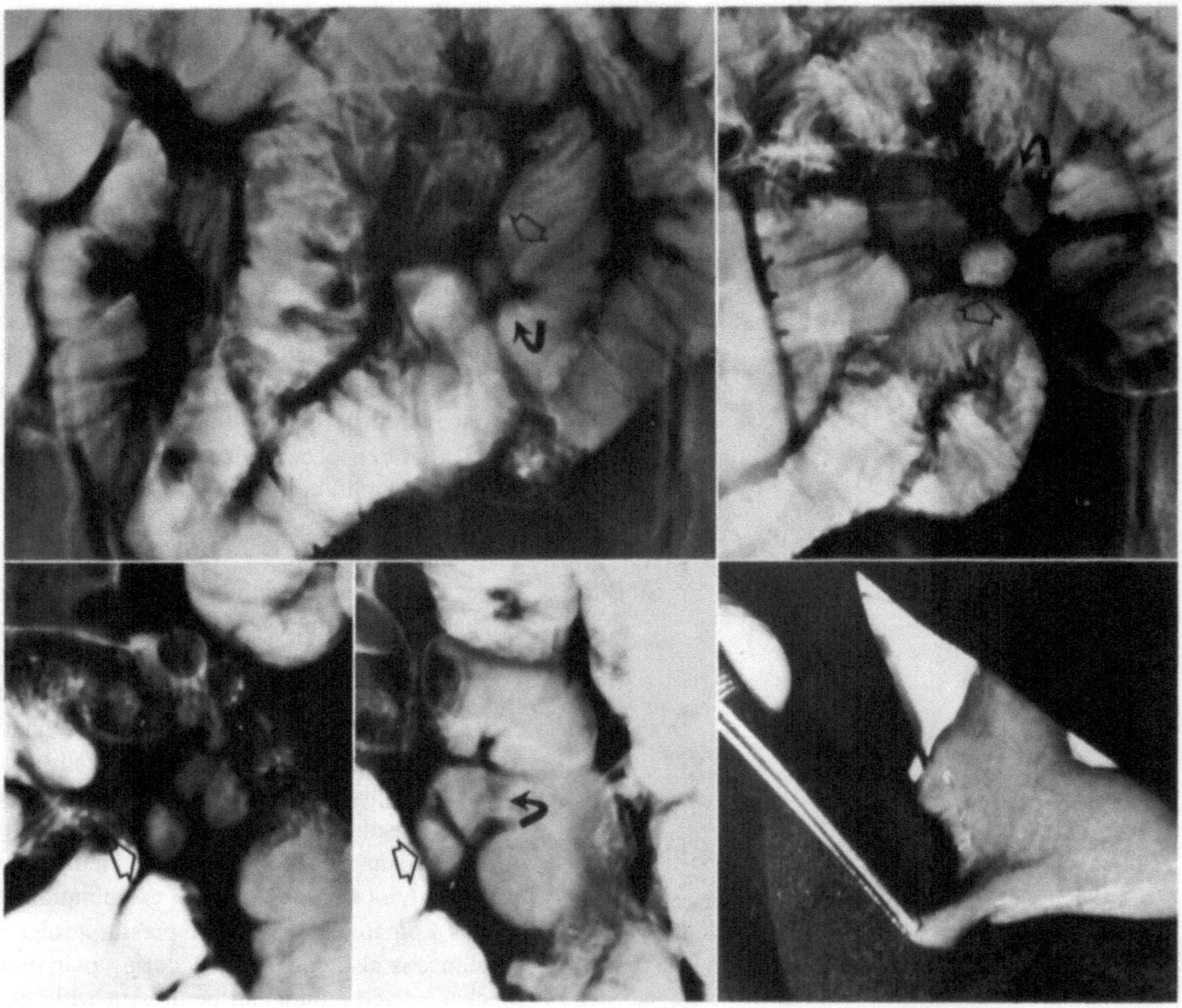

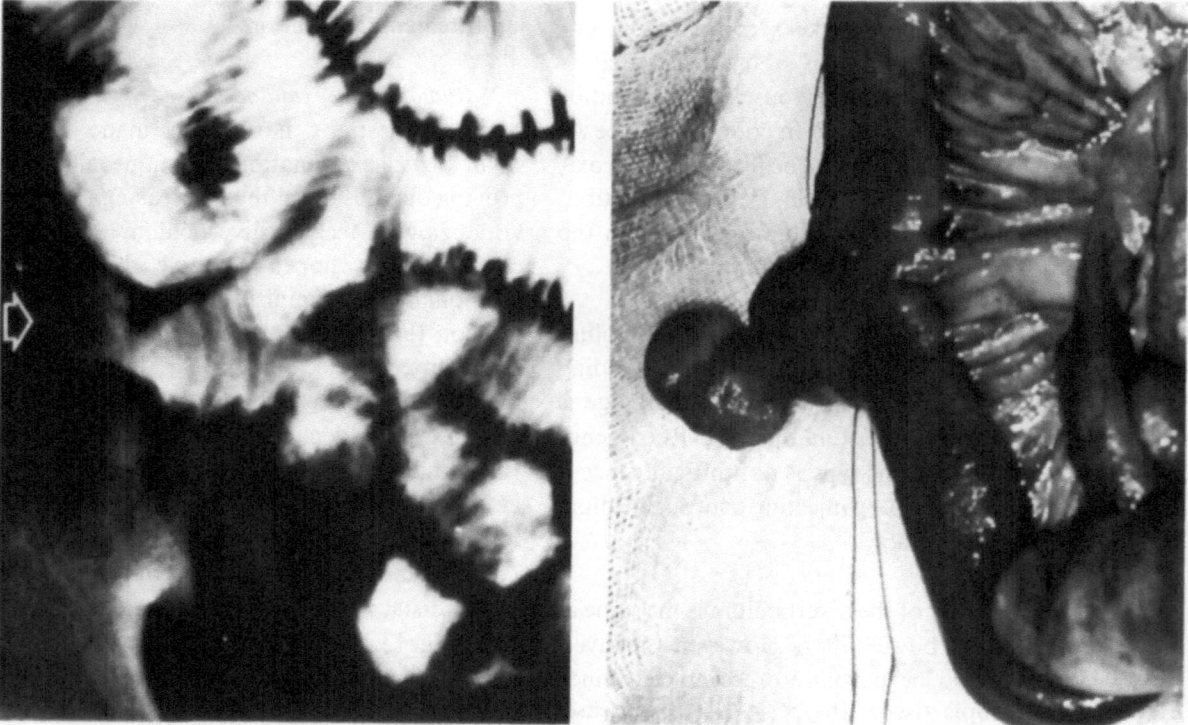

*Fig. 13.30*A. Small Meckel's diverticulum that is not or barely visible on the detail from the spot film (upper left) can be seen on the spot films taken with the compression technique. To the right below the surgical preparation.

*Fig. 13.30*B. Small Meckel's diverticulum with a short omphalomesenteric duct.

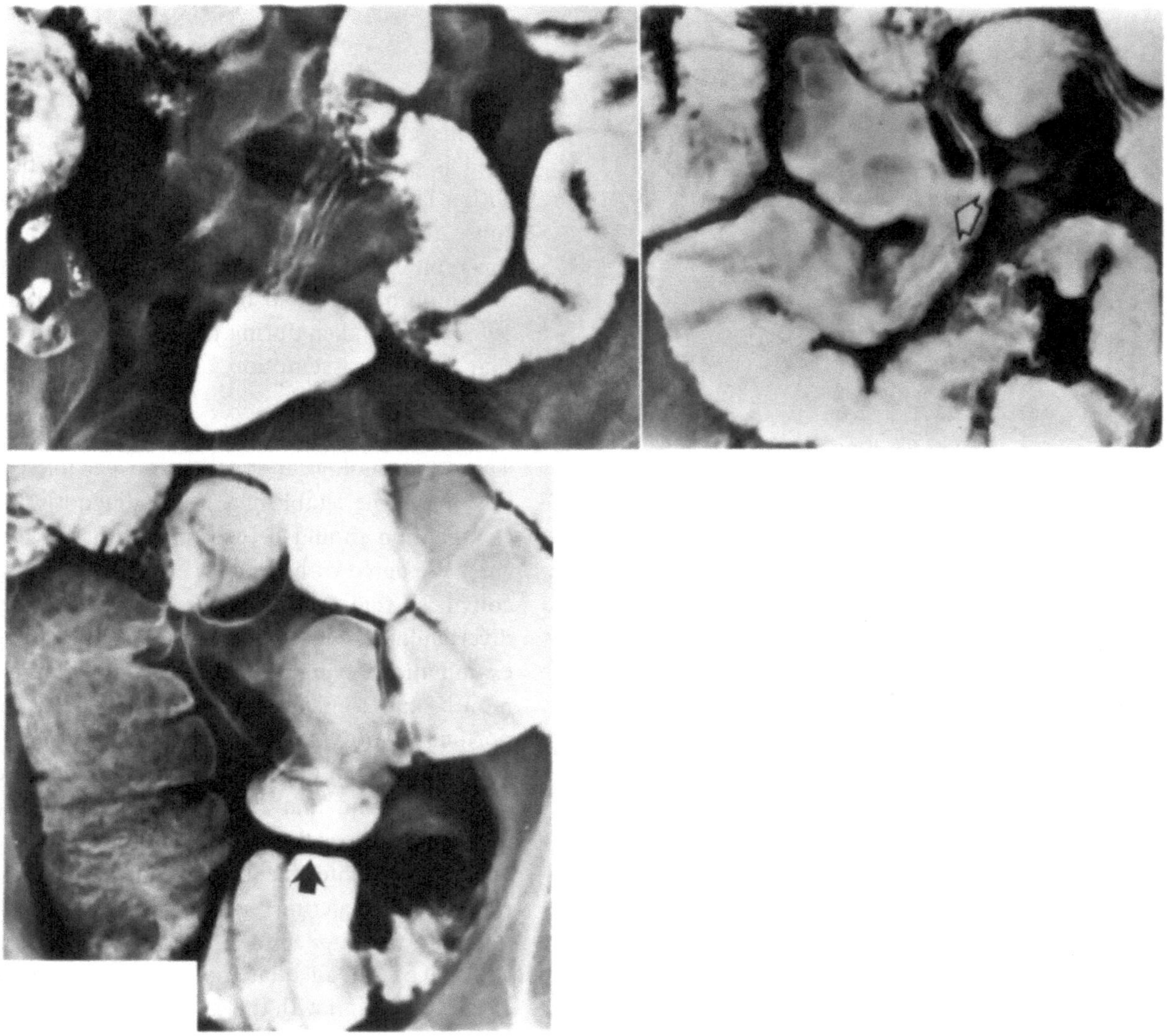

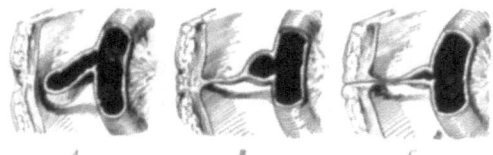

Fig. 13.31. Three medium-sized Meckel's diverticula. Also Crohn's disease in one of these cases (bottom).

Fig. 13.32. The three types of Meckel's diverticulum (Arey 1947). (A) Moving freely in the abdominal cavity. This type is by far the most common. (B) Attached by means of a band to the navel. (C) The lumen of the omphalomesenteric duct is not yet completely obliterated.

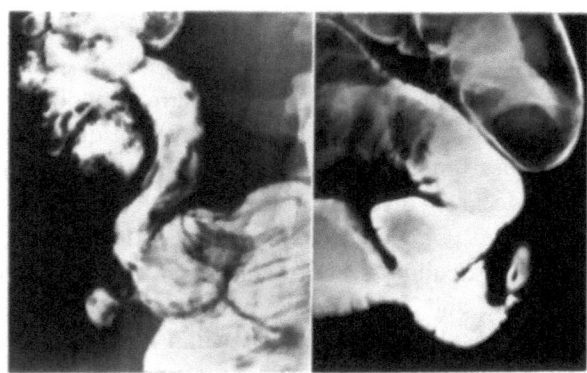

Fig. 13.33. A Meckel's diverticulum that changed position markedly. During one examination it was in the lower left quadrant; during a subsequent examination it lay to the right.

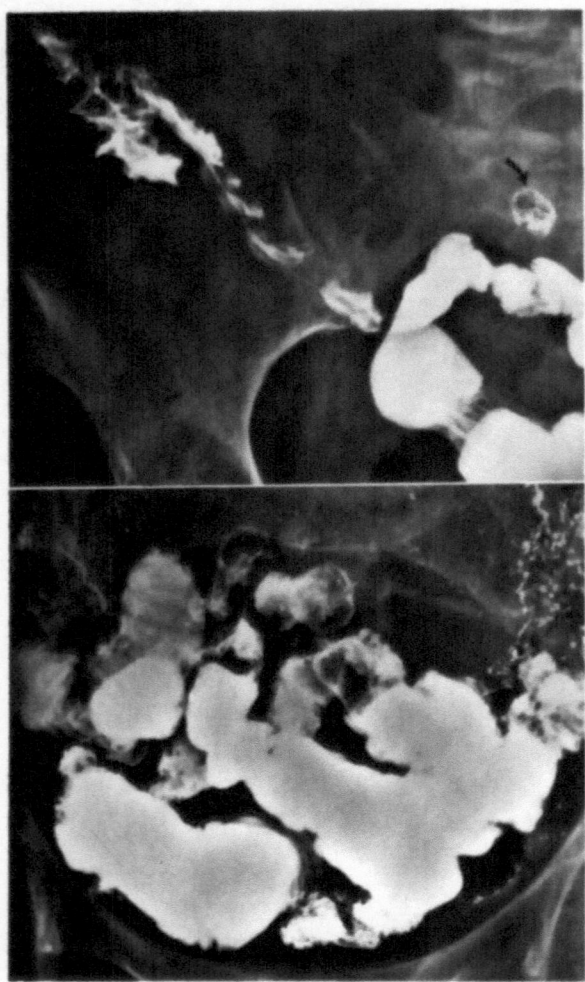

Fig. 13.34. Diagnosis of Meckel's diverticulum in the manner propagated in the past; retrograde filling of the small intestine via a colon enema (top). The diverticulum was not recognized during the conventional examination (bottom).

will in general be well filled because the contrast fluid is probably retained longer. A diverticulum with a large mouth will indeed fill more easily but subsequently will also empty quickly. Because of this rapid filling they are interpreted from the films as a loop of the small bowel (Alvary 1951; Berne 1959). Films taken during fluoroscopy have shown that the latter assumption is indeed true in most of our patients.

The roentgenological examination occupies a key position in the establishment of a diagnosis, so this examination should be executed with the greatest care. We agree with Dalinka et al. (1973), who are convinced that the failure to recognize a Meckel's diverticulum is mainly because of an inadequate examination technique. If a diverticulum has a wide mouth, and can therefore be well filled, it is important to provide such an abundant supply of contrast medium that this filling does indeed occur. We have found that for this purpose the entero-clysis technique is the only method for examination of the small intestine that is quick and certain. Merely administering the contrast fluid through a tube into the duodenum is in itself not a sufficient guarantee of an adequate radiological examination. The examination with the enteroclysis method must be carried out accurately. In order to discover a Meckel's diverticulum, it is essential that several spot films be made of the diverse ileal loops in different projections by using a good compression technique. During the examination these films must be studied carefully so that further detailed studies can be carried out in the case of doubt. If this is not done, then one can be sure that most of Meckel's diverticula, even the large ones, will be overlooked and not diagnosed (fig. 13.35A). In particular the presence of a diverticulum should also be suspected if suggestive configurations are visualized that show no signs of mucosal ridges (fig. 13.35B).

If a triangular shadow, as seen in fig. 13.36, is encountered anywhere in the mucosal patterns of the intestinal loops, then one can be sure that this is the junction with the omphalomesenteric duct. A Meckel's diverticulum is therefore present, even if it cannot be visualized further on the x-rays.

A frequently encountered misleading pattern is the round diverticulum shadow that is in fact an axial projection of an intestinal loop (fig. 13.37).

diverticulum. But even with these methods most radiologists were convinced that numerous Meckel's diverticula were still overlooked. If a diverticulum is inflamed and the mouth is swollen by edema, it is logical that closure can occur. The number of such cases will, however, be quite small. It does not explain the failure to identify the many Meckel's diverticula that are present but never cause complaints. Some contend that because the diverticulum is contractile, it is not continuously filled and is therefore overlooked on the roentgenograms (Elias et al. 1950; Lewitan 1953; Berne 1959). The presence of feces or intestinal contents could also prevent filling with contrast medium. Alvary (1951) believes that diverticula with a small mouth

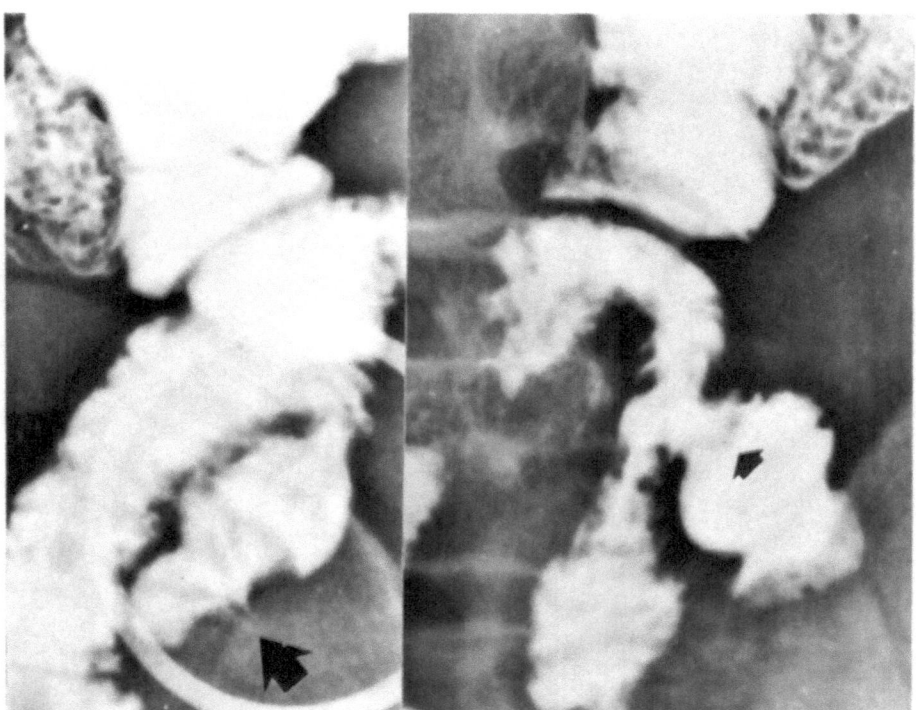

*Fig. 13.35*A. Bleeding Meckel's diverticulum containing an ulcer with mucosal folds radiating outward. The diverticulum was not demonstrated until a second radiological examination was carried out, in spite of the fact that the enteroclysis examination performed a few weeks before included numerous spot films. Angiographic examination and a technetium scan, as well as endoscopic and radiological examination of the stomach and colon, failed to reveal the cause of the melena.

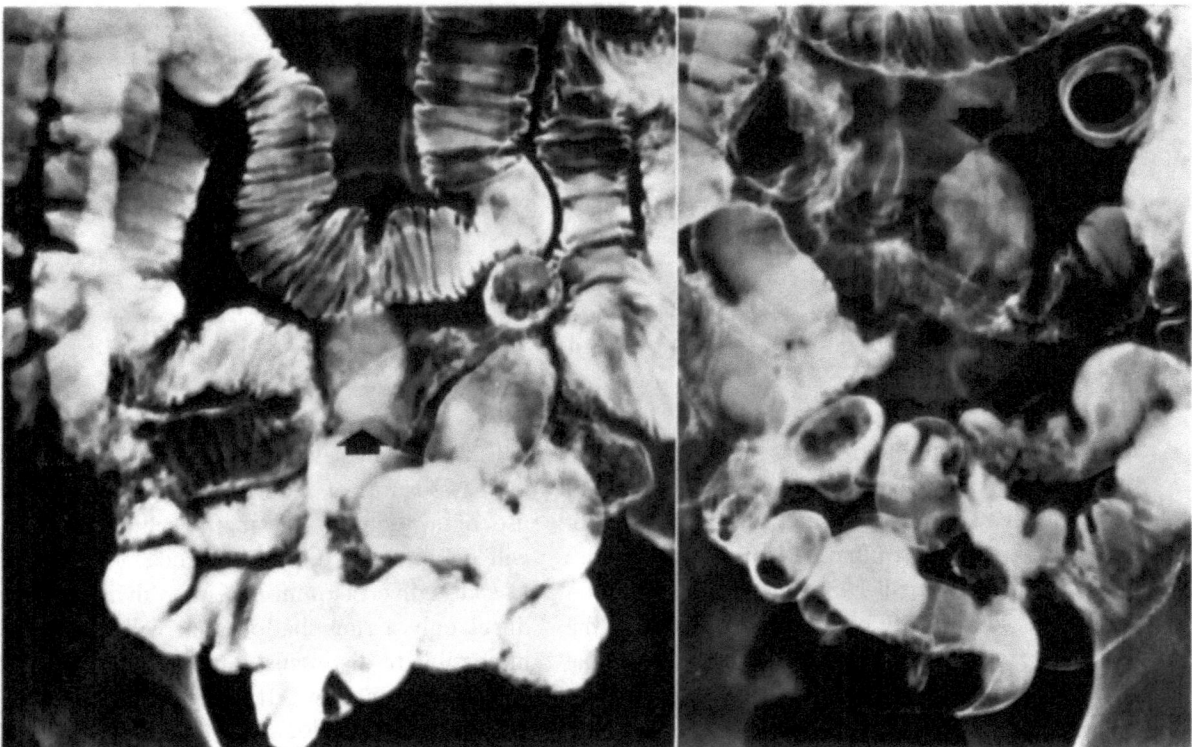

*Fig. 13.35*B. This Meckel's diverticulum (arrow) was not recognized on the survey film of an enteroclysis examination performed elsewhere (left). The spot films taken later also clearly showed a round shadow with no signs of mucosal folds (right). There is an approximately 6-cm-long omphalomesenteric duct (on the photo to the right below the diverticulum, although poorly visible).

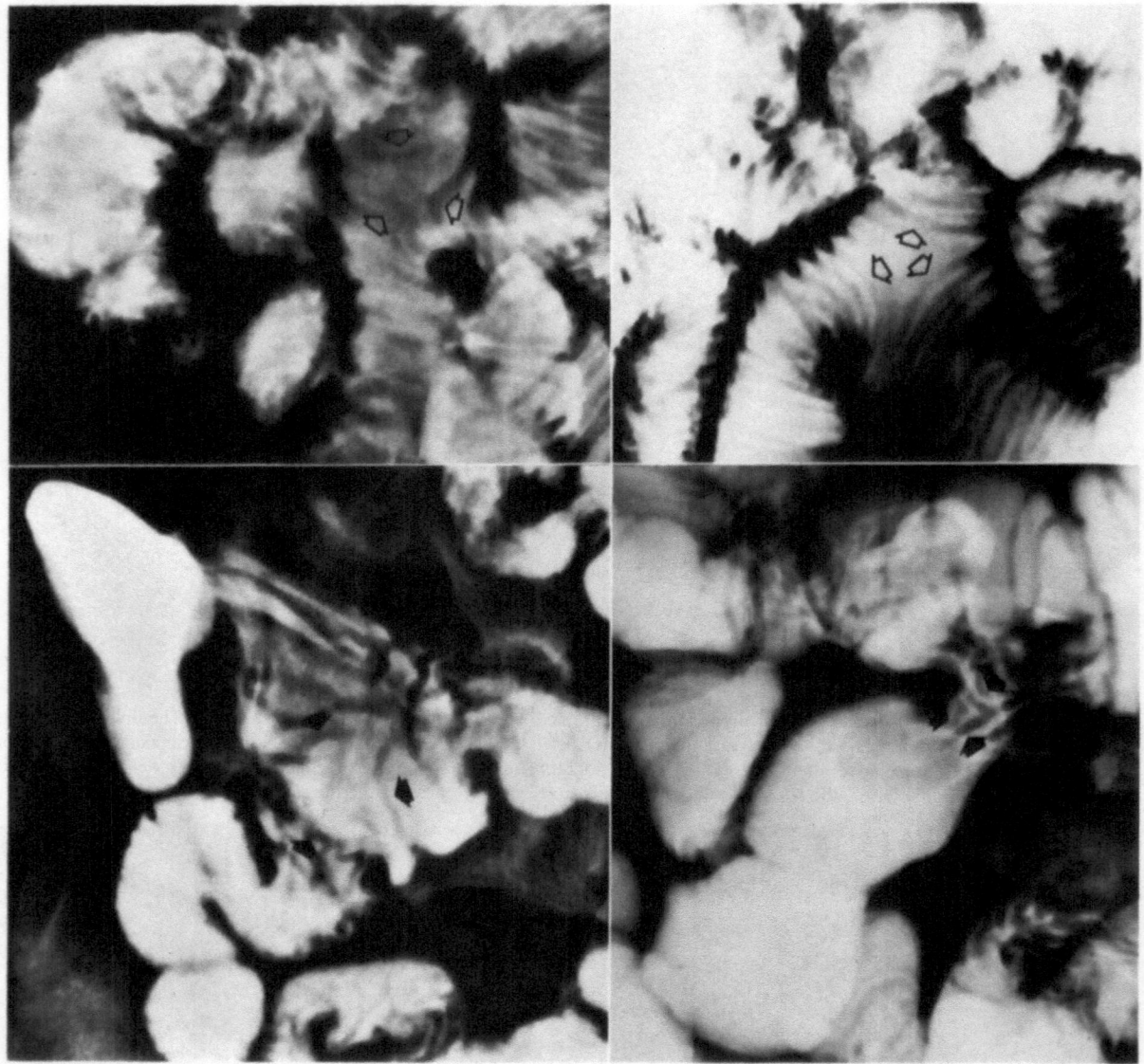

Fig. 13.36. Four different cases of Meckel's diverticulum, all more or less recognizable. The triangular plateau between the mucosal folds indicates the site of the exit of the omphalomesenteric duct.

Another misleading pattern is the configuration that resembles a blind sac but is actually the front of the advancing column of barium suspension. Moreover, in this apparent blind sac, mucosal folds are often missing. This is because of the disintegration and increased viscosity of the contrast fluid at the front as a result of the mucin and juices in the intestinal lumen (fig. 13.38).

A most unusual misleading pattern is seen in fig. 13.39 where a configuration resembling a small diverticulum is caused by the partial superposition of two intestinal loops.

Finally it must be emphasized that double-contrast exposures of the distal ileum, with either the use of air-contrast or methylcellulose technique, will definitely reduce the chance of identifying a Meckel's diverticulum. An empty diverticulum produces only a ring shadow that will be difficult or impossible to distinguish among the other line and ring-shaped shadows. It is also recommended that the air configurations on the abdominal survey exposures be studied carefully. Only in this manner can important conclusions be drawn or suspicious patterns detected (fig. 13.40).

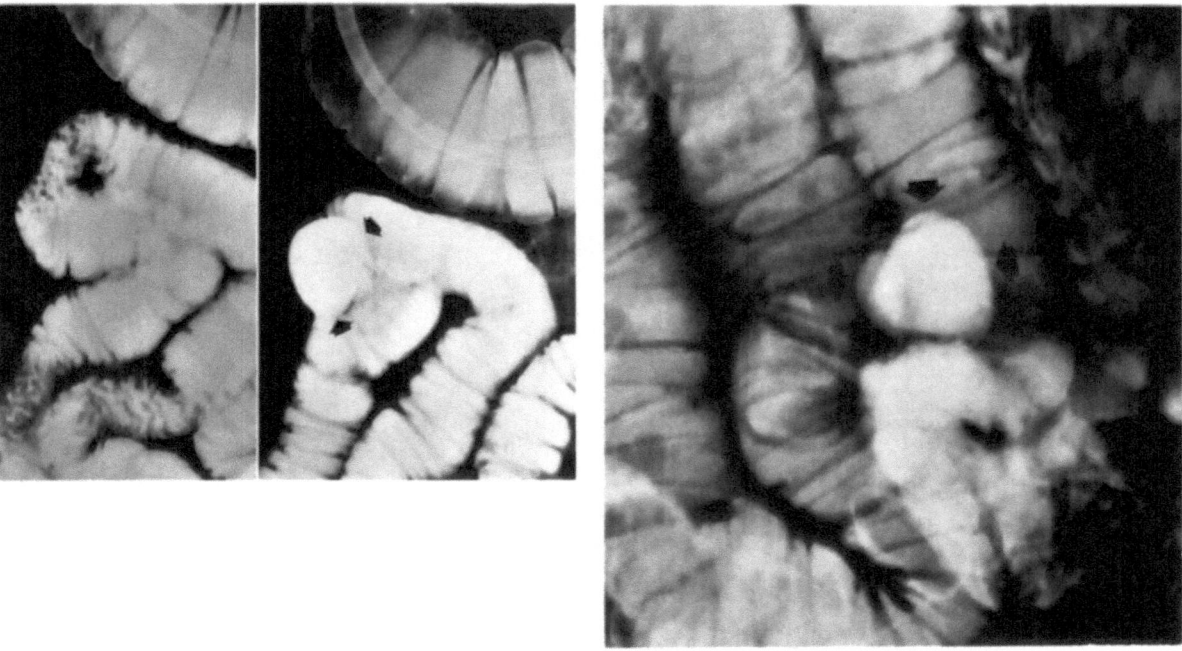

Fig. 13.37. Two patients with a diverticulum-like shadow in the mass of intestinal loops that is from an intestinal loop taken in axial projection. To confirm this, a repeat examination was necessary for the patient in the right photograph.

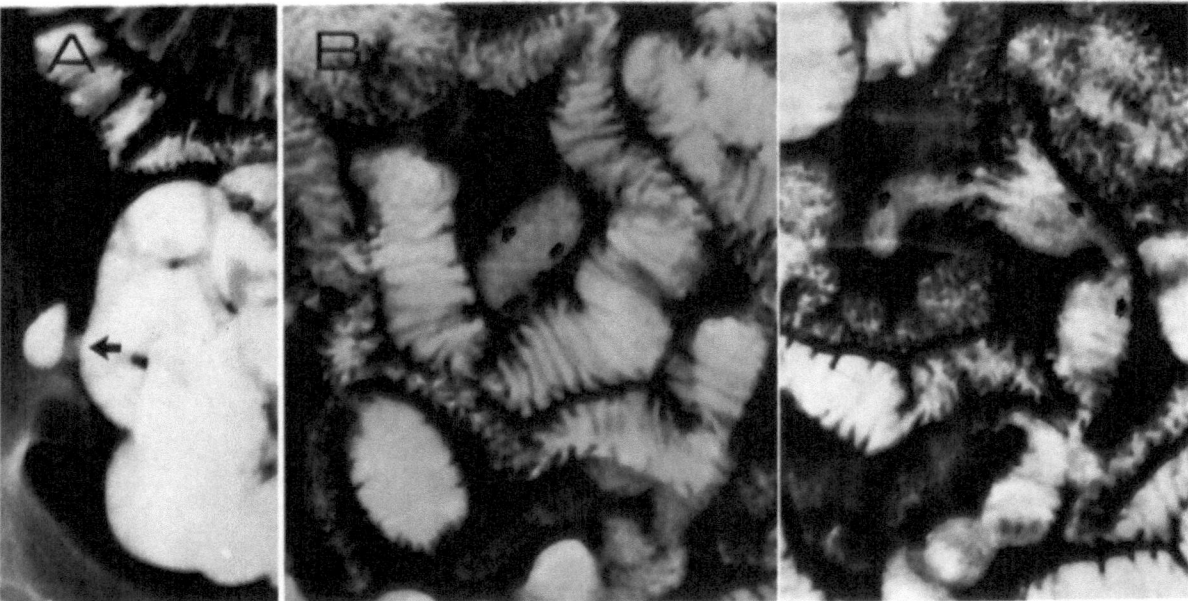

Fig. 13.38. Two patients with a misleading pattern suggesting a (Meckel's) diverticulum. In both cases this is the front of the contrast column. In patient B, disintegration of the contrast fluid is clearly visible. The photograph of this patient on the left shows an isolated round shadow similar to that seen in fig. 13.55. A second exposure taken almost simultaneously revealed that it was a normal segment of the intestine.

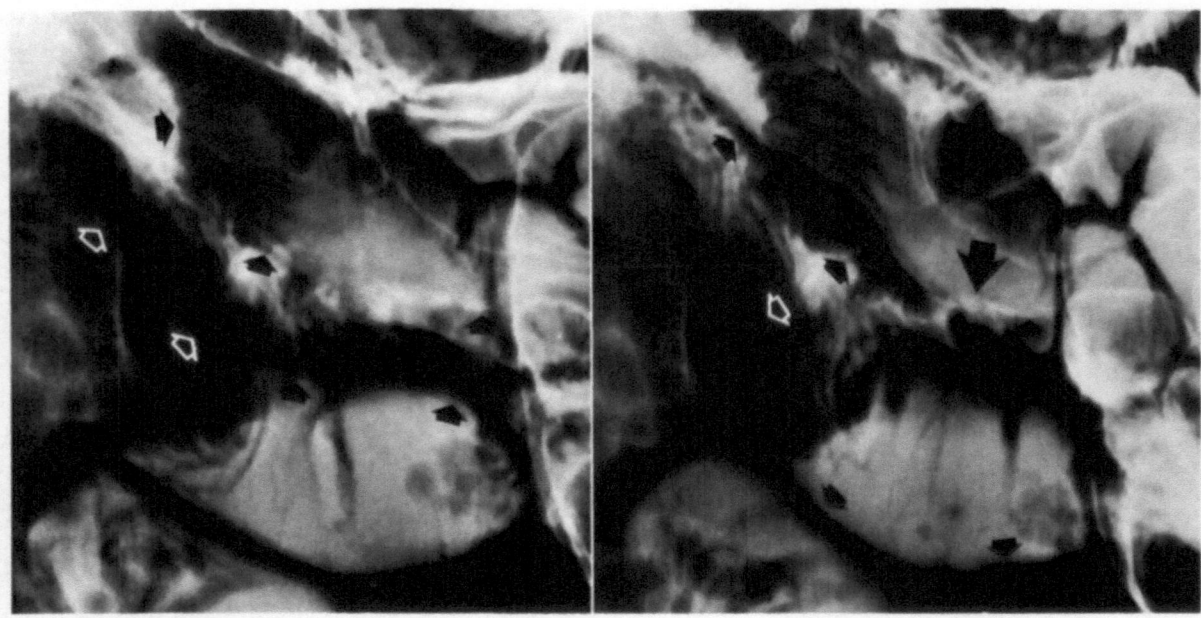

Fig. 13.39. Misleading pattern suggesting a small (Meckel's) diverticulum because of an air bubble and the partial superposition of two intestinal loops. As often occurs a second exposure taken almost simultaneously provided the explanation.

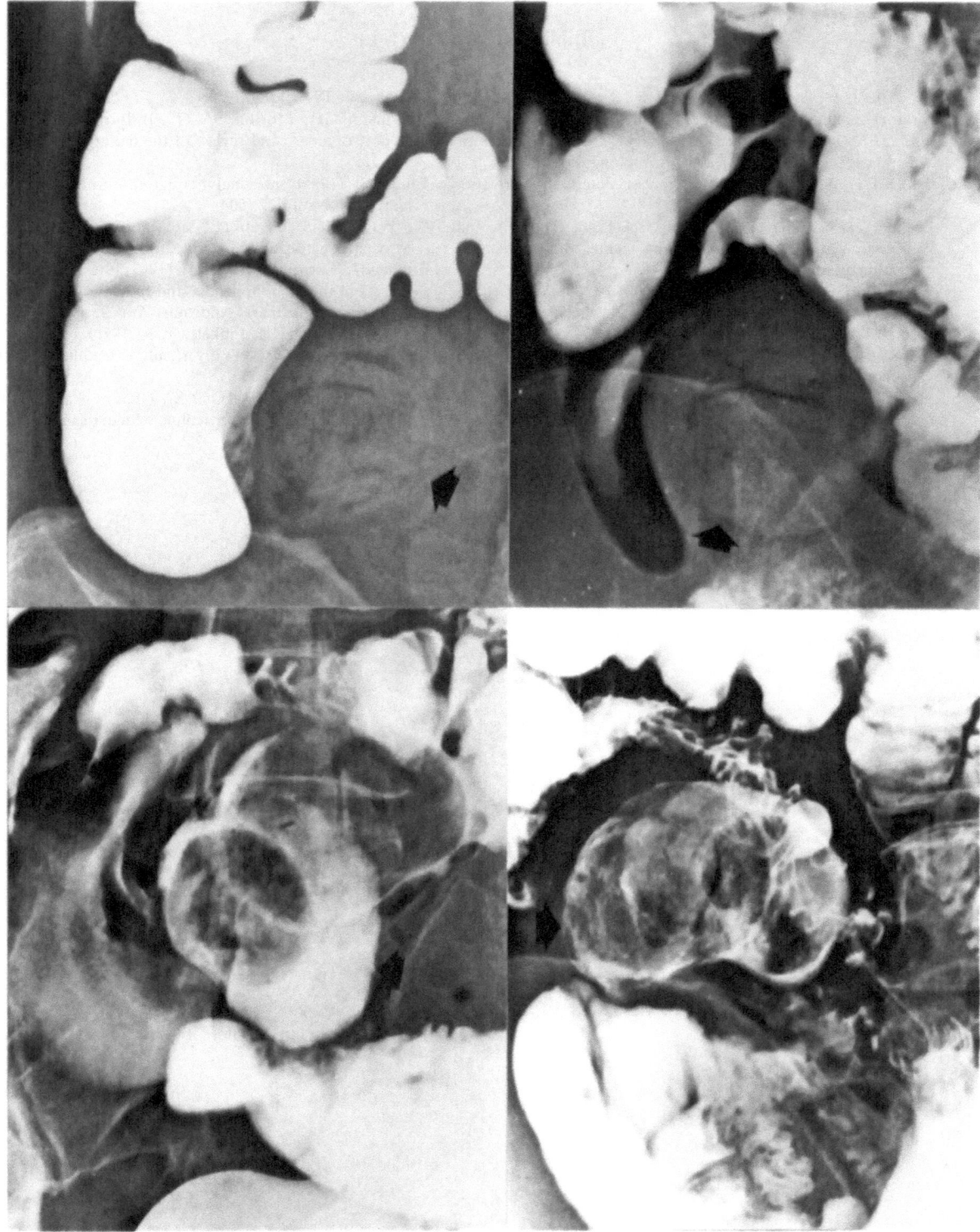

Fig. 13.40. Large Meckel's diverticulum rather distal in the ileum. Its existence was suspected from a previous colon examination on the basis of the air configurations suggesting retention (top). There are, in addition, a number of ordinary diverticula in the distal ileum.

Bibliography: chapter 13

Arey LB (1947) Developmental anatomy. A textbook and laboratory manual of embryology. Philadelphia: Saunders.

Bischoff ME, Stampfli WP (1955) Meckel's diverticulum with emphasis on roentgendiagnosis. Radiology 65: 572.

Cutler GD, Scott HW (1944) Transmesenteric hernia. Surg Gynecol Obstet 79: 509.

Dalinka MK, Wunder JF (1973) Meckel's diverticulum and its complications, with emphasis on roentegenologic demonstration. Radiology 106: 295.

Duszynski DO, Jewett TC, Allen JE (1971) Tc99m Na pertechnetate scanning of the abdomen with particular reference to small bowel pathology. Am J Roentgenol 113: 258.

Grossman JW, Fishback CF, Lovlace WR (1950) Hemorrhage from a Meckel's diverticulum as a cause of melena in infancy. Radiology 55: 240.

Fiddian RV (1961) Herniation through mesenteric and mesocolic defects. Br J Surg 49: 186.

Henke F, Lubarsch O (1929) Handbuch der pathologischen Anatomie IV/3: 158–179.

Hansmann GH, Morton SA (1939) Intraabdominal hernia. Report of a case and review of the literature. Arch Surg 39: 973.

King ESJ (1935) Intestinal herniation through a mesenteric hiatus. Br J Surg 22: 504.

Mock CJ, Mock HE Jr (1958) Strangulated internal hernia associated with trauma. Arch Surg 77: 881.

Rooney JA, Carroll JP, Keeley JL (1963) Internal hernias due to defects in the meso-appendix and mesentery of small bowel, and probable Ivemark syndrome. Ann Surg 157: 254.

Stein GN, Bennet HH, Finkelstein A (1958) The preoperative Rö-diagnosis of Meckel's diverticulum in adults. Am J Roentgenol 79: 815.

Wagner FB, Shallow TA, Eger SA (1955) Gastroenterological aspects of Meckel's diverticulum. Analytical review of 100 cases. Am J Gastroenterol 23: 195.

14. ILEUS – FUSION – BANDS – VOLVULUS – INTUSSUSCEPTIONS – INCISIONAL HERNIA

1. Ileus

When there is an obstruction in the small intestine, then even if no fluid is administered orally, the contents of the loops proximal to the stenosis will increase. This is a result of the secretion and exudation products from the intestinal wall. This fluid causes an increasing dilution usually accompanied by flocculation of the contrast fluid in the loops proximal to the obstruction. Dehydration, as generally feared, does not occur (fig. 14.1A). In all literature not one single publication concerning experiments with animals or patients can be found that reports thickening of the contrast medium in the small intestinal loops on the proximal side of an obstruction. As a result of the increased tone, the peristaltic movements are initially enhanced; if the obstruction persists, peristalsis decreases gradually.

Sloan et al. (*Radiology* 76: 407–414, 1961) carried out an excellent series of experiments with 60 dogs. They showed that the increased fluid and the distended loops proximal to a stenosis will develop within several hours. They also showed that the radiologist may only suspect a diagnosis of ileus when gas is also seen in these loops. This gas consists of 68% ingested air, 12% gas caused by bacteria, and 20% gas from the blood via the intestinal wall. During the same experiments it appeared that the length of the distended segment proximal to a stenosis increases gradually with time. The viscosity of the contrast fluid decreases. Several hours after an obstruction had been induced, the radiological diagnosis 'ileus' could be established more easily in well-hydrated dogs than in dehydrated dogs. At a later stage, significant differences between these two groups could no longer be seen.

About 1960, an attempt was made to use water-soluble iodine contrast media to localize the obstruction radiologically in what was assumed a safer way.

Many radiologists believed that Gastrografin would be ideal when barium failed due to flocculation or was contraindicated. The following indications are mentioned in the literature:

1) Atresia or fistulas in the tracheo-esophageal area (danger of aspiration).
2) Diagnosis of certain preoperative and postoperative disorders of the digestive tract such as bleeding ulcers, suture leakage or perforation.
3) Partial obstructions that the barium cannot penetrate or whenever dehydration and thickening of the barium suspension might occur.

It was found that Gastrografin is generally a satisfactory contrast medium as far as the reproduction of gastric mucosa is concerned. It was satisfactory too because of the greater ease with which a pyloric stenosis can be diagnosed or a fistulous tract filled. However, all authors discovered that dilution of the contrast medium in the small intestine was so great that morphological evaluation was absolutely impossible. In addition no one succeeded in making acceptable double-contrast exposures. Some authors reported that more than 50 ml can cause abdominal cramps, vomiting, and diarrhea. Reasonably satisfactory colon films can, however, be made because absorption of fluid causes an increasing thickening in this organ. Thus it was often possible to obtain good filling of the colon on the proximal side of a stenosis because the barium could not penetrate from the distal side. It remained impossible to localize tumors in the small intestine, although the diagnosis 'obstruction' could often be made from the presence of dilated loops.

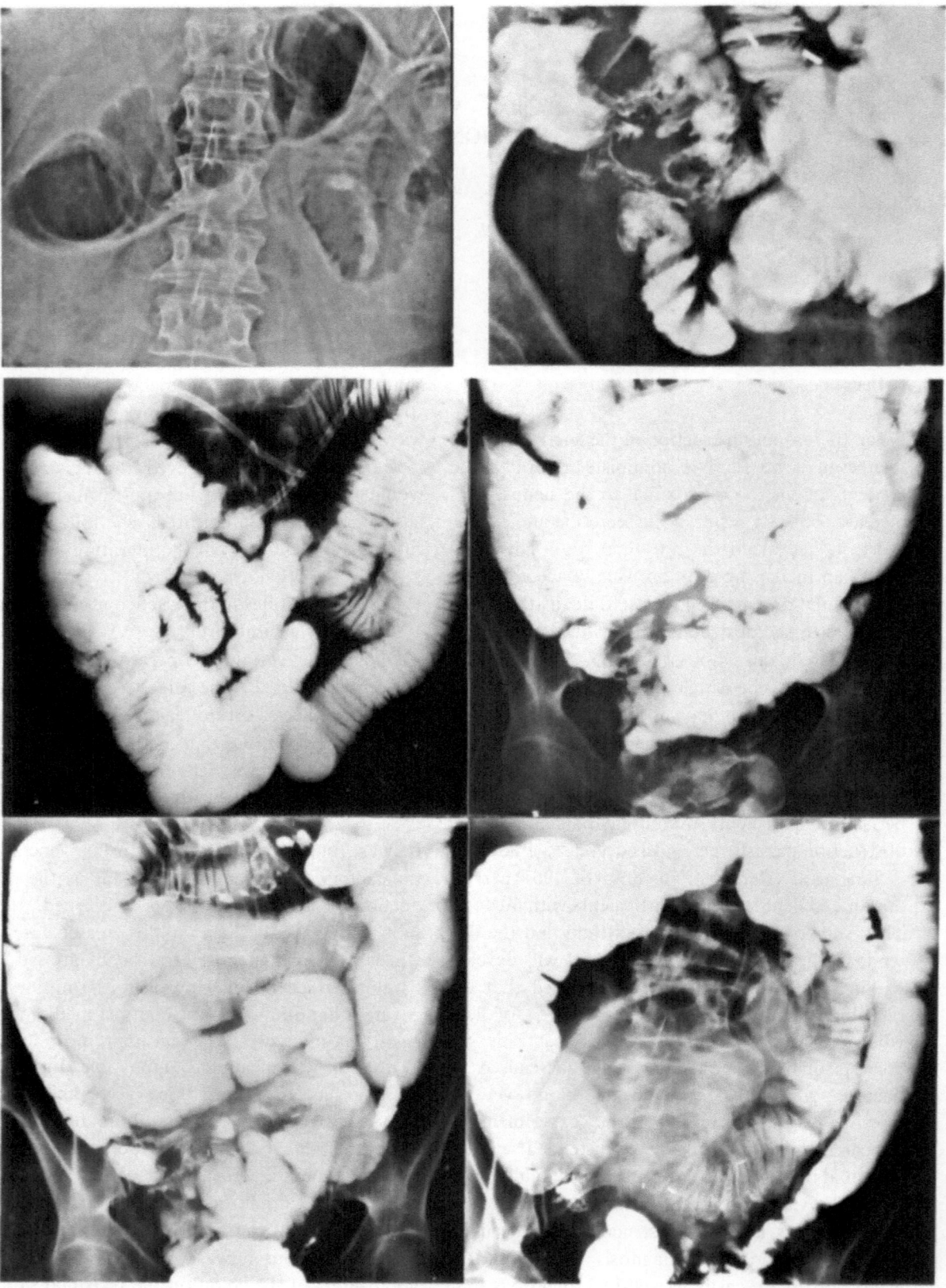

*Fig. 14.1*A. Pronounced obstruction in a patient with metastases of ovarian carcinoma in the lower right quadrant (top right). The gas configuration in the upper abdomen *seems* to indicate that the obstruction lies farther proximalward (top left). There was no peristalsis whatsoever (middle left). After administration of a total of 2500 ml contrast fluid and two doses of metoclopramide via the tube, the site of the obstruction was reached in about 3 h (middle right). One week later, most of the contrast fluid had left the small intestine (bottom left); three weeks after the examination the small bowel was practically empty (bottom right). One week later the contrast fluid had also disappeared out of the colon (not shown). This unique series of films demonstrated very clearly that the barium suspension does not thicken in the small intestine – thus demolishing a widespread and highly feared assumption.

Some radiologists believed that if Gastrografin had not reached the colon 4 h after oral administration, a postoperative ileus must be from an obstruction and not a paralysis. Gastrografin may, however, be visible in the colon within 15 min even when a definite obstruction exists in the small intestine. This thin liquid contrast medium can pass through a very narrow stenosis of 1 or 2 mm easily. In approximately 2% of the patients, some of the iodine contrast medium is excreted into the urine. This is believed by some to indicate the presence of an obstruction, perforation, or other pathological condition in the digestive tract. Surgical confirmation has often supported this line of reasoning, and Tosch (*Fortschritte R* 95: 189–222, 1961) has shown with radioactive Gastrografin that it can indeed occur. However, disappointment and false-positive diagnoses have also been reported.

Gastrografin has strong hyperosmotic characteristics and this may be dangerous in cases of intestinal obstruction. The osmotic pressure of 50 ml 70% Urokon is equal to that of 15 g magnesium sulfate. A dose of 6 ml/kg body weight can cause such excessive fluid withdrawal that the circulating plasma volume can be reduced by 15%–30%. The osmotic pressure of Gastrografin in isolated intestinal loops can be so great that the circulation in the intestinal wall is seriously disturbed. In addition, vomiting and diarrhea caused by Gastrografin can further disturb an already critical electrolyte balance. It has therefore become crystal clear that, in the event of a suspected obstruction in the small intestine, Gastrografin is most unsuitable as contrast medium. If for extremely unusual conditions, it is still considered desirable, then it must in any event be handled with extreme caution. It may be used only when the clinical condition of the patient does not form a contraindication. Gastrografin does not adhere easily and reliable morphological information can only be obtained when the loops are well filled. In addition, Gastrografin is such a thin liquid that fistulous tracts or perforation may not be discovered. This is because the contrast medium flows past such abnormalities so rapidly that there is not enough time for penetration. In 1960, Shehadi wrote that the introduction of the aqueous iodine contrast medium could be considered a milestone for diagnosis involving the digestive tract (*Am J Roentgenol* 83: 933–941). Fortunately

since then the use of Gastrografin has lost much of the ground it had taken by storm. A new landmark in digestive tract diagnosis will be reached when use of this medium is only a rare exception.

The development of an adequate diagnostic technique for patients with ileus has been continuously impeded by the exaggerated value attributed to Gastrografin. It has also been impeded by a second factor that appears to be equally as insurmountable. The majority of almost all referring colleagues from other disciplines still believe that, when an ileus is suspected, the most adequate approach is an abdominal survey film with horizontal beam. Although there is no danger in this method and even the inexperienced clinician can easily see the fluid levels on such films so that his clinical suspicion is confirmed, their value can be considered dubious. It is apparently not or insufficiently realized that:

1) An ileus can exist without visible fluid levels. As described above this is certainly true in the beginning stages when there may as yet be insufficient gas. The intraabdominal pressure may be so high that the accumulation of gas is greatly retarded or even prevented.

2) Fluid levels form as a result of the presence of gas and thin fluids in the digestive tract. This combination is not at all rare! It is pronounced in patients with diarrhea, or malabsorption accompanied by hypersecretion, or retarded resorption. Erect abdominal survey films of patients who for some reason have been allowed to eat before the examination are not often encountered. Therefore it is understandable that many will have acquired little or no experience in recognizing this particular phenomenon (fig. 14.1B).

3) Even the presence of fluid levels together with dilated intestinal loops need not necessarily indicate an ileus. This combination can also be encountered in a number of the diseases discussed in chapter 6, such as drug-induced atony, scleroderma, amyloidosis, or certain forms of celiac disease.

4) An x-ray of an erect patient taken with a horizontal beam may demonstrate the presence of free intraabdominal air below the diaphragm. Actually such films should not be considered adequate for this purpose. Often the film is assumed to be satisfactory if the diaphragm is just visible along the

416

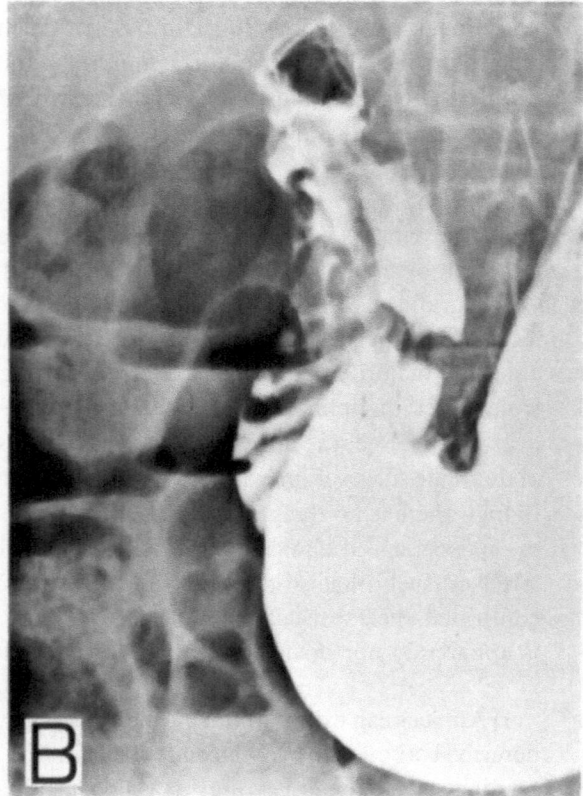

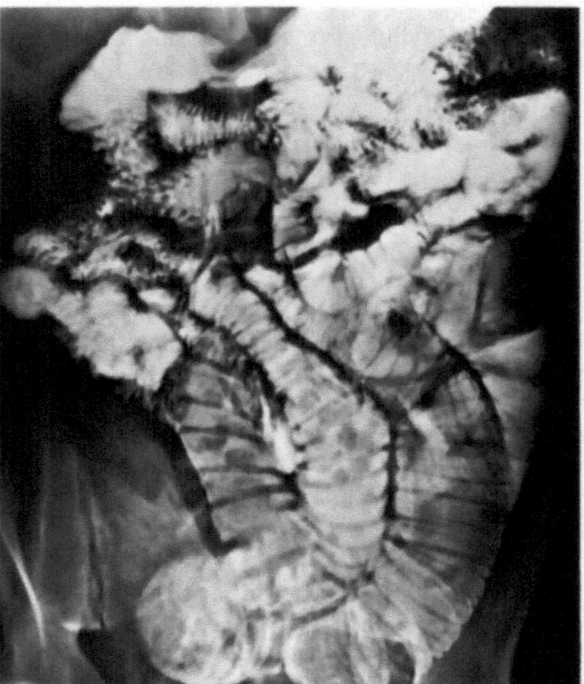

*Fig. 14.1*B. Multiple fluid levels in the ileocecal region in the upper right quadrant; the patient had had something to drink about 1 h before the gastric examination. There were no indications at all of an ileus or any other abnormality in the small bowel.

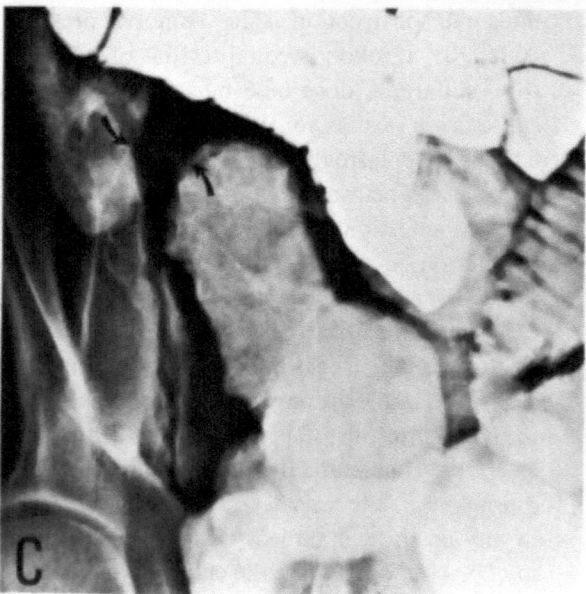

upper edge of the roentgenogram. It should be remembered, however, that only larger quantities of gas will be seen on such films. Small and therefore narrow sickle-shaped pockets of air between the liver and the diaphragma are not visualized by an oblique beam. It is always necessary to demonstrate the presence of smaller gas accumulations below the diaphragm! The diaphragm should lie at the level of the central beam, thus in the middle of the roentgenogram.

5) Dilatation of intestinal loops filled with gas can be established much more easily on an exposure taken with a vertical beam. The gas in the lumen spreads out over a much larger area when the patient is lying down, and gives much more information.

Experienced radiologists certainly do not need fluid levels to establish a diagnosis of ileus.

An ileus characterized by dilated loops filled with

*Fig. 14.1*C (see also page 214). Patient with ileus due to an obstructing stenosis in the distal ileum (Crohn's disease). In the jejunum peristalsis is still active. Distalward, however, the loops become dilated and the peristaltic movements diminish. In spite of the administration of 1800 ml contrast fluid. it was still possible to take adequate exposures with the compression technique.

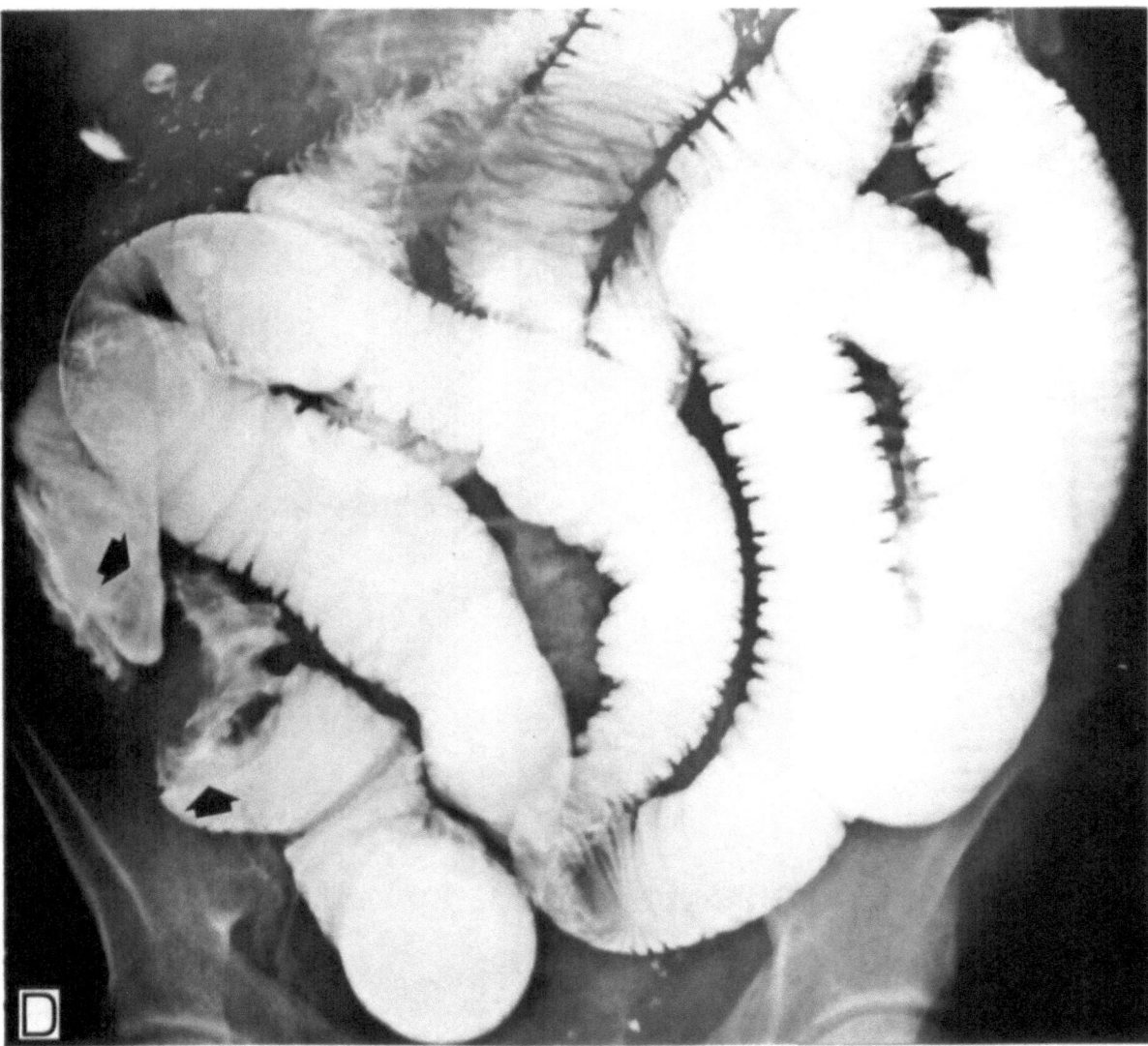

*Fig. 14.1*D. Obstruction from a tumor in the distal part of the ileum. Total dose of contrast medium was 1600 ml; water infusion superfluous in this case.

large quantities of gas is difficult to differentiate only from more or less similar patterns. These are patients with atony of the intestine, scleroderma, Naish syndrome, or amyloidosis, when the ileus is a result of any one of these diseases. If there is no nonobstructing or pseudo-obstructing ileus in conjunction with the above mentioned diseases, then the intestinal loops will show no hairpin-like configurations. The air accumulation will be highly local or will alternate with more or less normal segments. If the ileus is more advanced, then the peristaltic movements in the segment most proximal to the obstruction will be greatly disturbed. A second x-ray taken several minutes later will show

that the gas pattern in the intestine has barely changed. This local 'stillness' will not be observed in conjunction with one of the above-mentioned diseases, even if the intestinal motility is greatly disturbed. This local but total absence of peristalsis is identified by lack of change in and sometimes the persistence of a single dilated intestinal loop filled with gas. This can be considered highly significant for diagnosis. It almost certainly indicates a local obstruction or paralysis (fig. 11.2). At this stage, only a subileus is involved and often it has not even been recognized clinically. However, further analysis of the nature of the disease is exceedingly worthwhile. The establishment of a correct or

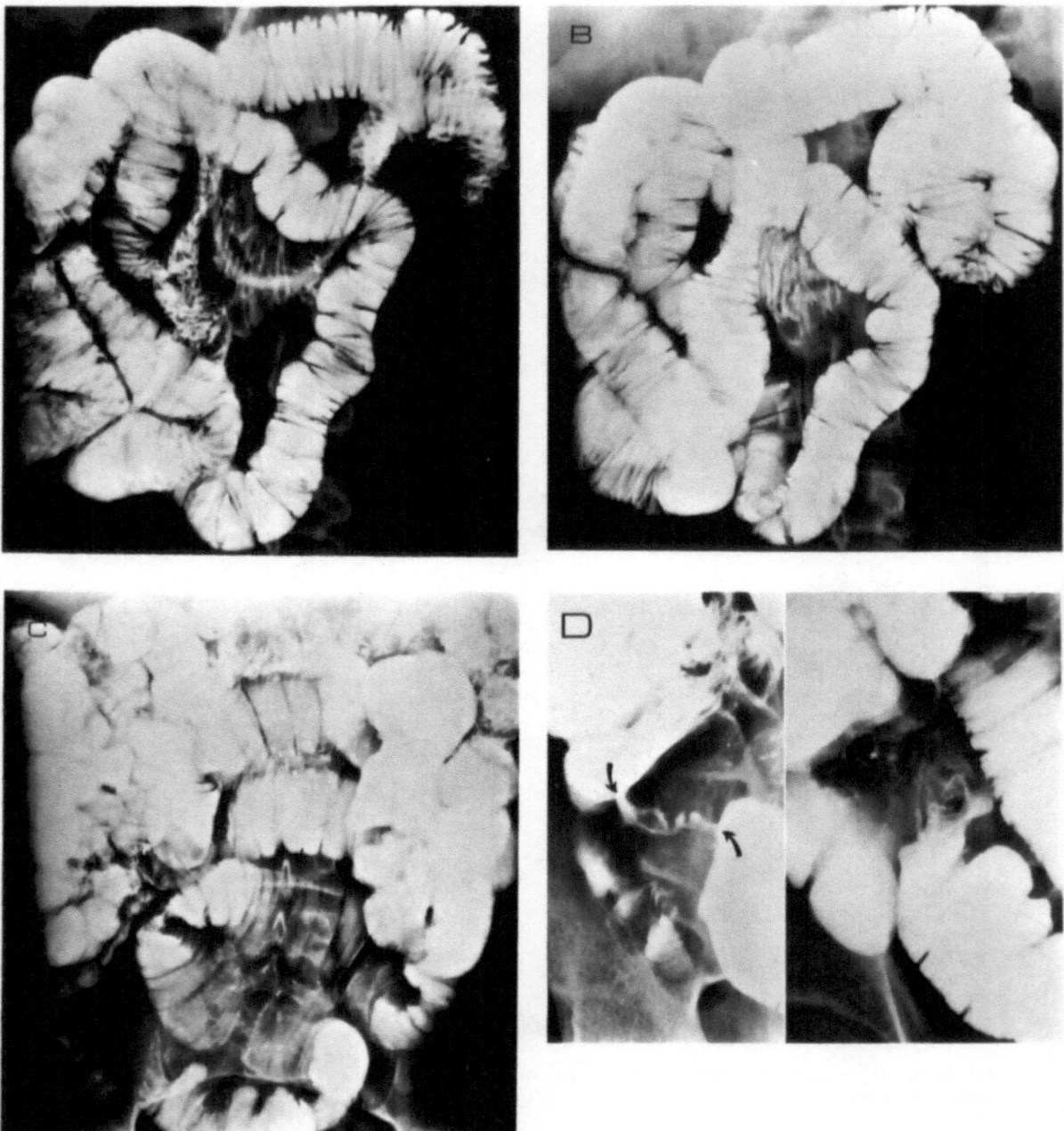

Fig. 14.2. A series of exposures of a patient with a tumor causing marked stenosis in the distal ileum. (A) Survey film after 600 ml barium suspension. (B) Survey film after 1200 ml barium suspension. (C) Survey film after 2400 ml barium suspension. (D) Spot films with compression technique after administration of 2400 ml barium suspension showing the tumor in the region of Bauhin's valve.

probable diagnosis is almost always possible.

Only a barium suspension can be considered as contrast medium for the diagnosis of ileus, as is true in every other enteroclysis examination. The total amount of contrast medium required for the examination is variable. It is highly dependent upon whether the obstruction is in the proximal or distal ileum, the stage of the ileus, and the degree of motility still present. In general much more than an initial dose of 800 ml must be administered; a total

dose of 2400 ml is, however, never exceeded.

As the amount of contrast fluid administered to patients with ileus increases, peristalsis decreases in a fairly long segment as stretching of the intestinal wall continues.

In order to retard this so-called 'inhibitory' reflex mechanism, it is recommended that the flow rate of the contrast medium must be decreased gradually during the examination. As in all other cases when large quantities of contrast fluid must be adminis-

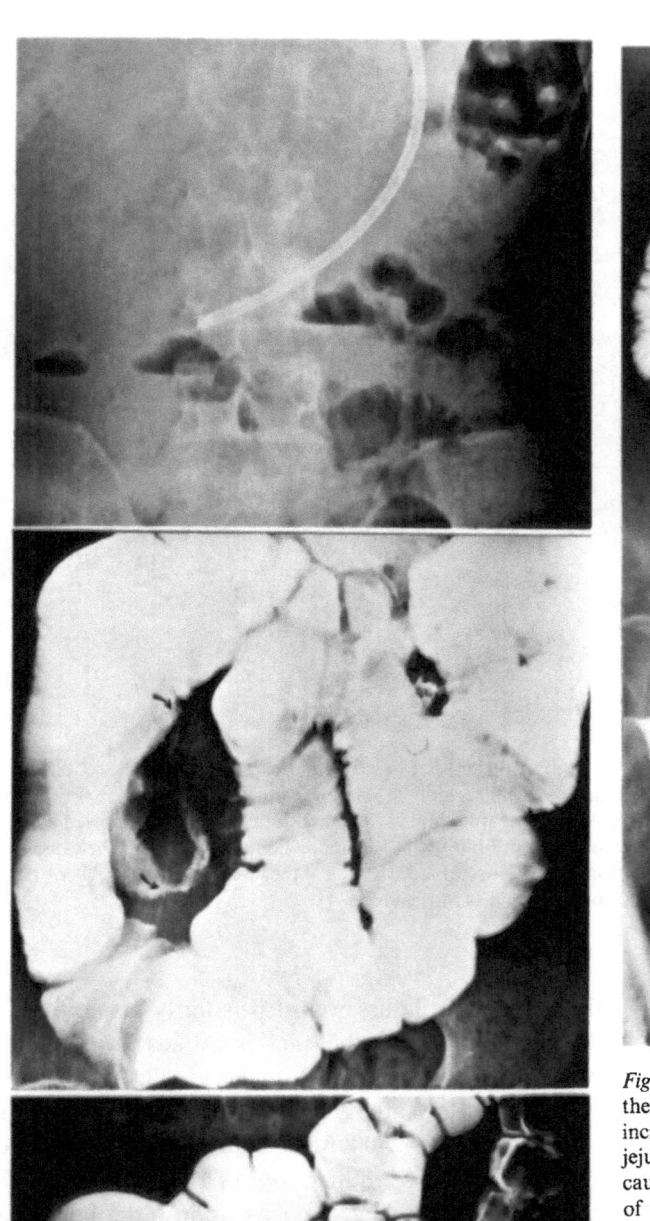

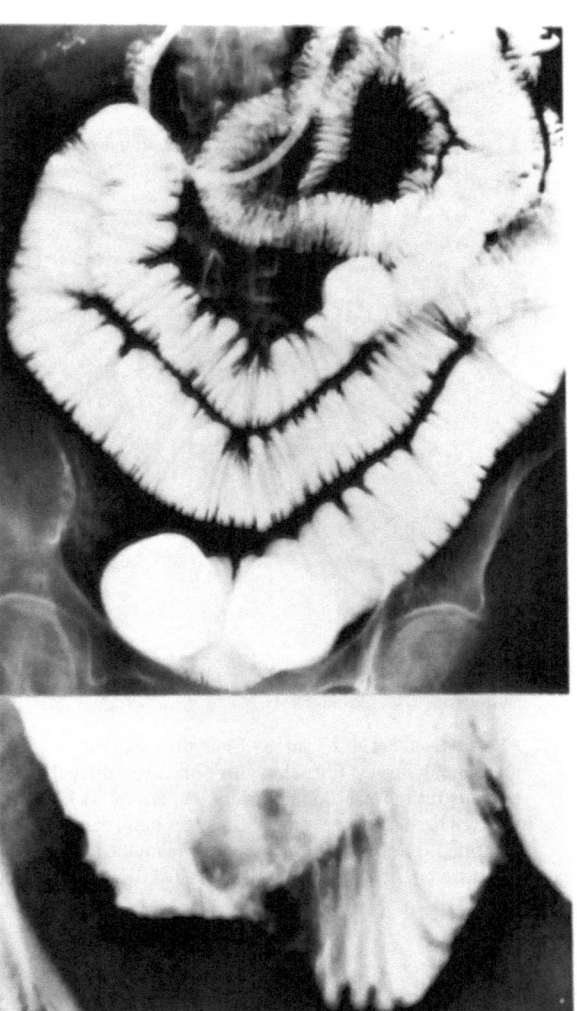

Fig. 14.3B. Mechanical obstruction from Hodgkin's disease in the ileum in the lower abdomen. Note the dilatation that increases distalward and the normal motility in the proximal jejunum. On this basis, the possibility of a nonobstructing ileus, caused by certain drugs could be eliminated within the first 60 s of the examination.

tered, here too the specific gravity of the next dose of 800 ml barium suspension is decreased with respect to the preceding dose. In practice this gives the following dose schedule:

1) dose of 800 ml
   s.g. = 1.30; rate of flow 75 ml/min
2) dose of 800 ml
   s.g. = 1.15; rate of flow 40 ml/min
3) 30 ml metoclopramide through tube, to enhance peristalsis.
4) dose of 800 ml water
   rate of flow 25 ml/min

Obviously it is essential to know beforehand how high the infusion bag must be suspended in order to

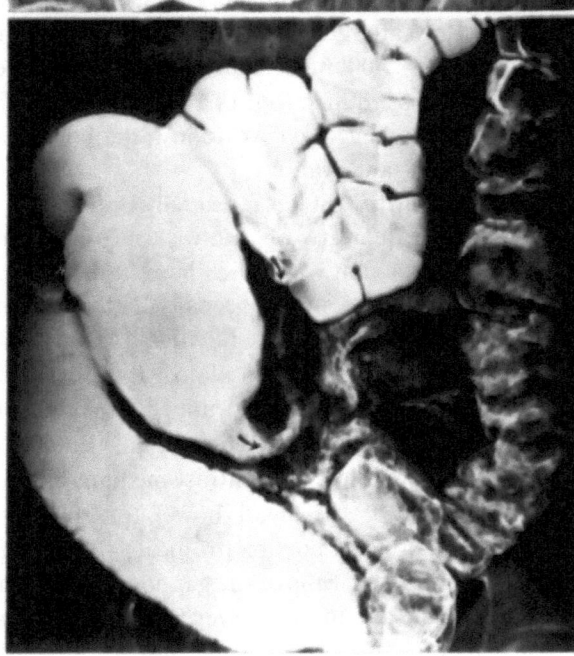

Fig. 14.3A. Ileus due to recurring stenosis in a patient with an ileocolic anastomosis and a 'short bowel' (Crohn's disease). In spite of the use of 1800 ml contrast fluid, the small bowel was almost empty within 3 h.

420

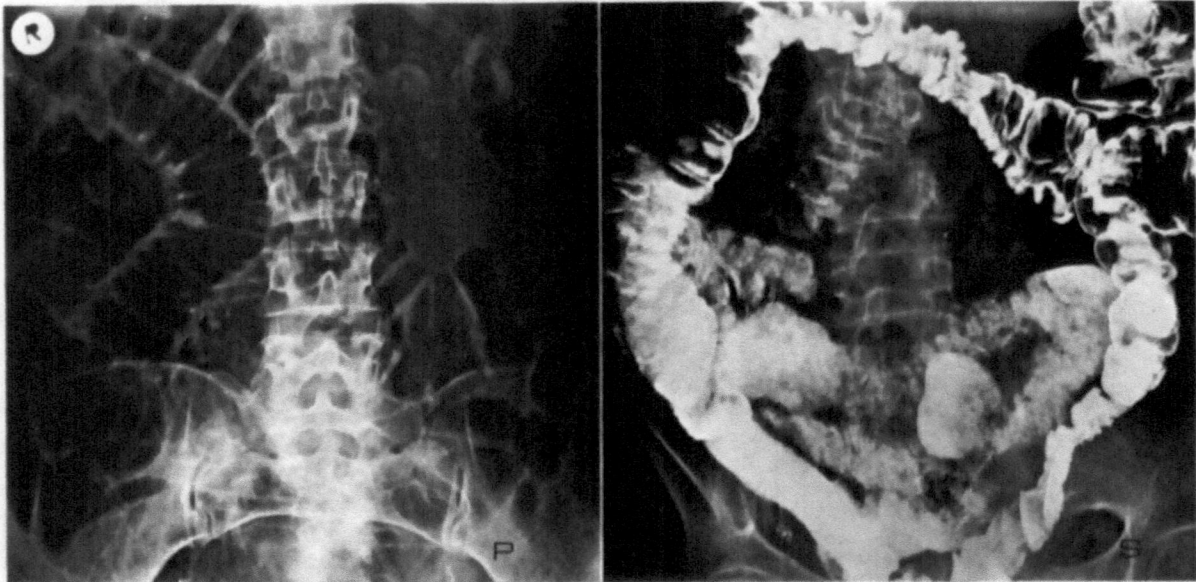

*Fig. 14.4*P–S. Series of survey films of a stenotic process in the distal ileum that developed after a minor ileal resection. (P) Plain abdominal survey film showing numerous dilated intestinal loops filled with an overabundance of gas. (Q) Survey film after administration of 1200 ml barium suspension. (R) (see page 422) Survey film after 1200 ml barium suspension followed by 1200 ml water. The stenosis, several centimeters long, was visualized on the spot films with the compression technique, but the cause was not identified. The obstruction was solely from the narrow anastomosis with pronounced edema of the intestinal wall. (S) About 10 h after the start of the examination, that lasted 1 h, most of the contrast fluid is in the colon.

obtain the correct rate of flow for each phase of the examination When uncertain, it is preferable to be on the safe side and choose a rate that is too low.

In most cases the obstruction site is reached in

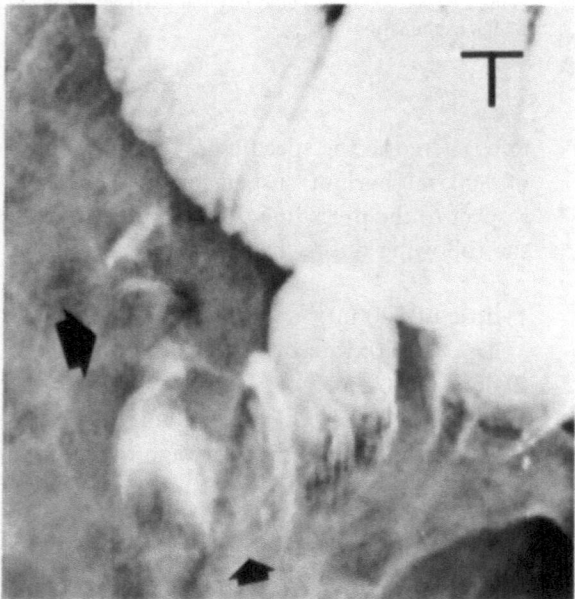

*Fig. 14.4*T. Compression detail of the stenosis in the case of fig. 14.4QR. (See also pages 421 and 422.)

about an hour, even if it is fairly pronounced and rather distal in the small intestine (fig. 14.1CD). It is certainly possible to make excellent compression spot films after administration of this maximum dosage of 2400 ml – but a careful and precise technique is required (fig. 14.2). If the obstruction is not yet reached, then we follow the conservative approach – and wait.

To our surprise it has repeatedly been shown that this large quantity of contrast medium usually reaches the colon within 6–8 h, even in the case of very pronounced stenoses located in the distalmost part of the small intestine (see figs. 14.3A and 14.4). In a few patients with an almost total obstruction the colon was not reached until the next morning (24 h later). It can in such cases take one to three weeks before all of the contrast medium has disappeared out of the small bowel (see fig. 14.1A). Occasionally it is possible to locate the site of the obstruction by means of the gas contours on one or more of the abdominal survey films. In other cases, signs of a space-occupying infiltrate are clearly visible in the lower right quadrant. Partly on the basis of other factors such as age and clinical course, the diagnosis of an 'appendicular infiltrate'

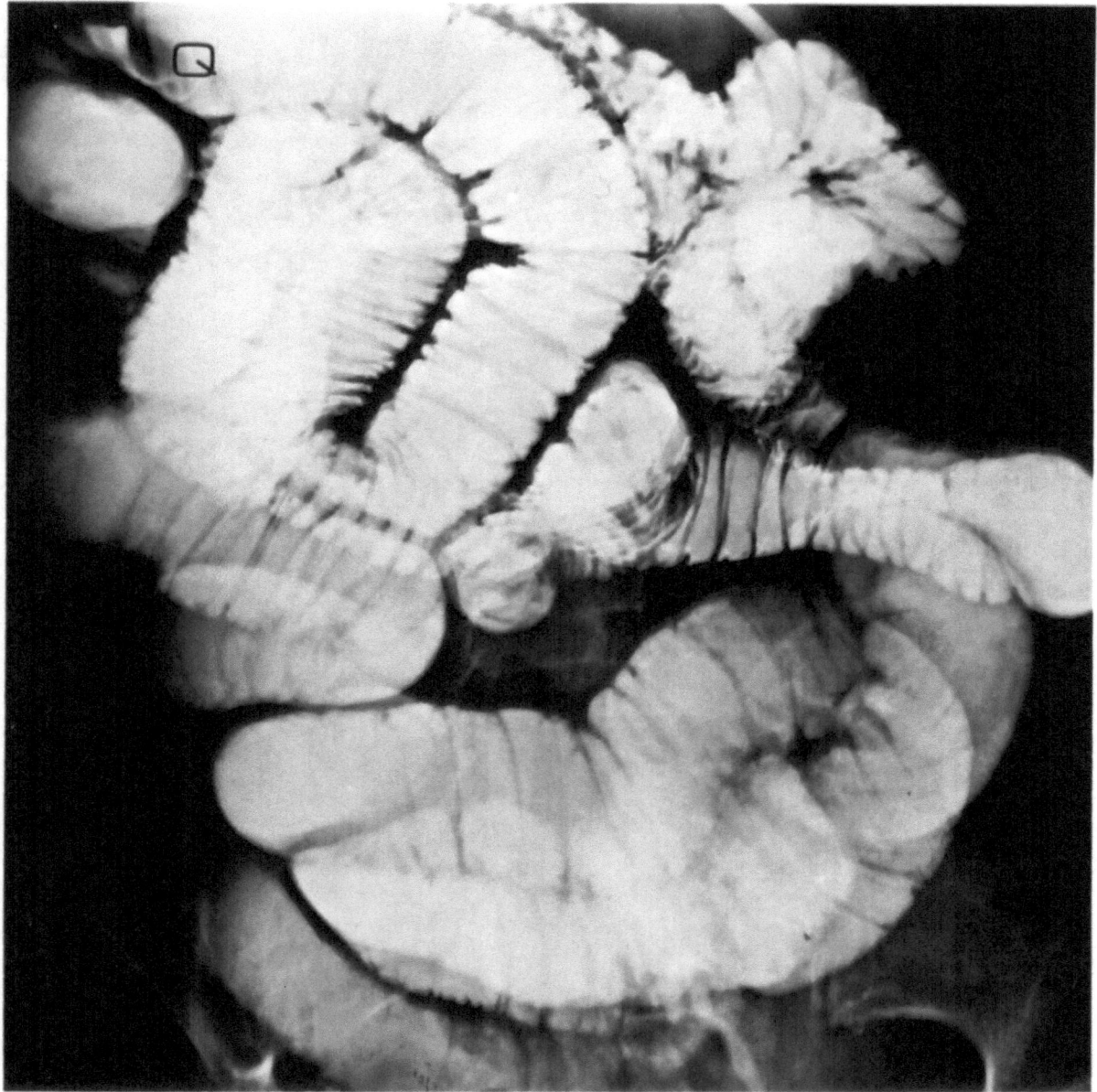

*Fig. 14.4*Q. See legends on page 420.

can easily be made without using a contrast medium. It must be stressed that extensive preoperative diagnostic techniques serve little purpose when the chest and abdominal films have already revealed the diagnosis. The abdominal films may show the presence of extensive bands, an ileus from gall stones, perforation of the digestive tract and indicate when surgical intervention must not be delayed.

It should be mentioned that an enteroclysis examination may be carried out only after it has been determined that the obstruction is *not* located in the colon. Usually this is easy from the survey films.

Carefully evaluate the abdominal survey films taken before the barium examination. Remember that the site of the obstruction usually lies further distalward than is presumed from the gas configurations on these films!

In the case of a stenosis in the *colon*, there is dehydration of the contrast fluid proximal to the site of the obstruction. The barium suspension becomes so thick that barium stones develop, causing an evental subileus to become a manifest ileus.

422

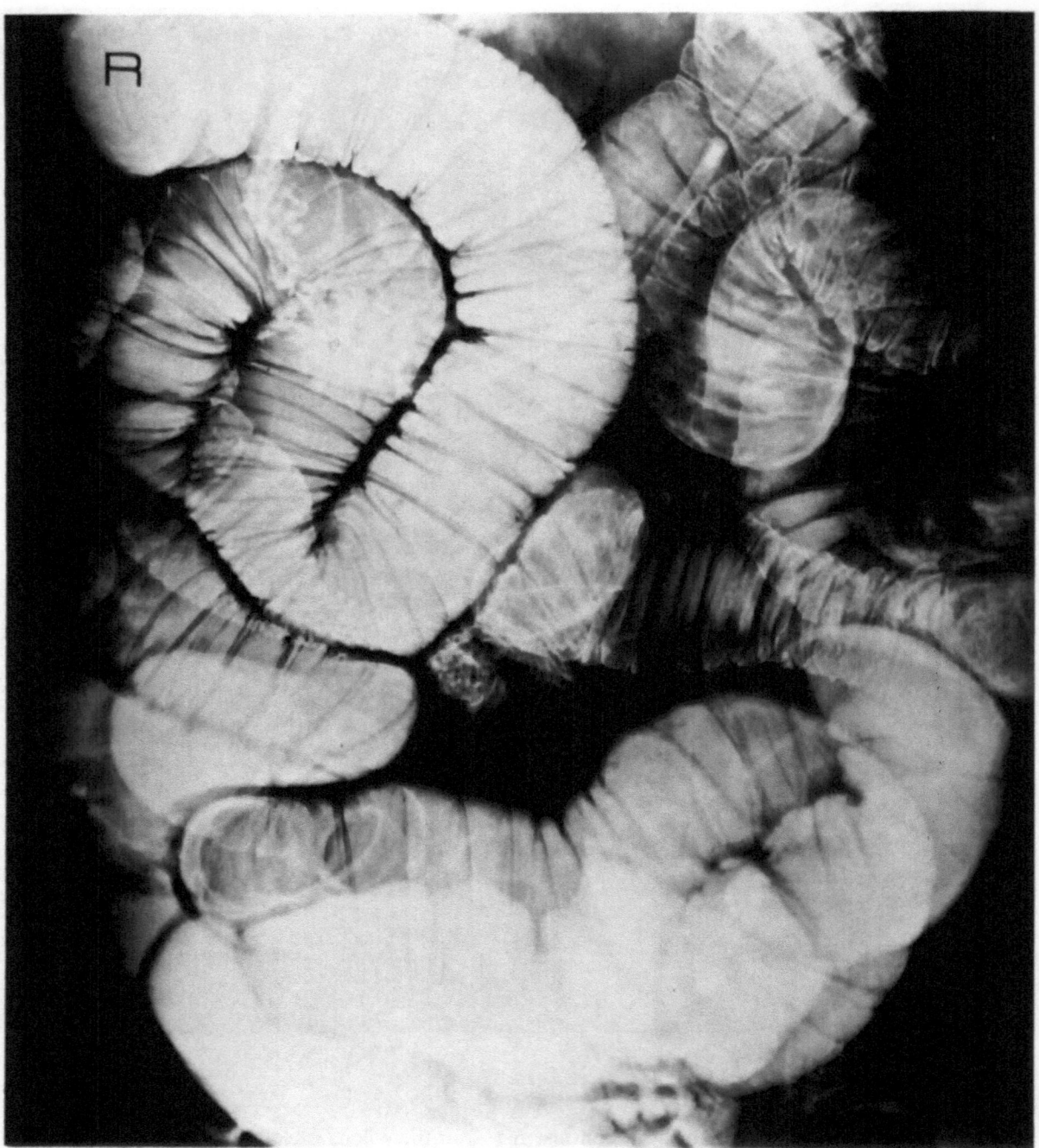

Fig. 14.4R. See legends on page 420.

In the event of doubt as to the location of the ileus, a retrograde enteroclysis examination may also be considered (fig. 14.5).

When a patient with ileus is examined by using enteroclysis, it is important to note during the first minute of the examination whether active peristalsis exists in the proximal jejunum. Important conclusions can be based on this finding! If peristalsis is active in the beginning, then a drug-induced non-obstructing ileus can be eliminated (fig. 14.3B). In the event of a mechanical ileus, peristalsis may be active at first and then gradually decrease during the course of the examination. This is true also in the most proximal part of the jejunum. If there is no peristalsis in the proximal jejunum from the immediate beginning of the examination, then either a

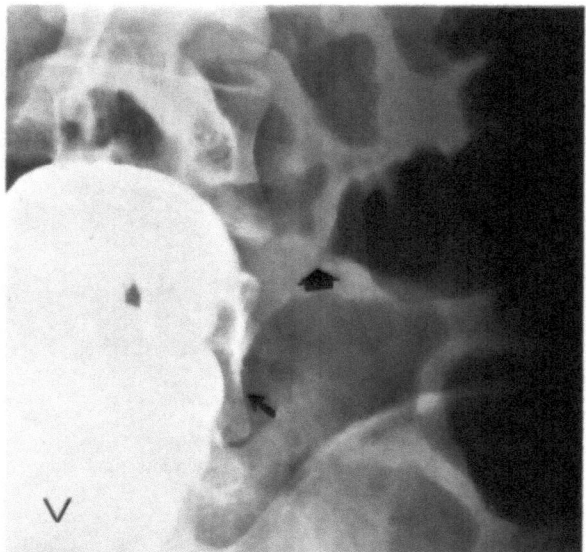

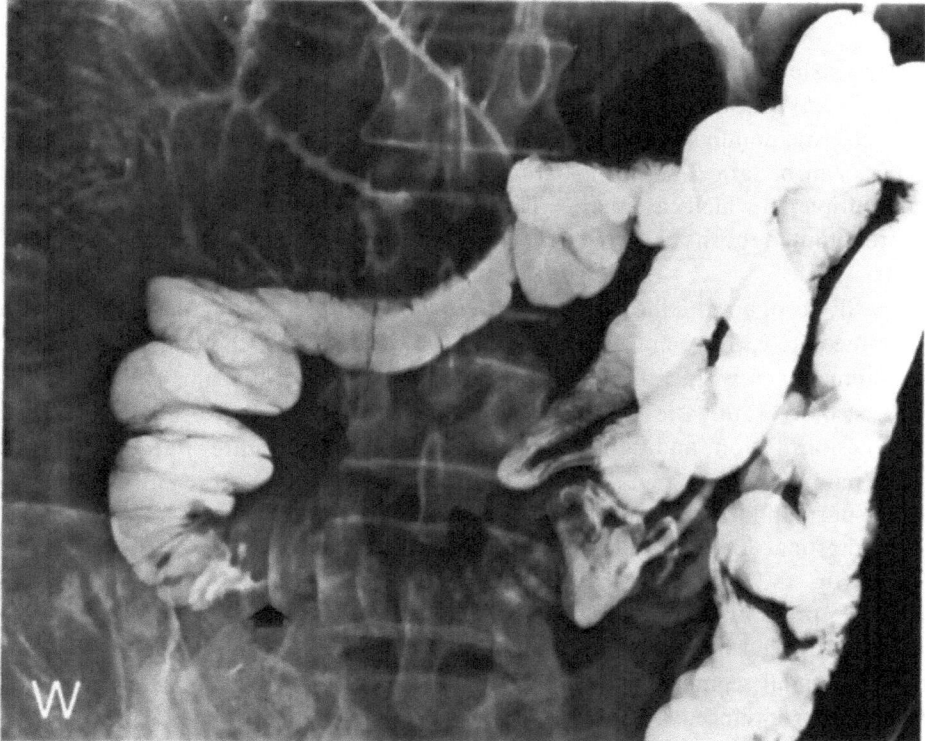

Fig. 14.5. (v) Ileus that was found during surgery to be from constriction by a band. The survey films without contrast fluid showed a cone-shaped shadow (thick arrow). By means of retrograde enteroclysis, the site of the obstruction (thin arrow) was approached from the distal direction. (w) Total obstruction due to metastases in the intestine. The site of the obstruction (arrow) could be approached only from the distal side. Highly swollen jejunal loops filled with air.

paralytic ileus, or a long-term, or severe mechanical obstruction is possible and likely.

2. Fusion – Bands

Bands are almost never demonstrated by a radiological examination. Because of this and prob-

ably also as a result, guidelines for the identification of bands cannot be found in textbooks of roentgenology.

Bands are often multiple; they can develop after surgical intervention although other causes are certainly also possible. Small bands between adjacent loops can be considered more or less as local adhesions. The x-rays often reveal highly elongated

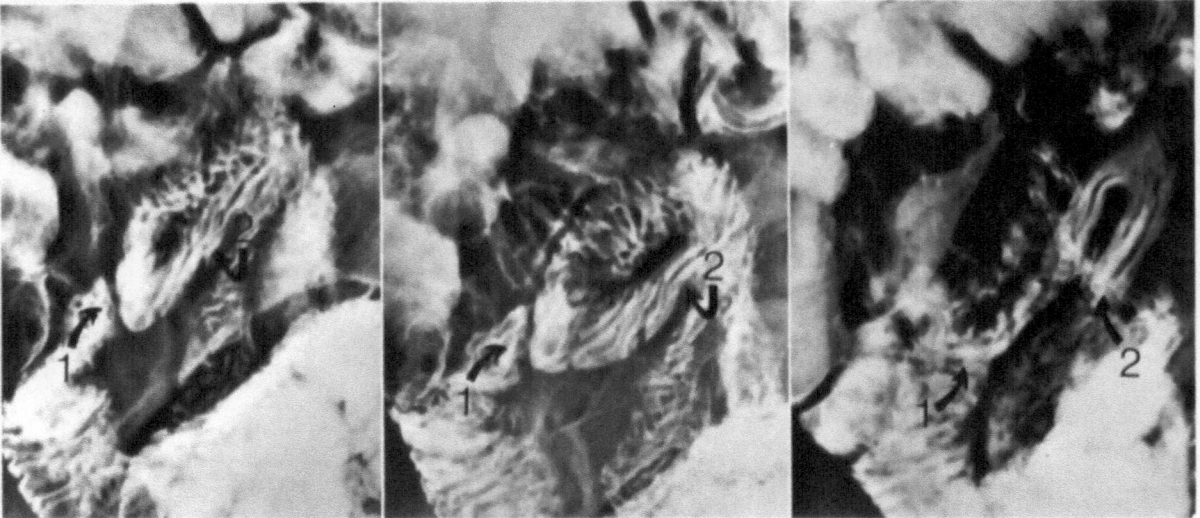

Fig. 14.6. Stretched mucosal folds extending along the length of the intestine (2) and local adhesion of two intestinal loops (1) (see elsewhere on this page).

mucosal folds locally that extend parallel to the length of the intestine (fig. 14.6). In other cases the band causes highly characteristic pointed bulges on the intestine. These bulges can be large and single (fig. 14.7) or small and multiple, in which case they generally appear as several pointed thorns clustered close together (fig. 14.8).

However, even these easily recognized adhesions are not demonstrated immediately. They are usually only visible on spot films taken with compression during careful fluoroscopic examination. The complaints caused by adhesion, fusion, and bands consist mainly of periodic pain in the abdomen that can be either colic-like or sharp and thrusting. This is not only because the intestinal loops are elongated or have sharp kinks (fig. 14.9), but probably also from the often quite pronounced motility frequently visualized (fig. 14.10). This hypermotility can encompass a large or a small segment of the intestine. It is often most pronounced after a copious meal, and presumably develops as a result of a temporary anoxia in some of the intestinal loops. The complaints arising from adhesions and fusion usually are not severe enough to require surgery. They do, however, increase gradually in the course of time.

The patients suffer more from the long bands that cross several intestinal loops. Sometimes these bands may be visualized on the abdominal survey films as long thin ribbon-like dense streaks that extend straight across the air-filled abdomen. Bands are highly constricting and, in contrast to ad-

hesions, quickly give rise to complaints of obstruction. In intestinal loops filled with contrast fluid, the bands are easily identified by the indentations that they cause in the intestinal lumen (fig. 14.11). These indentations may be only on one side or may extend across one or more intestinal loops. This depends upon whether the loop is in the center or at the periphery of the abdominal cavity. It also depends on the course of the band with respect to the direction of the x-ray beam.

The diverse findings described above often appear in combination. In figures 14.6–14.8 and 14.11, these findings are numbered as indicated below:

1) Local adhesion of two loops.
2) Highly elongated mucosal folds extending along the length of the intestine.
3) Pointed bulge from local adhesion.
4) Several small thorn-like bulges from local adhesion of the intestinal wall to the surroundings.
5) Indentation of the intestinal loop by a band.
6) Long band traversing several intestinal loops.
7) Hypermotility.

As mentioned at the beginning of this section, bands and adhesions receive little or no attention in textbooks on radiology.

Although extremely common, this phenomenon is often not listed in the radiological reports. For this reason several x-rays of six patients (A–F) are shown on pages 429–436 to illustrate clearly the characteristic signs of this abnormality.

425

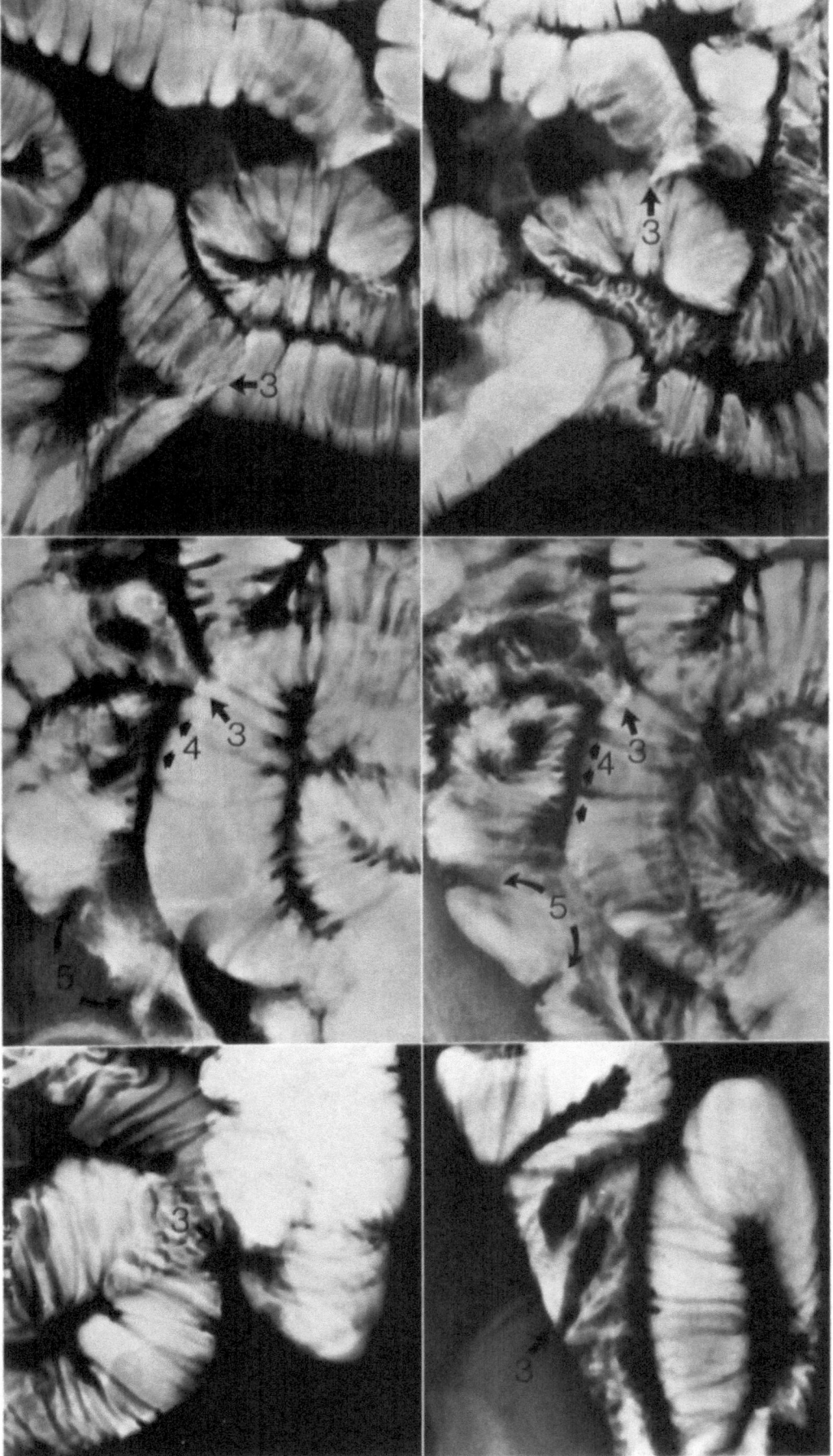

Fig. 14.7. Pointed bulges on elongated intestinal loops (3) due to fusion. Also visible are several indentations (5) as well as slight elongation of the somewhat thorn-like spaces between mucosal folds (4).

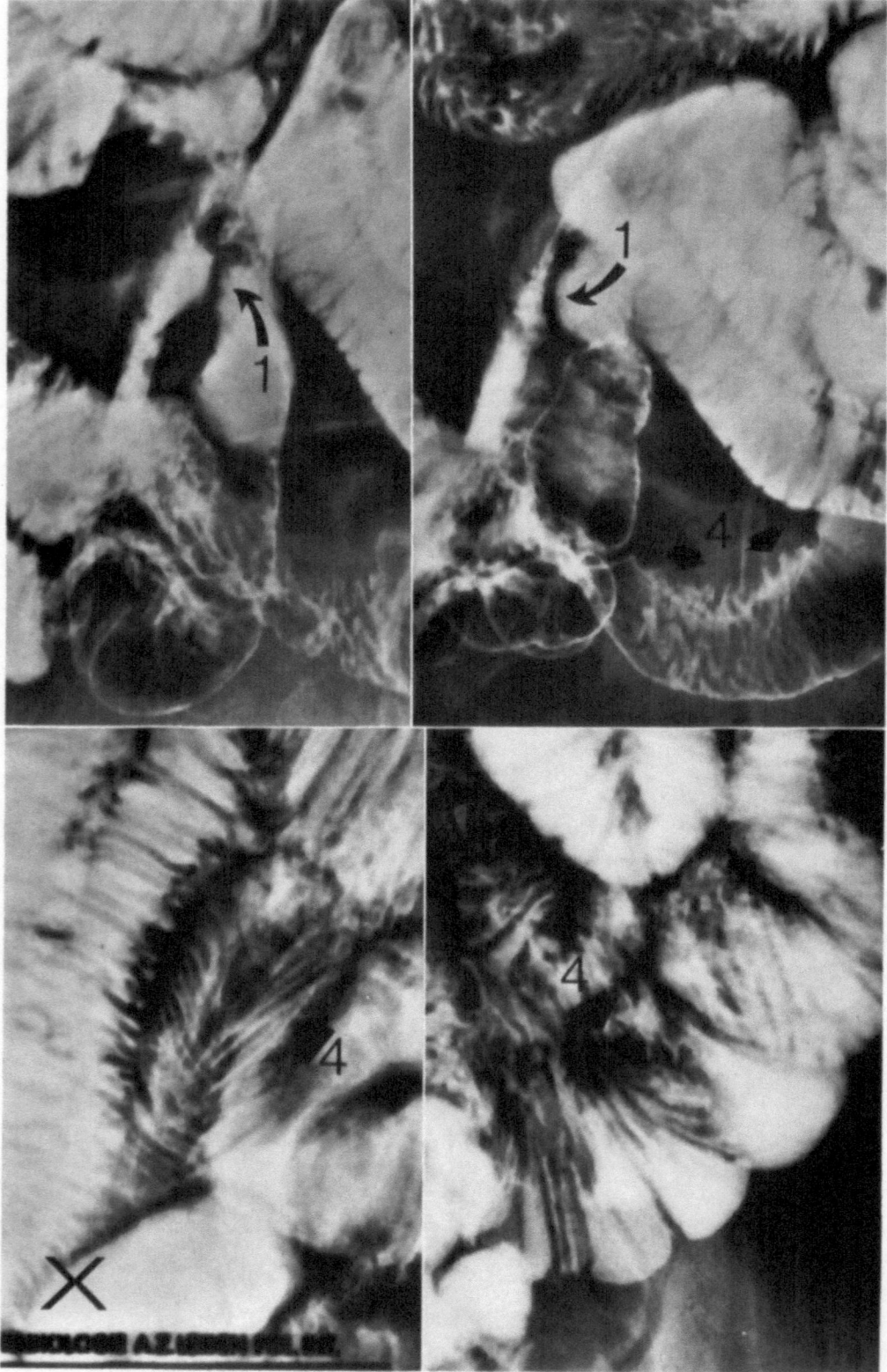

*Fig. 14.8*x. Pointed elongated mucosal folds from local fusion of the intestinal wall with the surrounding tissue (4); local adhesion of two loops (1).

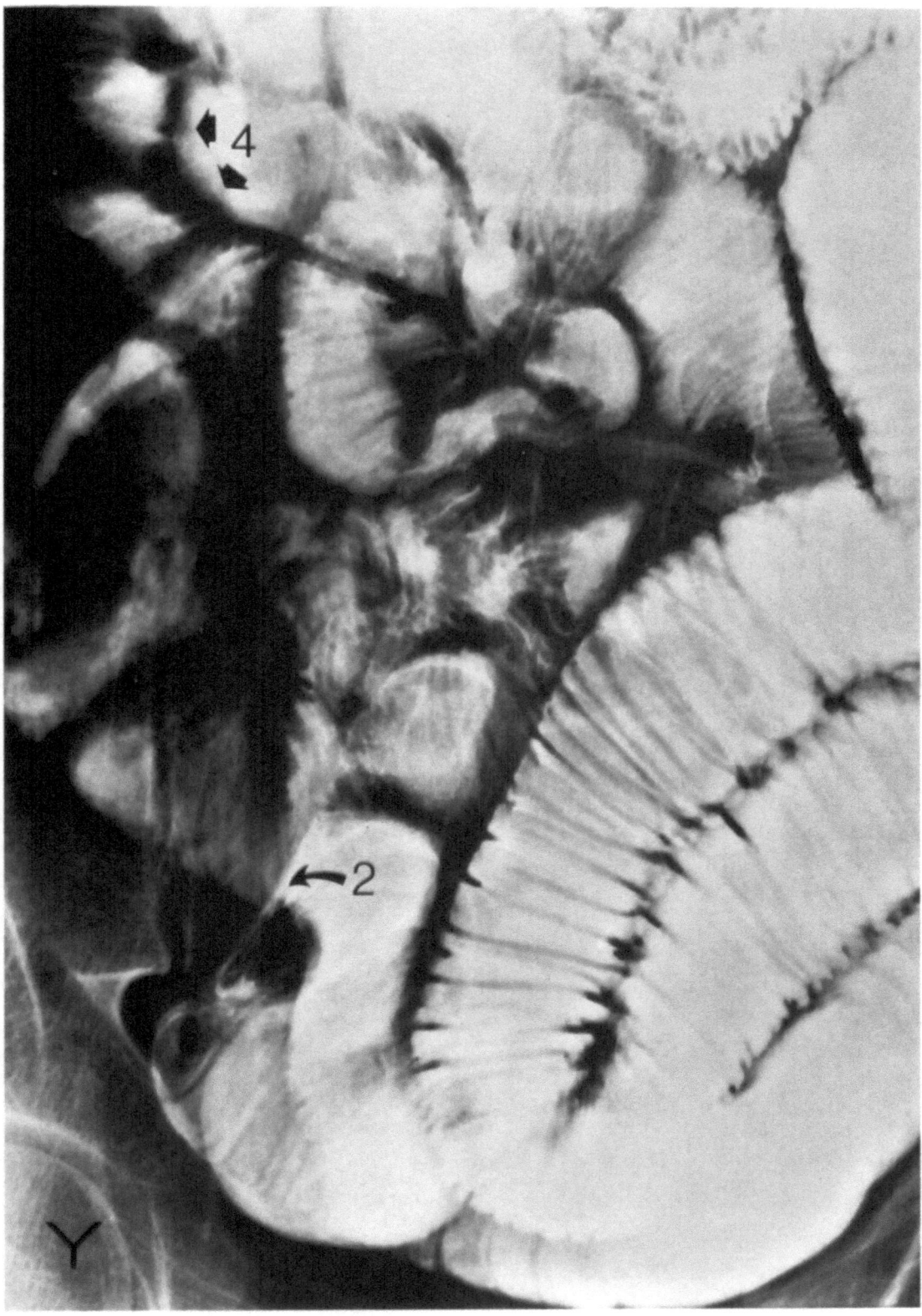

*Fig. 14.8*Y. Mucosal folds elongated in the lengthwise direction (2) in a patient with complaints of ileus. Extensive fusion throughout the entire left half of the abdomen. (For an explanation of the numbers, see page 424.)

428

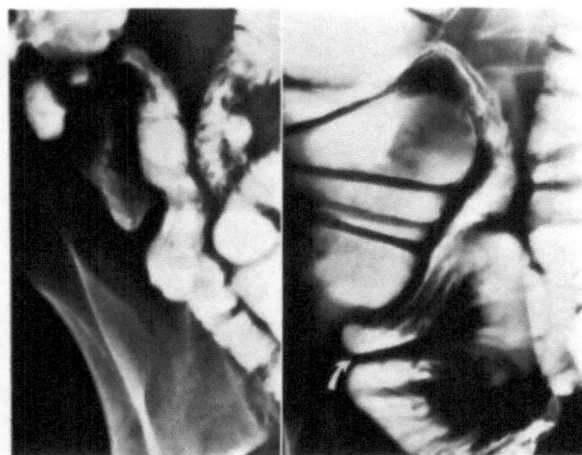

Fig. 14.9. Patient with periodic colic-like abdominal pains that developed only during the day. They were possibly caused by the kink in the distal ileum that is fused with the lowest part of the cecum. Transit would be impeded at this point when the patient stands erect and the cecum is well-filled (right).

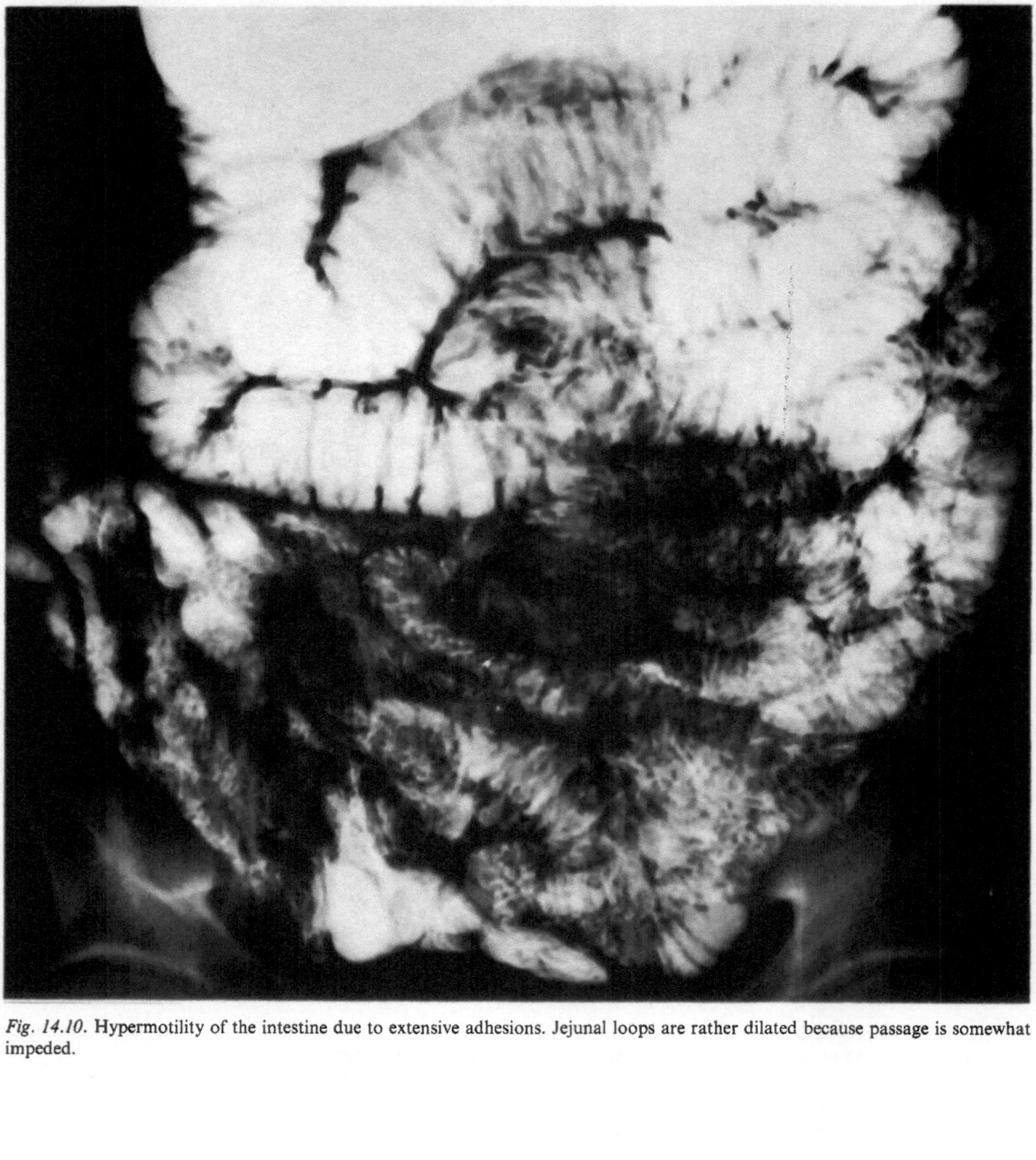

Fig. 14.10. Hypermotility of the intestine due to extensive adhesions. Jejunal loops are rather dilated because passage is somewhat impeded.

429

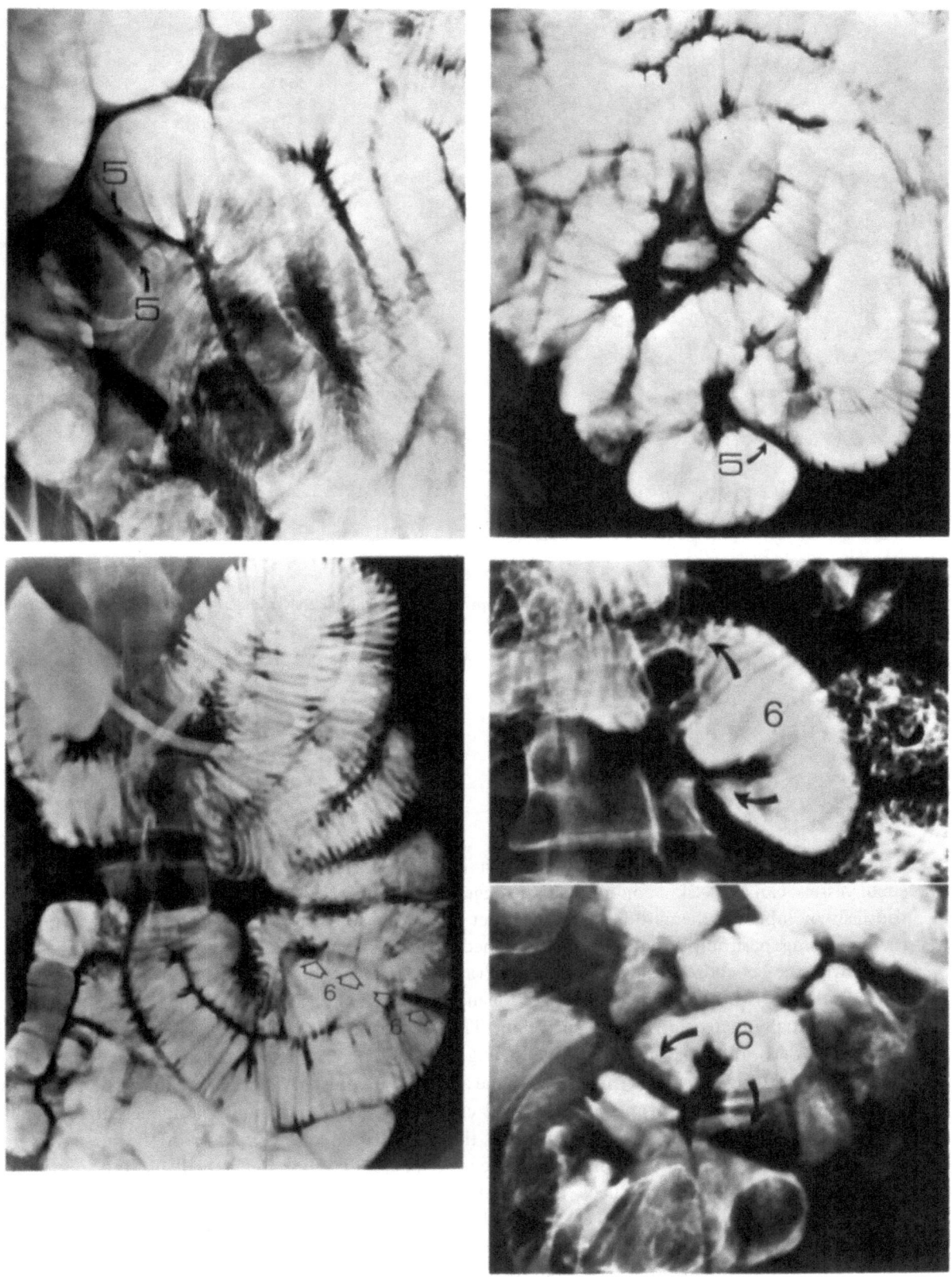

*Fig. 14.11*A. Several examples of indentations in the intestine due to bands (5), some of which cross several loops (6).

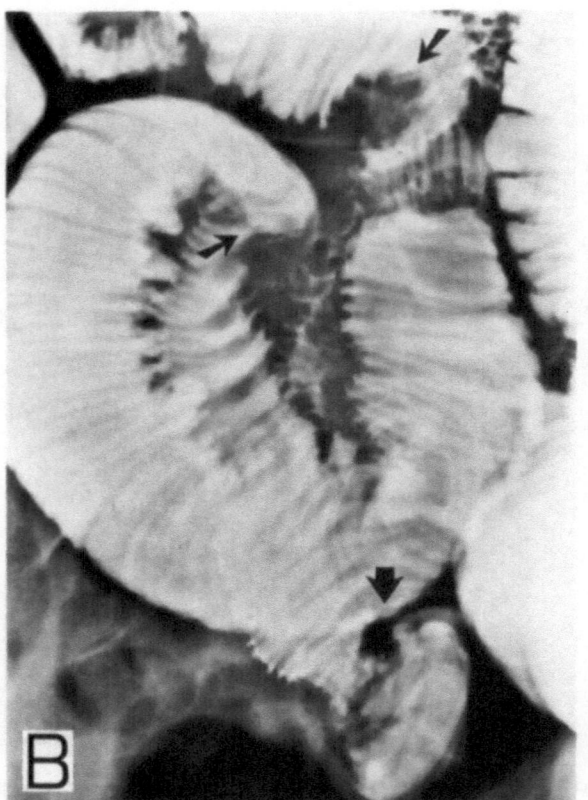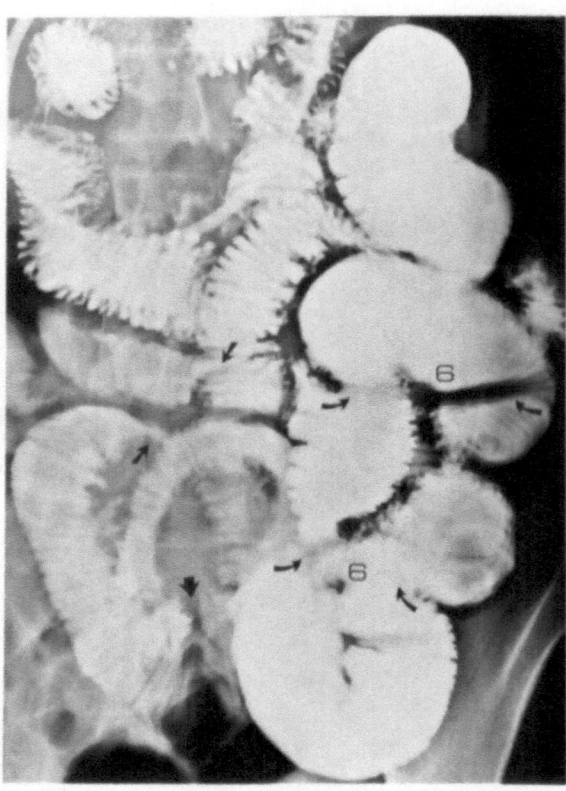

*Fig. 14.11*B. Multiple bands crossing several intestinal loops in a patient who had never undergone abdominal surgery. The bands were a livid blue and possibly congenital in origin.

A certain disorder, probably from occlusion of small vessels, can cause skin conditions that suggest psoriasis or lupus erythematodes. This disorder is the sclerosing peritonitis that results from medication with the beta adrenergic blocking drug Practolol. Both the visceral and the parietal peritoneum show a gradually increasing fibrous shriveling. The entire mass of loops of the small intestine is caught as it were in a strong net, and is forced to assume an increasingly central position in the abdominal cavity. Although transit can be seriously impeded, the intestinal loops are not able to dilate. This means that the radiological diagnosis 'ileus' is masked. It has been noted, however, that these loops show numerous widely scattered indentations suggesting bands or abrupt kinks. It is possible then to establish the diagnosis – if the possibility is considered (fig. 14.12).

3. Volvulus

Because of their constricting nature, bands sometimes cause a volvulus of the intestine. On the roentgenogram the point of torsion of the volvulus can often be identified. This is shown by concentric rings of mucosal folds in the dilated intestinal loop that decrease in size toward the center (fig. 14.13).

Volvulus of a mass of intestinal loops can be caused by a particularly long mesentery. It can also be caused when fixation of the mesentery to the posterior abdominal wall is too short or inadequate. A good example of the latter is shown in fig. 14.14. It can be seen that the mass of intestinal loops changes position easily and as a result can cause intermittent complaints. If in patients with unexplained colic-like abdominal pain a positional anomaly is demonstrated, the possibility of a vol-

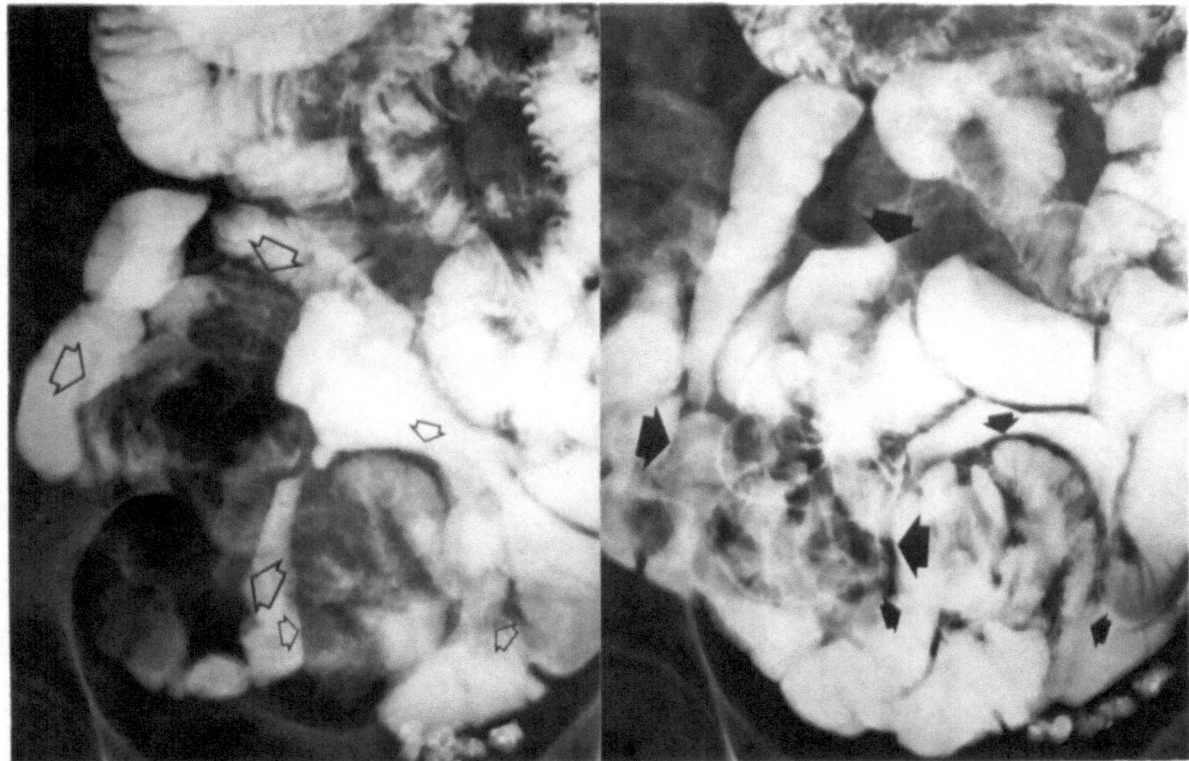

Patient A. Massive fusion of the entire mass of intestinal loops in the lower abdomen as a result of irradiation of a suspected Crohn's disease 30 years ago. At the beginning of the examination (left), large oval defects (open arrows) appeared in the mass of intestinal loops. They later filled with contrast fluid (right). The position of the intestinal loops (compare, open and solid arrows) does not change. Such a situation indicates extensive fusion – even without verification by means of compression.

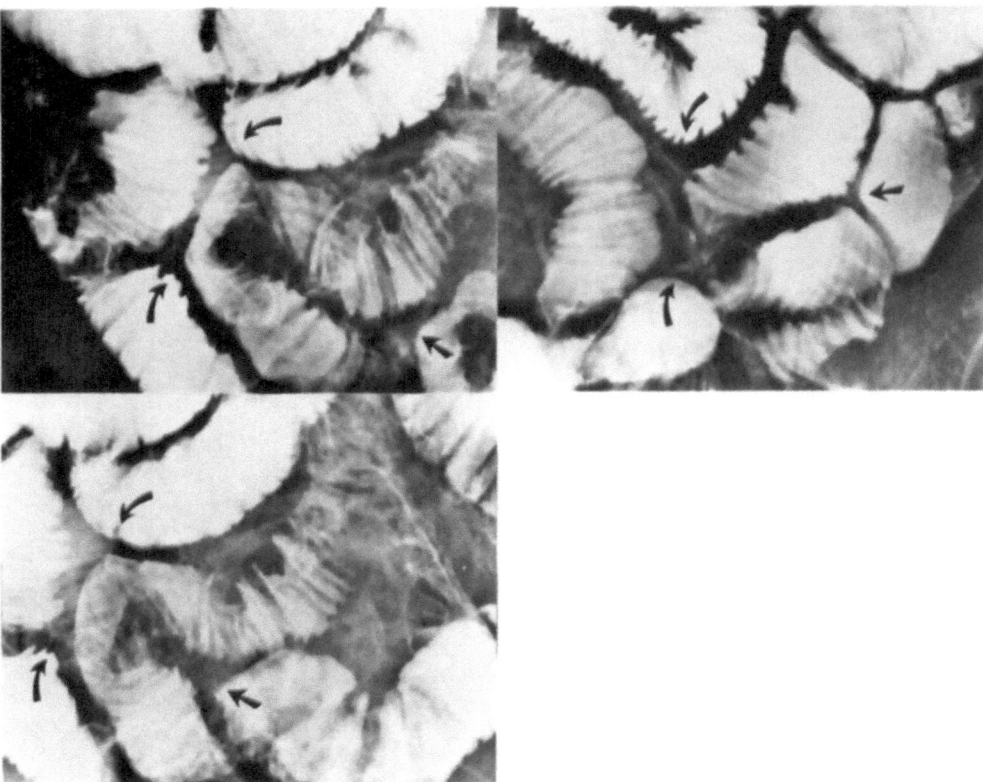

Patient B. A characteristic of adhesions is that specific sections of the intestine (see three different arrows) are always located in the same position with respect to adjacent loops. If a loop contracts, the loop that adheres to it will undergo passive stretching in width and the mucosal folds will follow a stretched course even when the loop is not wellfilled.

432

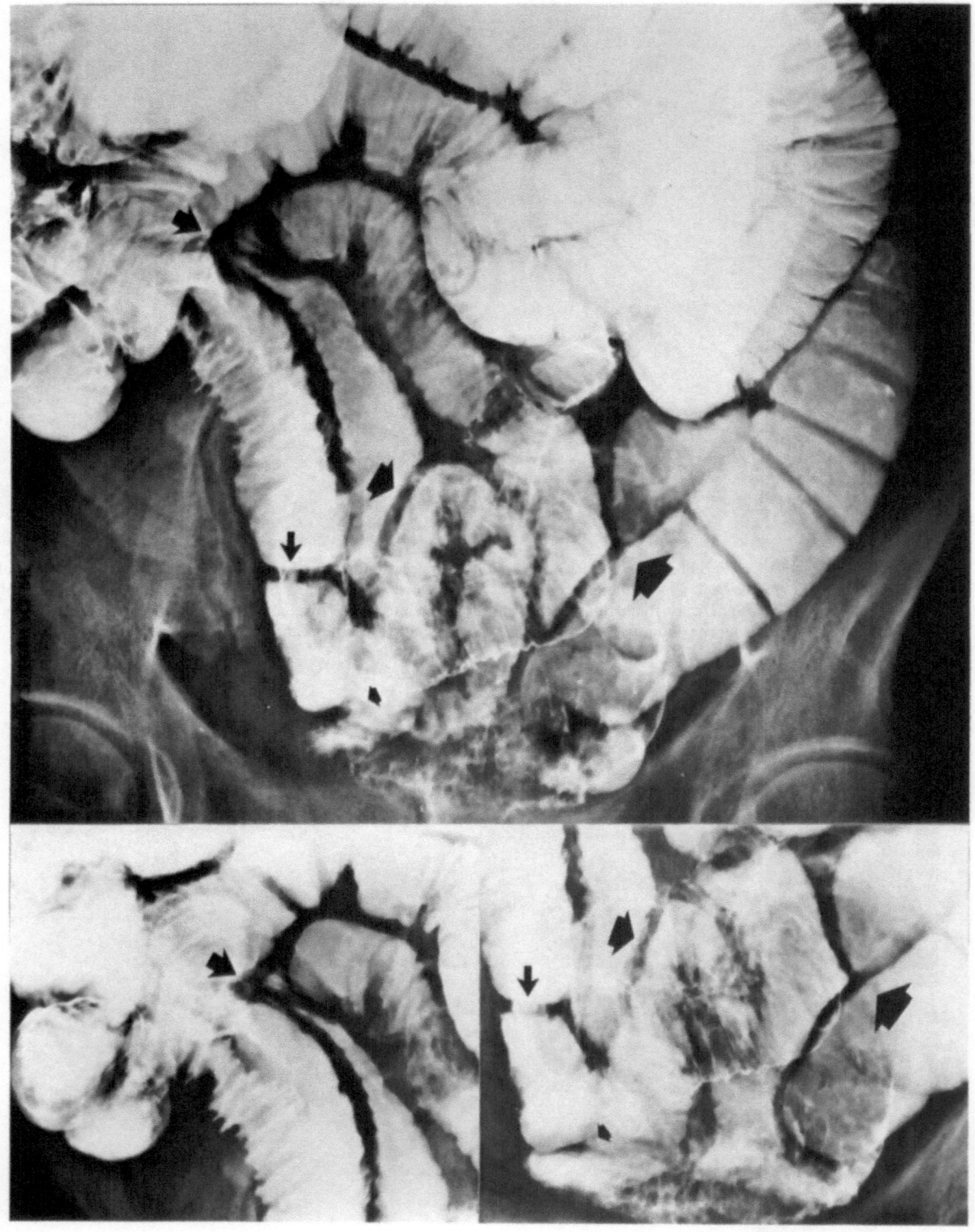

Patient C. Patient with complaints of obstruction. The roentgen examination revealed multiple fusions in the lower abdomen and on the right, next to the navel.

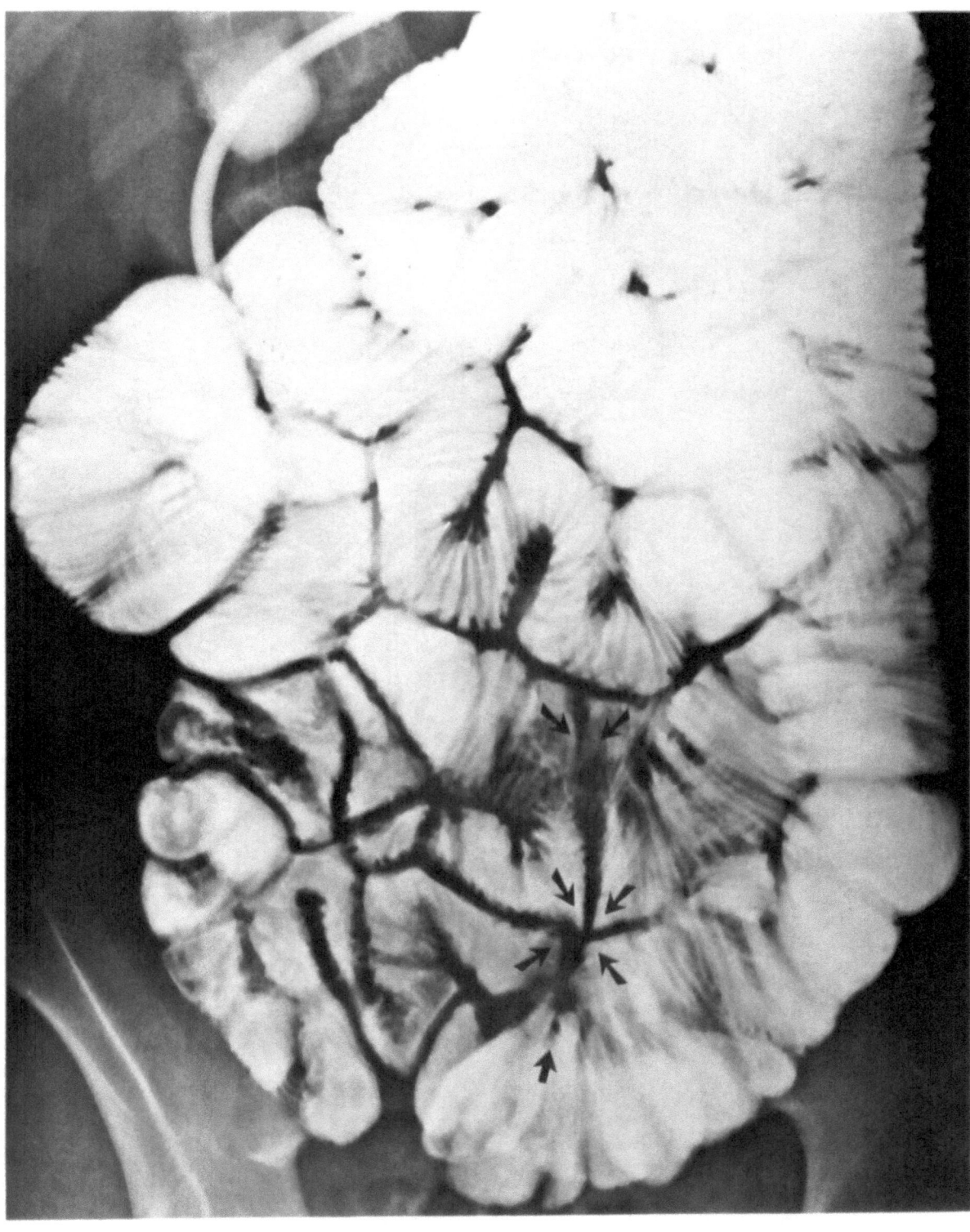

Patient D. Numerous fusions and bands in the lower half of the abdomen. This patient complained of obstruction after a Douglas pouch abscess had developed subsequent to gynecologic surgery.

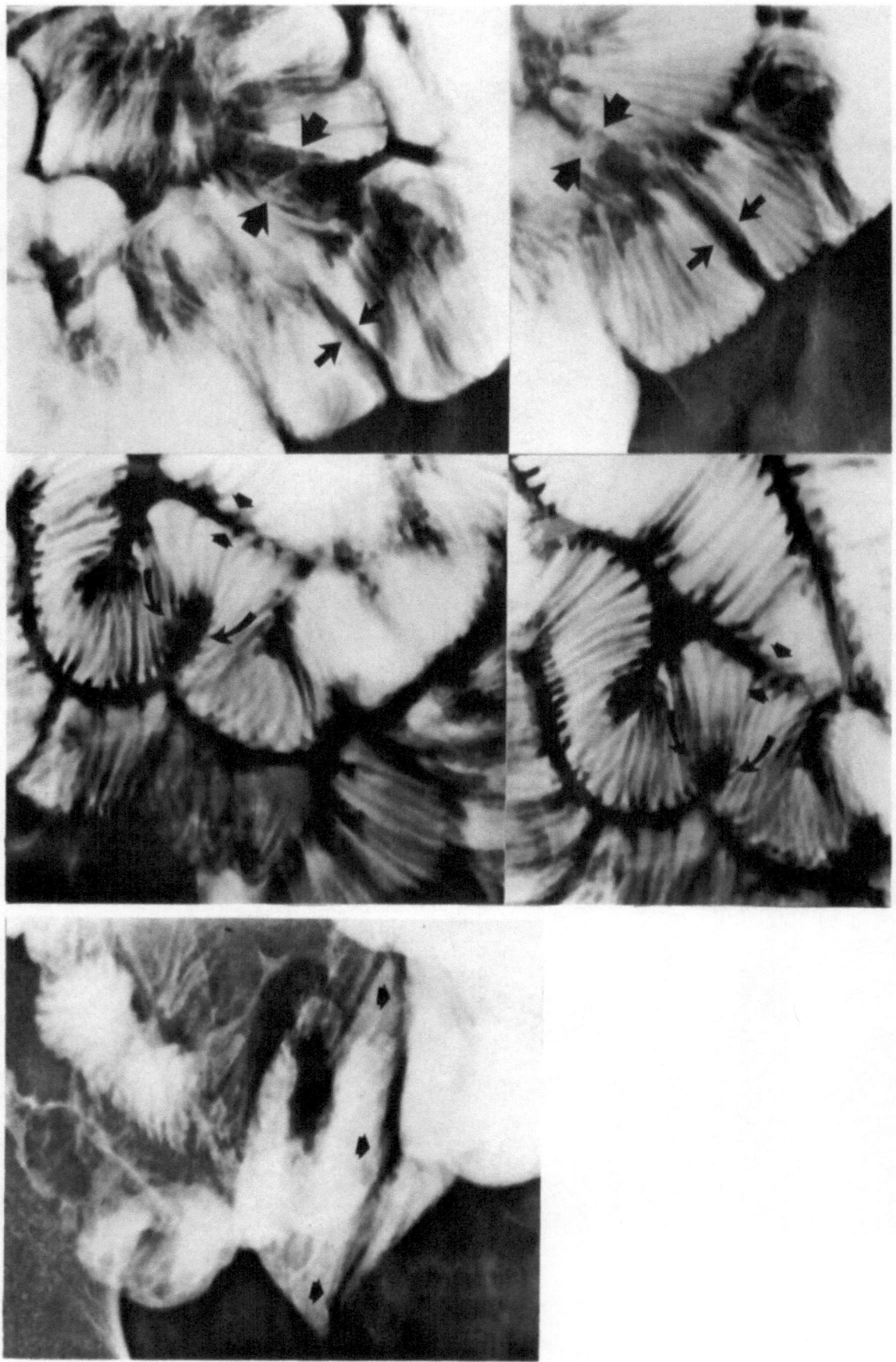

Patient E. Extended line of clarification, characteristic of a band crossing the mass of intestinal loops.

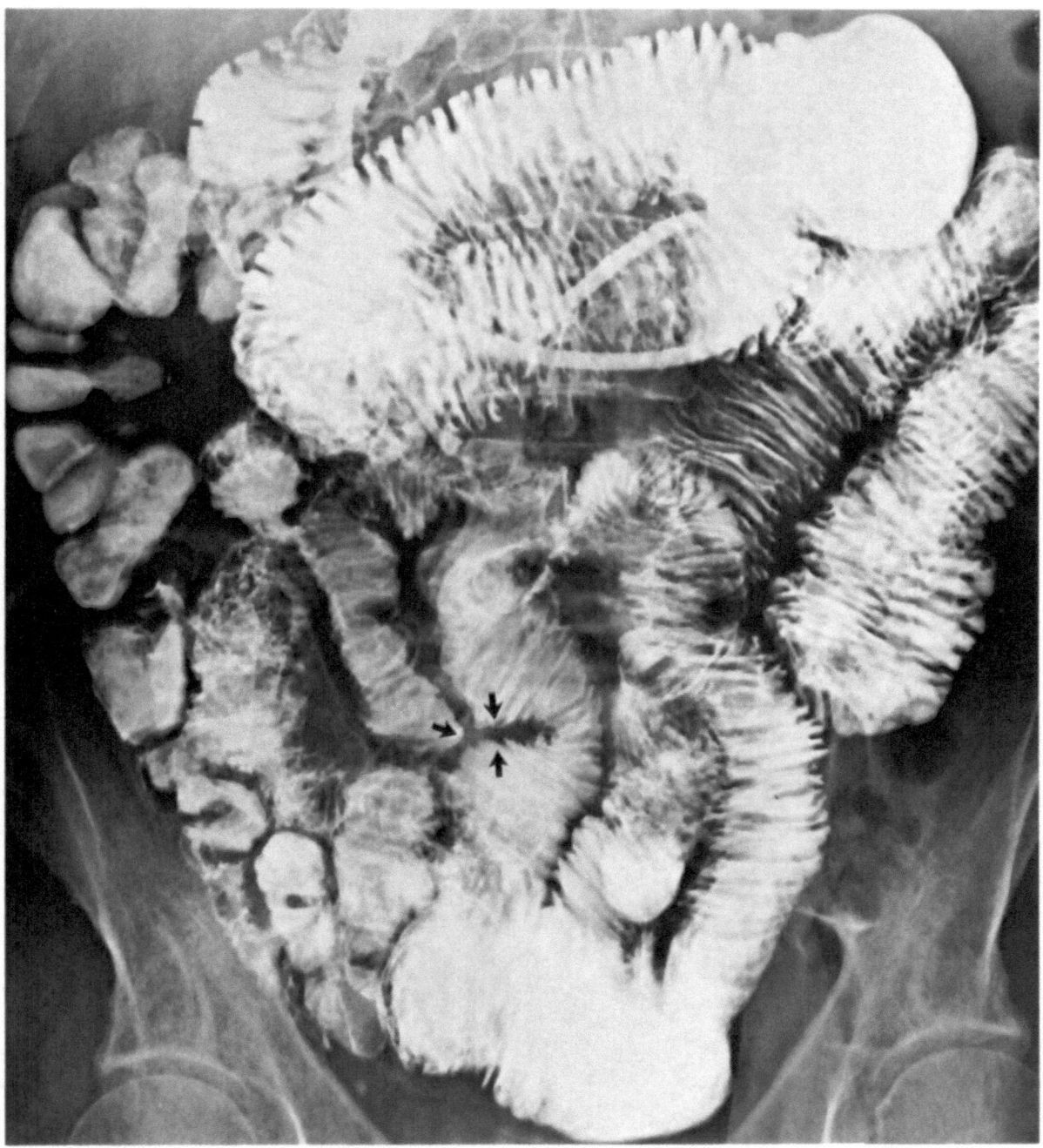

Patient F. Extensive fusion between the loops of the ileum and the distal jejunum. Enteroclysis examination several weeks after patient suffered severe abdominal pain and a state of subileus following a copious dinner. Presumably this is a case of temporary ischemia (severe intestinal angina) resulting in a coat of fibrin on the intestine. A follow-up examination one year later showed that the fusions had disappeared entirely and that the caliber of the intestine was once again normal. (See also page 436.)

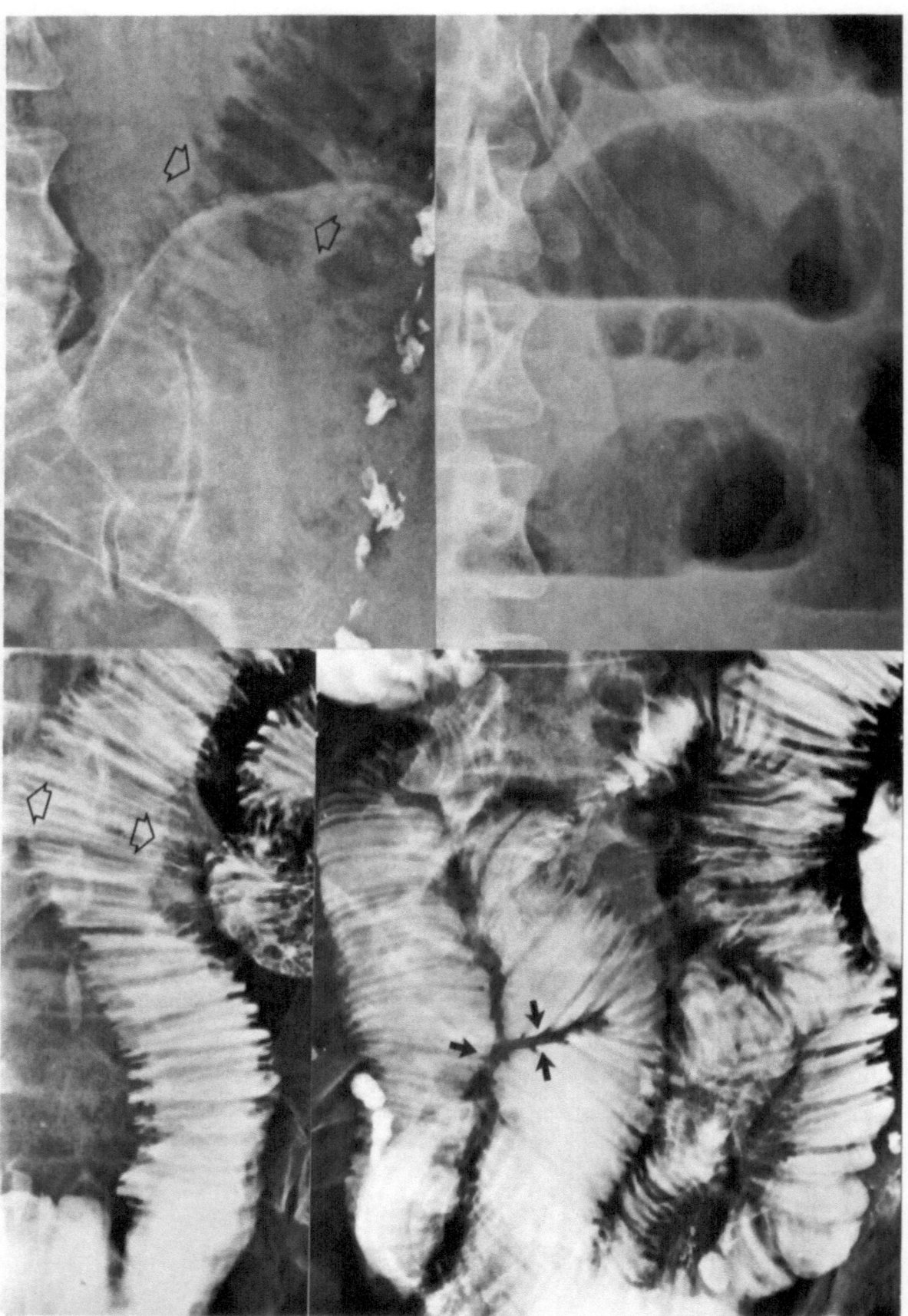

Patient F. See legend on page 435.

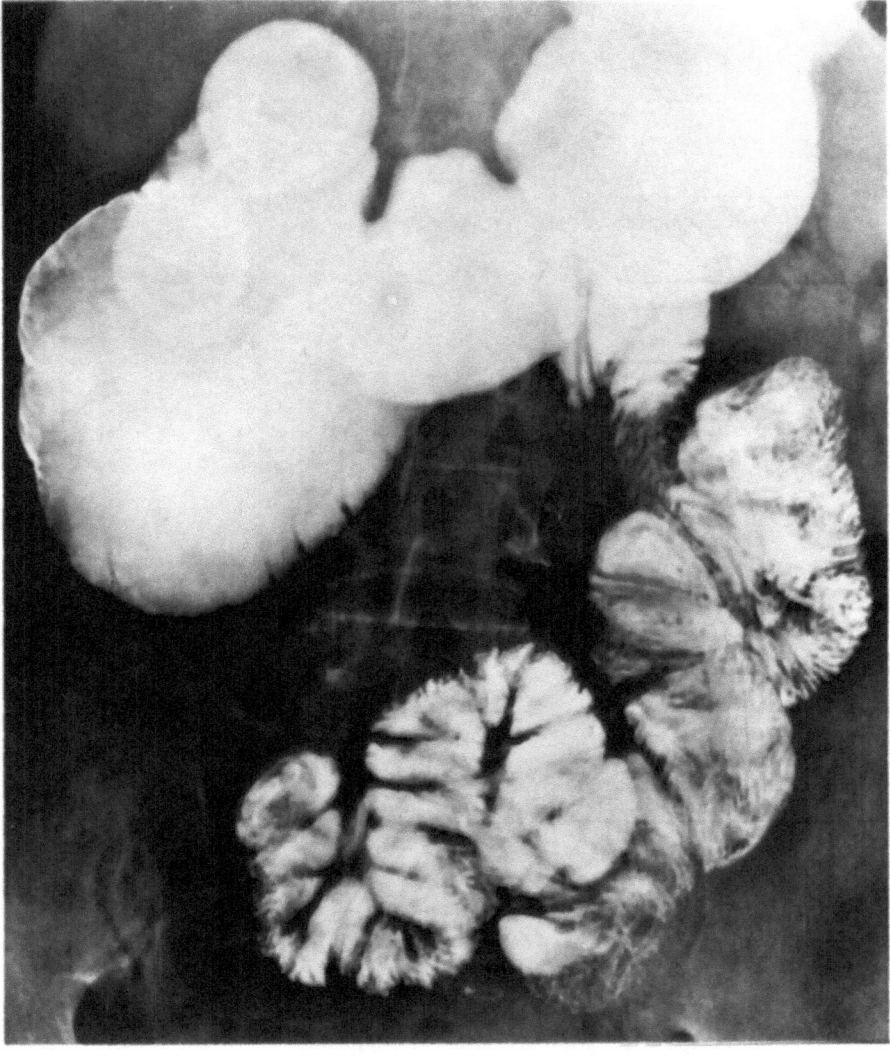

Fig. 14.12. Two examples of so-called 'sclerosing peritonitis' whereby the mass of intestinal loops becomes more or less wedged in a continuously shriveling peritoneal sac. The intestinal loops show multiple indentations like those seen in fig. 14.11. Markedly dilated duodenum in the patient on the left; only slight dilatation in the patient on the right. The normal ileus pattern is masked because the intestinal loops are not able to dilate. (See also page 438.)

vulus should always be considered (fig. 14.15). Often in volvulus the circulation is greatly disturbed in the involved intestinal segment. There can then be signs of mucosal swelling due to elevated venous pressure as well as hyperperistalsis due to anoxia of the intestine (fig. 14.16).

4. Intussusceptions

Small intestinal intussusceptions are often not recognized, but it is interesting that in the literature this diagnosis is also often based on insufficient evidence. This also supports the statement sometimes made, but not really obvious, that intussus-

ception in the small bowel can occur without causing symptoms and may be found accidentally.

An intussusception is seldom demonstrated, in spite of the more active peristalsis during an enteroclysis examination. A filling defect or radiolucency in the contrast column will be observed more readily with the enteroclysis examination than with conventional methods. On the latter, generally less than 500 ml contrast medium is administered at a much lower flow rate. In celiac disease in particular the intestinal loops are often dilated. The minute volume of the propulsive peristalsis may be greater than the stomach is able to pass on through the pylorus to the intestine. Large filling defects, sometimes due to air, may be seen then in the contrast

438

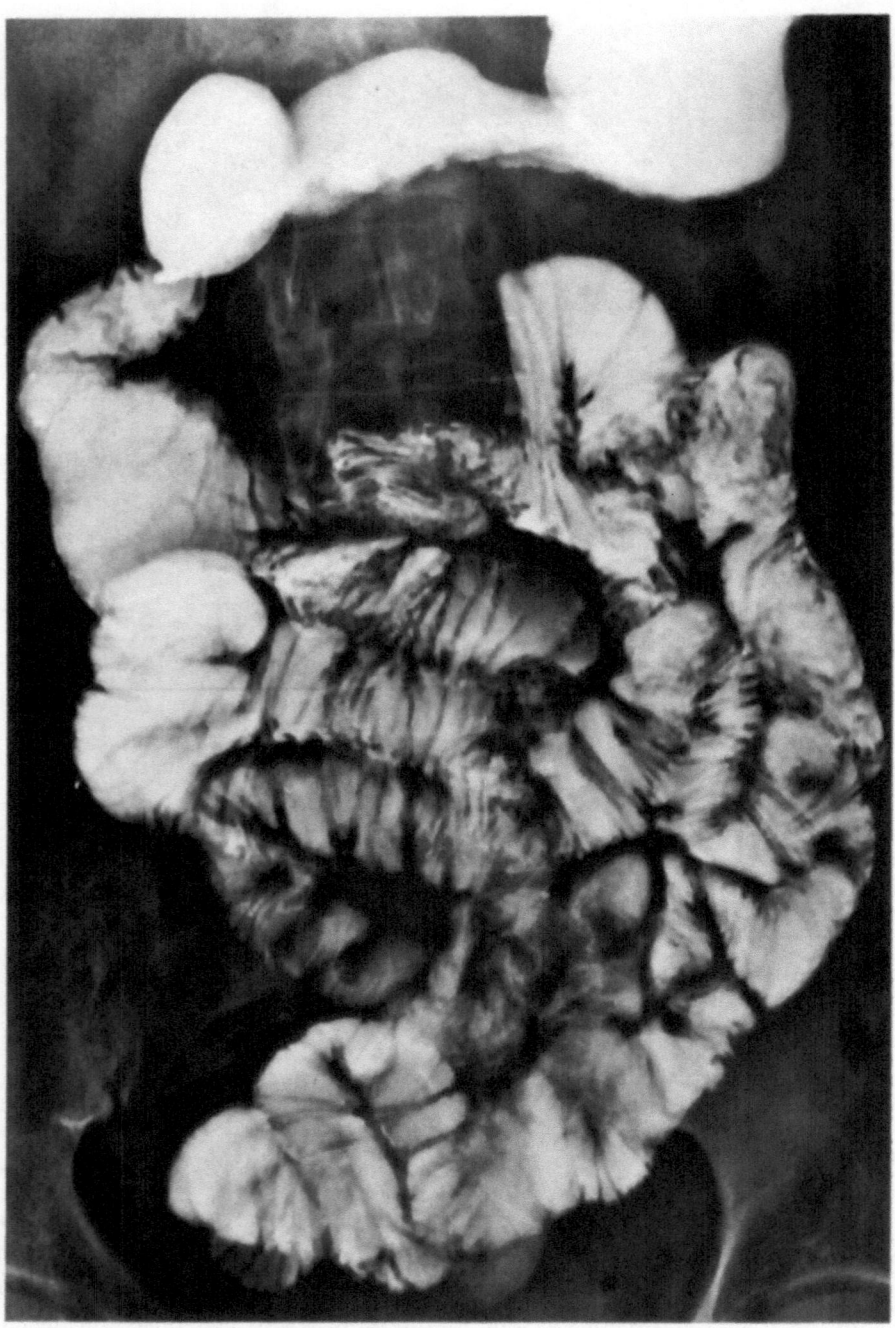

Fig. 14.12. See legend on page 437.

439

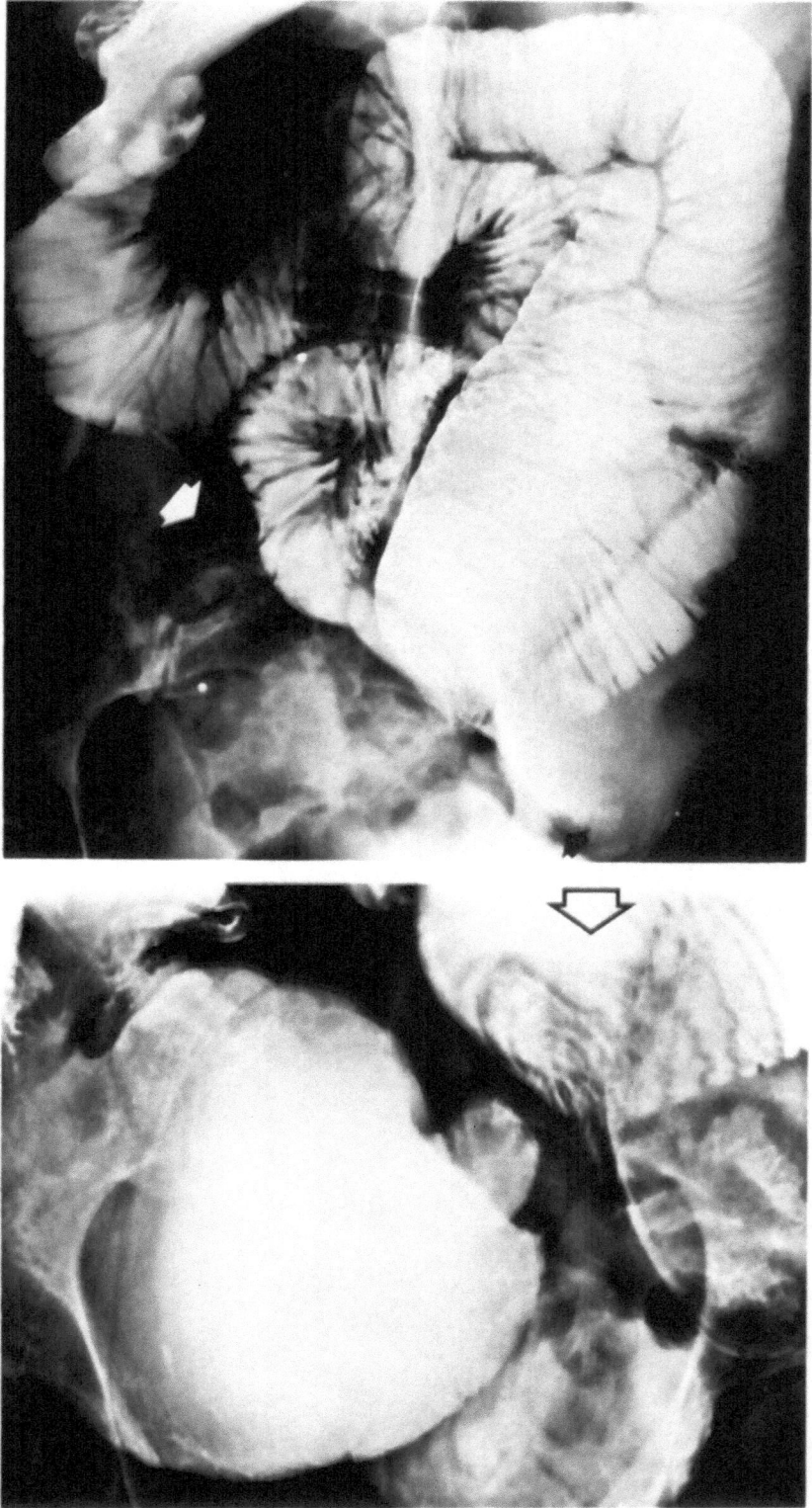

Fig. 14.13. Almost total obstruction of the small intestine because of a band that runs from the upper right to the lower left quadrant (solid arrows) in a patient with a 'short bowel' (Crohn's disease). This band constricted one loop completely and another quite markedly, thus causing a volvulus. Survey film after administration of 1200 ml contrast fluid. Subsequently the site of obstruction was approached from the distal direction by filling of the colon. The point of torsion can be recognized on this roentgenogram by the mucosal folds that form concentric rings (open arrow).

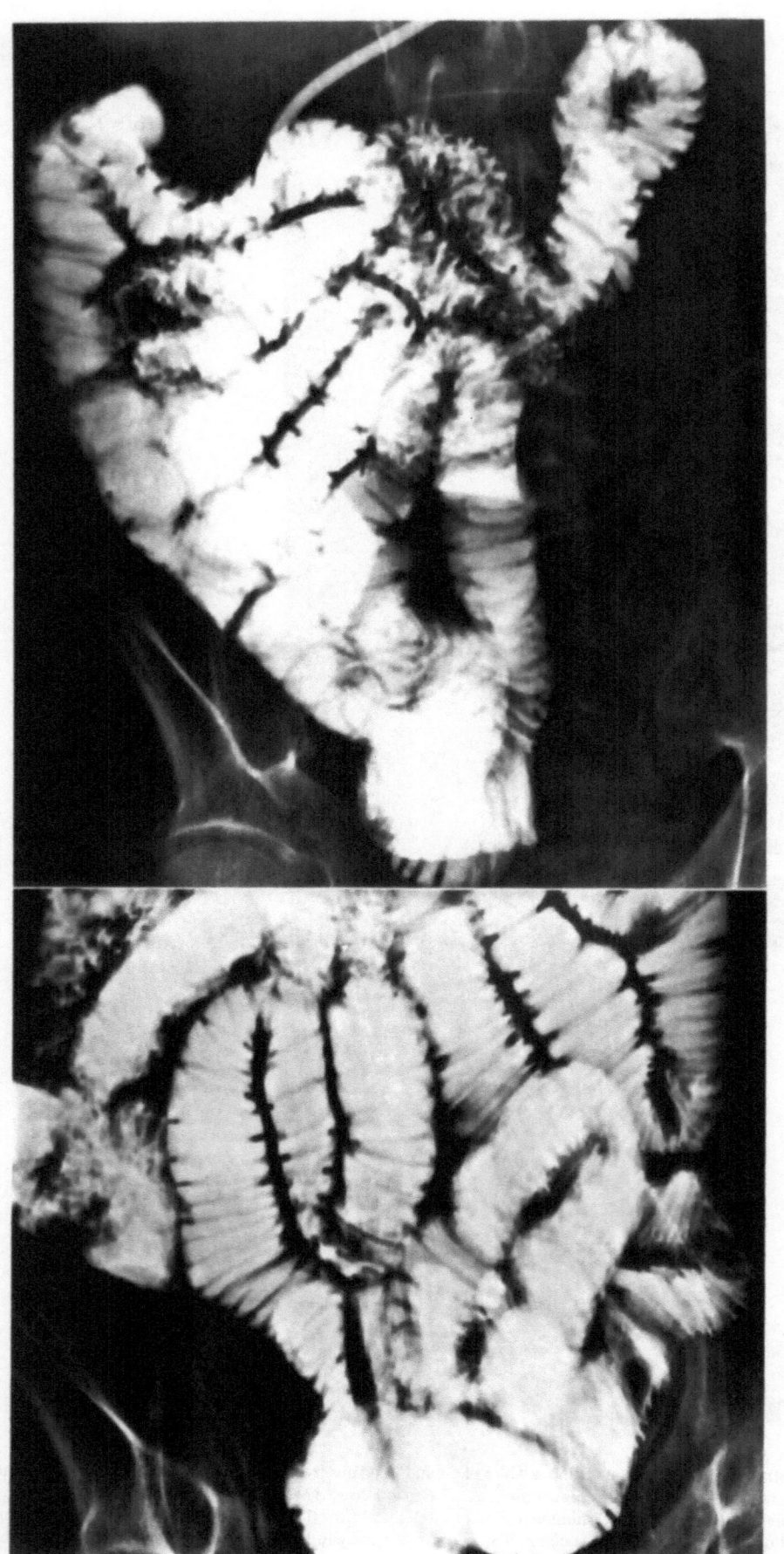

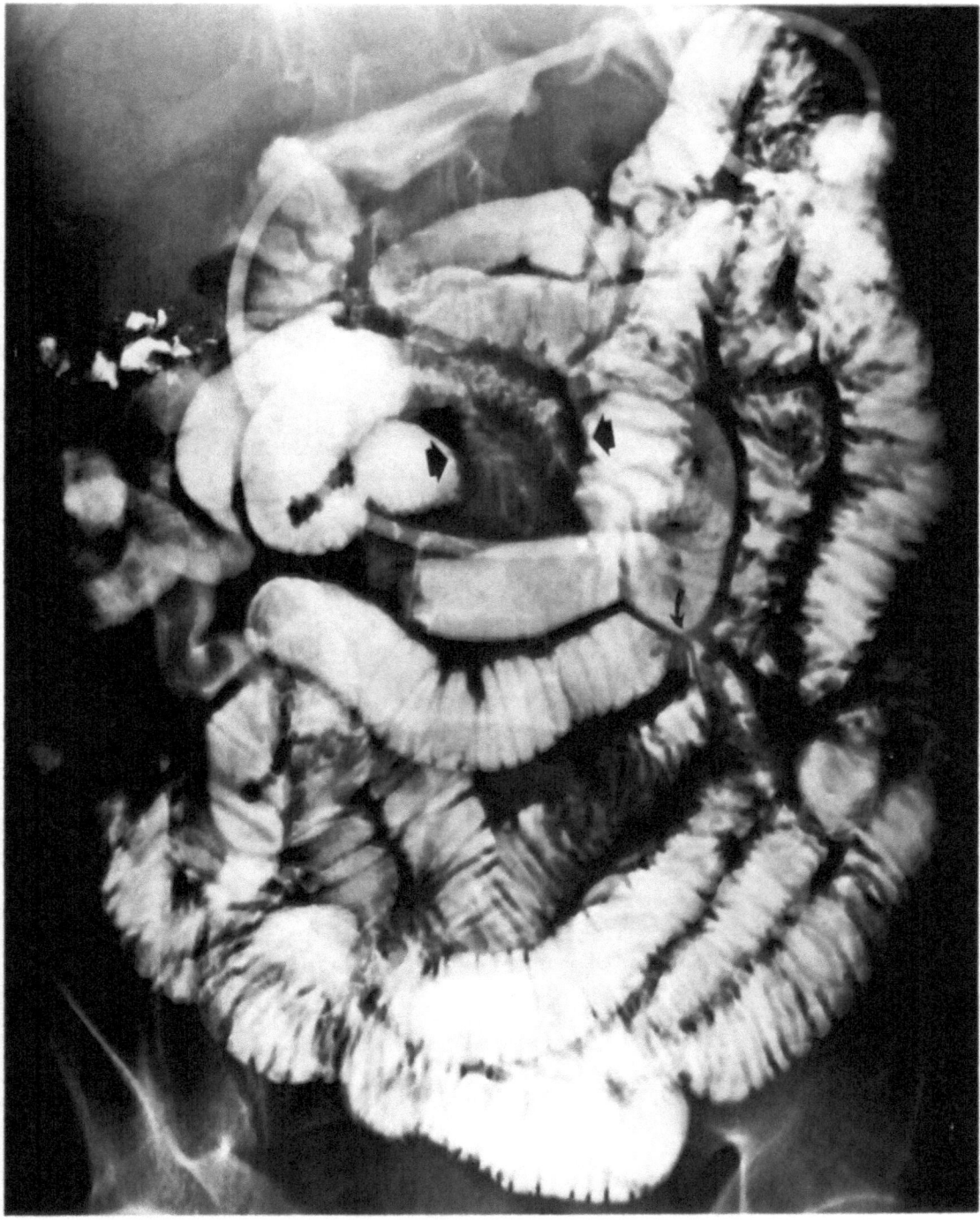

Fig. 14.14. Volvulus of the small intestine because the attachment of the mesentery was too short. The attack could be provoked by having the patient bend over as far as possible. The jejunum is in the upper right quadrant, the ileum in the lower left. The moderately dilated ileal loops show multiple indentations and the mucosal folds are stretched perpendicular to the axis of the intestine (left page). During periods without complaints the jejunum lies in the lower left quadrant and the ileum in the upper right. The mass of intestinal loops is therefore rotated through a 45° angle with respect to the normal position. To the left of the navel is an elongated intestinal loop with a pointed bulge (thin arrow) probably caused by a band. Local hypermotility with mucosal folds stretched in the perpendicular direction above the navel (thick arrows) (on right page).

442

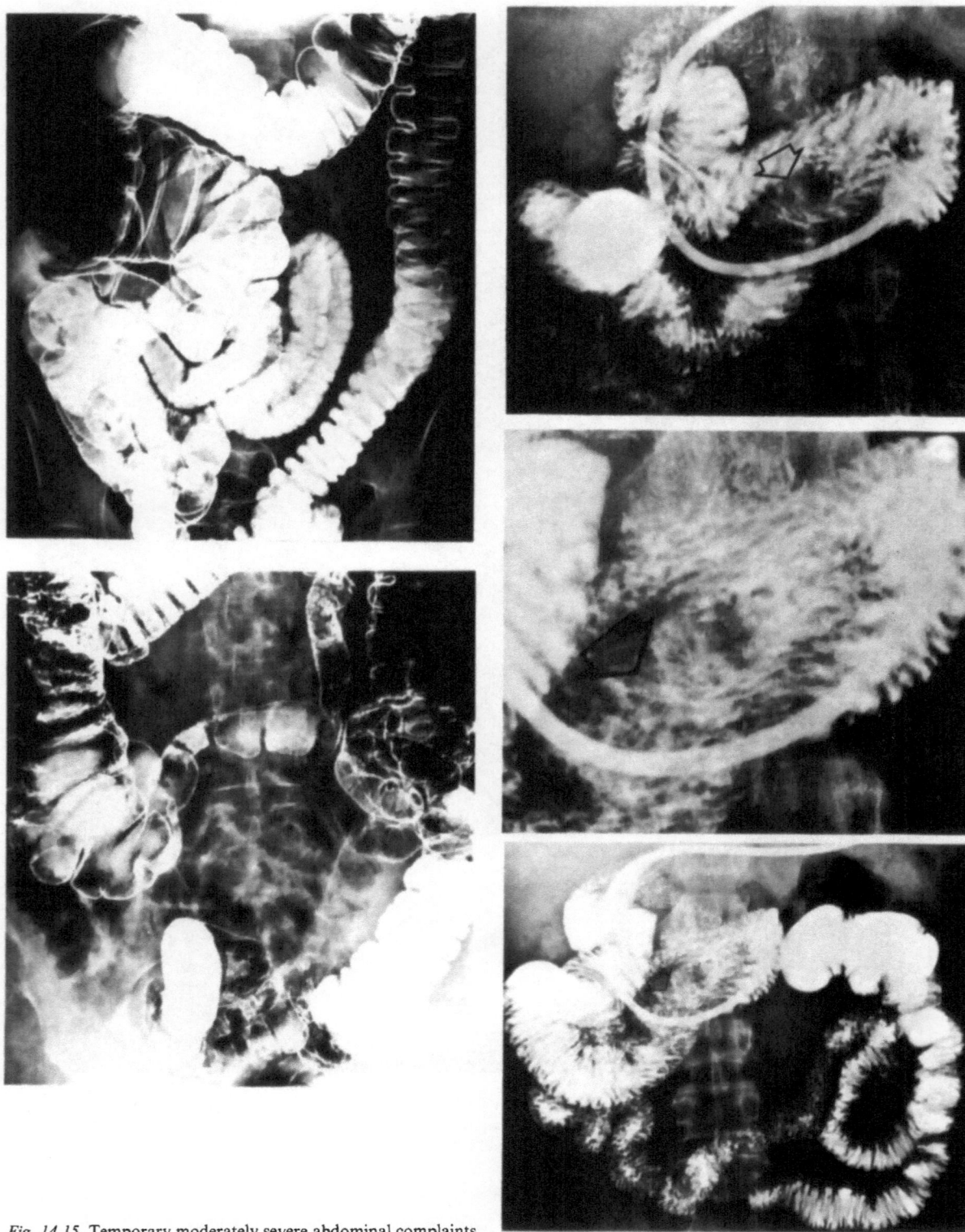

Fig. 14.15. Temporary moderately severe abdominal complaints connected with a change in the position of the ileum. The distal half of the mass of ileal loops is changed from the lower right (bottom) to the upper left (top) quadrant. Under all conditions the jejunum was to the left and in the center in the upper half of the abdomen. The proximal half of the ileum was in the middle in the lower abdomen. Probably this anomaly is because that part of the mesentery is too long.

Fig. 14.16. Intermittent moderately severe attacks of abdominal pain presumably connected with slight torsion of several proximal jejunal loops in the right upper quadrant. Locally there was quite strong hypermotility (arrows) so that it was not possible to visualize this segment of the intestine in a well-filled state.

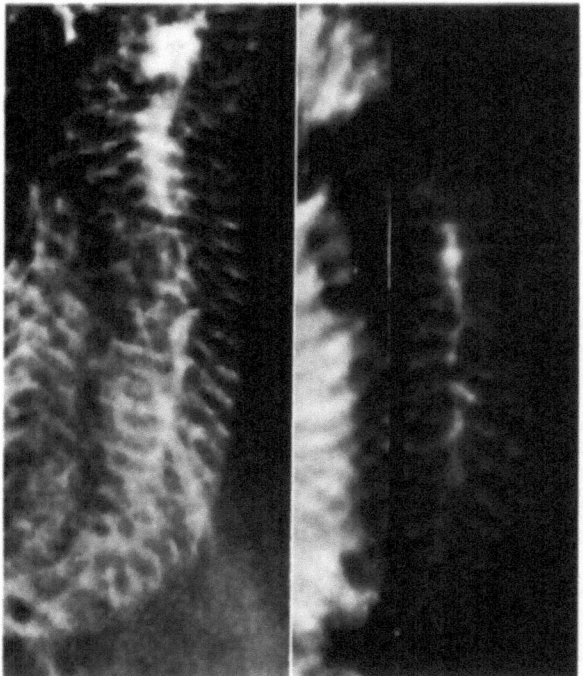

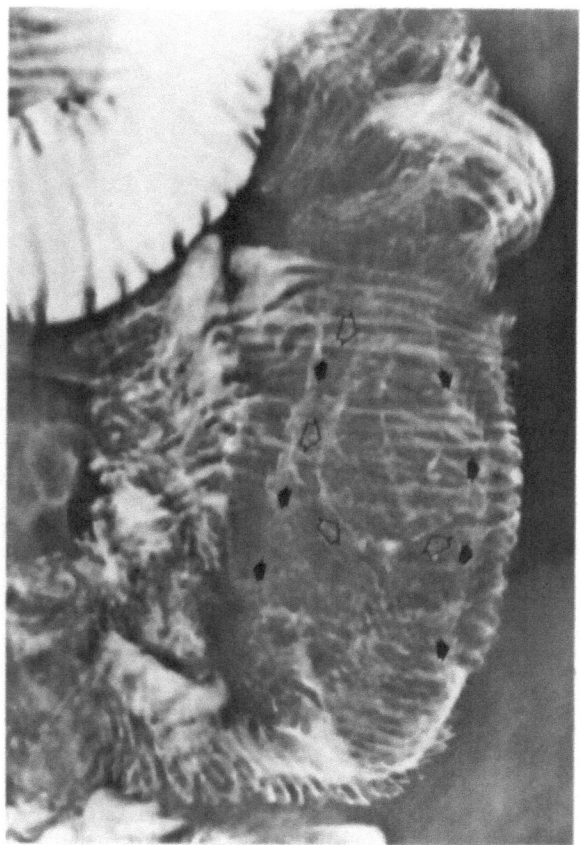

Fig. 14.17. Two barium streams in the middle of an intestinal loop as seen in cases of hypermotility. This misleading pattern suggesting an intussusception can develop in particular when the lumen of the intestine is greatly dilated and disintegration of the contrast fluid has occurred (as seen in some cases of celiac disease).

column. This must be carefully differentiated from an intussusception. Because there are usually large quantities of fluid in the intestine in celiac disease, the barium suspension often flocculates during a conventional examination. Under these conditions, barium 'streamers' may become visible in the center of the intestinal lumen where the rate of flow of the fluid is the greatest. These central streams may suggest an intussusception (fig. 14.17). As mentioned previously, films should not be used for diagnosis if the intestinal loops are inadequately filled or if signs of flocculation are detected.

The roentgen pattern of an intussusception is complete if an otherwise well-filled intestinal loop shows a distalward portio-like well-defined radiolucency with a barium stream in the middle. In the intestinal loops containing the intussusception (the so-called intussuscipiens), the mucosal folds are pressed flat against the wall and therefore are not or just barely visible (figs. 14.18 and 14.19M). Understandably, circulation in the intussuscipiens will be severely disturbed leading to marked mu-

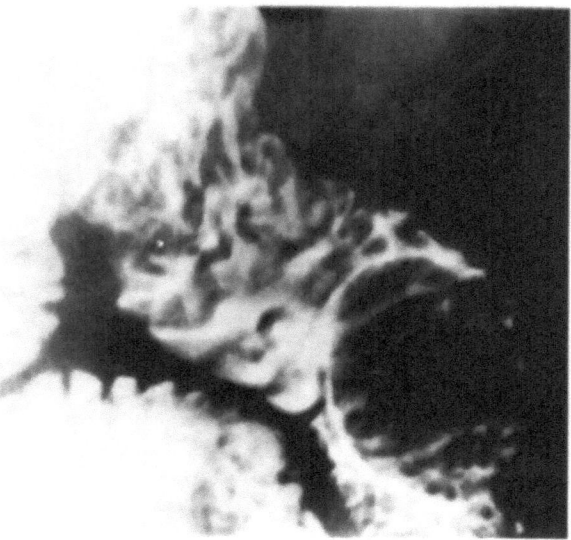

Fig. 14.18. Intussusception of jejunum into jejunum, caused by a lipoma ±2 cm in diameter (bottom); the latter can be seen in the intussuscipiens (solid arrow). The mucosal surface of the intussuscipiens is also just visible (open arrows) about 0.5 cm inside the wall of the enclosing intestinal loop (top).

444

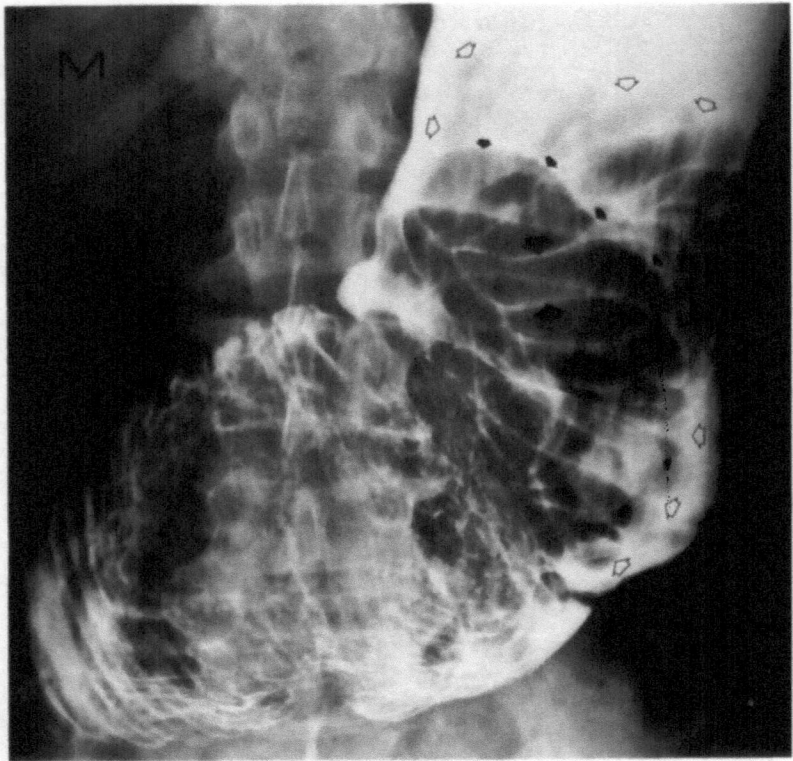

*Fig. 14.19*M. Greatly swollen mucosal folds (arrows) in a large intussuscipiens after a BII gastrectomy. This was a complicated intussusception consisting of the afferent loop into the efferent loop and then a retrograde intussusception of both into the residual stomach. The wall of the intussuscipiens is clearly visible next to the inner wall of the stomach.

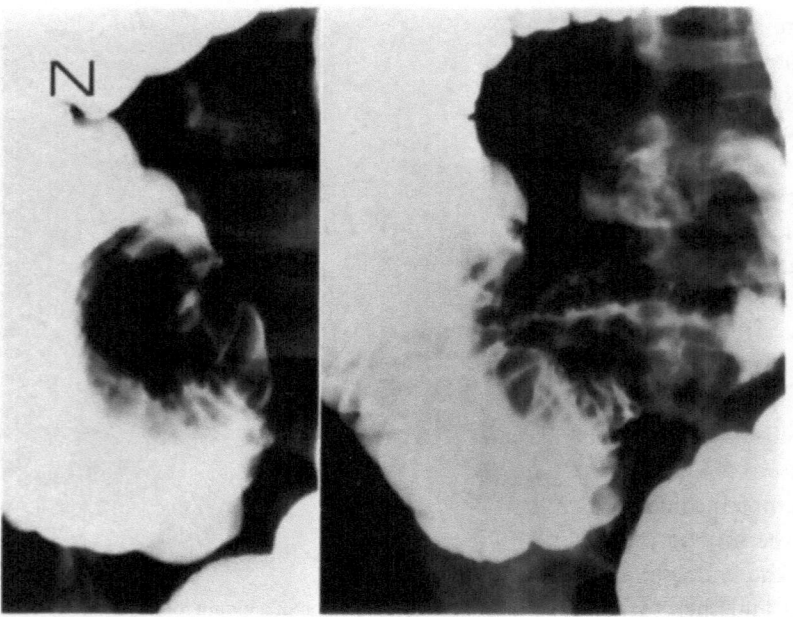

*Fig. 14.19*N. Edematous swelling of the mucosa in the distal ileum and Bauhin's valve immediately after reduction of an intussusception (of several days' duration). This intussusception had extended to the left flexure of colon. Since the complaints were only moderately severe, it was decided to try a conservative reduction in spite of the prolonged duration of the intussusception.

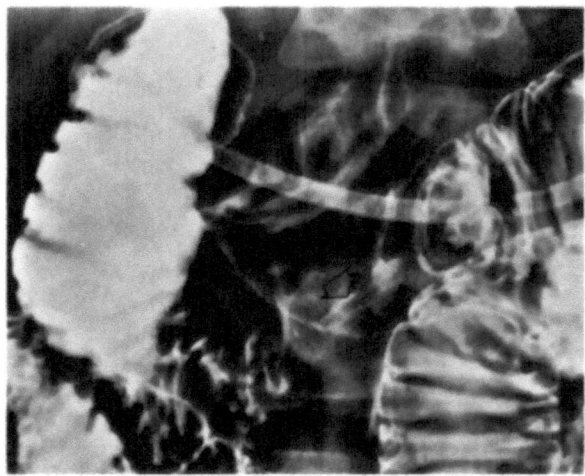

Fig. 14.20. Temporary subileus phenomenon. The examination taken after hypotonia was induced showed a stream of contrast medium ±5 cm long in the distal duodenum that started abruptly and ended in a portio-like configuration. Since the complaints disappeared and abnormalities were no longer seen during a follow-up examination, surgical intervention was not required.

cosal edema, especially if the intussusception has existed for some time. The trio of phenomena that indicate the diagnosis of 'intussusception' is a portio-like configuration, a central barium stream, and visualization of a double intestinal wall. This is, however, certainly not always (and in fact is usually not) complete. Unfortunately one must be satisfied with less. The abnormality may be temporary and occur only once so that a surgical indication is no longer present. Confirmation then of the radiological diagnosis, however probable it may be, is not always available (fig. 14.20).

In adults, an intussusception is almost always caused by a polyp or tumor of the intestinal mucosa. It is found most frequently near the ileocecal junction where these abnormalities commonly occur (fig. 14.21).

Recently, intussusceptions in children, not readily reduced by the usual techniques, have been aided by the use of glucagon (0.5–1.0 mg i.v.). Surgery has therefore been avoided in several cases.

5. Incisional hernia

The presence of a mass of intestinal loops in an incisional or congenital inguinal hernia is a frequent finding (fig. 14.22A). If the hernial opening is small, then an incarcerated hernia can develop that requires immediate surgery. When constriction occurs the venous circulation will be disturbed first and the most severely. If obstruction of venous flow is not total or is intermittent, then it is possible that mucosal hematomas will not become so large that they cause acute obstruction. Moreover a transient and increasingly pronounced fibrosis during the recovery phase(s) can apparently prevent the development of necrosis. As discussed in chapter 10, after some time the results of a disturbance in venous circulation can no longer be differentiated radiologically from a disturbed arterial flow nor from Crohn's disease, or conditions after radiotherapy.

A good example of an obstruction to venous flow (in the rest phase) that proceeded so gradually that the history was in fact 'clean' is seen in fig. 14.22A. There is a large hernial sac that developed in the incision of a previous kidney operation. The patient could report only that the hernial sac was much smaller in the beginning. It was not until later that he could force the intestinal loops in the sac back through the hernial opening into the abdominal cavity. The rigid and stiff intestinal loops were easily palpable through the thin flabby wall of the hernial sac. By this means it could be established that the most lateral loops were fused with the wall of the hernial sac.

446

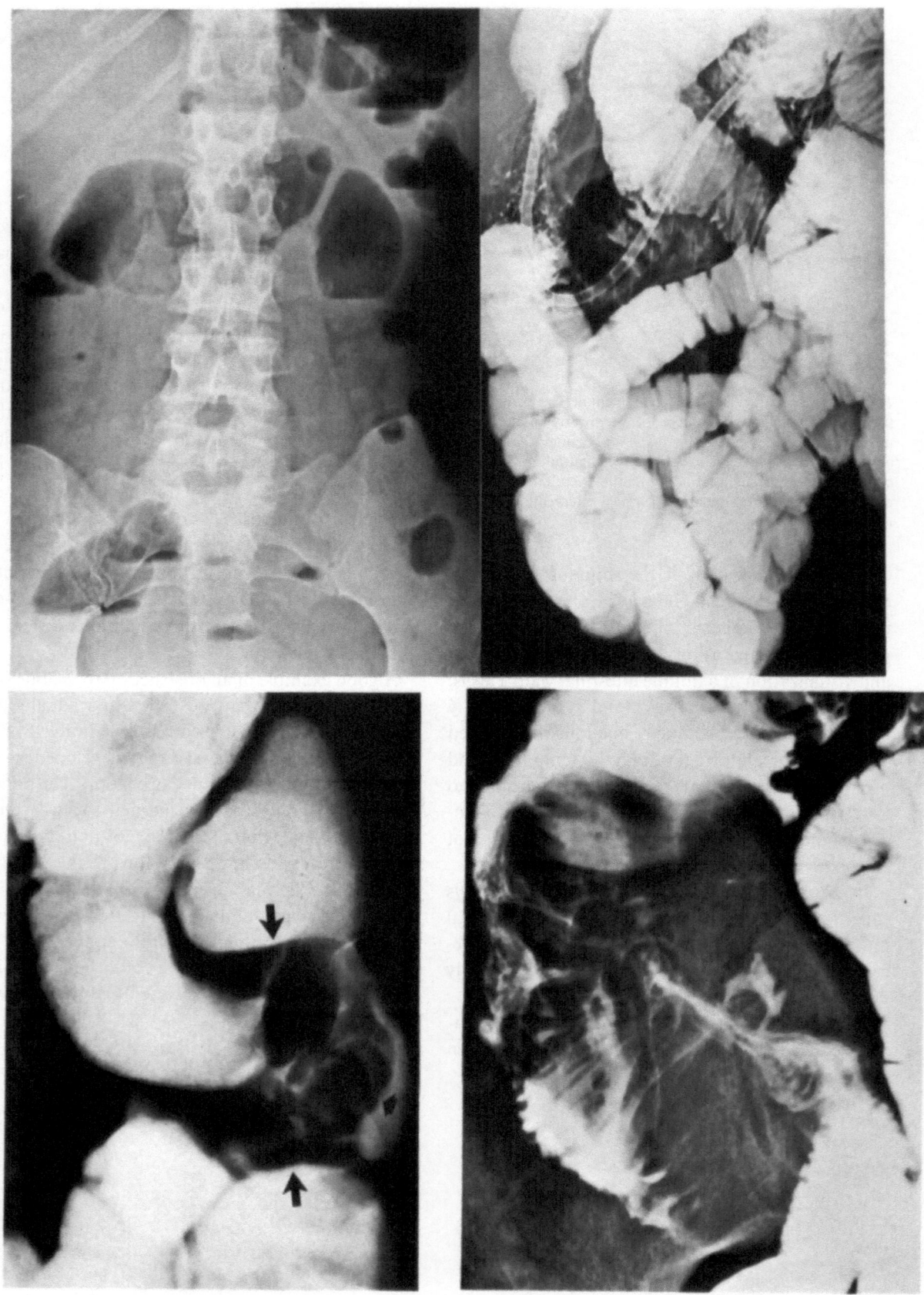

Fig. 14.21. Tumor in Bauhin's valve causing an intussusception in the cecum.

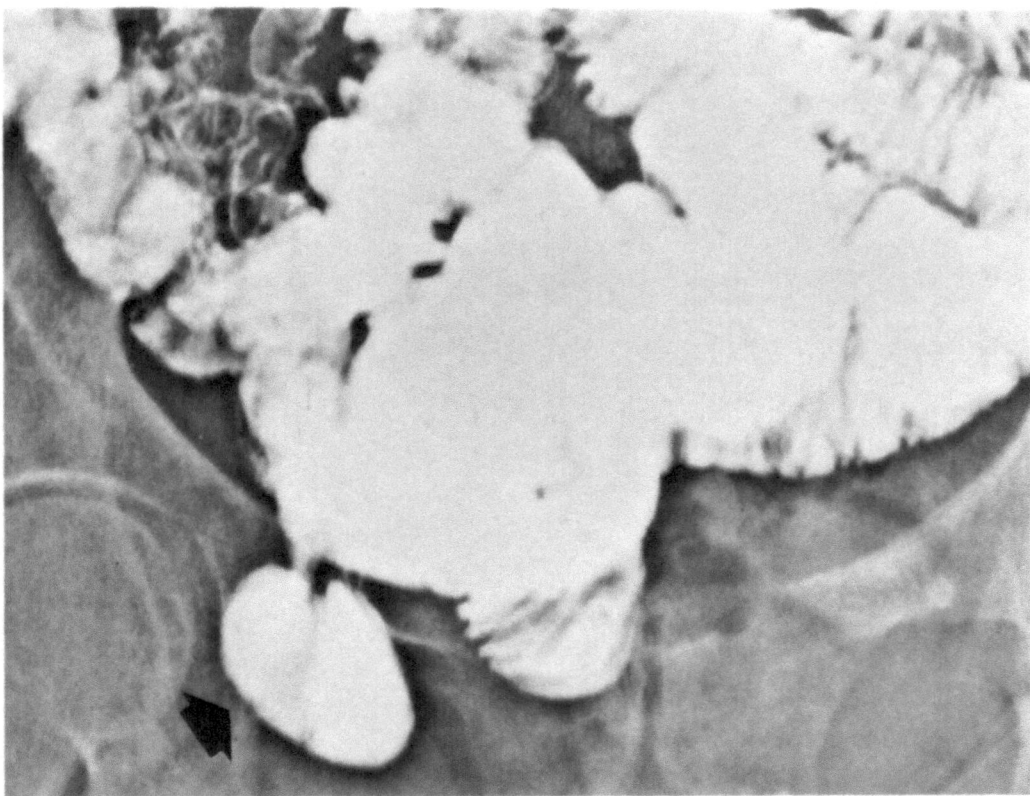

*Fig. 14.22*A. Right inguinal hernia.

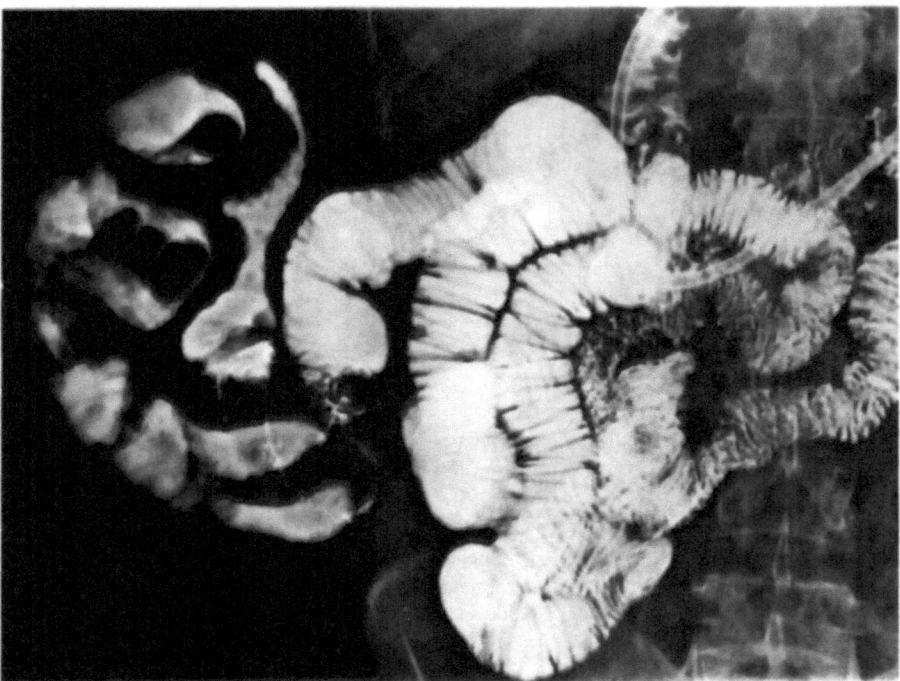

*Fig. 14.22*B. Lateral hernia through the abdominal wall after previous kidney operation. The hernial sac contains part of the ascending colon and a mass of jejunal loops that show the results of a disturbed venous flow. The abnormalities, consisting of multiple longitudinal ulcerations, asymmetric and circular shriveling, a markedly thickened intestinal wall, and frequent spasms cannot be differentiated from those in Crohn's disease or radiation enteritis. (For detail, see page 448.)

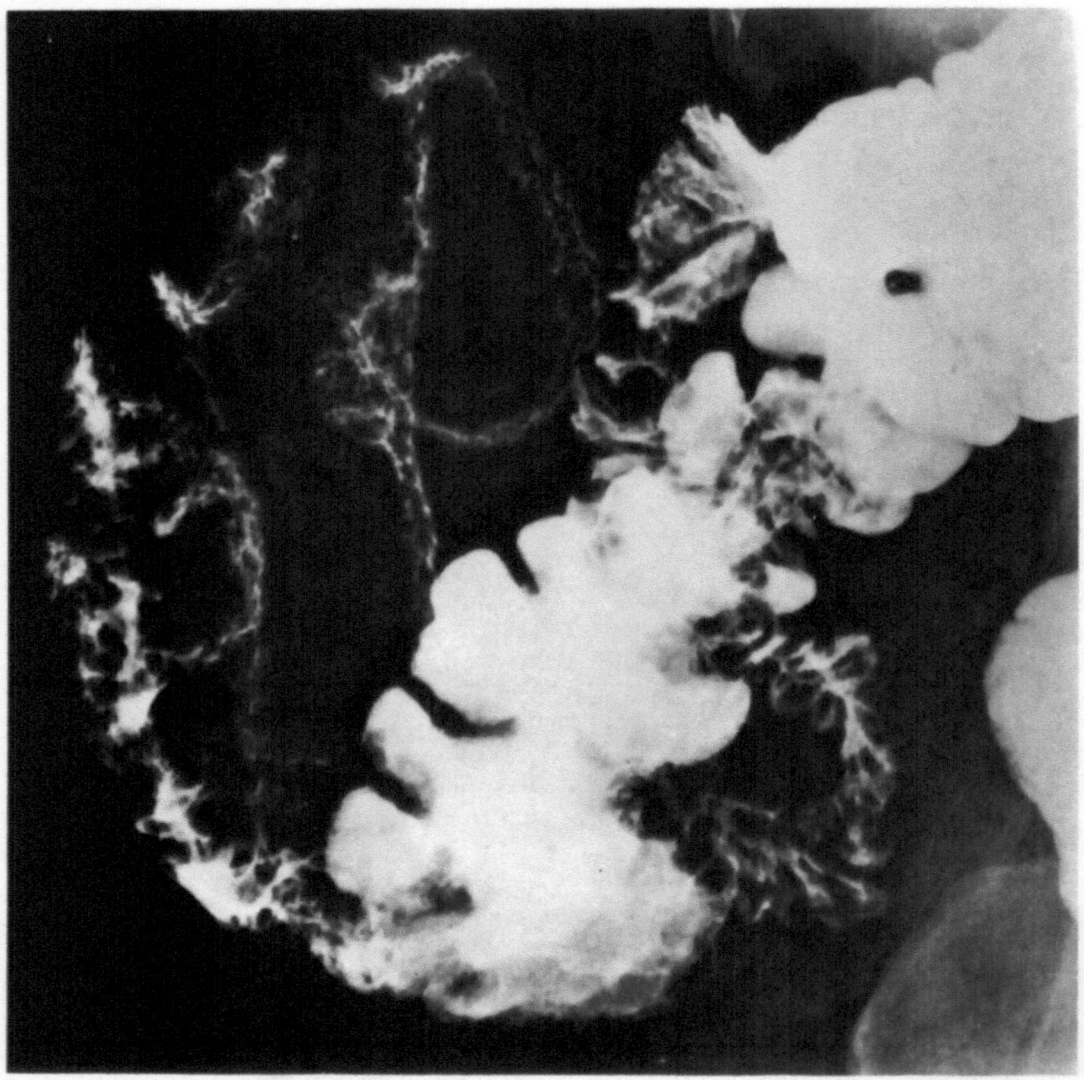

*Fig. 14.22*B. See legend on page 447.

Bibliography: chapter 14

Brown P et al (1974) Sclerosing peritonitis, an unusual reaction to a beta-adrenergic-blocking drug (Practolol). Lancet 2: 1477–1481.

Bryk D (1972) Functional evaluation of small bowel obstruction by successive abdominal röntgenograms. Am J Roentgenol 126: 262–275.

Donhauser JL, Kelly RC (1950) Intussusception in the adult. Am J Surg 79: 673.

Kerr WG, Kirkaldy-Willis WH (1946) Volvulus of the small intestine. Br Med J 1: 799.

Moss AA, Goldberg JH, Brotman M (1972) Idiopathic intestinal pseudo-obstruction. Am J Roentgenol 115: 312–317.

Moretz WH, Morton JJ (1950) Acute volvulus of small intestine. Analysis of 36 cases. Ann Surg 132: 899.

Riccabono XJ, Haskins RM (1970) Gastroduodenal intussusception: report of 2 cases. Gastroenterology 38: 995.

Saidi F (1966) The high incidence of intestinal volvulus in Iran. Gut 10: 838.

Talbot CH (1960) Volvulus of the small intestine in adults. Gut 1: 76.

See also the nos. 66, 173, 174, 221, 236, and 246 of the bibliography on pages 164 and following.

15. THE ENTEROCLYSIS EXAMINATION OF INFANTS

In fairly recent literature, it is stated that air is an excellent contrast medium for the digestive tracts of children and that, in addition, it is very cheap ([41], page 46). It cannot be denied that a careful study of the gas shadows on one or more abdominal survey films can sometimes lead to useful conclusions. This fact certainly does not apply to children alone. However, it has been explained clearly in chapter 4–6 why air is not a useful contrast medium for the visualization of the intestinal lumen. This is true for children as well as adults.

Air, however, is no worse than a barium suspension when a conventional follow-through examination is carried out. The illustrations in this atlas should be sufficient proof that the preceding statement must be considered a testimonium paupertatis for the conventional transit examination. It does not apply at all when the barium suspension is used for an enteroclysis examination. To date, a good barium suspension is the most suitable contrast fluid, both for children and for adults.

As is already mentioned in chapter 4.8.4, Gastrografin definitely is not a suitable contrast medium for children. In fact, because of its marked hyperosmotic properties, it may be dangerous. As a result of the rapidly increasing dilution, the mucosal relief in the duodenum and most proximal part of the jejunum may be visualized without danger of flocculation, but further distalward this is impossible.

As in many areas, certainly also in radiology, the procedures developed for the examination of adults cannot be applied directly to small children. This is also true for enteroclysis. In particular the enteroclysis examination of babies and infants between 0 and 3–4 years of age is without doubt much more difficult than the examination of adults. Therefore new prerequisites and procedures have been determined experimentally and will be described here.

1. Preparation

The younger the child the greater the tendency toward rapid flocculation of the contrast fluid. The precise reason for this is still unknown. It could be because of the larger quantities of mucus and especially lactic acid present in the small bowel. This is particularly true during the period that the child receives a milk diet, whether from its mother or not. It should be obvious after studying this book, that flocculation can be prevented only by administering a large dose of contrast fluid quickly, i.e. relatively more and faster than for an adult. As a result the degree of small intestinal filling will be relatively greater than in an adult. In addition, there is much less chance of obtaining spot films by using compression because of the fragility and minute size of the intestine. The problems arising from excessive filling of the ileal loops in the lower abdomen can be limited by ensuring that the contrast medium flows smoothly to the cecum. In other words, the colon must be thoroughly cleansed. Here too, as in adults, a rectal cleansing enema is not recommended. A satisfactory oral laxation procedure for children between 1 and 15 years of age is as follows:

7.00 a.m. – 1 g magnesium sulfate powder for each kg of body weight, dissolved in 200 ml water; 1 Ducolax tablet.

9.00 a.m. – 300 ml (2 large cups) of tea with sugar. 30 g (1 slice) of white bread with 30 g (1 slice) of cheese; 1 boiled egg.

11.00 a.m. – 300 ml lemonade.

1.00 p.m. – 200 ml beef tea.
cooked fish or chicken without skin;
no potatoes, fruit or vegetables!
200 ml soda water.
3.00 p.m. – 300 ml lemonade or tea with sugar.
5.00 p.m. – 200 ml beef tea.
30 g white bread with one slice of cheese.
7.00 p.m. – 1 g magnesium sulfate powder for each kg of body weight, dissolved in 200 ml water; 1 Dulcolax tablet.
9.00 p.m. – 300 ml lemonade or tea with sugar.

For the preparation of babies under 12 months of age, the radiologist should contact the pediatrician or the dietician of the children department. The day before the examination the milk food should contain less fat than usually and the overnight fasting period must be rather long.

There is another aspect of the preparation of the baby and small child that is clearly different from that of adults. A child younger than four to five years of age is sedated just before the examination. In spite of the unfavorable effect of sedation on intestinal motility, this procedure is necessary for successful intubation and for effective performance of the examination itself. If the decrease in intestinal motility is marked, some compensation can be obtained by disconnecting the bag of contrast fluid and administering a few ml Primperan (metoclopramide) via the tube. This step must be carried out as soon as possible after hypomotility is demonstrated, since reflux into the stomach has by then probably not occurred. Most of the Primperan then will enter the duodenum and thus the effect will be achieved as rapidly as possible.

2. Duodenal intubation

For adults, duodenal intubation is carried out by the staff of the radiology department. In contrast, for babies and small children the tube should be inserted as far as the stomach by a member of the pediatric staff who knows the child. The easiest route is via one of the nostrils since less resistance will be encountered than when the mouth is used. Furthermore, fixation of the tube with adhesive tape is easier. If the child is more than two years old, the Bilbao or Sellink tube can be used. For younger children the Bilbao tube is much too stiff. It is better to take a thinner, more flexible, lead-rubber tube or a plastic tube with a marker line. In all cases the end of the tube should be closed and rounded. The openings should lie only along the side of the tube. Maneuvering the tip of the tube, merely by turning the child, can be facilitated considerably by inserting ±1 cm of tin solder into the tip of the tube. In this way the tip becomes heavier and as a result of its own weight will sink to the lowest part of the stomach. The lead-rubber tubes with metal olive available today are not suitable for babies since they are too thick. The olive in particular does not pass easily through the pyloric canal and certainly not through the child's nostril. When the tip of the tube is somewhere in the stomach, the child is brought to the radiology department. There, under fluoroscopic control, and using a thick Seldinger angiographic guide wire, the tube is pushed through the pyloric canal into the duodenum. Only when the child is two to three years old may the much stiffer Bilbao guide wire be used for this purpose. Obviously this second phase of the duodenal intubation of babies may not be carried out at a distance (telecommand). The physician should do it himself from the head of the table while fluoroscopy is regulated by a colleague or technician. For this procedure, only an exceedingly low radiation dose is required for fluoroscopy.

3. The contrast fluid

It is unreasonable and stupid but also true that there are radiologists who still use the same contrast fluid for every examination! It has the same density or specific gravity, for normal adults, for babies, for children and, to mention the other extreme, for extremely obese patients! If such an approach is ever to produce hopeless results, then that is certainly true in babies. We have found that the densities listed below for the contrast fluid are the most suitable.

0–12 months s.g. = 1.15 = 19% wt/vol
(i.e. 1 part 85% barium suspension diluted with $3\frac{1}{2}$ parts water)
1–3 years s.g. = 1.17 = 21% wt/vol

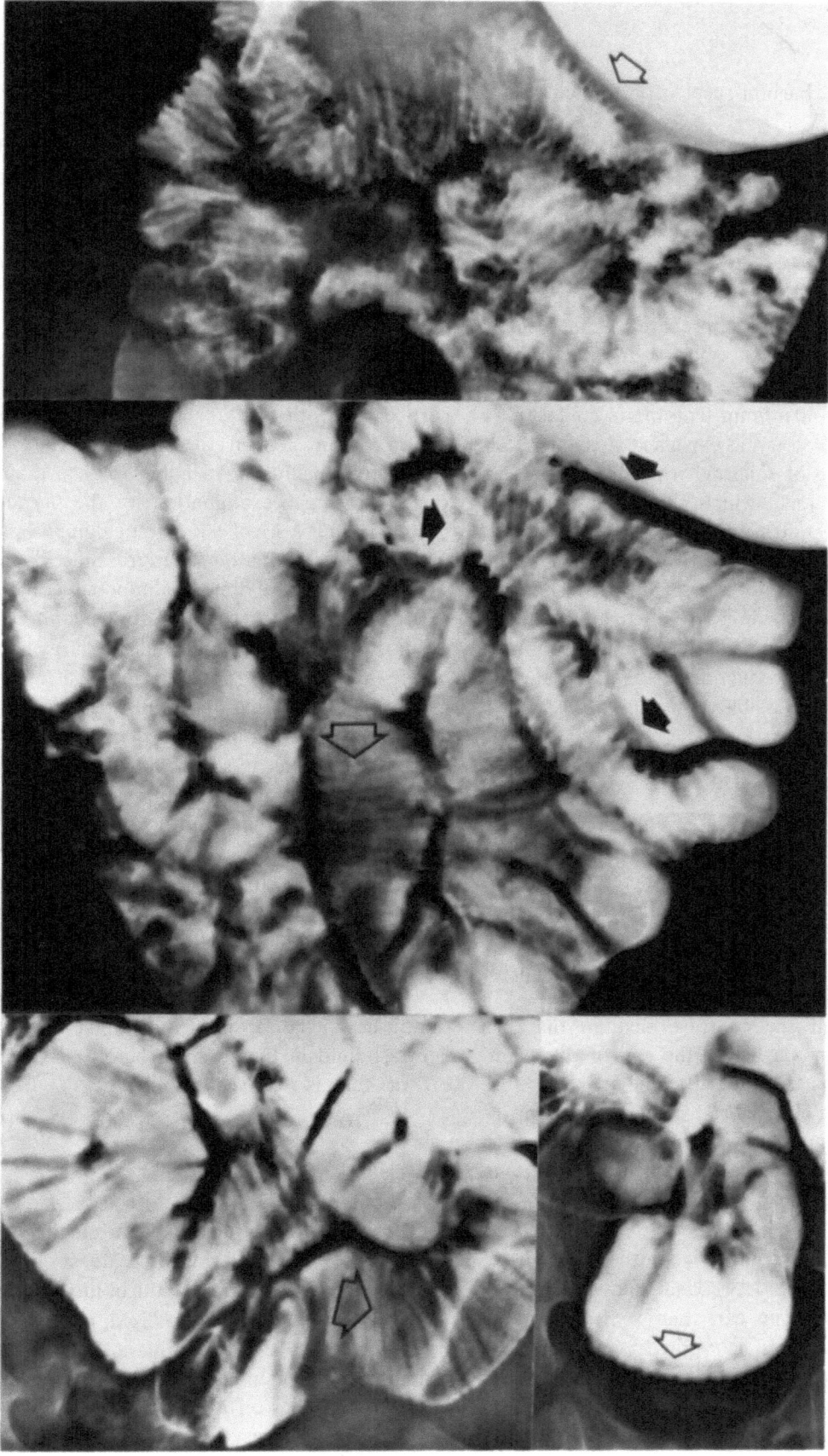

Fig. 15.1. Shallow but easily recognized mucosal folds in an eight-week-old baby. In the ileum in particular the folds are only visible as minute ridges. For some unknown reason the ileum shows adhesions and is therefore dilated.

452

(i.e. 1 part 85% barium suspension diluted with 3 parts water)

3–12 years s.g. = 1.2 = 24% wt/vol

(i.e. 1 part 85% barium suspension diluted with 2½ parts water)

Although doses of 200, 300, and 400 ml, respectively, are sufficient for these age groups, more contrast medium must be prepared. Some usually ends up in the stomach, and may or may not be vomited. For all three age groups listed above, the rate of flow is ±40 ml/min. This may seem fast for a baby but it is necessary, as explained in chapter 15.1. The importance of this high rate of flow is seen clearly in fig. 15.1, which illustrates that flocculation of the contrast medium begins as soon as the flow decreases or stops. Even more convincing proof of the necessity of a rapid flow is seen in fig. 15.2AB. Here, celiac disease caused an unusually strong tendency toward flocculation of the contrast medium so that reproduction of the mucosal relief seemed almost impossible.

4. The examination

The flow of the contrast medium is relatively faster in children, and, in addition, there is a greater tendency toward retroperistaltic movements than in adults. Because of this, there will practically always be a more or less pronounced reflux of the contrast medium into the stomach. In numerous cases the child will vomit the contrast medium that has entered the stomach before the end of the examination – that lasts only 5–10 min! It is therefore wise to turn the child's head to the left or right as soon as the stomach starts to fill. This is best left to a nurse from the pediatric department who, wearing a lead apron and lead gloves, should stand at the head of the table. A good alternative to be considered is to insert a second tube via the other nostril into the stomach (fig. 15.9). Using a hypodermic or a suction pump, one can then try to keep the stomach empty. This can prevent vomiting and avoid the inherent danger of aspirating the barium suspension. The danger of aspirating the barium suspension into the lungs must not be overrated; to date, we have never observed this phenomenon during an enteroclysis examination.

In contrast to adults who, using telecommand equipment, lie prone during administration of the contrast fluid, children must always lie on their backs. This is because it is absolutely necessary to take spot films as quickly as possible, irrespective of whether compression is used or not. After all, as soon as the flow of fluid decreases due to reflux or vomiting or is terminated for any reason, disintegration of the contrast fluid begins. Further exposures are no longer possible! It should be emphasized once again that compression must be carried out with the greatest possible care. Adequate compression in the minor pelvis can be considered an illusion in babies of less than one year. A roentgen examination for the purpose of demonstrating a Meckel's diverticulum, in particular, in babies of this age is absurd. Since compression of the lower abdomen is impossible, it is just as ridiculous to try to take double-contrast exposures with air. This will result in a large number of extremely confusing curved lines that will yield no diagnostic information at all. Because the tendency toward vomiting and flocculation of the barium suspension is so pronounced, a water infusion is just as bad. As soon as enough contrast fluid has reached the cecum to obtain the desired degree of filling, and several survey films as well as spot films have been taken, the examination can be terminated. Because of rapid disintegration there is no chance of taking supplementary exposures (at least in children less than one year old) after the first have been evaluated. The tube is pulled back until the tip lies in the cardia of the stomach. After the contrast fluid in the stomach has been suctioned off, the tube is removed entirely.

5. Results

This was previously mentioned in chapter 3. All claims that the small intestine does not show mucosal relief in the first months of life, or that the mucosal relief cannot be visualized, can now truly be relegated to the land of fables. The enteroclysis examination has demonstrated that, although these folds are thin, they certainly can be visualized (figs. 6.2 and 15.1). Autopsy studies have shown that the mucosa slides easily over the underlying layers. The folds disappear quickly when the intestinal lumen is

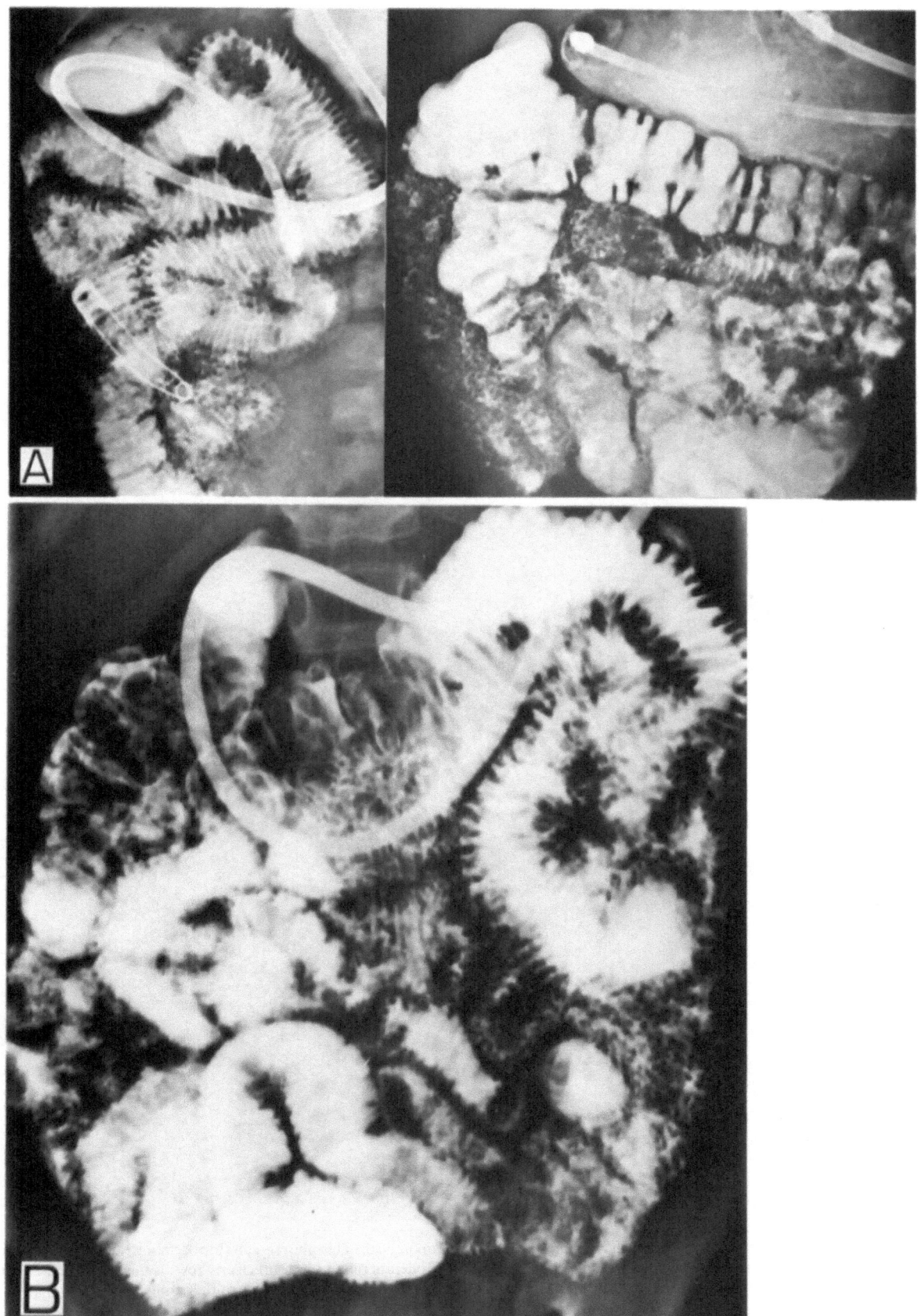

*Fig. 15.2*AB. Two different four-year-old children with celiac disease and an unusually marked tendency toward flocculation of the contrast fluid. The mucosal folds that are somewhat coarse and bulbous in the jejunum were visible only during the infusion.

454

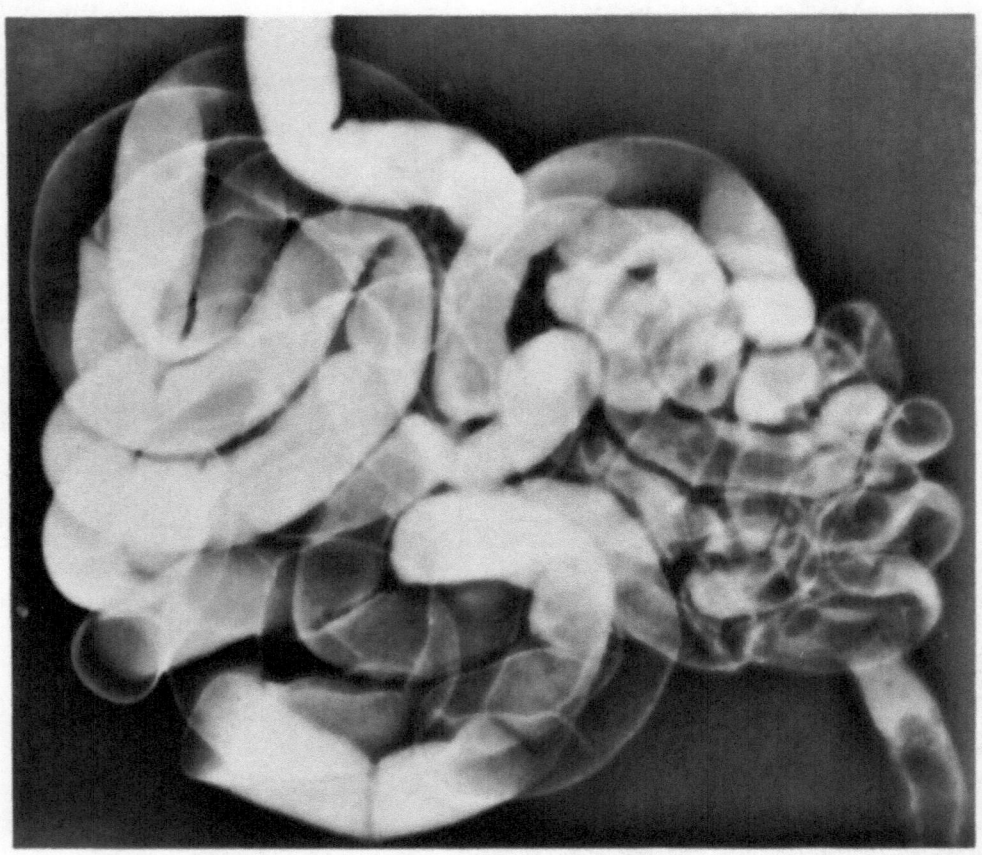

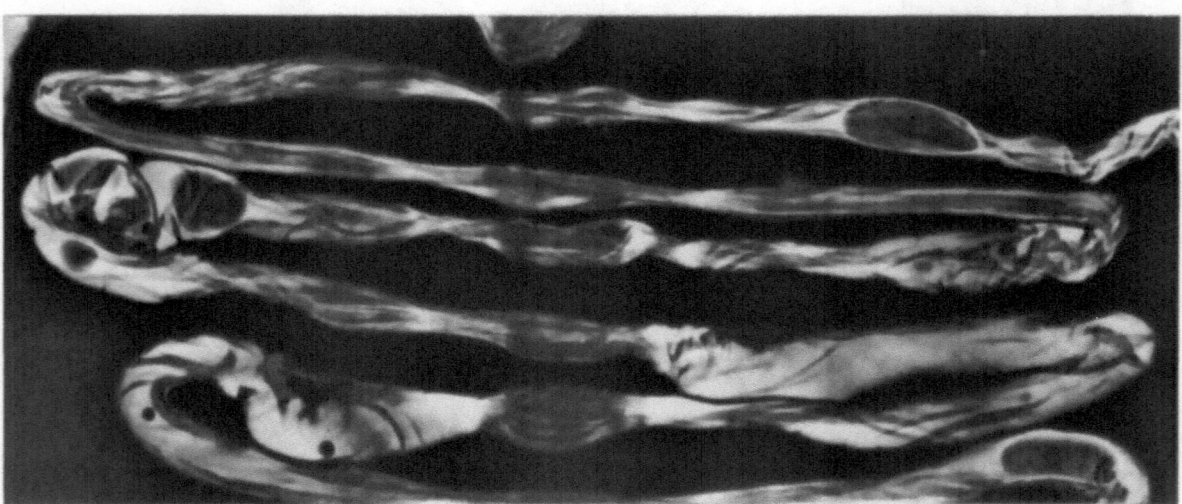

Fig. 15.3. Contrast medium in the small intestine of a baby dead upon birth. This photograph (top) demonstrates vividly that a high degree of filling produces a smooth intestine without wrinkles. Moderate filling (bottom) clearly reveals mucosal relief, despite the complete loss of tone in this case. The folds are of normal thickness regardless of the course they follow.

455

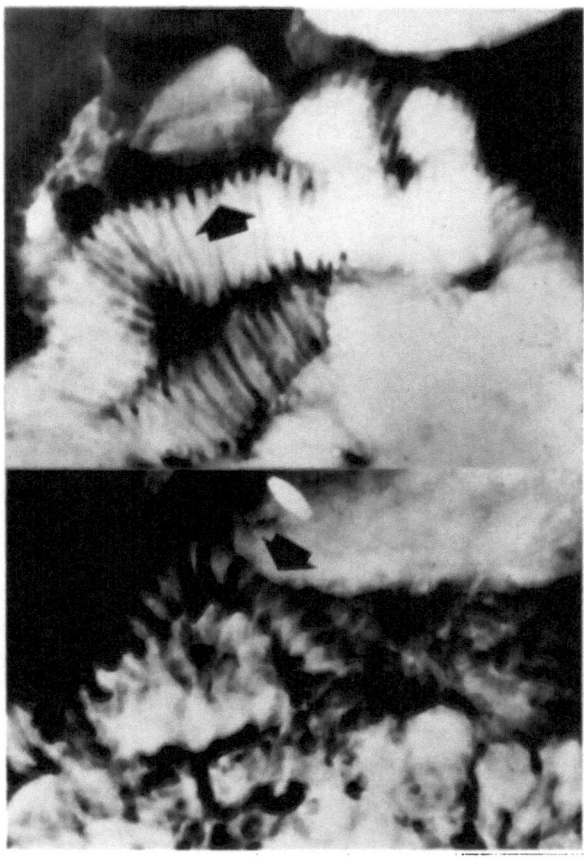

Fig. 15.4. There are as yet no signs of degeneration of the contrast medium in this child with hypoalbuminemia. It is immediately obvious that the folds in the proximal jejunum are much thicker when the loops are only moderately filled (bottom). When they are well filled, they appear entirely normal (top).

stretched slightly. The folds may be visible along the intestine's length or in any other direction just as easily as in the normal way perpendicular to the axis (fig. 15.3). It can be assumed that the muscular tone in the longitudinal direction is responsible for the transverse folds while the circular muscular tone accounts for the longitudinal folds.

An edematous swelling of the mucosal folds can be observed much more easily when the intestine is moderately filled than when it is well filled. This is true in adults, but even more so in children. The folds appear to swell more markedly and more easily than in an adult, presumably because of

either the greater elasticity or the loosely meshed connective tissue. On the other hand, these pronounced bulbous folds disappear easily as the lumen is stretched (fig. 15.4).

The mucosa in children probably swells temporarily as a result of absorption of fluid from the hypotonic contrast medium. The extent of this phenomenon is not yet clear and certainly should be investigated further. So far, however, we have only observed bulbous swelling of mucosal folds in those cases in which a clinical cause could also be demonstrated (e.g. hypoalbuminemia).

Because of the greatly improved film quality brought about by better filling of the intestine and elimination of flocculation, we could establish several diseases more frequently. Such diseases as Crohn's disease (fig. 15.5) and *Yersinia EC* infection (fig. 15.6) occur much more frequently than formerly assumed – at least after three years of age. In even younger patients we often see hyperplastic lymph follicles and Peyer's patches together with thickened mucosal folds; the cause is usually never ascertained. Massive fusion of almost all of the intestinal loops after a laparotomy, a highly unusual phenomenon, is shown in fig. 15.7. As a result of our observations, we have come to the conclusion that massive fusion does indeed occur sometimes shortly after surgery; it subsequently often disappears spontaneously in a later stage – except in the minor pelvis. Such a fusion seldom or never leads to obstruction. Unfortunately it is not always possible to arrive at a specific diagnosis in spite of the greatly improved quality. One example, seen in fig. 15.8, concerns an eight-year-old boy with markedly retarded growth obviously from disturbed resorption in the small intestine. Another example is a one-year-old child with a recurrent ileus that could not be explained, even after a laparotomy. The radiological examination showed highly dilated intestinal loops with moderate peristalsis and occasionally also retroperistaltic movements. A mechanical obstruction was definitely excluded so that a Naish syndrome or some other innervational disorder had to be considered (fig. 15.9).

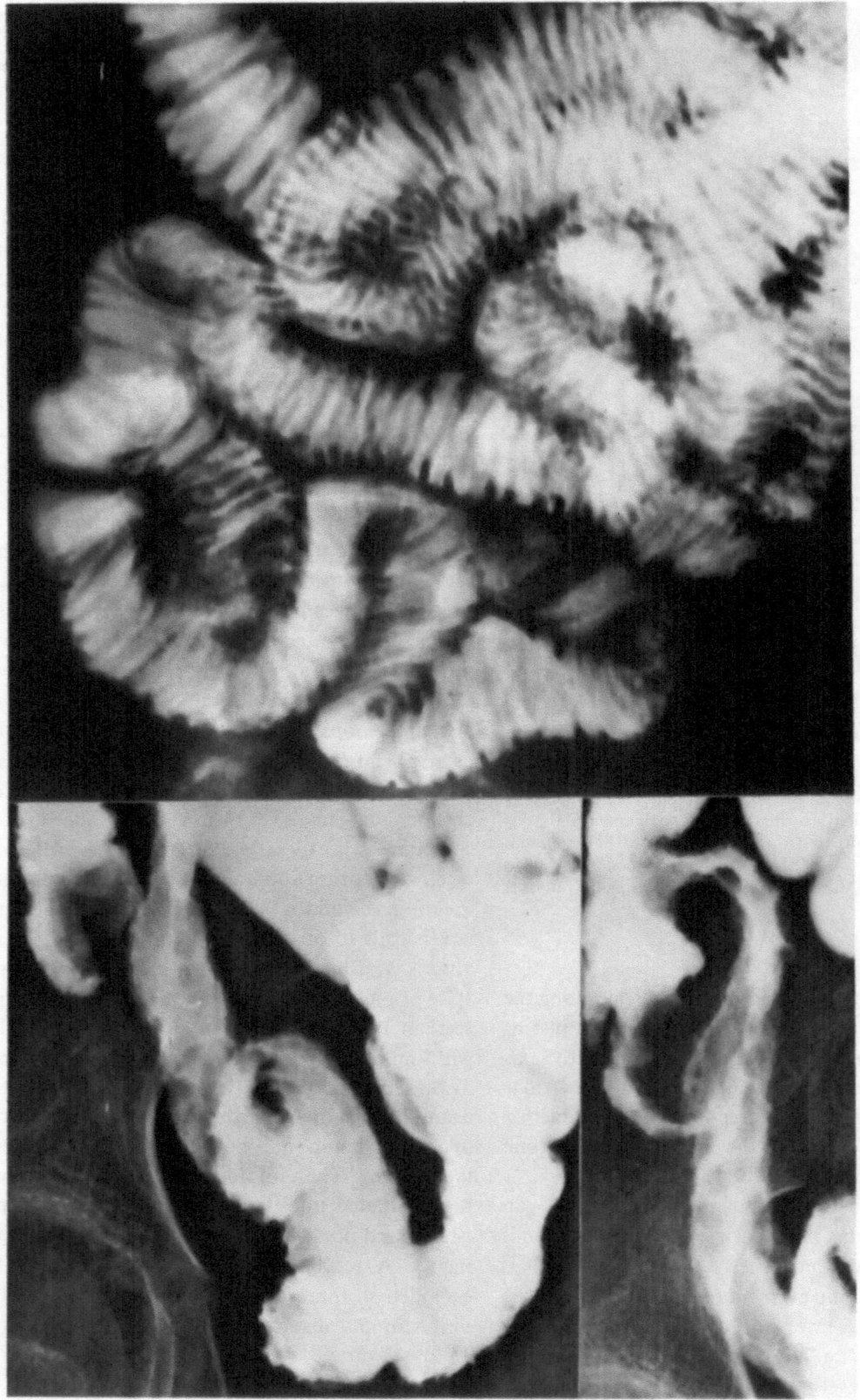

Fig. 15.5. Extensive Crohn's disease involving a segment 30 cm long in a four-year-old child. The mucosal folds are markedly thickened; cobblestones and numerous ulcers are visible.

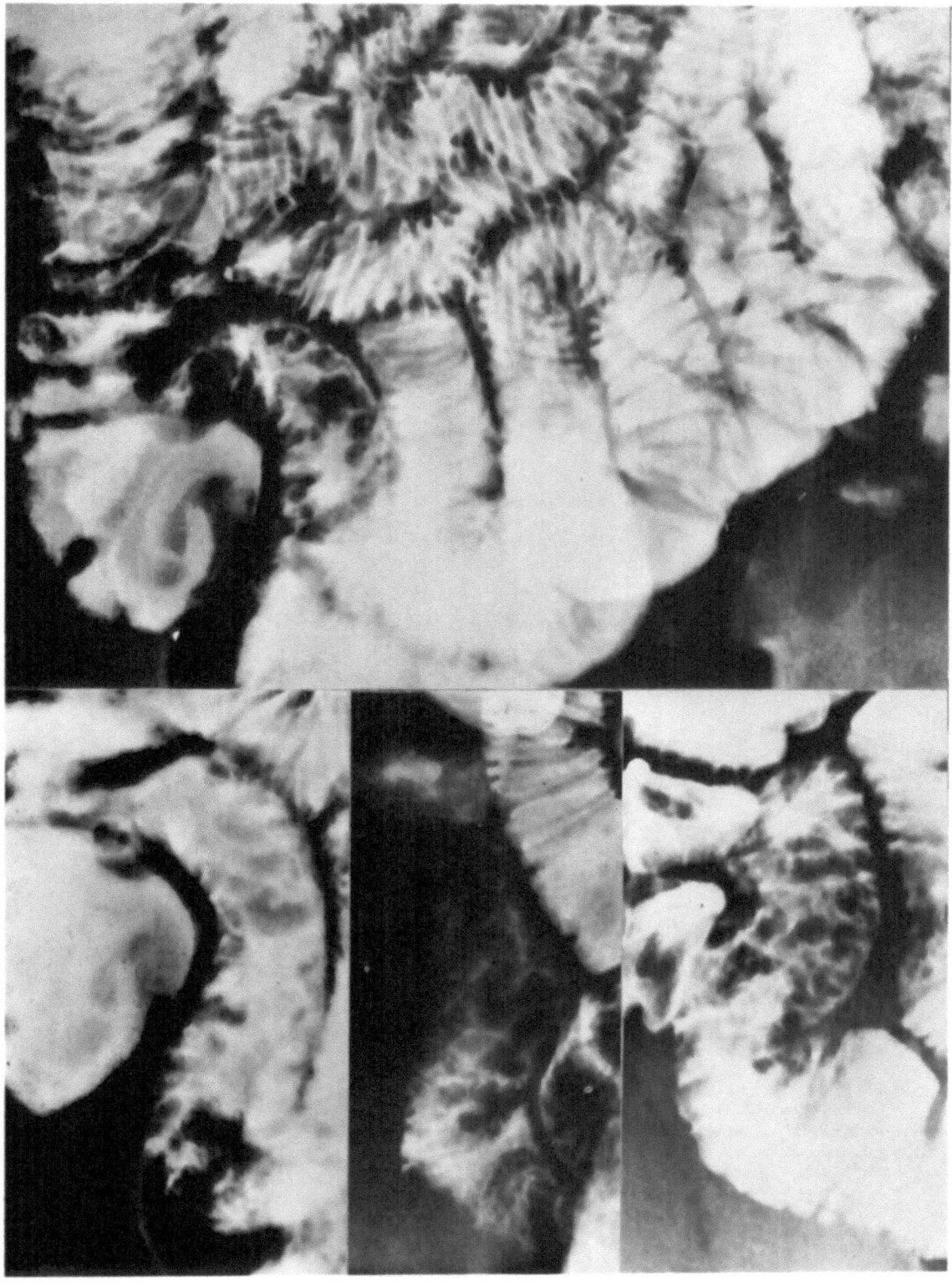

Fig. 15.6. Yersinia EC infection in a five-year-old child with thickened erratic folds in the last 8–10 cm of the distal ileum. Because there are so many folds, the presence of enlarged lymph follicles is not easily established.

458

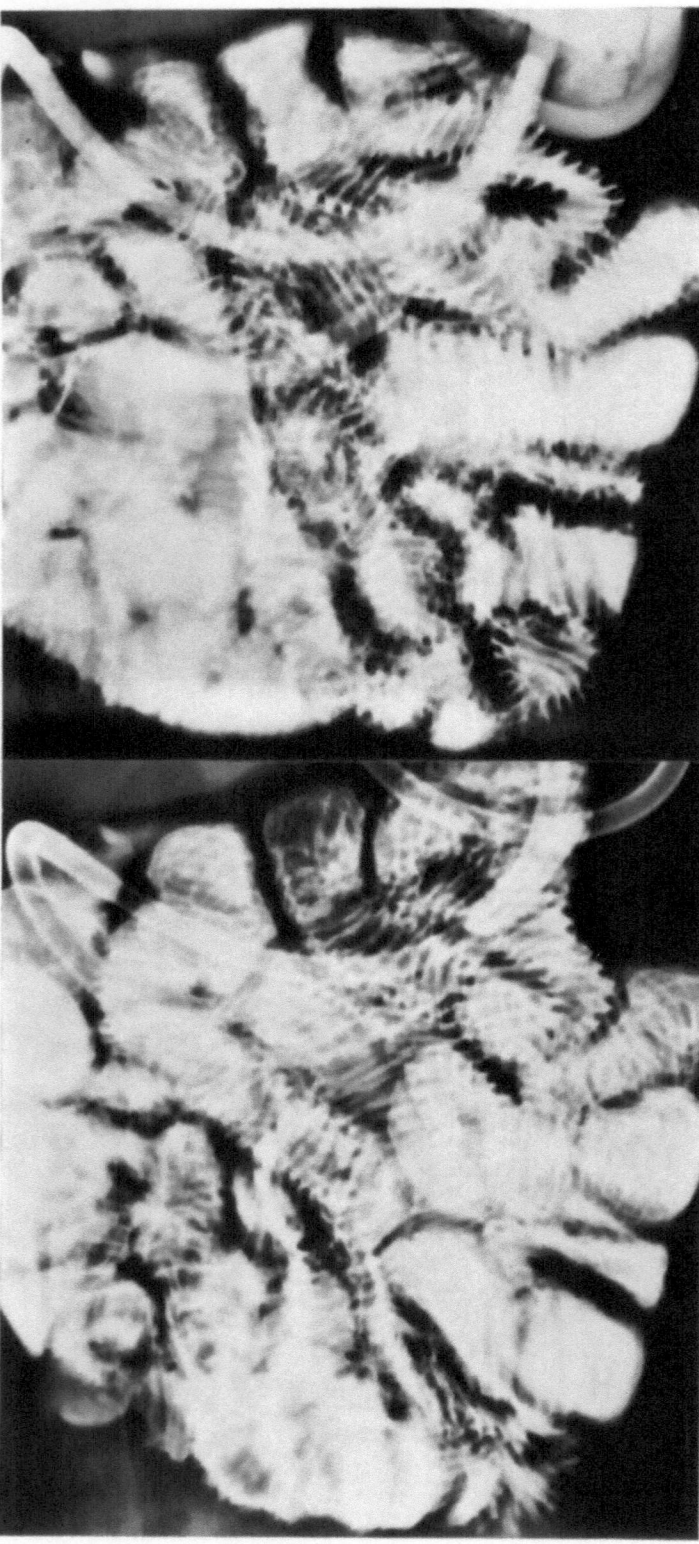

Fig. 15.7. A one-year-old baby with massive fusion of all intestinal loops after a laparotomy carried out because of melena. The position of the intestinal loops remains the same on all exposures (most obvious in the left half of the abdomen). The upper exposure shows thickened folds in the upper and lower left quadrants. On the lower exposure, it can be seen that fusion has caused the folds to be highly stretched in the left lower quadrant. The cause of the melena could not be identified.

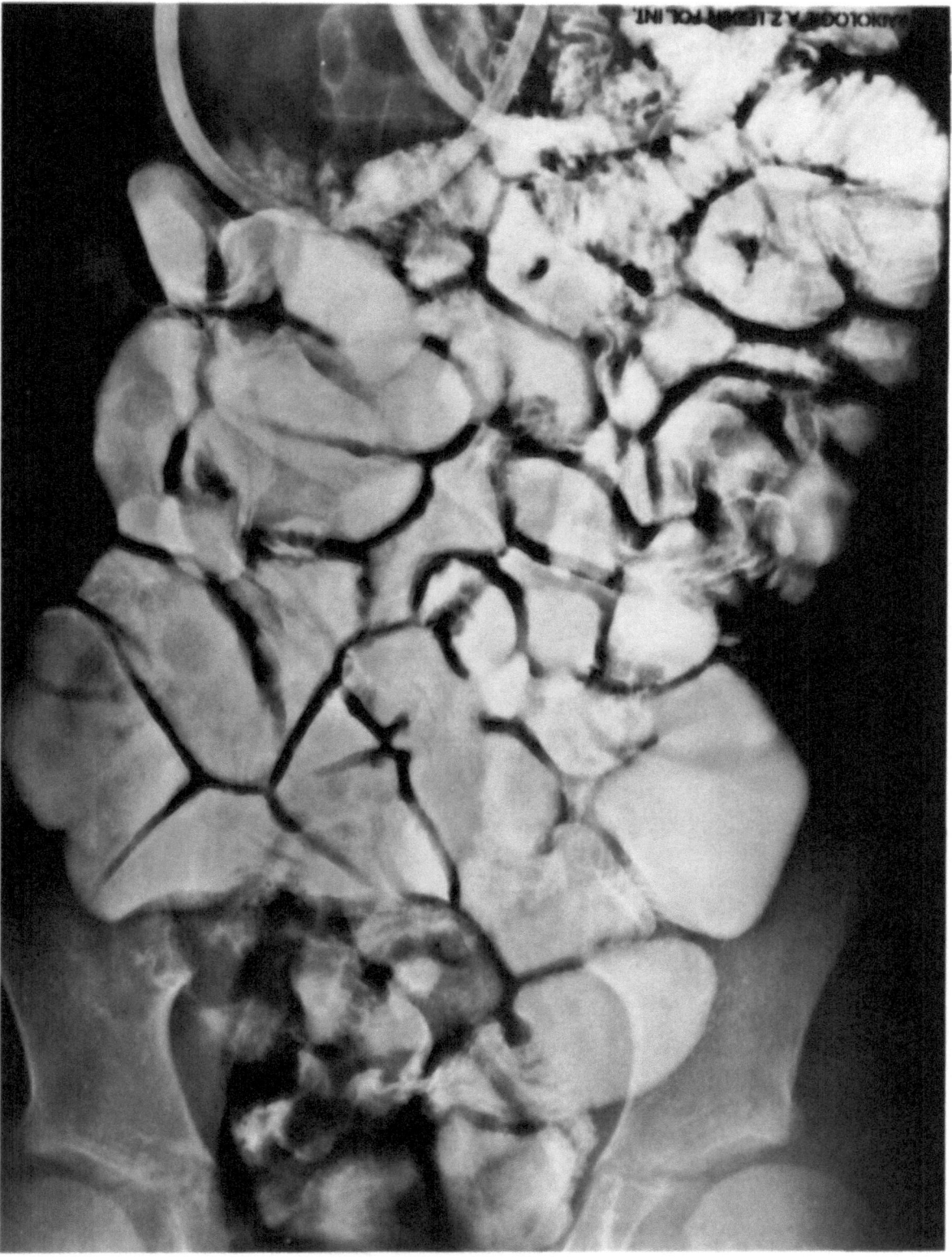

Fig. 15.8. An eight-year-old boy with a growth deficiency of several years' duration. The roentgenogram showed pronounced mucosal atrophy. In the ileum no folds can be seen at all. In the jejunum they are noticeably shortened. Moreover, there is an increased tendency toward flocculation of the barium suspension and a marked dilatation of the ileum. The nature of these abnormalities that have caused a disturbed resorption is unknown. It is definitely not celiac disease, but possibly some similar abnormality is involved, for example tropical sprue. (See also page 460.)

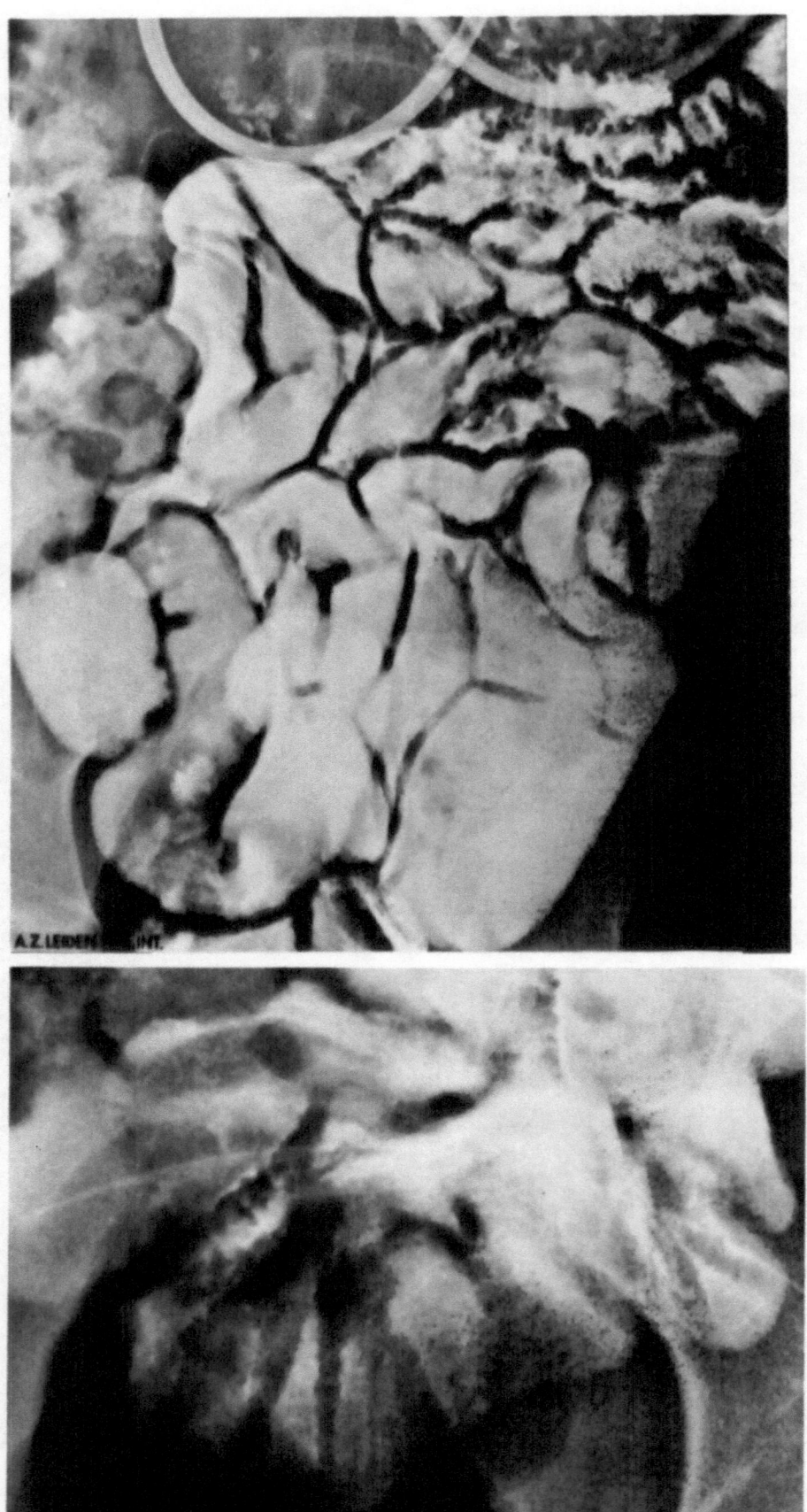

Fig. 15.8. See legend on page 459.

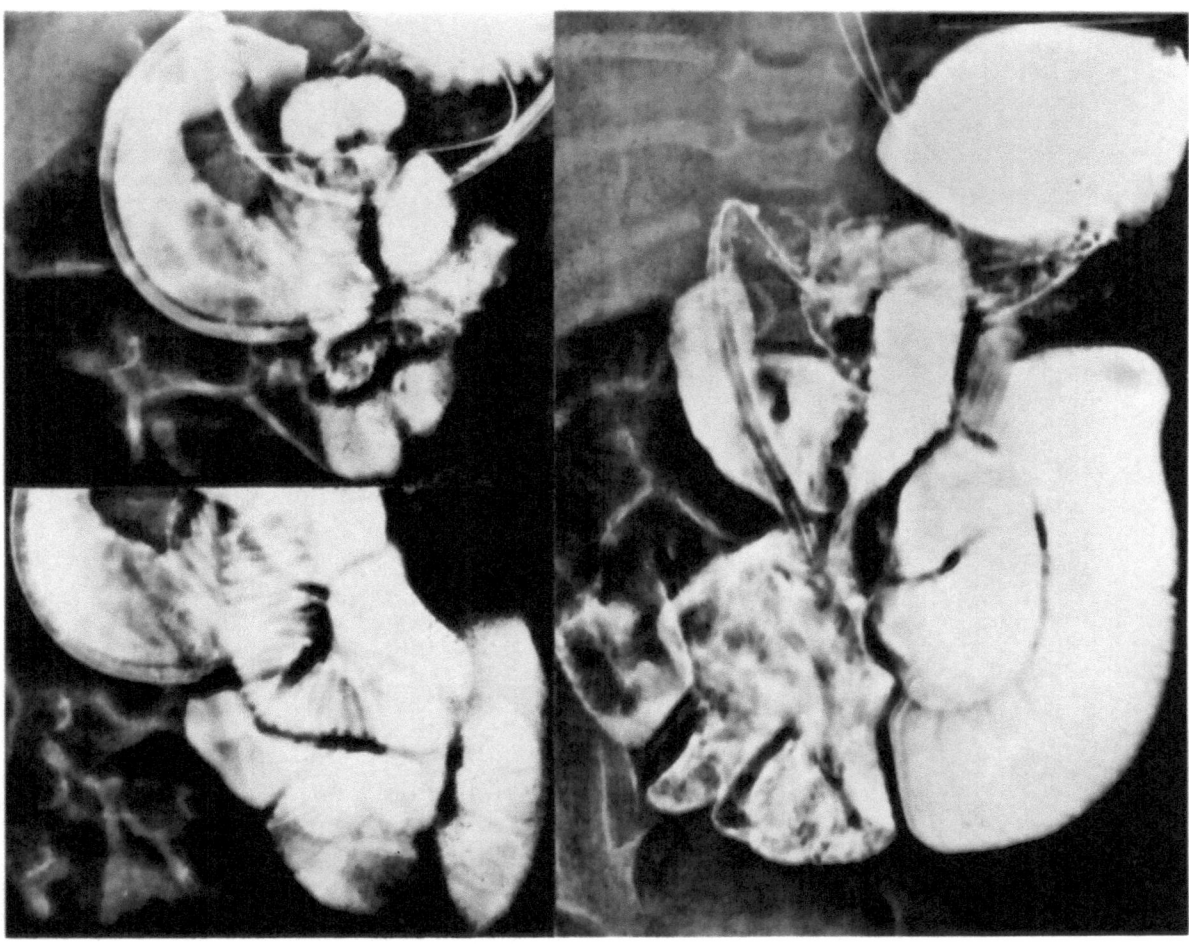

Fig. 15.9. Enteroclysis examination of a one-year-old baby with recurrent nonobstructing ileus due to disturbed innervation of unknown origin. During the examination, most of the contrast fluid ended up in the stomach due to reflux; a second tube was introduced via the nostril to enable constant suctioning off of this contrast medium.

16. COMMON ERRORS AND FAILURES

Ten years of reviewing unsuccessful examinations made elsewhere have proven that unfortunately there are numerous ways to completely ruin an enteroclysis examination! In many cases the results are such that it would have been better for the patient if a conventional follow-through examination had been carried out. Indeed, the results of a poorly executed enteroclysis examination can be much worse than those of an inadequately performed conventional examination. Although these failures are frequently attributed to the method itself, or to the company producing the contrast fluid, neither are in fact responsible. It was been found repeatedly that the physician conducting the examination was convinced of one false fact. He believed that the only difference with respect to the conventional approach is the manner in which the contrast medium is administered, i.e. through a tube directly into the duodenum instead of orally. Apparently many are not willing to take the time to read the literature on enteroclysis. Otherwise, they would learn about and understand the reasoning behind all of the other factors that, together with the contrast medium infusion, are essential for optimum results.

We have received numerous telephone calls requesting information about the technical execution of an enteroclysis examination. The attentive reader of this book will realize that this is truly a most absurd question. We cannot read this entire book over the telephone! Frequently these poor results originate from a marked lack of interest and an unwillingness to change routine procedures that have been in use for years. Often the gastroenterologist or the internist has been the first to hear or see of the results and existence of the enteroclysis technique. Subsequently he requests the radiologist to increase his diagnostic yield for the examination of the small bowel by trying this method. Some-

times it seems that the radiologist is highly irritated because a colleague has intruded into his field and has urged him to improve his results. He then prefers a failure in order to prove to himself and his colleagues that his old trusted method is the best after all. He can then state that the new method gives striking results only in incidental or rare cases. He is sure that these are the only ones published or demonstrated in lectures! Clumsy attempts at duodenal intubation, a result of not carefully studying the available literature, is likewise a fairly common reason for condemning the infusion technique. He bitterly condemns it after trying it only a few times. The attempt and the results in these instances are never approached with enthusiasm and knowledge.

The most common errors and their causes will be discussed systematically.

1. Preparation

1.1. Colon not thoroughly cleansed

In numerous cases it has been found that before the examination the colon was not cleansed. The essential importance of this step has been explained in chapter 7.1. It is striking that in these patients passage proceeds quickly through the jejunum but becomes greatly retarded further distalward, especially near the contaminated cecum. The examination then takes a long time and the contrast fluid thickens in the ileum such that exposures of this region are of poor quality. A water infusion after administration of the contrast medium can force filling of the distal ileum (the so-called water push). However, the caliber of the loops then increases so greatly that compression cannot be used, and minute changes in the mucosal relief can barely be seen.

464

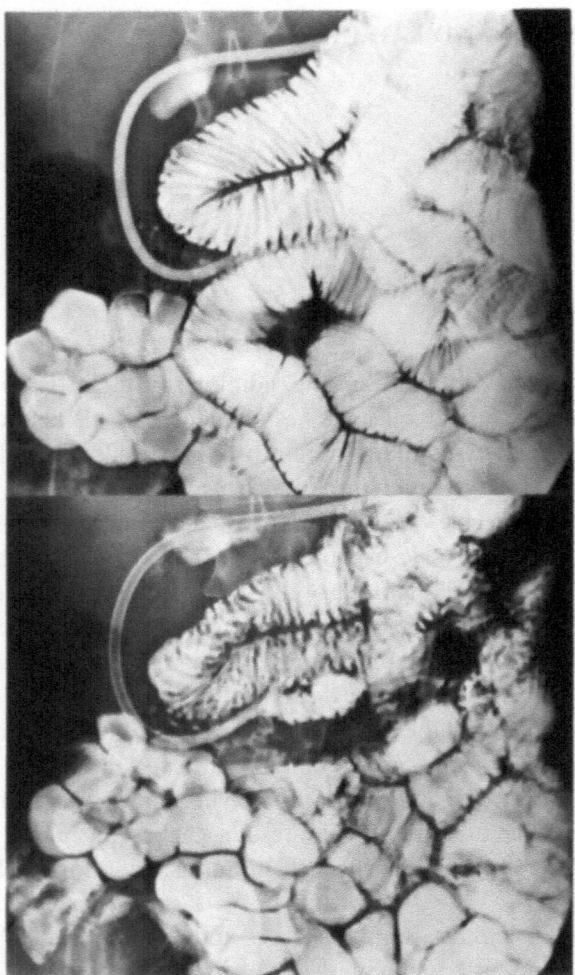

Fig. 16.1. Hypomotility and dilatation due to the long-term use of antispasmodics. Cecum not yet reached ater 1200 ml contrast fluid (top). Within 2 min after the i.v. injection of Primperan (metoclopramide) there is an increase of muscular tone and peristalsis and the cecum is reached (bottom). It will be clear that it is much easier to make compression details under these latter circumstances because it is less full in the abdomen.

1.2. Colon cleansed by means of a rectal clysma

The actual cleansing of the colon obtained in this manner is certainly as good as that resulting from the diet we prescribe (page 81). However, the former method is definitely not to be preferred. Frequently there is reflux of clyster fluid into the ileum and therefore considerable mixing occurs with the contrast fluid flowing from the proximal direction. The troublesome disadvantage of clyster fluid in the small intestine can be avoided by postponing the enteroclysis examination until 1 or 2 h after the clysma. Then, of course, a 'quick' examination is out of the question.

1.3. Drugs not discontinued

Another frequent error is that treatment with tran-quilizers, sedatives, and antispasmodic drugs has not been discontinued before the examination. Because of marked reduction in motility, drug administration (see chapter 12) leads to a marked increase in the amount of contrast medium required and therefore prolongs the examination. Furthermore there is less chance of obtaining good spot films by using compression (fig. 16.1).

1.4. Contrast medium too warm or too cold

The technician usually receives no instructions about the temperature of the contrast fluid. He often either tends to be motivated by brotherly love or follows the procedure for a colon examination. In other words, the barium suspension is mixed with warm water. It is well known that a cold contrast fluid enhances motility and a warm fluid does not. Furthermore, a cold contrast fluid causes the pyloric canal to close more tightly than a warm one. Cold suspensions thus reduce the chance of reflux into the stomach. On the other hand, an icy contrast fluid causes nausea and vomiting, at least when administered in large quantities. Therefore ice-cold suspensions also cause reflux into the stomach as well as the possibility of regurgitation of the infusion tube. Experimental studies have shown that a temperature of $10°-15°$ C is the best. It is then possible to reach the cecum with the lowest dose of contrast medium in the shortest possible time and with the best chance of projecting the loops freely and adequately. Measurements have shown that the temperature of the contrast fluid is about $5°$ C higher when it enters the duodenum than in the infusion bag.

1.5. Specific gravity of the barium suspension too high or too low

All too often the technician asks the physician what the dilution of the contrast fluid should be before he has even seen the patient. He apparently believes that this factor is dependent upon his personal whims. However, although there are some excep-tions, such as a scheduled double-contrast exam-ination, the radiologist must try to keep to the specific values listed in chapter 6 (page 53). If the contrast fluid is either too dense or too radiolucent, the results will be unacceptable. If the specific gravity is too high, much more radiation will be required to obtain exposures that are even slightly useful. In fact this compensation usually appears to be an illusion rather than reality (see fig. 4.19, page 53). If the specific gravity is too low, the contrast medium will generally be fairly thin and fluid, and there will be excessive filling of the intestinal loops. The contrast will not be sufficient to visualize details such as aphthoid ulcers. In particular if the specific gravity is too low and the voltage too high, the films are easily overexposed. The results can only be called tragic (fig. 16.2).

2. Execution of the examination

2.1. Tube is not far enough into the duodenum
This mistake can often be attributed to the radiologist who is careless or leaves it to his technician and orders Bilbao tubes that are too short for many patients. It has been pointed out repeatedly that, for enteroclysis, longer Bilbao tubes have been produced for the radiologist (125–135 cm). Furthermore, these new tubes are safer because the guide wire cannot pass through the side openings. Once the tube is in the duodenum, it is usually easy to push the tip further toward the ligament of Treitz. If problems should develop, for instance in extra-thin patients, do not keep trying to push the tube further. It is highly likely that the tube then will curl in the duodenum. If the tip should end up in the duodenal bulb, the obvious result will be reflux of the contrast medium into the stomach (fig. 7.8A, page 88).

2.2. Rate of flow of the contrast medium too low
If the flow rate of the barium suspension is less than 75 ml/min, there will be insufficient stretching of the duodenum, peristalsis will not be strong, and the examination will be prolonged. In addition, the degree of small intestinal filling will be similar to the conventional transit examination and the advantage of forced flow will be lost. Mild cases of celiac disease will certainly not be recognized. Prestenotic dilatations will not develop as easily and the differences between hypermotility and hypomotility will disappear. A sluggish flow will produce the same pattern in the small bowel as hypermotility when the flow is fast (fig. 16.3). The importance of a

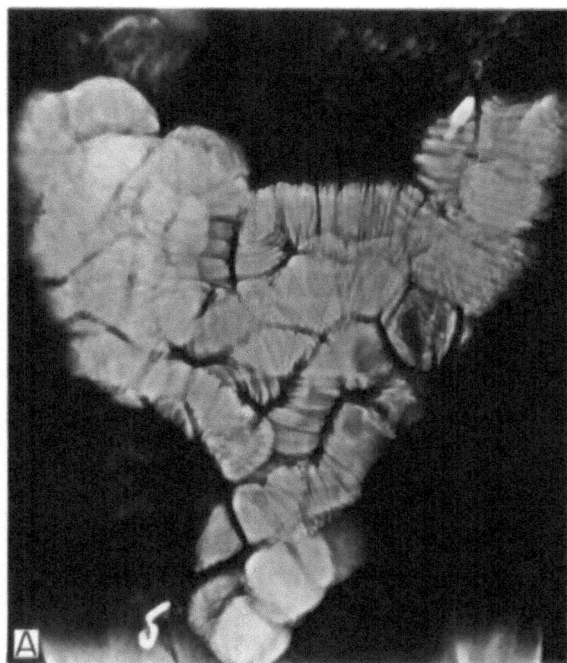
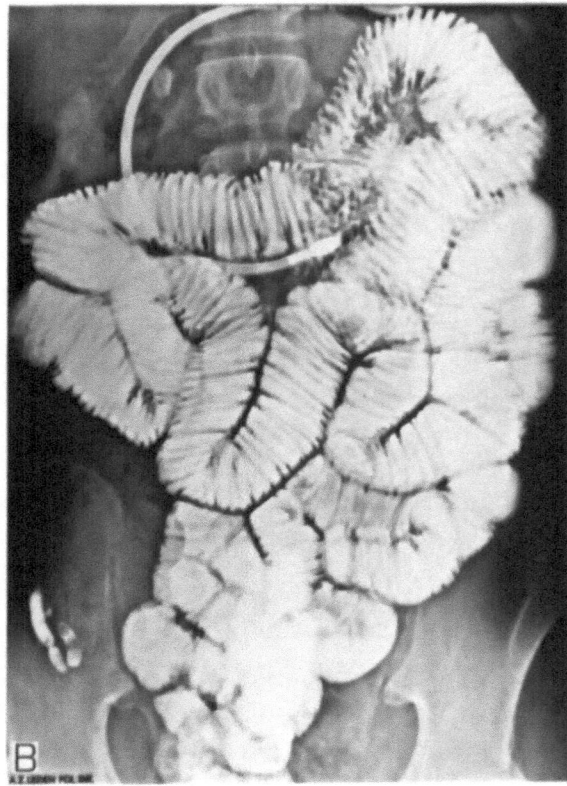

Fig. 16.2. Overexposured film and density of the contrast medium too low (top). Besides that, 150 kV was used! In order to try to compensate for the low specific gravity of the contrast medium, the result would have been better in this case if 90 kV was used. The degree of filling of the bowel is too great. The speed of administration of the contrast fluid must have been too high – probably because the barium suspension was diluted too much. A completely different result was obtained with a repeat examination a few days afterward (bottom).

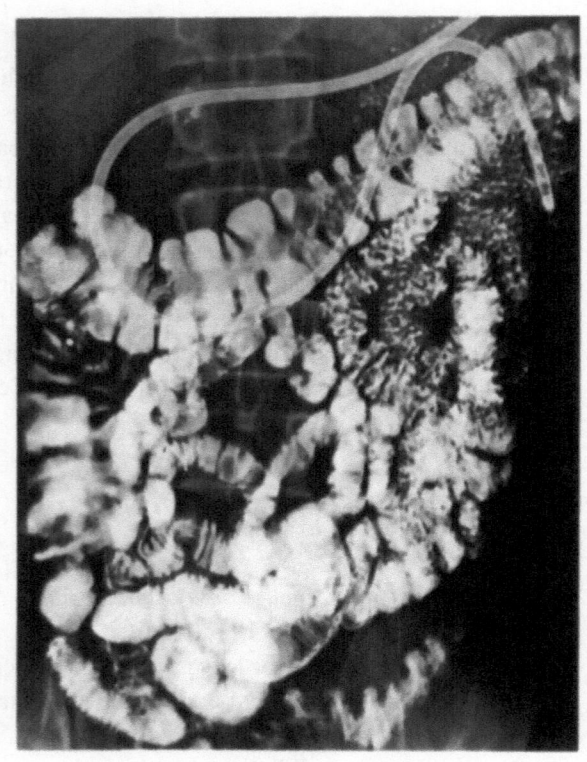

pattern will also hinder identification of polyps and Meckel's diverticula unless the loops can be projected free from one another. Constrictions caused by bands are visualized much more clearly when the intestinal loops are filled with barium suspension instead of air. Reproduction of slight abnormalities of the mucosa is better in air contrast, especially if a dense contrast fluid is used. However, a double-contrast examination means that the total diagnostic information is reduced. The only exception is when air is used to facilitate visualization of the mass of ileal loops deep in the minor pelvis.

2.6. The routine use of the water-push technique only

Stenosis of the intestine as well as constrictions and impressions are most easily discovered when the intestine is well filled. An edematous swelling of the mucous membrane is, on the other hand, seen only when the degree of filling is moderate. This latter state is also preferable for compression of individual loops. It is essential for the discovery of aphthoid ulcers as well as small Meckel's diverticula. If a water infusion is to follow the barium suspension, it is necessary to wait until the contrast column has reached the cecum. This is essential so that survey exposures and spot films of all areas of the small intestine can be completed first. In the event of ileus, serious stenoses, or greatly reduced motility, this waiting is not feasible. Water administered too soon leads to the previously mentioned situation (see 2.3 above) in which the motility of the intestine cannot be evaluated. The intestine may even more or less be paralyzed. Furthermore, after water infusion, flocculation of the barium suspension always develops quickly; thus it ruins all chance of detecting malabsorption. Finally, a large number of patients will be distressed by a rapid water infusion. This often results in the development of reflux into the stomach with nausea and vomiting. In our experience the administration of air or water following the barium suspension is worthwhile in, at the most, only one out of every ten cases.

2.7. Incorrect decisions during the examination

Frequently, the reasons leading to a decision to use air insufflation (fig. 16.7A), or a water infusion (fig. 7.33, page 110), are completely wrong. Often the

contrast medium infusion is terminated too soon. In case of hypomotility or obstruction, the physician frequently does not dare to administer more contrast fluid. He believes wrongly (usually owing to incorrect information in the literature) that the total dose would be too high.

Occasionally the contrast medium infusion has been allowed to run too long. If the colon is well cleansed, excessive filling of the rectosigmoid can develop quickly. Adequate compression of the ileum is then out of the question. The only alternative in such cases is to try to save the situation by emptying the rectosigmoid by using a cannula or by allowing a quick, short defecation! Air then is insufflated with the patient in the prone position.

Finally, an error that is much too common is to forget to give Primperan once hypomotility has been established. This is especially true after a large quantity of contrast fluid has been administered. When Primperan is given as an injection or via the tube, it is essential to wait 5–10 min before proceeding further. The useful effect of a Primperan injection is illustrated in figs. 12.11 and 16.1.

3. General mistakes and failures

3.1. Not enough exposures

Unusual or suspicious configurations of the mucosal relief or the contrast column should be recorded at least twice and more often if possible. This should be done especially when in doubt. It is therefore useful to take two exposures of the same region within a short time as a matter of course. This is because the position of the intestinal loops has then not yet changed and it facilitates comparison. We have been astonished to see cases in which the entire small bowel was covered by only two survey films!

3.2. Lack of or too few spot films by using compression

The most common of all mistakes is the assumption that it is worthwhile to use compression only in the distal ileum. It is incorrectly believed that abnormalities will seldom be found elsewhere. Our experience with thousands of patients, however, has shown that many more abnormalities are found in the much longer segment proximal to the 20-cm-

468

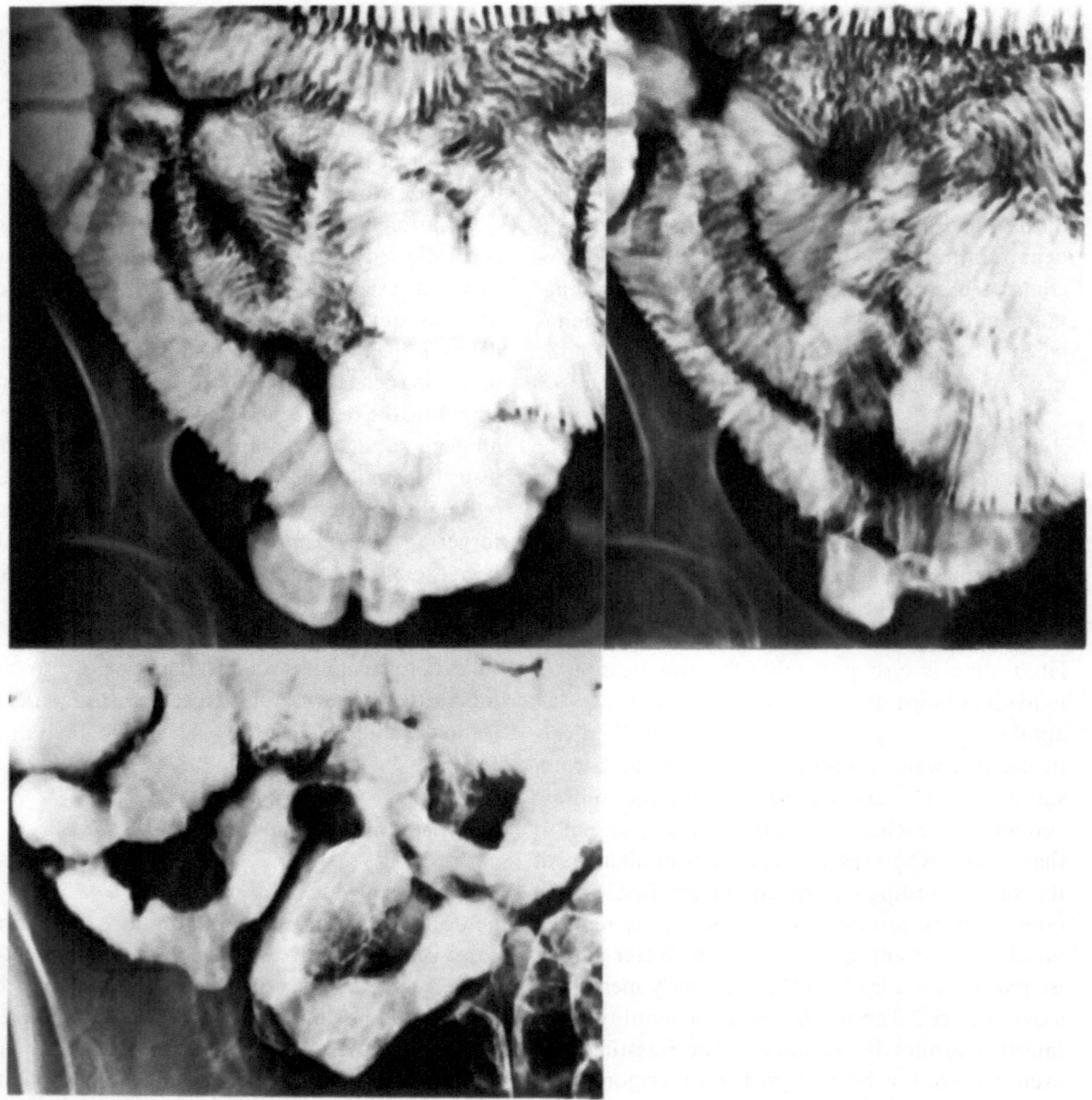

Fig. 16.4. Spot films of the lower abdomen that in our opinion showed pathological mucosal relief over a length of ±10 cm (top). One week later a repeat examination, whereby compression was carried out with even greater care, revealed Crohn's disease involving a segment 60 cm long (bottom).

long distal ileum. In our experience, 12 compression spot films spread out over the entire small intestine is considered the absolute minimum. Even if spot films of a mass of ileal loops in the minor pelvis have been made, one should not be satisfied too quickly (fig. 16.4). Spot films without compression are also an essential part of the examination, but they do not render compression superfluous (fig. 16.5).

3.3. Voltage too low

In too many radiology departments, the voltage used during the entire examination of the digestive tract is too low – especially for the well-filled intestine. Figs. 4.6 and 16.7A show that this is a serious mistake. The specific gravities recommended in this book are based on a voltage of 125–150 kV. A lower voltage, even if compensation is achieved by reducing the density of the barium

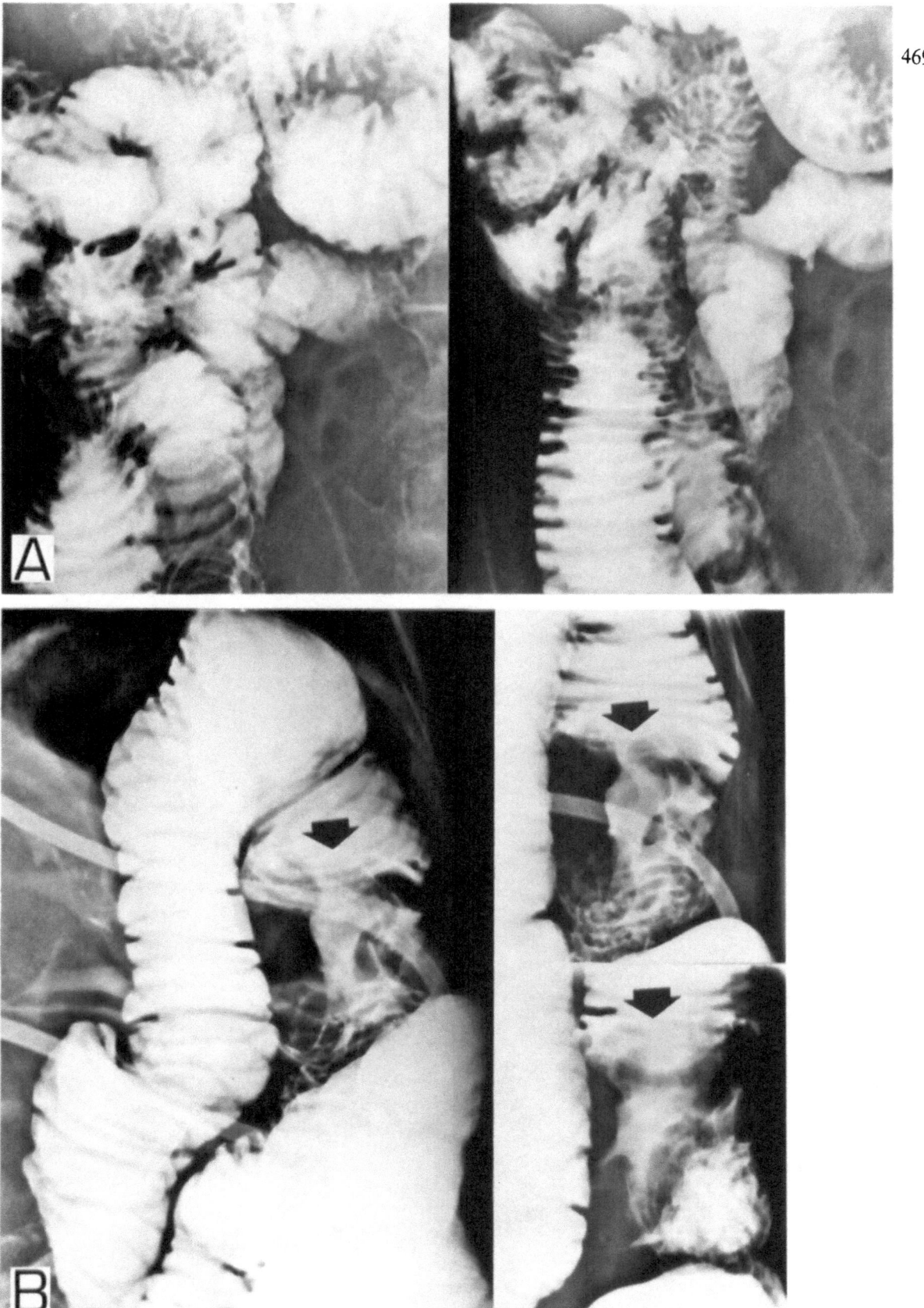

Fig. 16.5. (A) Spot films of the right upper quadrant in a psychiatric patient with anal bleeding. Except for a positional anomaly of the jejunum and suspected adhesions in this region, no peculiarities were seen. (B) One week later, the examination was repeated to verify the previous results. The jejunal loops are now in the left upper quadrant. Furthermore, careful compression revealed that there were no adhesions in this region, but instead a tumor (adenocarcinoma) that had not been detected during the first examination.

470

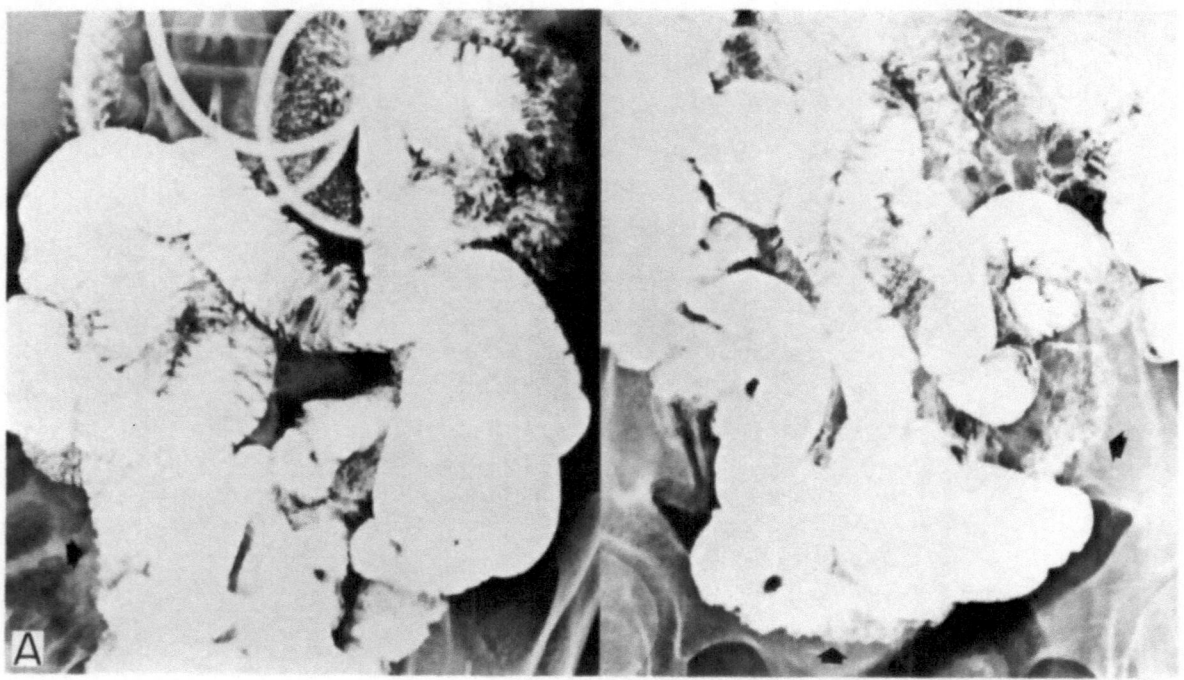

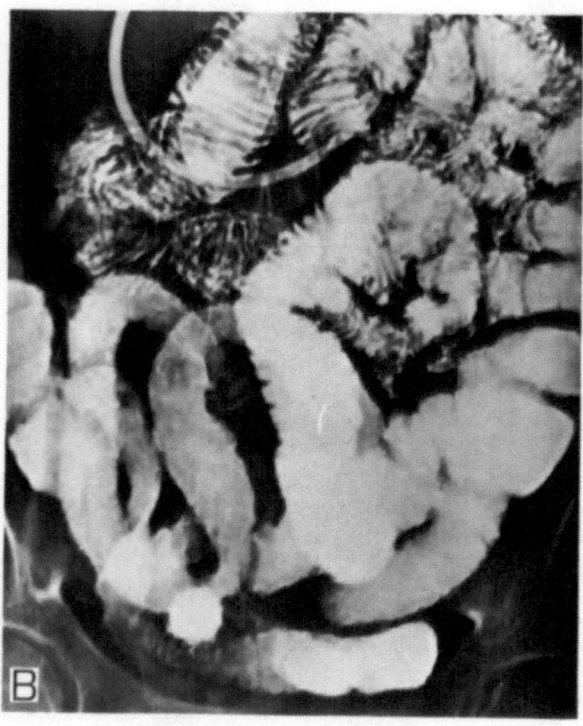

Fig. 16.6. (A) Example of a useless and misleading enteroclysis examination showing a pronounced underexposure. These films were reported as normal but in reviewing them there are irregular margins at different places (arrow). (B) Repeat examination of the patient of fig. 16.6A several weeks later reveals an extensive Crohn's disease.

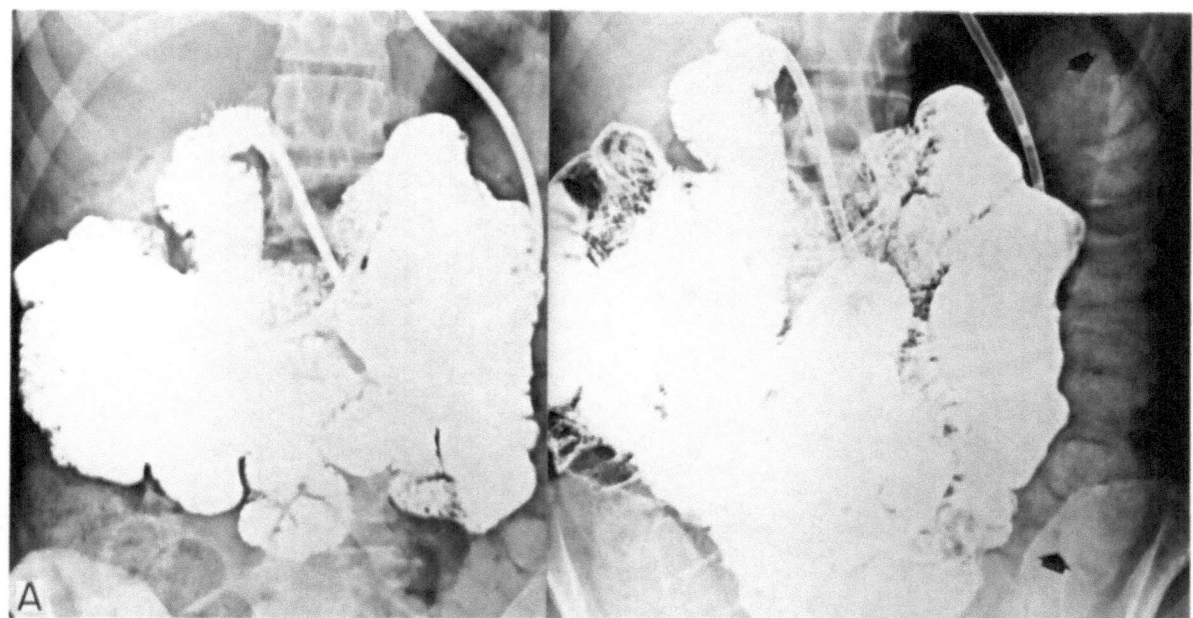

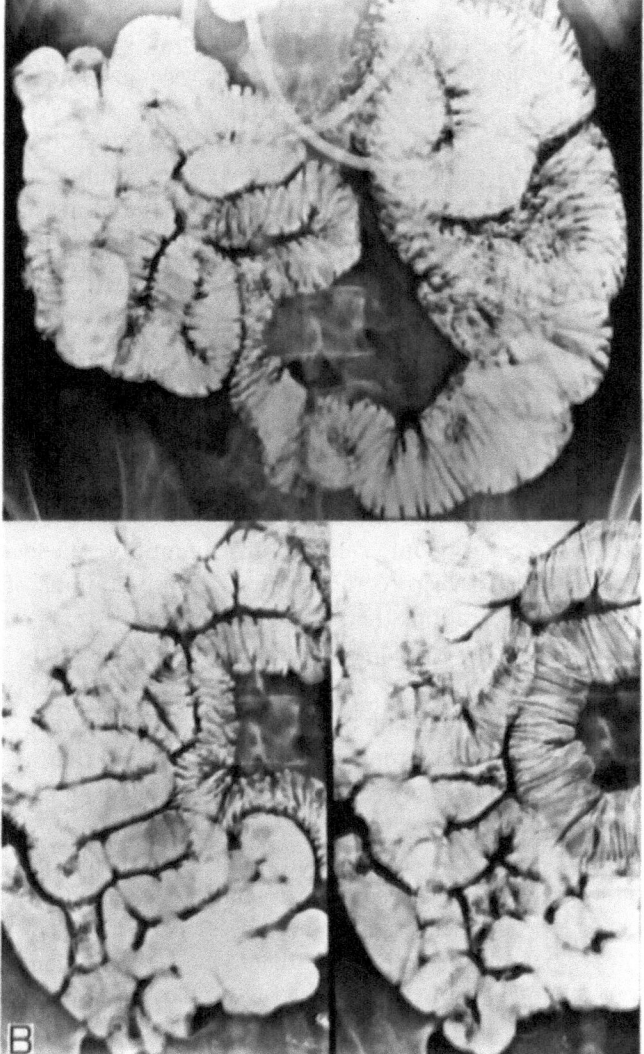

Fig. 16.7. (A) Useless and misleading enteroclysis examination, showing a clear underexposure of the films. The colon was not cleansed at all and therefore a considerable amount of contrast fluid was needed to reach the cecum. Finally air was insufflated through the tube without any rational indication and without any chance to be successful. (B) The result of the repeat examination, performed one week afterward. There were no abnormalities indeed!

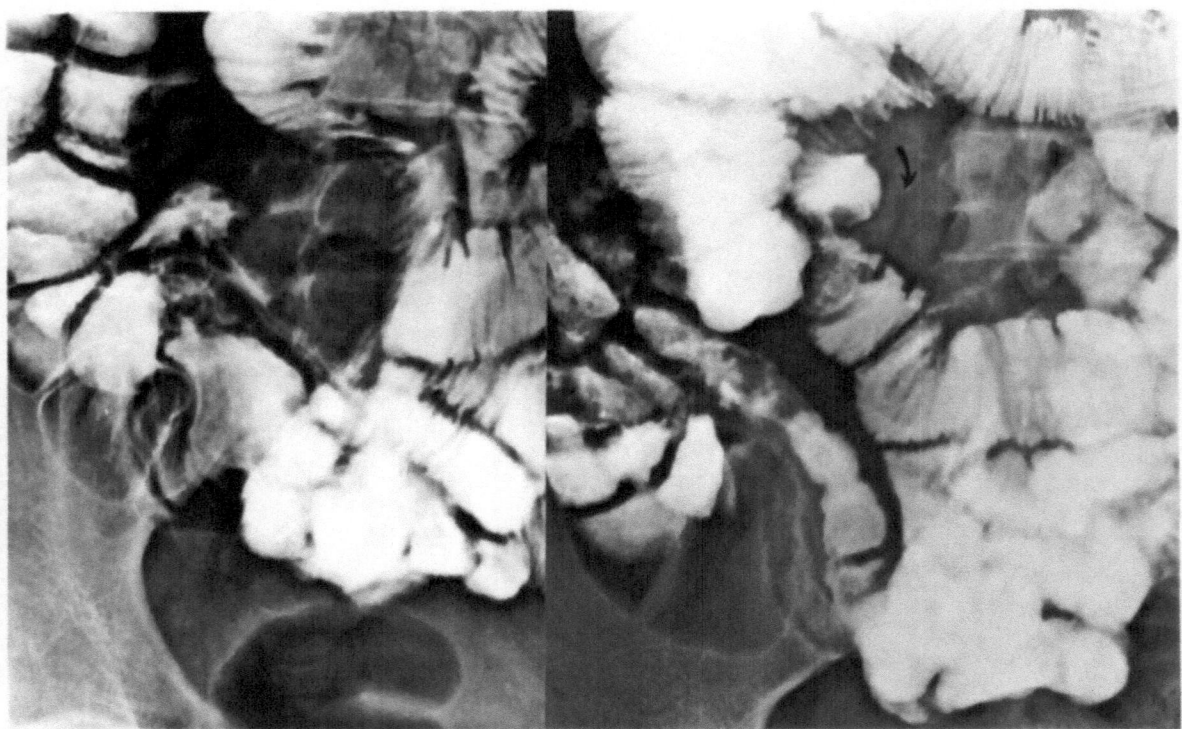

Fig. 16.8. Space-occupying defect in the ileocecal region attributed to an infiltrate or mesenteric tumor (left). A repeat examination was necessary to convince the radiologist conducting the examination that the colon was causing an impression on the intestinal loops (see the haustra pattern on the right film).

suspension, means that the patient is subjected to increased exposure.

3.4. Films underexposed or overexposed
A striking example of pronounced underexposure can be seen in fig. 16.6A. These two exposures were the only ones taken and – with considerable courage or ignorance – the findings were pronounced normal. Several weeks later we carried out a repeat examination that revealed extensive Crohn's disease (fig. 16.6B). In retrospect this can be seen along the edges of the contrast column on the first exposures (arrow).

Figure 16.7A shows two exposures of another patient's examination performed elsewhere. Here again the films are severely underexposed and were, as the above, evaluated as normal. One of these two exposures shows that the colon had not been cleansed at all before the examination. Furthermore, without any reason and without any chance of obtaining good results, possibly in desperation, air was insufflated. A repeat examination produced completely different results because the correct technique was used (fig. 16.7B).

Overexposure is less serious than underexposure since a bright light can compensate for this problem

to some extent. If, however, in addition to overexposure, the specific gravity of the contrast fluid is too low and the voltage is 150 kV, then the problems of evaluation will indeed be enormous (fig. 16.2A).

3.5. Mistakes in evaluation
All too often, abnormalities that are not known are also not observed on the roentgenograms, even when they are there. A common example of this type of situation is edematous swollen folds, mucosal atrophy, and disturbed motility. The tendency is to keep to the incorrect interpretations of configurations that have been in use for years and are persistent in the literature. Unfortunately these incorrect evaluations are not based on reality, but on misleading patterns. A common example of this are those conventional examinations that, according to many radiologists, show coarse and certainly pathological mucosal folds. When a subsequent enteroclysis examination does not show the coarse folds, the radiologist tends to conclude that the enteroclysis examination is inadequate. It is not able to reproduce this so-called 'pathology'. The cause of this so-called fold coarsening is described in chapter 8.7, page 169. Frequently the radiologist

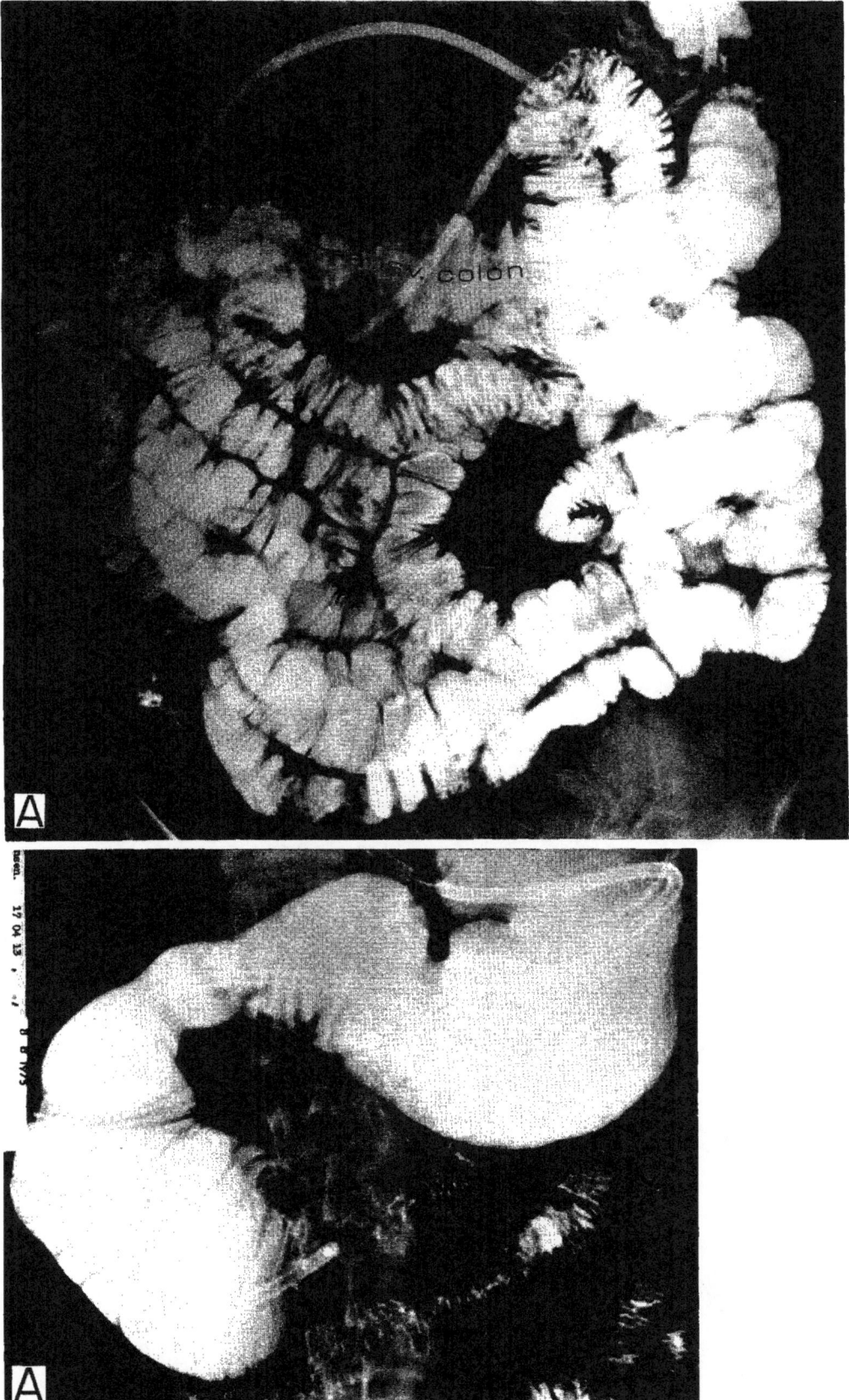

Fig. 16.9A. Completely normal small bowel examination of a patient with loss of blood from the digestive tract. The gastric examination, however, clearly showed tumor growth in the duodenum. Apparently it was possible to pass the stenosis with the infusion tube.

474

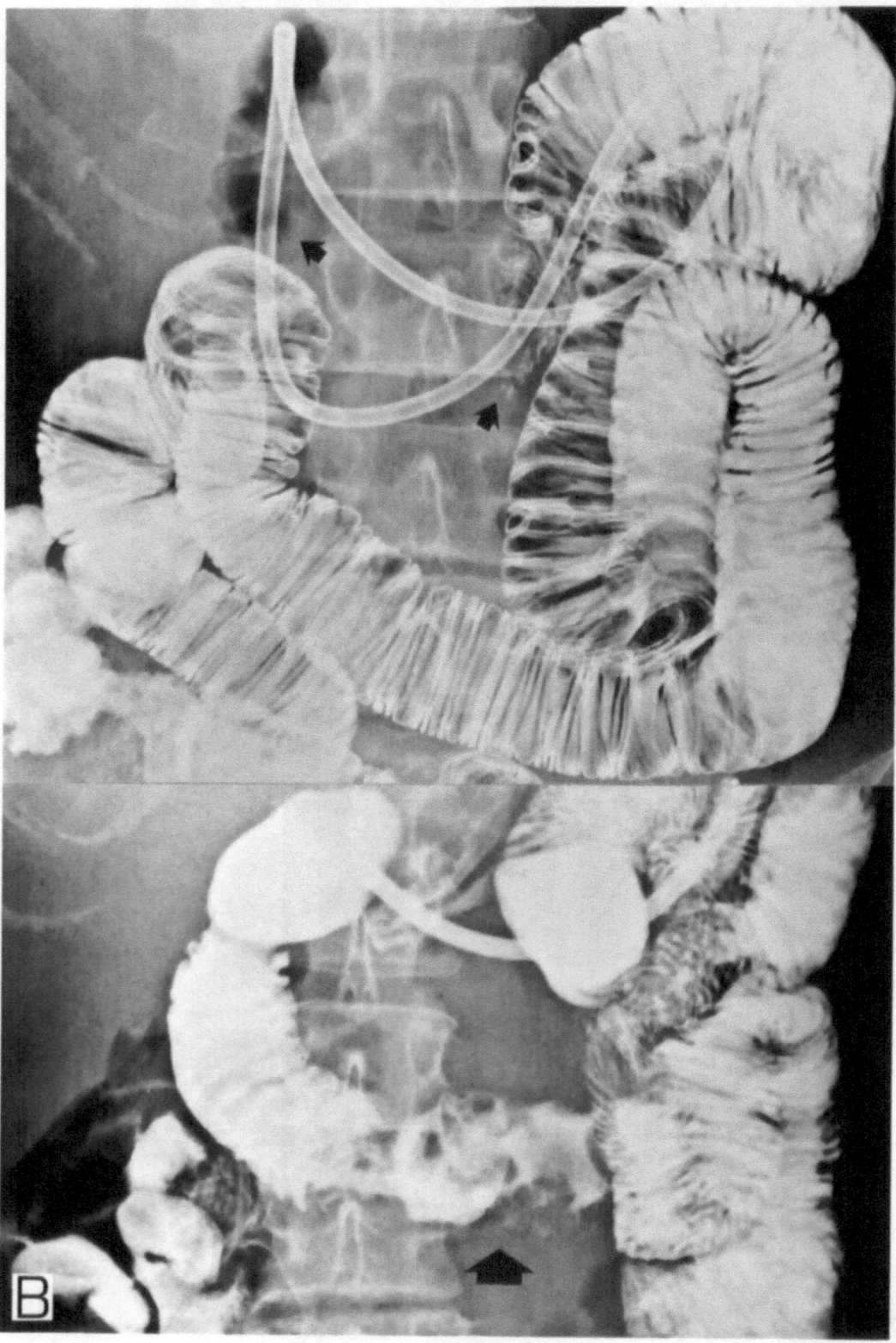

*Fig. 16.9*B. Duodenal tumor that was not visualized because the tube extends beyond the tumor (top). In this case, the examiner should have noted that, in spite of marked filling of the jejunum and total paralysis of the motility, reflux into the duodenum did *not* occur. Moreover the air configuration ends abruptly in the proximal duodenum. During a second examination carried out a short time later, the tumor was demonstrated because the tube could no longer be pushed past it (bottom).

does not even know the most basic and characteristic signs of pathology. Moreover he is also liable to report abnormalities when the only patterns present are normal ones (fig. 16.8).

It is also most important to be aware of the limits of an enteroclysis examination. The duodenum is certainly not always visualized. In such cases the report should contain the explicit statement that only the jejunum and the ileum were evaluated. Striking examples of this are seen in fig. 16.9AB, where the infusion tube passed a duodenal tumor that consequently was not visualized on the films.

When evaluating a series of x-rays, every radiologist has the irrespectable tendency to think only in terms of the patient's complaints. Regularly, therefore, abnormalities located elsewhere or of an entirely different nature are completely overlooked, even when they are clearly visualized on the films. A striking example of this is the enteroclysis examination shown in fig. 16.10A, which was evaluated by about ten individuals as being normal. None of them noted that reflux of the contrast fluid into the stomach caused a configuration in that organ that was highly indicative of tumor growth, a diagnosis that was confirmed several days later during a gastric examination (fig. 16.10BC).

Finally it has come to our attention that sometimes the physician's knowledge of small intestine pathology is seriously deficient. One of the most tragic examples of this was a telephone call from a colleague working in a large regional hospital. He requested information about the signs, symptoms, and nature of Crohn's disease – a disease that he had never heard about.

Some may wish to review quickly the possible causes of a complete or partial failure in their enteroclysis examination. A short summary follows of the most frequent failure problems. The technical errors listed in section 3 are presumed to be sufficiently well known by now so that failures because of one or more of these factors are not included.

1) Reflux to the stomach
Tip of the tube not far enough into the duodenum.
Tube may be too short or may have coiled in the stomach.
Temperature of the contrast fluid is too low or too high.

Flow rate of the contrast medium is too high.
Nausea of patient enhanced by excessive movement of the table, by rotating the patient, or by excessive palpation.
Patient under the influence of drugs that produce atony.

2) Much more contrast medium is needed to reach the cecum than is listed in this book
Colon not cleansed beforehand or rectal cleansing clysma given.
Drugs that induce atony were not discontinued.
Flow rate of the contrast medium too high.
Temperature of the contrast medium too high.
Reflux into the stomach.
Patient ate breakfast.

3) Mass of ileal loops appears too compact on survey exposures
Too much contrast medium administered (see 2).
Specific gravity of contrast medium too high.
Water infusion administered after barium suspension without specific indication.

4) Highly confusing mass of ileal loops in lower abdomen
Dose of contrast medium too large (see 2).
Water infusion contraindicated because of clump of ileal loops in small pelvis.
Patient examined in supine position only.
Examination took too long so that density of the contrast fluid in the ileum gradually increased.

5) Examination lasts longer than expected
Difficulties with intubation procedure.
Necessary equipment (water bag, compression apparatus, or insufflation equipment) not prepared beforehand.
Too much contrast medium required (see 2).
Survey exposures and compression spot films must be taken on different tables, or even in different rooms.

6) Examination too long for the radiologist
Although this is never a valid objection, the time that the radiologist needs to carry out the work properly can be shortened by using a good technician. He can do the intubation, give the contrast medium infusion, and take the survey films (patient

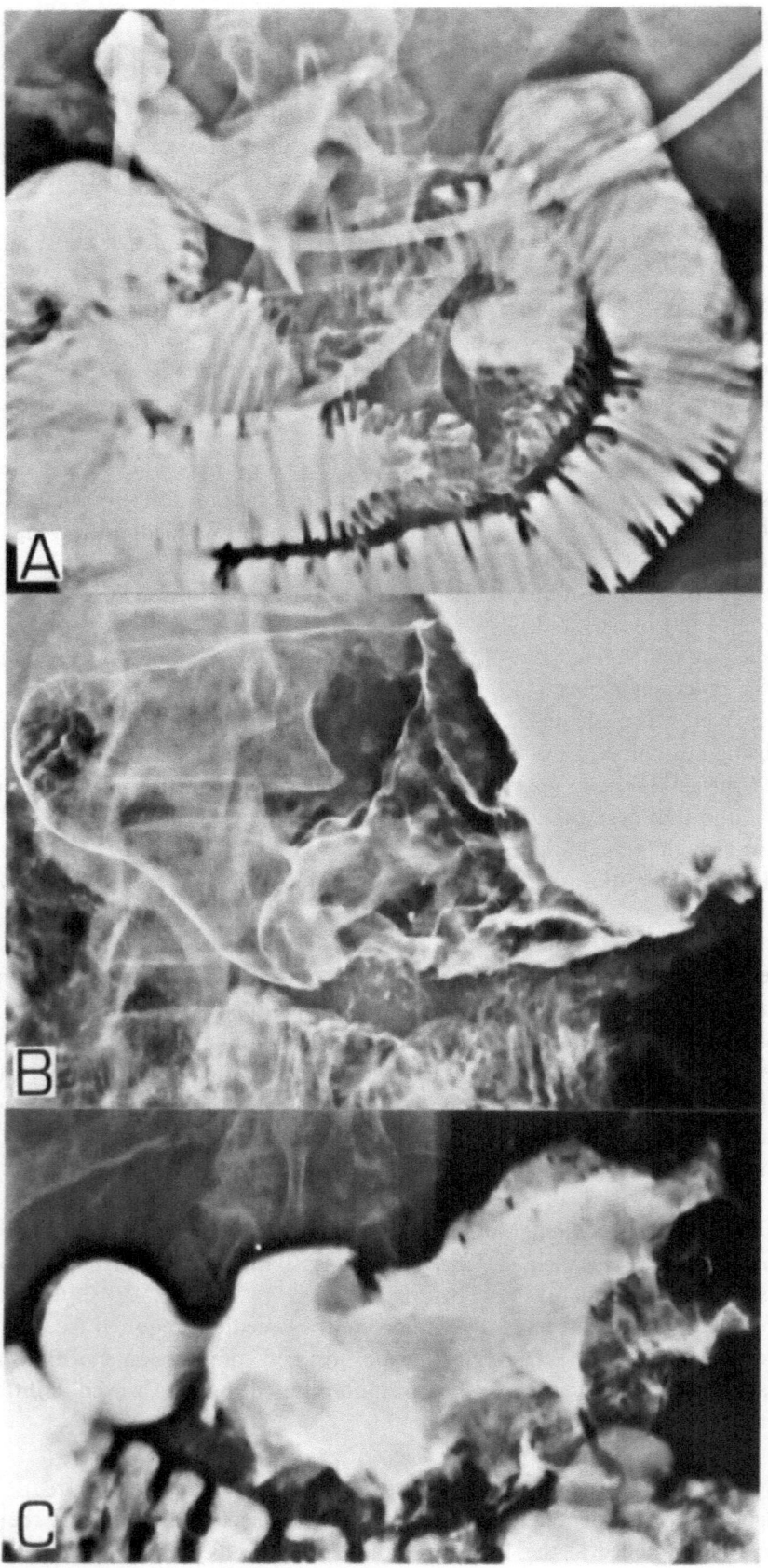

Fig. 16.10. (A) One of the films of an otherwise normal enteroclysis examination showed that reflux of the contrast fluid into the stomach caused a configuration indicative of a tumor; this was almost overlooked. (BC) A gastric examination carried out several days later confirmed the findings of the enteroclysis examination. The tumor was a lymphoreticular malignancy.

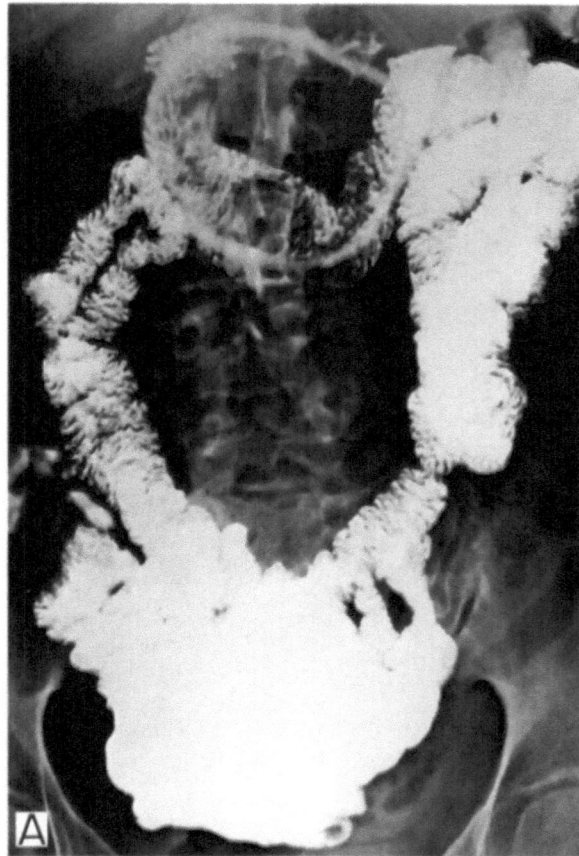

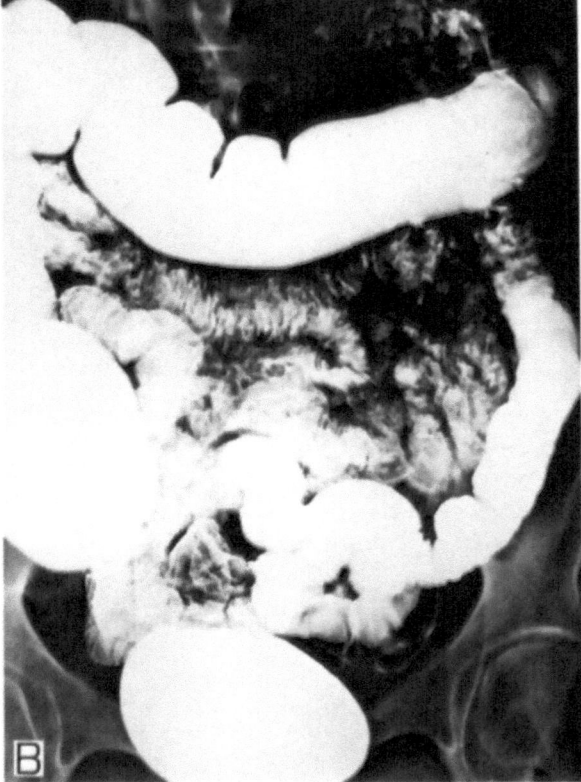

on his stomach). The radiologist can then concentrate on the spot films and the use of compression. This can even be carried out in two stages: jejunum after 600 ml, ileum at the end of the examination.

7) Disappointing results that are difficult to describe
An attempt has been made here to group the possible causes of errors in an enteroclysis examination under separate headings; this is not always possible. Often, several mistakes are made during one examination. This will produce a disappointing result that is more complex and therefore more difficult to describe. One example is the examination seen in fig. 16.11 that illustrates the following combination of errors:

a) Specific gravity of the contrast medium much too high.
b) Voltage too low.
c) Rate of flow too low (in this case because viscosity was too high) so that the degree of filling was inadequate.
d) Although the ileal loops in this case demanded rectal and possibly oral air insufflation, water was administered. The phase when the ileal mass must have been the biggest was not recorded. The high degree of colon filling, and the degree of contrast medium disintegration in the ileal loops proves that this exposure was taken late near the end of the examination. Note that the rectosigmoid, filled with water instead of air, has forced the ileal loops upward to such a degree that they are now accessible for compression. Thus it can be assumed that in this case oral air insufflation would have been superfluous.

Bibliography: chapter 16

Miller RE, Sellink JL (1979) Enteroclysis: the small bowel enema. Gastrointest Radiol 4: 269–283.

Fig. 16.11. Disappointing results because a combination of errors was made: (1) density too high, (2) kV too low, (3) viscosity too high and therefore rate of administration too low, (4) water infusion afterward instead of rectal and possibly also oral air insufflation.

SUBJECT INDEX

Page numbers in italics indicate general information on a particular topic